思考中药
The *Tao* of Chinese Formulas and Medicines
英汉对照本
English – Chinese Version

唐 略 著
Written by Tang Lue

张干周 译
Translated by Zhang Ganzhou

学苑出版社
Academy Press Limited Company

图书在版编目（CIP）数据

思考中药英汉对照本　汉文、英文/张干周译．—北京：学苑出版社，2021.12

ISBN 978 – 7 – 5077 – 6352 – 2

Ⅰ.①思… Ⅱ.①张… Ⅲ.①中药学 – 基本知识 – 汉、英 Ⅳ.①R28

中国版本图书馆 CIP 数据核字（2021）第 280141 号

责任编辑：黄小龙

出版发行：学苑出版社

社　　址：北京市丰台区南方庄 2 号院 1 号楼

邮政编码：100079

网　　址：www. book001. com

电子邮箱：xueyuanpress@ 163. com

销售电话：010 – 67601101（销售部）、010 – 67603091（总编室）

印 刷 厂：北京兰星球彩色印刷有限公司

开本尺寸：710mm × 1000mm　1/16

印　　张：68.75

字　　数：1126 千字

版　　次：2021 年 12 月第 1 版

印　　次：2021 年 12 月第 1 次印刷

定　　价：498.00 元

Forward about English Translation

In the middle of the 17th century, John Dryden (1631 – 1700), the British royal poet laureate, divided all the translations into three categories: metaphrase, paraphrase, and imitation. The so – called metaphrase refers to word for word and line for line translation, basically corresponding to the literal translation that is also the most used method by all translators. However, the biggest challenge in the transition between different languages is cultural translation. After the source language is converted into the target language, the readers and the source language that bears the weight of specific culture and the target language have undergone fundamental changes. It is indeed not an easy work to ensure that the readers of the target language can understand the culture and professional information contained in the source language completely in the same way as the readers of the source language. The paraphrase of translation refers to a flexible translation with certain freedom adopted by the translator according to the sense or information of the source language. The translator should strictly follow the real sense or implications behind the words used by the original author rather than the words themselves. Therefore, paraphrase involves the change of words, roughly corresponding to the translation of "information to information". The third type of translation is imitation by which the translator abandons the meaning of the original words and tries to use his own wisdom and creativity to create a new sense of beauty for the inevitable loss of beauty in the process of translation. Such a translation is basically a process of adaptation, which only extracts the major information of the original text and abandons some minor information.

Roman Jacobson (1896 – 1982), Russian born American linguist and Slavic-language scholar, from another perspective (1959/1966: 233), divides translation differently into: intralingual translation, interlingual translation, and intersemiotic translation. Intralingual translation refers to the process of interpreting language signs with another set of language signs in the same language. For example, ancient Chinese is first converted into modern Chinese before ancient Chinese is translated into English. Interlingual translation refers to the translation between two different languages, that is, using the signs of the target language to explain the source language, which is usually referred to as "translation", such as English-Chinese translation. Intersemiotic translation refers to interpreting linguistic signs through nonverbal sign systems or using linguistic signs to interpret nonverbal signs, such as using pictures, gestures, mathematics, movies, or music to express linguistic signs.

Many linguists and translators at home and abroad have illustrated the strategies and methods of translation from different perspectives. For example, many translation theorists take delight in talking about the "dynamic equivalence" proposed by American translation theorist Eugene Nida (1914 – 2011), the father of dynamic equivalence. The semantic translation and communicative translation by Peter Newmark (1916 – 2011) are also well known to translation learners in China. Lawrence Venuti, American translation theorist, put forward the strategy of domestication and foreignization in The Translators' Invisibility in 1995. These translation theories provide valuable guidance for language translators.

On the standard of translation, different people have different opinions. In the history of Chinese translation, apart from the standard put forward by Hsuan-tsang in the Tang Dynasty, the most famous translation standard should be Yan Fu's "faithfulness, expressiveness and elegance". Yan Fu once said, "Translation has to do three difficult things: to be faithful, expressive, and elegant. It is difficult enough to be faithful to the original, and yet if a translation is not expressive, it is tantamount to having no translation. Hence expressiveness should be required too. The Book of Changes says that the first requisite of rhetoric is truthfulness; Confucius says that expressiveness is all that matters in language. He adds that if one's language lacks grace, it won't go far. These three qualities then are the criterion of good writing and, I believe, of good translation too. Hence besides faithfulness and expressiveness, I also aim at elegance. " But no matter what translation strategy or method or translation criteria are to follow, the ultimate goal of translation is to put the culture and information contained in the source language into the target language, which is then understood and accepted by target language readers, as the Guidelines for Translators of UNESCO describes the translation purpose: after understanding the meaning that the author of the original works wants to convey, translators should put this meaning into English, and try to make the impression produced by English to English readers the same as that produced by the foreign language readers corresponding to the original text.

Following the Wuxing Doctrine (Theory of the Five Elements) of Chinese culture, this book selects the five most representative types of Chinese herbs, taking wood, metal, water, fire and earth as the typical representative symbols. Based on the four properties (i. e., warm, heat, cool and cold) and five tastes (i. e., sour, sweet, bitter, pungent and salty) of the traditional Chinese medicine (TCM), this book describes the characteristics, traits and effects of the five categories of Chinese herbs. In the meantime, this book illustrates the boring theory and principles in formulas and medicines in an easy, vivid, and interesting way like telling a story, which is rich in knowledge and information about TCM, and highly readable. I believe it will bring unexpected surprises and gains to the TCM learners and those who are interested in TCM at home and abroad.

Based on the above-mentioned theories on translation methods, translation standards and the contents of this book, the translator of this book starts from Roman Jakobson's intralingual and interlingual translation, and completes the English translation of this book by adhering to the translation criteria of faithfulness, expressiveness, smoothness, standardization, accuracy, and conciseness. "Faithfulness" refers to the faithful conversion of the information contained in the source text completely and accurately, for which the translator does not change, distort, omit, or add the sense and principles stated in the original text. TCM works, from the perspective of language, have very special linguistic characteristics, involving a lot of Chinese traditional culture factors, like astronomy, geography, history, literature, etc. in addition to the professional knowledge regarding principles of medical science, pathology, and pharmacology.

"Faithfulness" in TCM translation means to be faithful to the original text, to express the content of the original text accurately, completely, and scientifically, and not to distort, add, delete, omit or falsify the content of the original text. At the same time, it is necessary to make the translation fully agree with the original text, not only in the respect of the grammatical structure, and the meaning of the word, but also the logical relations in the sentences and paragraphs of the context, so that the translation accords with the target language, and avoid Chinglish as much as possible. In the process of translation, considering the great differences between English and Chinese languages, the amplification method in translation is also adopted. However, the purpose of such a method is only to make the translation more consistent with the English expression, but not to change the semantic meaning of the original text. "Expressiveness" means to have a thorough understanding of the source language of the book, and then accurately translate it into English language. In the early 19th century, the German literary critic Hillegher said, "A rigorous translator who can not only transplant the content of a masterpiece, but also know how to preserve the beauty of its form and original impression is the messenger of genius." For translation, if "faithfulness" is a simple transplantation of the content of a masterpiece, then "expressiveness" can be said to be the pursuit of content and form of beauty and original impression. The criteria of "expressiveness" here mainly refers to the thorough expression of the sense or implied meaning of words, sentences, and texts. "Smoothness" simply means "to follow the rules so that the text in English translation can be clear and consistent in the syntactic, literary and rhetorical style for the target readers' interest. Otherwise, the essence and meaning of the original text may not be conveyed correctly. In brief, "smoothness" is to follow the language rules of the target language based on being faithful to the original text, so that the target language readers can understand it clearly and smoothly without any sense of difficulty and obscureness. In order to ensure the smoothness of the translated text, the translator here tries his best to play the dual role of both translator and reader, and faithfully conveys the meaning of the original text. In addition, the translator also attaches great importance to the logic of the translation. In short, in the process of translation, the translator first faithfully reproduces the original text, that is, complies with the most fundamental principles of "faithfulness" and "expressiveness", and at the same time, tries his best to follow the grammatical rules of the target language so that the target readers can read and understand it. "Standardization" here refers to the norms that should be followed in translation, including terminology translation, choice of semantic meaning, sentence structure and so on. Translation norms, to some extent, can be taken as the product of the translator's choice between two different languages, cultures, and textual traditions. The norms of translation are often instructive, suggesting so that among the many possible choices, only one of them can be accepted and considered correct by readers. From the perspective of translation function, the first concern of translation is whether the target text can be accepted in the target language. No matter what strategies are adopted to deal with and solve translation problems, the role of norms in the target language system should not be ignored. The norm defines the semantic scope of a word or term and its collocation. Any arbitrary amplification, deletion or mistranslation of the semantics may be resisted by the target language. Therefore, translation norms can affect the behaviors of translators, and they are binding and mandatory to a certain extent and must be followed. In English and Chinese language expressions, there exist different norms in language usages, and it is hard to realize full equivalence, therefore, the translator here tries every possibility to narrow the differences and makes the sense of English translation equivalent to that of the source language in order to guarantee English readers to understand the translation with maximum likelihood in the same way as the Chinese readers understand the original Chinese text. The TCM translation criteria should include the standardization of terminology, choice of word and sentence structures. In short, the translator tries his utmost to follow the structural norms of both English and Chinese languages and convey the information contained in the text. "Accuracy" mainly refers to the accurate and exact conversion of the source language to the target language, that is, Chinese to English referred to here. On the one hand, it is faithful to the "accuracy" of the original text; on the other hand, it is the accuracy of the translation itself without equivocal or ambiguous expression. Accuracy is the "soul" of TCM translation. The translator needs to express the content of the original text accurately and completely without distortion, falsification, omission, or mistranslation to ensure that the content in the translated text is consistent with the original text. "Conciseness" refers to the information contained in the original text should be totally and completely expressed as possible in the most concise expressions and sentences. Therefore, in the TCM translation, in addition to meeting the standards of faithfulness, expressiveness, smoothness and standardization, the translator also tries his best to use direct, accurate, and concise expressions for translation.

As for translation of the names of Chinese medicines, in principle, for the first appearance of the name in the context, they will be translated in Chinese Pinyin plus bracketed translation equivalents in English. The subsequent appearance of the same medicine in the same volume or section will normally be translated in Chinese Pinyin only, but it does not rule out the translation of medicine names in the way of "Pinyin plus bracketed English names" irregularly in the following sections/passages in order to make it easier for readers to understand and avoid the trouble for readers to refer to the previous bracketed English names over and again. In addition, the medicine names, or special terms in the preceding volume, when they appear again in the new volumes, are first translated in Pinyin plus bracketed English names for the convenience of the readers, for example, the translation of Cangzhu (Rhizoma atractylodis) in the third volume is still translated in the same way of Cangzhu (Rhizoma atractylodis) in the fourth and fifth volumes for the first time when it appears, and in Pinyin Cangzhu only when it appears again in the following text.

Regarding the analyses of formulas and medicines in the book, each herb contained in all the formulas in this book, regardless of its appearing in the context or not, will be translated as Chinese Pinyin plus bracketed English name to ensure that readers can have a better understanding of the formulas. For instance, in the fourth volume, when the formula of Longdan Xiegan Tang is analyzed, all the ingredient herbs are translated in the way of Pinyin plus bracketed English equivalents: Longdancao (radix gentianae), Chaihu (radix bupleuri), Huangqin (scutellaria baicalensis), Zhizi (fructus gardeniae), Zexie (rhizoma alismatis), Mutong (akebiaquinata), Cheqianzi (semen plantaginis), Danggui (angelica sinensis), Sheng Dihuang (radix rehmanniae recen), Raw Gancao (raw licorice). Besides, among all these herbs, Huangqin (scutellaria baicalensis) repeatedly appears in the second, the third and the fourth volumes, however, it is still translated as Huangqin (scutellaria baicalensis) in its first appearance in the fifth volume, and its different chapters in the same volume. The purpose of such a translation way is to ensure the clarity and integrity of the formulas and facilitate English readers to be more familiar with the formulas. In addition, Tang, San, Yin and Pill are used respectively as the translation for the different forms of Chinese Medicines "汤"(Tang), "散"(San), "饮"(Yin) and "丸"(Pill) involving formulas or prescriptions. The frequently used special TCM terms, such as "阴", "阳", "上焦", "中焦", "下焦"and "三焦", are translated as Yin, Yang, the Upper Jiao, the Middle Jiao, the Lower Jiao, and the Tri-Jiao respectively.

Entrusted by Tang Lue, the author of the original work, and Academy Press Limited Company, Zhang Ganzhou, an English teacher at Qianjiang College of Hangzhou Normal University, Zhejiang Province, China, completes the English translation of the whole book. In the process of translation, Ms. Mickey Mi and Mr. Yang Jingbang, an Australian TCM practitioner have done a lot of work on the translation of the first draft of Volume I and Volume IV respectively. During the painstaking translation process, my wife, Ms. Huang Meijuan, has been silently contributing a lot and helping me to consult TCM classics and provided me with a lot of valuable TCM basic guidance for my translation work. I would like to express my heartfelt thanks to all of them. At the same time, I would like to express my heartfelt thanks to the author of the original work, Mr. Tang Lue for his hard work and providing the readers with a valuable book on the *Tao* of Chinese formulas and medicines, which is suitable for TCM learners and those who are interested in TCM culture at home and abroad. Last but not the least, all the constructive suggestion and kind advice on the English translation of this book from readers will be highly appreciated.

By the Translator
Hangzhou, China
June, 2021

英译前言

　　17 世纪中叶，英国王室桂冠诗人约翰·德莱顿（John Dryden，1631 – 1700），将所有翻译分为三类，即：逐字译、意译、拟作。所谓的逐字译也就是逐字逐行的翻译，与大家所熟悉的直译基本对应，也是翻译者最为常用的一种方法。但是，不同语言之间的转换，最大的挑战莫过于文化的翻译。一种语言文字转化为另外一种语言文字之后，原来承载一个特定文化的语言和译文的读者都发生了根本性的变化，如何保证译入语读者能够原汁原味地理解源语言所包含的语言、文化和专业信息，着实不是一件容易的事情。第二类意译是指译者根据源语言的信息而采取具有一定自由度的灵活翻译，译者严格遵循原作者所用词语背后的真实语意而不是其所用的词语本身。因此，意译就涉及词语的变更，与“意对意”的翻译大致相对应。第三类拟作，即译者摒弃原文词语的意思，对于翻译中无法避免的美的丢失，运用译者的智慧与创造力去创造出新的美感，这样的翻译基本上属于编译性质，译文最终只摘取了原文的主要信息，舍弃了一些次要的信息。

　　语言学家罗曼·雅可布森（Roman Jakobson）则从另外一个角度，将翻译分成三种类型：语内翻译、语际翻译、符际翻译。语内翻译是指同一语言中用一些语言符号解释另一些语言符号，如在古汉语英译前，首先将古代汉语翻译成现代汉语的过程。语际翻译是指两种语言之间的翻译，即用另一种语言的语符来解释一种语言的语符，也就是人们通常所指的“翻译”，如英汉互译。符际翻译是指通过非语言的符号系统解释语言符号，或用语言符号解释非语言符号，如把语言符号用图画、手势、数学、电影或音乐来表达。

　　关于翻译的策略和方法，国内外许多语言学家和翻译家分别从不同的角度进行过诸多的论述，如美国翻译理论家尤金·奈达提出的“动态对等"，常常为翻译论者所津津乐道。皮特·纽马克的语义翻译、交际翻译也为国内翻译学习者所熟知。美国著名翻译理论学家劳伦斯·韦努蒂（Lawrence Venuti）于1995年在《译者的隐身》中提出来归化与异化翻译策略。这些翻译理论为语言翻译者提供了很有价值的翻译指导。

针对翻译的标准，可谓仁者见仁、智者见智。在中国翻译史上，除唐玄奘之外，最为著名的翻译标准应属严复所阐述的"信、达、雅"三字标准。严复曾讲道："译事三难信、达、雅。求其信已大难矣。顾信矣不达。虽译犹不译也。则达尚焉。……易曰修辞立诚。子曰辞达而已。又曰言之无文，行之不远。三者乃文章正轨，亦即为译事楷模。故信达而外，求其尔雅。"但无论是采用什么翻译策略或方法，以及遵循什么样的翻译标准，译文的最终目标是将源语言中所包含的信息原原本本地翻译到译入语中，并为译入语读者所理解和接受，正如联合国教科文组织的《译员指南》中对翻译目的的描述：译者理解原文作者"想表达的含义"之后，应该把这一含义译成英语，且"尽可能地使英文对英语读者所产生的印象与原文相对应的外语读者所产生的印象相同"。

本书从中国的五行学说出发，选取最具代表性的五种中药材，分别以五行中的木、金、水、火、土作为典型的代表符号，基于中医的四气五味，讲述五大类中药材的特征、性状和功效。语言浅显易懂，生动有趣，将原本枯燥的中医医学像讲故事一样讲给读者，具有很丰富的知识性和很强的可读性，相信会给国内外中医爱好者带去意外的惊喜和收获。

基于前人有关翻译方法及翻译标准的论述和本书的内容，在翻译过程中，译者从语言学家罗曼·雅可布森（Roman Jakobson）的语内翻译、语际翻译出发，坚持信、达、顺、度、准、简的翻译标准完成了本书的英译工作。信，即忠实原文的信息，完整准确地反映原文内容，对原文中所叙述的事实、阐述的道理等无改变或歪曲、无遗漏或增减。传统中医药的著作，从语言角度看，具有非常特殊的语言特征，除了涉及主体内容医理、病理和药理专业知识外，还涉及大量的中国传统文化内容，包括天文、地理、历史、文学等。

中医翻译中的"信"就是要忠实于原文，准确、完整、科学地表达原文的内容，不任意对原文内容进行歪曲、增删、遗漏和篡改。同时，还要使译文合于原文，不仅要全面正确地理解原文的语法结构，正确理解词义，不随意引申，还要理顺原文长句乃至段落中的逻辑关系，使译文符合译入语的表达习惯，尽可能地避免中文式的英语。翻译中，考虑到英汉语言的巨大差异，采用了增词法翻译，但是增词法翻译的目的只是让译文更加符合英语的表达习惯，而不改变原文的语义。"达"，就是要对所译题材源语言彻底地理解，然后准确地在译入语中传译出来。19世纪初德国文艺批评家希勒格尔说："一个严谨的译者不仅会移植一部杰作的内容，并且懂得保存它的形式的优美和原来的印象，这样的人，才是传达天才的信使。"对于翻译，如果说"信"是停留在简单地移植一部杰作的内容的话，那么"达"可以说是在追求内容以及形式的优美和原来的印象。这里所讲的"达"字标准主要侧重于词、句、篇信息含义的透彻表达。"顺"，简单地说，就是"遵循规律而行"。翻译中的"顺"是指翻译时因应译文句法文理、修辞文风，则文通理明，使读者受益。若违背了文理，则无法正确地传达原文的本旨要义，所以，"顺"是要在忠实原文本旨基础之上，实现遵循译语的语言法则，使人读起来明晓通顺，文理顺畅，没有任何拗口和晦涩之感。为了保证译文的通顺，译者努力发挥自己既是译者也是读者的双重身份作用，忠实传达原文语义。另外，翻译要顺达，必须重视译文的逻辑性。通过分析原文的逻辑关系，然后再根据英语的逻辑思维习惯，进行组句翻译。总之，翻译过程中，译者首先把原文做忠实地再现，即符合"信""达"这一最根本原则，同时尽最大可能遵循译入语的文法规则，使译文的受众看得懂、读得通。这里的"度"是指翻译中应遵循的规范。"翻译规范在某种程度上可说是译者在两种不同语言、文化、篇章传统规范之间取舍的产物。"翻译的规范往往具有指导作用，可以暗示多种可能的选择中，只有一个结果能够被某个社会群体共同接受，并认为这是正确的。从翻译的功能看，翻译首先需关注译文在译入语中能否被接受。无论采用什么样的策略来处理和解决翻译问题，都不可忽视译入语体系中规范的作用。规范限定了词语或者术语的语义范围及其搭配方式，任何语义的随意增减或误译，都可能受到译入语的抵制。因此，翻译规范可以影响译者的行为，具有一定的约束力和强制性，必须遵守。在英汉语言的表达上，存在各自的形式规范，翻译中很难实现形式上的完全相同，所以，译者尽可能根据两种语言的形式规范，找到英语和汉语最大可能的彼此呼应，使原文与译文之间的差异性降至最小化，保证英文读者对原文的理解与中文读者对译文的理解尽可能地相同或相似。传统中医翻译的规范应该包括术语统一规范、词义选择规范、句子结构规范。总之，翻译是要遵循英汉语言各自的结构规范，准确表达语义。"准"，主要是指内容的准确性，一方面是忠实于原文的"准确"，另一方面是译文本身表达的准确，不含糊其词。准确是中医翻译的"灵魂"，译者需要准确完整地表达出原文的内容，不得有歪曲、篡改、删节、遗漏或误译等现象，保证译文表达的内容与原文一致。"简"，即用最简洁的词句表达尽可能多的信息，所以，在传统中医翻译中，除了要满足信、达、顺、度、准等标准外，译者还尽可能地使用直截了当、精确无误、简洁明了的语言进行翻译。

关于药名的翻译，原则上首次出现的药名，采用了汉语拼音，并在拼音后面加括号标出英文药名的方式翻译；同一卷或章节下文中再次出现同样的药名时，则仅采用汉语拼音，但不排除为了方便读者理解，前文出现过的药名，在下文中不定位置处在汉语拼音之后再次用括号标注英文药名，从而避免读者向前翻书查找汉语拼音所代表的英文含义的麻烦。另外，在前一卷里出现过的药名或术语，下一卷又出现时，第一次出现用拼音并加括号标注出英文以方便读者理解，如第三卷出现的 Cangzhu（rhizoma atractylodis），在第四卷首次出现时，仍然采用 Cangzhu（rhizoma atractylodis）翻译，后面再次出现时，则仅使用拼音 Cangzhu 翻译。

书中涉及药方分析时，对每一个药方中的每一味药，无论上文中是否出现过，均采用汉语拼音并在后面加括号标出英文药名的方式处理，确保读者更好地理解药方，如在第四卷中，龙胆泻肝汤药方中包含龙胆草、柴胡、黄芩、山栀子、泽泻、木通、车前子、当归、生地、生甘草，其中黄芩在第二卷和第三卷中均多次出现，但在翻译第四卷分析龙胆泻肝汤药方时，仍然把黄芩翻译为 Huangqin（scutellaria baicalensis），而非仅仅用拼音 Huangqin；同样，在第五卷中黄芩这味药也是多次出现，在首次出现和不同章节中均翻译为 Huangqin（scutellaria baicalensis），这样处理的目的在于保证药方的清晰和完整性，便于英语读者更好地熟悉药方。另外，翻译中涉及方药的汤、散、饮、丸的翻译，分别采用了 Tang, San, Yin, pill 来统一处理。对于传统中医文化中特有的术语如阴、阳、上焦、中焦、下焦、三焦等则沿用医药书中常用的翻译，分别译为 Yin, Yang, the Upper Jiao, the Middle Jiao, the Lower Jiao, the Tri-jiao，特此说明。

本书译者中国浙江省杭州师范大学钱江学院英语教师张干周受原著作者唐略先生和学苑出版社委托，负责该著作的英文翻译工作。翻译过程中，米奇女士和澳洲中医师杨靖邦先生分别对第一卷和第四卷的初稿翻译做了大量的工作；在艰苦的翻译过程中，我的夫人黄美娟女士一直在背后默默地奉献并协助查阅中医典籍，帮助熟悉中医药知识，为我的翻译工作提供了许多很有价值的中医基础指导，在此特表示由衷的感谢。同时，也要特别感谢原著作者唐略先生的辛勤付出，为我们提供了一本内容翔实的中医药著作。本著作适合于国内外广大传统中医学习者和中医文化爱好者阅读，并在此恳请广大读者对英语译文提出建设性批评意见。

译者
2021 年 6 月
于中国杭州

Preface

In 2012, I began to give lectures about "The Tao of Chinese Formulas and Medicines" in Qing Aixuan's network classroom. After three – year revision and polishing, the manuscript of the lectures was finally published.

Time is the best teacher, and especially the knowledge about traditional Chinese medicine (TCM) need time for accumulation. Now, when looking back to examine the lectures, I do feel the content of my lectures appears insufficient. After all, the knowledge of TCM is boundless, and the magical effect of the TCM formulas and medicines is boundless, too. Therefore, we must keep on studying to comprehend the medical experience accumulated and left to us by the ancient sages and the finest men of the ancient times. This book is unable to cover all the TCM knowledge, but as the book of introduction to TCM formulas and medicines, it is more than sufficient. After reading this book and laying a foundation, the readers and the TCM learners will be able to better comprehend the ancient wisdom. Therefore, this book was finally given the title of "The Tao of Chinese Formulas and Medicines ".

It is stated, "He who has ten thousand books in his mind and has no stereotype to follow can then start to write his own book, which tells us that it is not an easy work to write a book. Also, he who is learning TCM should not rush to write books about TCM until he is over 60 years old when he has reached high degree of professional proficiency in the field of TCM. Otherwise, what he does may mislead the coming generations. " I dare not say that I have "ten thousand books in my mind". Moreover, even if I had ten thousand books in my chest, I still must travel ten thousand miles as the Chinese proverb goes. Especially, for the knowledge concerning TCM, books may at most contain half of the related knowledge only, and the other half will have to be tacitly understood and acquired from the clinical practice. Writing books has always been a great mission of the sages and men of virtue to impart knowledge. Any mistake even in one word would spread the fallacy and mislead the people. Therefore, in the past time, few people dared to write books. However, we are now in an age of information explosion, the sense of writing a book is different.

This book starts with lectures, which is also an indispensable link in the process of pursuing studies since the ancient times. Through lectures, we can practice our thinking and exchange ideas so that learnings will be deeply integrated into our own life instead of loading one's mind with hackneyed phrases without originality. In particular, the conception of traditional Chinese learnings needs such repeated practices.

This book tries to reflect those practices. First, the classification of the TCM formulas and medicines is done based on the Wuxing Doctrine (about the five elements of metal, wood, water, fire and earth), which is the essential model of the traditional Chinese way of thinking. The Confucian classic "Book of History – Hong Fan" listed the five elements on the top of the "Hong Fan Nine Categories", and summarized their basic characteristics as: "Water is characterized by moistening and downward flowing; fire characterized by flaring up; wood characterized by growing freely and peripherally; metal characterized by clearing and changing; and earth characterized by cultivation and reaping." It also suggests the thinking mode of analogical association: "water moistening and downward flowing comes to the taste of salt (this concept stems from the salty seawater); fire flaring up comes to the bitter taste (this concept stems from the fact that all things will become bitter after they are burnt); wood growing freely and peripherally comes to the sour taste (this concept stems from the fruits growing out of wood); metal clearing and changing comes to the pungent taste (this concept stems from that melting and casting of metal will produce a kind of smell of pungency that is neither bitter nor sour); and cultivation and reaping comes to the sweet taste (this concept stems from Chinese Baijiu brewing)". The book of Principles of Wuxing says: "all things have their own constitution, and the saint gave them the names respectively according to their images and classification... before all the other things come the first – the five elements with their forms and functions being endowed by nature. Isn't that they were named first, and then their functions were known to all?" All things in the world are classified into five categories, namely wood, fire, earth, metal and water, based on which their properties and their mutual relationships are concluded and cognized. Or through imitating objects to compare species, human beings carry on reasoning of species, conjecture boldly, practice repeatedly to link their similarities, verify them cautiously, make the best choice and finally make the perfection more perfect. Since the ancient times, Chinese ancestors and people today have been trying to follow such means to understand the traditional medicines. This book is more inclined to let the readers experience the process of understanding, but is not eager to indoctrinate pharmacological potency.

The way of thinking in traditional Chinese learning is the foundation of TCM. Chinese people have been following such thinking mode for thousands of years. Unfortunately, this kind of thinking has been marginalized and even ridiculed under the influence of the western thinking. Therefore, a lot of ideas in my book might be disapproved of, but it doesn't matter. Just because of the different way of thinking, the true gentlemen ought to seek common ground while reserving the differences, and let the harmony exist in diversity.

I would like to express my heartfelt thanks to the friends of Qing Ai Xuan working group. They come from all walks of life, with the love of Chinese medicine, gathering through the network, taking their precious time every day to transcribe the recording into text, which is really a hard work, every five – minute recording usually taking an hour to reproduce in script. In particular, I would like to give my special thanks to Fang Haiping, Shen Minling, Gao Shang, Dong Jie, Zhang Meng, Cai Xiaoqiu, Chen Linyan and other friends, who also undertook the post – editing work. With their assistance, I do feel warm in my heart.

Tang Lue

Autumn, 2016 in Beijing, China

自　序

　　2012 年，我开始在清艾轩的网络讲堂讲方药，课程的名称叫"方药之道"，蒙听众们的厚爱，课程的录音被整理成文字稿，我再加工润色，成为本书。整个加工整理工作，持续了三年多。

　　时间是最好的老师，像中医这样的学问，更需要时间的积淀。如今再看这个讲座，内容已经略显单薄。毕竟中医学海无涯，方药妙用无穷，古圣先贤积累下来的经验还有待我们长期不断地学习、领悟，本书也无法穷尽这些知识，但作为学习中医方药的入门之书，让大家树立中国传统学问的思维方式和认知方式，这本书还是绰绰有余的。有了这个基础，我们再去接受古人讲的东西，就势如破竹了。所以，和学苑出版社的黄小龙兄商议，决定把本书的书名定为《思考中药：纯中医思维下的方药入门课》。

　　有人说："胸中有万卷书，笔底无半点尘者，始可著书。可见著书之难。中医不到 60 岁之后炉火纯青，不可著书，否则，必将贻误后人！"我不敢说自己"胸中有万卷书"，而且，即使胸中有万卷书，也是不够的，还得行万里路呢！尤其是像中医这样的学问，书本中能承载一半，还有一半在无言的实践中，只能心领神会。著书，历来圣贤用于传道授业，一字不慎，则谬种流传，误尽苍生，所以过去人们是不敢轻言著书的，但在今天这个信息爆炸时代，著书的意义又有所不同。

　　这本书，源于讲习。讲习自古就是治学过程中不可或缺的一个环节，通过讲习可以操练思维，交流思想，使学问不再是寻章摘句式的严谨，而是融入自我生命的深情。尤其是中国传统学问的思维，是更需要这种反复操练的。

　　这本书体现了这种操练。首先，在方药的分类上，我们以五行为依据。五行是中国传统思维方式的基本模型。儒家典籍《尚书·洪范》将五行列为"洪范九畴"之首，并概括了它们的基本特征："水曰润下，火曰炎上，木曰曲直，金曰从革，土爱稼穑。"还提示了其类比联想的思维模式："润下作咸，炎上作苦，曲直作酸，从革作辛，稼穑作甘。"《五行大义》云："夫万物自有体质，圣人象类而制其名，……从革作辛，稼穑作甘。"《五行大义》云："夫万物自有体质，圣人象类而制其名，……五行为万物之先，形用资于造化，岂不先立其名，然后明其体用？"人们把万事万物按木、火、土、金、水分成五大类，去归纳它们的性质，认识它们的关系，甚至通过取象比类，纵情联想，大胆猜测，再在反复的实践中小心翼翼地验证，精益求精地取舍。自古以来，人们对中药的认识，也经历着这样一个过程。本书更倾向于让大家体验这个认识的过程，而不急于灌输教条式的药理药性。

中国传统学问的思维方式是中医的根本，几千年来，中国人都是这样的思维，只可惜在西方思维的影响下，这种思维已经边缘化了，甚至被人嘲笑。所以，在当今，我这本书中的很多内容也会被人不认可。不认可不要紧，只因为思维方式不同，君子可以求同存异，也可以和而不同。

感谢清艾轩整理小组的朋友，他们来自各行各业，怀着对中医的热爱，通过网络集结在一起，每天抽出宝贵的时间进行将录音转录成文字的工作。五分钟的录音通常需要一个小时才能翻录完成，这是一项艰巨的工作。尤其是要感谢方海平、沈敏玲、高尚、董捷、张萌、蔡晓秋、陈林炎等朋友，他们还承担了后期编辑整理工作。有这么多志同道合的朋友的协助，我心里感到温暖。

唐略
2016 年秋于北京

— 2 —

Contents

目　　录

— 1 —

Volume 1
Introduction of Chinese Formulas and Medicines

Chapter 1　About the Tao of Chinese Formulas and Medicines

Let us start the journey of learning Chinese Medicine.

While talking about Traditional Chinese Medicine (TCM), one cannot focus on medicines only because the clinical formulas are also a critical and inseparable part of TCM. Meanwhile, the starting point of the journey hereof about TCM is the Chinese dialectical materialism of philosophy, i. e. Wuxing Doctrine (the Five Elements doctrine, referring to principles about the elements of metal, wood, water, fire and earth). Therefore, this book is named as *The Tao of Chinese Formulas and Medicines*.

Learning of "One Principle Running through All"

The western knowledge system tends to break up things into subjects so that students can study them one by one. The so-called "science" was literally translated into Chinese as "the study of subjects". However, the traditional Chinese knowledge is different—it focuses on the integrity, i. e., one principle runs through all.

In fact, certain knowledge can be acquired as an individual subject, but some cannot. For example, a complicated machine can be designed and assembled by different teams. However, one cannot do the same to the intellectual, organic, harmonious things such as human body. It is impossible to assemble human bodies like dismantling and re-installing a head. Some organs might be transplanted, but they cannot be as good as the original ones.

Therefore, for such an intellectual, organic, and harmonious human body, we need a medical science. So far, perhaps only TCM is able to reach such an extent. Definitely, there is no doubt that the other medical sciences are developing very rapidly so they can be divided into different branches for learning, but TCM cannot and it can only be learnt as a whole.

In modern universities, however, medicines and formulas are instructed and learnt separately. In teaching Chinese medicines, it is all about the properties of the medicines; in teaching the formulas, it is all about the analysis of different formulas with the properties of medicines inevitably at the same time. Why cannot medicines and formulas be put together to instruct the students in the classroom?

Drawbacks of "Inconsistency of Learning from One Expert"

To be worse, these two branches might be instructed by different teachers who have different manners of medication, or even different concepts for medical treatment. Then the students will feel lost somehow.

A living human body cannot be knocked down, and TCM cannot be knocked down, either. If TCM is divided into different disciplines as Chinese pharmacology, formulas of Chinese medicine, basic theories of Chinese medicine, internal medicine, surgery etc., all of which are to be taught by different teachers with different styles and modes of thinking, students finally may find themselves nowhere and at loose ends.

Once a beginner of TCM came to visit me and said that he had interviewed many TCM experts, which I don't quite approve of since he just acquired fragments of knowledge from some or the others. In *Huangdi Neijing (The Inner Classic of Huangdi)*, there is a term called "inconsistency of learning from one expert", which means one can never thoroughly learn from any teacher. If one tries to learn TCM in such a way, he or she may never acquire the genuine knowledge of TCM. In fact, as a beginner, one should start well and end well, i. e., to follow one expert to learn his complete conception regarding TCM before visiting other experts for broadening his horizon and learning more clinical expertise. At the beginning when one doesn't have even the most fundamental knowledge about TCM, he starts to visit many different experts and may easily get lost when he hears of some viewpoints from every Tom, Dick and Harry.

My Way of Stating the *Tao* of Chinese Formulas and Medicines

One cannot study Chinese medicines without learning formulas. Similarly, one cannot study formulas without learning medicines. Also, medicines and formulas cannot be understood without learning TCM theories and clinical practices. They all must be well integrated. Therefore, while I am discussing medicines and formulas, I will definitely not neglect the TCM theories and clinical practices in this book. I will illustrate TCM basic theories and methodologies of medical treatment by the way of focusing on medicines and formulas, i. e., to explain TCM theories from the perspective of medicines and formulas. In fact, it is about the *Tao* of traditional Chinese medicine, i. e., the idea of "one principle running through all" in Chinese philosophy. Therefore, this book is titled as ***the Tao of Chinese Formulas and Medicines***, for which I do not intend to confine it to one subject only.

Basics about Chinese Medicines and Formulas

Interpretation of the Chinese Character "药" (Yao, Medicine)

The Chinese characters are pictograph writing, which is very poetic and inspiring for imagination. The pronunciation, form and meaning of Chinese characters imply rich information. Whenever seeing a Chinese character in the course of learning TCM, one should use an associating way to understand the implied meanings. That is very helpful to train one's way of thinking.

Let us look at the character "药" (Yao in Pinyin, medicine in English), written as "藥" or "葯" in its original complex font. However, the form "藥" is most commonly used while "葯" has another implication in addition to the meaning of "medicine".

In the character "藥", the upper part (艹) means "grass" or "herb", and the lower part (樂) means "happy". When put together, the character means herbal medicine that can bring about happiness. How can herbs bring about happiness? One can imagine that herbs can cure diseases and maintain one's health, or even improve one's health conditions. When one recovers from illness and becomes healthy, he or she surely will become happy.

However, herbal medicines can bring about happiness, and they can bring about pains as well. If they are used properly, they bring about happiness; if used improperly, they aggravate the illness and even cause death. In such cases, they will be no longer medicines but pain makers.

Therefore, herbs are not unconditional medicines. Only when herbs are in the hands of a good doctor, can they become medicines. Otherwise, they are just grass roots, tree barks, dried bones or insensate stones. If they are used wrongly, they could even become poisons. Therefore, the talk of medicinal properties or toxicities of certain herbal medicines does not make any sense if without considering the specific circumstances of disease treatment.

Even in its simplified or variant form, the character "药" (Yao, medicine in English) also has its implied meaning. Its upper part (艹) means "grass" and its lower part (约) means "brief" or "economical". This character implies that one ought to use medicines moderately, not abusively. One essential principle in TCM is to cure diseases in the shortest time with least and mildest herbs at the lowest cost. It reflects the principle of thrift in terms of time, money and material resources, for which all the TCM doctors of all dynasties in the history of China have been trying their utmost so that TCM practices usually impress people with its unique advantages of being simple, convenient, effective and inexpensive.

Interpretation of the Character "方" (Fang, Formula)

Some people call a prescription written by a TCM doctor "a list of herbs", which appears superficial. In essence, it is called "formula".

In Chinese, the character "方" (Fang) means "method", signifying ways to cure diseases. Doctors in the history of China have passed down a lot of formulas, which reveal their experiences and methods to cure diseases. While one is studying formulas, he or she should not just try to memorize and use them mechanically. The key is to learn the conception implied in them, since TCM doctors give the treatment of diseases in line with certain concepts and philosophy. Reading books makes one sensible, and similarly, reading formulas helps to understand the implications.

Besides, the character "方" has another meaning of "orientation". A formula can guide the human body to a certain direction. For instance, following the principle of "warming the cold", one can use warm or hot medicines for cold symptoms, that is, to guide the body towards the direction of getting warm or hot. In this sense, the effectiveness of a formula mainly depends on whether it is in the right direction. Specific choices of herbs are secondary considerations. I have a small medicine cabinet at home to store some commonly used medicines such as Shigao (gypsum), Dihuang (rehmannia), Lugen (rhizoma phragmitis), E-jiao (donkey-hide gelatin) and Muli (concha ostreae) and so on, and totally, there are over 100 kinds of herbal medicines. Basically, they are enough for normal uses. Sometimes, I don't have a specific medicine at hand, but I can use the medicines available to substitute for it, which always proves quite effective since the right orientation to set can help to achieve the medical effects.

Pedagogical Formulas and Clinical Formulas

When one reads the TCM books written by ancient doctors, he or she often feels puzzled since in the books, the ancient doctors always gave lots of formulas to illustrate the functions with definite evidence; however, in the recorded cases of their clinical practices, different formulas were used instead of the corresponding ones in the books.

Antient doctors have left so many formulas; but those are seldom used if without any modification in clinical practices. These can be seen in books such as **Linzheng Zhinan Yi'an(Guideline to Clinical Practice With Medical Record)** by Ye Tianshi (a well-known medical expert in Qing dynasty, one of the most famous scientists of epidemic febrile disease school in Chinese history), the overwhelming majority of his formulas recorded from his clinical practices are not those passed down from the ancient doctors.

Another typical example is **Shibing Lun (Treatise on Seasonal Diseases)** by Lei Shaoyi (a famous medical expert on Seasonal Diseases). At the beginning of this book, the author described that certain diseases should be treated with certain formulas, however, in the following parts about the recorded cases of clinical practices, many modifications were done with additions or subtractions of medicines to/from the formulas, and some of them were even totally different.

What are the reasons for all those modifications to the given formulas? Actually, it is a matter of differences between the pedagogical formulas and the clinical ones.

Pedagogical formulas are those to be used by the teachers to expound certain rules of medication, to illustrate the right direction of a specific disease treatment, or to provide the dosage for the learners' reference. However, in clinical practices, it is necessary to do some modifications according to the patients and the symptoms of their diseases. Therefore, the best way to use those formulas is "to follow the underlying principles without being confined by the specifications".

Therefore, the formulas listed in *Yifang Jijie (Collection of Formulas with Notes)*, or in textbooks about formulas of Chinese medicine, are in reality all for teaching purposes; while the formulas in the ancient medical cases and those taken down by students accompanying the teachers in clinical practices are all clinical formulas, both of which can be learnt or used as references, but they are not dead rules to follow. Otherwise, the real essence of TCM will be totally lost if the practitioners do not understand how to make appropriate modifications.

In this book, a great number of pedagogical formulas will be included, for which more importantly, some flexible modification methods will be introduced and practiced.

Classic Formulas and Current Formulas

It might be asked whether the formulas included in this book are of classic formulas or current formulas? Some readers even ask me which medical school I belong to, the school of classic formulas, or school of current formulas?

In fact, such an idea is rather a human element classification. Formulas are intended to cure diseases, not to create debates. Doctors are expected to treat diseases with any proper means, not to stand in schools.

The so-called schools are usually used to describe typical features of some doctors' treatment of diseases. For example, Li Dongyuan (the representative of spleen-stomach theory) is regarded as a medical expert of "the school of invigorating spleen", Zhang Zihe (one of the four greatest medical masters in Jin-Yuan dynasty) is regarded as a medical expert of "the school of aggressive purgation", and Ye Tianshi is regarded as a medical expert of "the school of epidemic febrile diseases" etc.. I suppose that they all would strongly disagree with such labels marked on them.

There are also some doctors who use certain schools to show off, like "the school of classic formulas" as a typical example. They label the formulas in *Shanghan Zabing Lun (Treatise on Febrile and Miscellaneous Diseases)* by Zhang Zhongjing as classic formulas(Zhang Zhongjing, about 150 ~ 219 AD, who is respected as "the Saint of TCM". He wrote the book of *Shanghan Zabing Lun*, the first and most important TCM clinical guide for using herbal medicine formulas based on syndrome differentiation). In clinical practices, they would mainly use those classic ones, or even use those classic formulas only. Some even boast of using the "original formula with original dosage". This is largely influenced by doctors of kampo medicine from Japan (Kampo medicine: TCM practiced in Japan).

They admire the classic formulas so much so that they would reject all the other formulas that they take as the current formulas with an attitude of disdain.

Such attitude is inadvisable. Great doctors are those who have a spirit of inclusiveness, just like a sea welcoming all the rivers. Take Ye Tianshi as an example. He is usually regarded as an expert of the school of current formulas, or the school of febrile diseases, because most of the formulas he used are not classic ones. But in fact, he was far better in understanding and application of the classic formulas than those who call themselves as doctors of the school of classic formulas. From his book, *Linzheng Zhinan Yi'an(Guideline to Clinical Practice with Medical Record)*, one can also find many case studies using classic formulas. A book *Classical Formulas Prescribed by Ye Tianshi* written by Zhang Wenxuan, says that Ye Tianshi was not only very skillful at using the classic formulas, but also very good at modifying the classic formulas by adding or subtracting herbs to/from the classic formulas. He used the classic formulas in both direct or indirect ways. Many of his formulas were originated from the classic formulas, but could not be easily recognized by the ordinary learners. Such a state represents the highest realm of understanding the classic formulas.

Therefore, all the formulas, including the classic and current formulas, should be studied carefully and earnestly. This book will show respect to both the classic and current formulas without any differentiation of the schools.

Secret Formulas and Forbidden Formulas

From some TCM related novels and movies, or in the daily life, one may often hear about the term "ancestral secret formula". Then what are the secret formulas? What are they different from the formulas that are usually talked about?

As a matter of fact, the so-called secret formula is nothing but a formula that is not disclosed to the others. Keeping a formula as a secret is not just because of selfishness, but it is more about some rules that TCM follows to pass on the traditional heritage. It is a human nature that people tend to neglect the things that are easy to obtain, and treasure the things that are difficult to obtain.

Therefore, a teacher might give a hint that he or she has a secret formula in order to guide a learner to study hard to learn TCM. Afterwards, the learner will value every secret formula that he or she may obtain or acquire. Gradually such formulas become more valuable in the clinical practices, and thus, the true essence of TCM is also inherited from generation to generation.

Otherwise, the learners might take a formula as a negligible prescription, and then, will never realize the true values of the formula, or even ignore it gradually. With such a seemingly conservative way, some may worry about losing those secret formulas. In fact, more and more secret formulas are publicized. For example, the frequently used **Guifu Dihuang Pill** is originally named as **"Cui's Eight-ingredient Pill"**, which means it is an ancestral secret formula passed down from a Cui's Family. However, there are still so many people who know the secret implied in this formula but do not know how to use it properly.

Similarly, many secret formulas passed on among the "hand-bell healers" (referring to those practitioners who walked along the streets to meet potential patients, usually holding a hand bell to announce their presence) were made public by a scholar named Zhao Xuemin in Qing Dynasty in his book **Chuan Ya (Treatises on Folk Medicines)**

I also have a book on my desk named **Collection of Secret Formulas by Ye Tianshi**. Although I am not so sure whether the book was really written by Ye Tianshi, most of the formulas covered are very valuable and potentially could be secret formulas.

The key point is how many people would value them after these formulas are made public? And how many people could use them properly? Not so many, indeed. Therefore, to know about the formulas is just nothing important, but to know how to use them properly is more important. That will depend on learning from the teachers through explaining, highlighting, and demonstrating in clinical practices. Without such a learning experience, the so-called secret formulas are merely a list of herbs.

Therefore, there are some ancient formulas that are explicitly noted that they are forbidden to use if without the corresponding learning from teachers. Such formulas are called "Forbidden Formulas", which is for the sake of safety to the health of patients and also an important threshold in TCM.

The key point of my book here is to focus on how to use the formulas and medicines. For every formula to be discussed in this book, I will try every possibility to corelate the formula and medicines in multiple aspects rather than the plain introduction of meanings, functions and treatments, which is to help the readers and learners to fully understand the formulas so that they may feel really "grasping" those formulas.

第一卷　方药导论

第一章　"方药之道"题解

大家好，从今天开始，我们一起来学习中药。

课程的名称，本来是想叫"中药学"，但考虑到讲中药就离不开方剂，讲方剂又会讲到药物，方剂和药物没法分开，所以改为"方药之道"。

"一以贯之"的学问

西方的学问喜欢把一个东西分割开来讲，于是有了一个一个的科，一个一个的学，分科而学，就是科学。可能当初东方人把 science 一词翻译成"科学"时，就注意到了它"分科而学"的特征。中国传统学问不是这样的，它讲究"一以贯之"。这跟"分科而学"恰好相反。

有的学问可以分科而学，有的却不可以。比如设计一个很大的机器，我们可以把它分成几个部分，每个组负责完成一个部件，最后由总工程师把它拼装起来，就大功告成了。制造机器是可以分工，然后组装的。而那些灵动的、有机的、圆融的东西则不然。比如人体，人体可以组装吗？脑袋卸下来了可以重新安上去吗？器官移植，还能有原装的那样好吗？不可能的。

面对这样一个灵动的、有机的、圆融的人体，就需要一门灵动的、有机的、圆融的医学。到目前为止，大约只有中医达到了这个境界吧，当然，其他医学仍在快速发展之中。所以，其他医学可以分科而学，中医不能。

现在的大学里，中药学和方剂学是分开讲的，先讲中药学，然后再讲方剂学。二者割裂了，讲中药的时候光讲中药什么性质，讲方剂的时候又讲某个方是什么方义，同时也不得不讲一些药性。为什么就不能把方和药放到一块讲呢?

"受师不卒"的弊端

更要命的是,如果这两门课程分属两位老师讲,他们用药风格不一样,甚至治疗思想也不一样,学生就会感到无所适从。

人体是不能割裂的,中医也不能割裂,你把中医分解成中药学、方剂学、中医基础理论、内科学、外科学这些学科,由不同的老师来讲,一个老师是一个老师的思维方式,一个老师是一个老师的体系。学生学到最后,无所适从,会看病才怪呢!

前不久有一位初学中医的人来拜访我,他说他参访了很多的名师、高人。我对此毫不以为然,因为一个名师讲一套,一个高人讲一点,你听到的只不过是一些浮光掠影的碎片。针对这种状况,《黄帝内经》提到过四个字,叫"受师不卒",就是你在一个老师门下,没有学到底,这是学不好中医的。必须善始善终,把这个老师所有的东西完完整整地学来。接下来,你可以去参访名师,拓宽见识,取长补短,这样才能有所成。你一开始还不懂什么,就去参访名师,没有跟他们交流对话的基础,张三老师说向东你就向东,李四老师说向西你就向西,最后你就失去了方向。

"方药之道"的讲法

方不离药,药不离方,方和药又不离医理,不离临床,必须放在一起讲。现在我们要讲方药,也不会离开医理,不会离开临床,而是以方剂和药物为核心,演绎中医的基础理论和治病的方法。因此,我们讲一遍方药,也等于又从方药的角度,演绎了一遍中医的基础理论,一以贯之,这就上升到了道的高度。所以,我们称之为"方药之道",而不是把它仅仅局限于一个学科。

对药和方的一些必备认识

药字解

汉字是象形文字,是很有诗意的,可以激发我们的想象。从一个字的音、形、义上,都能折射出很多内容。我们学中医,看到每一个字,都可以去联想一下它们背后的意义,这个对于训练我们的思维是很有好处的。

我们看这个"药"字,繁体写作"藥""葯"。"藥"字最常用,"葯"

字则另有意义，也可以用来指药，可以看成"藥"字的异体字。

藥，一个草字头，一个快乐的乐字，这意味着，药，是给人带来快乐的草。草为什么能给人带来快乐呢？因为它可以治病、养生，能解除我们的病痛，还能让我们的身体更好，可不是带来快乐吗？

只不过，能给人带来快乐，就能够给人带来痛苦。你用得对，它就能给人带来快乐；用得不好，加剧病情，甚至把人治死了，那就是给人带来痛苦，那就不是药了。

所以说，没有绝对的药。必须到了会用的人手里，它才是药，否则，就只是草根树皮、枯骨顽石。如果用错了，它就更不是药了，而是毒。脱离了具体运用，去谈某药有某用，某药有毒，都是不合理的。

就连简体或异体的"药"字，都有其寓意，从草从约，意味着，用药要有节制，不能滥用。中医的一个原则就是：用最少最平和的药、最快的时间、最少的钱，治愈疾病。在时间、金钱和物力上，都体现了"节约"二字。历代医家都在为此不懈努力，因此，中医中药给人的印象往往是"简便验廉"。

方字解

有些人把中医开出的方子叫"药单"，这是从表面上看的；从实质上看，我们把它叫"方"。

方，有"方法"的意思，它体现着治病的方法。历代医家传下来很多方子，其中都体现了他们治病的经验和方法，我们在学习方剂的时候，不要死记硬背，更不能生搬硬套，关键要学习其中的思想，因为中医是靠思想治病的，方子是思想的产物。读书明理，读方知义，是我们学习方剂的正确途径。

方，还有"方向"的意思。它会把你的身体往某个方向引导。比如，寒者温之，寒证用温热药，就是把身体往温热的方向引导。从这个意义上讲，方子治病，关键是要方向正确，用哪些药倒在其次。我家里有一个小药柜，会存放一些常用而又不容易生虫的中药材，比如石膏、地黄、芦根、阿胶、牡蛎之类，大约有一百来种。平时用这些，也就够了，可能某个药没有，但我可以用其他性质类似的药去代替，效果照样很好。因为只要把准了方向，就会有疗效。

教学方与临床方

我们看古人的医著，会发现一个问题：他们的方书，会列举出很多方子来，说明其功能主治，言之凿凿。但他们的医案，遇到这种病，用的却未必是他在方书中说的那个方子。

古人留下来的方子那么多，但我们看叶天士《临证指南医案》等经典医案著作，会发现，他们在临床中开出的方子，绝大多数不是古人现成的。

最典型的是《时病论》，前文说好了某病用某法某方，后面医案部分就变卦了，大多对原方进行了加减，有的甚至另起炉灶，重拟新方。

这是为什么呢？这就涉及教学方法和临床方的差异问题。

教学方，是老师用来教学生的方子。老师用这个方子，来说明某个道理，告诉大家某个病治疗的方向，甚至列出剂量，供大家参考。但真正到了临床上，还要根据具体的人、具体的病，进行加减，有的加减，甚至能使原方面目全非。所以，用这些方剂，最佳的境界是"师其法而不泥其方"。

像《医方集解》还有《中医方剂学》里列出来的方剂，其实都是教学用方；古人医案里的方，你跟着老师侍诊抄出来的方，都是临床方。二者都是用来学习，用来参考的，在你自己今后的临床中，都不能生搬硬套。否则，不知变通，那就不是真正的中医了。

我们这本书，会提到大量的教学方，更会告诉大家临床变通的方法，并且跟大家一起操练。

经方与时方

可能有人会问，你这本书里涉及的方剂，是经方还是时方呢？

甚至还有人会问：你是经方派还是时方派呢？

其实，"经方"和"时方"都是人们生造出来的概念，方子是用来治病的，能把病治好就行，分什么经方与时方呢？医生的目的就是要把病治好，在方法上勤求博采，哪里还有心思分什么门派？

所谓门派之说，很多都是旁观者用来形容某些医生的特色的，比如我们把李东垣叫补土派，把张子和叫攻下派，把叶天士叫温病派，只恐怕李东垣、朱丹溪和叶天士要是地下有知，也会棺材板啪啪作响，抗议这些封号。

也有的派别之名是某些人用来自诩的，比较典型的就是"经方派"。他们把张仲景《伤寒杂病论》中的方子叫经方，在临床中，他们以用经方为主，有人只用经方，甚至讲究使用原方原量。这很大程度源于日本汉方医学的影响。

因为如此推崇经方，所以很多人就对经方以外的方子产生排斥，于是将其命名为"时方"。有的人甚至一提到时方，就有点鄙夷的态度。

其实，这种态度是不可取的。必须兼容并包，海纳百川，才能成就真正的精诚大医。比如叶天士，很多人都认为他是时方派、温病派，因为他开的绝大多数方子都不是经方。而实际上，叶天士对经方的理解和运用水平，远远高于那些自称"经方派"的人。我们看《临证指南医案》，其中用经方的医案不在少数。张文选先生有本书叫《叶天士用经方》，就指出，叶天士不仅在经方的使用上非常纯熟，还擅长加减变化，他不仅直接使用经方，还间接使用经方。他使用的很多方法，都脱胎于经方，却了无痕迹，一般人看不出来。这才是使用经方的最高境界。

所以，经方要好好学，时方也要好好学。我们这本书，将不论经方时方，一视同仁。

秘方与禁方

我们看一些关于中医的小说或影视，或是在现实生活中，都常常会听说"祖传秘方"这个词，那么，到底什么是秘方呢？秘方跟我们平时讲的方子有什么不一样么？

其实，秘方也是方，只不过是秘不示人而已。秘不示人，并不完全因为自私，更多的，是出于中医传承的某些规律。人性本来就是这样，某个东西，得到得越容易，你就越不重视；越难得，你就越重视了。

所以，老师可能会暗示你：我有秘方，你要好好学，到时候我会传给你的。以后，每得到一个秘方，你都会视若珍宝，好好体会其中的意义，在使用中也会格外重视，这样的方子，以后使用起来会更顺手。这样一来，中医才算传承下来了。

如果不这样做，学习者反而会心生怠慢，那他永远体会不到这个方子的妙处，以后甚至不会用。这样做看似保守，有些人甚至担心这样会使这些秘方失传。其实，越来越多的秘方，都被公开了。比如，我们常用的桂附地黄丸，原名"崔氏八味丸"，可能就是某个姓崔人家的祖传秘方，后来就公开了呀，但知道它而不会用它的中医不仍然大有人在？

过去在铃医中口口相传，秘不示人的很多秘方，被清朝学者赵学敏变成一部书，叫《串雅》，完全公开了。

我案头还有一本《叶天士手集秘方》，是不是叶天士亲手编的，姑且存疑，但其中的方子都很好，有作为秘方的潜质。

但这些秘方公开后，重视它们的人有多少呢？会用它们的人又有多少呢？并不多。光知道方子是没用的，更重要的是要知道如何用。这就要靠老师口传心授、并且在运用中亲自示范了。如果没有人带你，你得到的所谓秘方，也只不过是一张张"药单"。

所以，古代就有一些方子，明言若无相应的传承，则禁止使用，这就是"禁方"。禁止使用，是为了安全起见，这也是中医的门槛。

方药如何使用，这也是我们这本书的重点。因此，我们在讲每一个方子的时候，并不机械地介绍其方义、功能、主治，而是尽可能地多方关联，让这些方子扎根在读者内心。这样，你才算真正拥有了这些方子。

Chapter 2   The Way that Chinese Medicine Cures Diseases

Integrity of Chinese Medicine

What is Chinese Medicine

To understand the way that Chinese medicine cures diseases, first, one needs to rule out a wrong concept that Chinese medicines contain certain substances that have certain targeting effects towards some specific diseases or bacteria, or supplement something to human body.

If one is thinking in such a way, he or she is not talking about Chinses medicine, nor using Chinese medicine in a proper way, but looking at Chinese medicine with the concept of the western medicine. What is Chinese medicine? Chinese medicine refers to the medicine prescribed under the guidance of TCM conception. Those so-called Chinese medicines, such as Huanglian (coptis chinensis), Duzhong (eucommia ulmoides), Shigao (gypsum), Guiban (tortoise plastron), in terms of material form, are merely tree barks, grass roots, stones or dried bones. They become Chinese medicines only because their functions and effects were found and proved under the guidance of TCM theory, and they are seemingly endowed with souls to function their roles in the TCM field.

Never Destroy the Integrity of Chinese Medicines in Analytical Ways

Thinking that "there's certain substance in certain herbs......" is a way to destroy the integrity, or the wholeness of herbs. Take Huanglian (coptis chinensis) as an example. Some studies say that Huanglian has the function of "clearing fire" since it contains berberine. So, berberine is extracted from the plant to treat the corresponding diseases. It works well for some time until human bodies developed medicine resistance. However, turning back to Huanglian, doctors find it still works well.

Similarly, Qinghao (artemisia apiacea), an indispensable anti-malaria herb.

Professor Tu Youyou has discovered and extracted artemisinin from the herb as a new medicine. But its effect is lost after certain period of clinical application. Professor Tu also expresses her concern regarding the medicine resistance to artemisinin during her speech at the news release as a Nobel Prize winner. What could be done then? Just use Qinghao, as it is still effective. This shows that Qinghao does not equal to artemisinin. Of course, one cannot deny the great contribution of artemisinin in treating malaria, and that it is a well-deserved Nobel Prize.

Take a metaphor of a very successful family as an example, one cannot say that the success is just because of one of the members in the family, and actually, it should be attributed to all the family members. One individual member may become nobody if he or she is separated from his or her powerful family.

From the perspective of composite analysis, one herb contains numerous substances. They are a family to function as a whole, and cannot be separated from each other. Huanglian works well as Huanglian is used as a whole. Qinghao works as a medicine in the same way. Each works as an intact function unit, not because of certain individual substances it contains. How exactly does the function take place? Well, one might never achieve an ultimate result if he or she uses a micro view to analyze their material compositions and chemical attributes. Therefore, this book will introduce the traditional "analytical method" that is unique in TCM theory. The first concept is about the "four properties and five tastes" of medicines.

Four Properties and Five Tastes of Chinese Medicines

In accordance with TCM theory, medicines are the products of nature. And from the perspective of traditional Chinese wisdom, everything should be understood in the context of the Heaven, the Earth and the Human Being. So, the medicines are regarded as having four properties from the universe, and five tastes from the Earth. The four properties refer to the coldness, heat, warmth and coolness of the four seasons in a year, which are endowed by the universe. The five tastes refer to the sour, bitter, sweet, pungent, and salty tastes, which come from the Earth. Thus, every medicine has its unique natural attributes in terms of its property and taste combined.

Properties and Tastes, Full or Partial

Is the nature absolutely impartial? No, it has obvious favoritism. It only gives partial properties or tastes to animals, or plants, or minerals. For example, it gives coldness to Shigao and Huanglian; it gives heat to Fuzi (radix aconiti carmichaeli) and Ganjiang (rhizome zingiberis); it gives warmth to Shanyurou (common macrocarpium fruit); it gives sourness to Baishao (radix paeoniae alba or white peony root); it gives bitterness to Huanglian and so on.

Some may argue that Wuweizi (fructus schisandrae chinensis) has all the five tastes. But this is a very rare example. Furthermore, Wuweizi only has warmth in terms of the four properties.

Many herbs grow in spring, and wither in fall. Some sprout around the winter solstice, and wither around the summer solstice. They won't experience the four seasons of a year. Some herbs only grow in the south, and some only in the north. Those are limited in specific areas, which is obvious that they only have partial properties or tastes.

In fact, only human beings get the full properties and tastes from the nature, and therefore, human beings are regarded as the "spirit of the universe". The life span of human is usually long enough to experience many cycles of four seasons of a year. And people travel to all the directions and adapt to different locations around the world. Hence, human beings gain the four properties and five tastes in full, which is essential to make human different from animals. Please do not regard human species as one kind of animal. There are similarities, but human beings are absolutely not animals. According to Buddhism, human beings and animals belong to different divisions in the wheel of karma (according to Buddhism, there are six great divisions in the wheel of karma: gods, demi-gods, human beings, animals, hungry ghosts and hell beings. The first three of them are the higher realms and the last three are the lower realms.) The human race lives in a much higher realm than the animals, and it is a very precious opportunity to become a human in the wheel of karma. The human beings are the beloved children of the universe, and they are so blessed by the nature with many things that have curing functions. The illness can be regarded as an imbalance among the four properties and five tastes inside the body, thus displaying certain partiality. So, the Chinese medicines could be used to correct or compensate such partiality by their specific properties and tastes. This is the first level of understanding regarding the four properties and five tastes.

Functions of the Four Properties and Five Tastes

The second level of understanding is about the effects of the four properties and the five tastes. If one is too cold in his or her body, warm or hot medicines can be used to warm up; if he or she is too hot, cool or cold medicines (Here the "cool, cold, warm, hot" are not just about simple concept related to body temperature. They are actually syndromes judged by TCM theories. Some situations could be very complex such as alternating chill and fever, etc.) would be used to clear the heat. This principle is called "treating the cold diseases with the hot medicines; treating the hot diseases with the cold medicines".

The effects of the five tastes can be briefly summarized as: pungent for dispersing, salty for softening, sour for astringing, sweet for relieving, and bitter for drying.

Scents and tastes can be classified as the thick and the thin. Their effects can be briefed as "medicines with thin scent promote dispersing; medicines with thick scent promote heating; medicines with thin tastes promote to breaking through; medicines with thick tastes promote discharging. "

These are some basic guidance in TCM, just like the fundamental theorems and axioms in mathematics. More explanations about these principles will be provided later when specific herbal medicines are to be illustrated so as to help further understanding of the practical cases.

Other Natural Properties of Chinese Medicines

The four properties and five tastes are the major guidelines of understanding Chinese medicines, and of course, they are highly emphasized. However, there are many more natural properties to be observed about medicines. As often mentioned by the ancients, observation of the nature involves "looking up and down", which means to look up to the sky and down to the earth, so as to thoroughly comprehend the properties of substances. In addition, the knowledge will be further verified again and again in practical applications. This is a very broad vision and also a very interesting process of understanding.

Next, let us take some examples of Chinese medicines to illustrate their differences in terms of natural properties.

Mahuang (Ephedra) vs. Congguan (Scallion)

Let us take Mahuang (ephedra) for example. In terms of four properties and five tastes, it is pungent and warm. So, it can disperse pathogenic Qi because of pungency, and can dissipate the cold because of warmth, that is, it can induce perspiration. There are so many medicines that are both pungent and warm, why does Mahuang have a stronger power for inducing perspiration? This is because of its some other properties. Look at its shape: Mahuang is a kind of green, thin, straw-like grass, with sectioned hollow leaves. Because it is hollow, it can promote circulation of Qi; and because it is thin, it can open the fine pores on the skin.

Another plant is the scallion. It is pungent and warm, too, with hollow leaves that are larger than those of Mahuang. Scallion also has the function of inducing perspiration, but less powerful than Mahuang. Because of its larger size, scallion functions less upon fine pores; but it functions more on nares, perhaps because the diameter of the scallion leaves is more comparable to that of nares.

The large tubed leaves can open the larger openings, and the smaller tubed leaves open the smaller openings. Is this imagination too whimsical? It is possible, but it has to be further verified. In many cases of nasal obstruction (snuffling) caused by a common cold due to the wind-cold, the patient often uses **Congchi Tang** (Scallion and Fermented Soybean Decoction). After drinking it, the patient may sweat a little, and the stuffy nose can be released right away. The formula of **Congchi Tang** is very simple: just scallion and fermented soybean, which are quite common in the kitchen of all Chinese families.

Many cases have proved the effectiveness of Mahuang and scallion, which also have verified our whimsical assumption again and again. Therefore, let us tentatively accept the theory about the causal association between the functions and shapes of plants.

Understanding Cicada Slough from Chirping Cicadas

The cicada slough is a layer of skin taken off from a cicada. It is described as sweet taste and cold in property in many books, and can dissipate wind-heat. It is sweet and cold because it comes out of the earth. According to *Souvenirs Entomologiques(Insect Records)* written by Jean-Henri Casimir Fabre, the larva of a cicada usually lives under the ground at least four years before it can sing on the trees. The temperature under the ground is in a state of relative equilibrium, neither too cold in the winter, nor too hot in the summer. The earth is neutral and inclusive. If buried under earth and given long enough time, the fire (hot) property of anything could be removed. Therefore, many herbal medicines processed by frying/parching, such as the fried Baizhu (white atractylodes rhizome) or the fried Cangzhu (rhizoma atractylodis) , need to be spread out on the ground for at least one night for removing the hot property after being fried, because these medicines get hot property when fried, and could be harmful to the human body. Spreading on the ground is a way to let the earth absorb the fire (hot property) . Since cicadas live under the ground for such a long time, the hot property is already removed. Thus, it is known as a medicine with cold property.

It is sweet also because it comes out of the earth and the earth tastes sweet. It attracts the sweet taste of the earth as like draws to like. Meanwhile, it can dissipate since it is a layer of skin, the superficial part of the body. Hence, it is related to the function of dissipating the superficial pathogens——the pathogenic wind-heat. For example, it can induce eruption, as eruption is a symptom of pathogen on the surface of body. Therefore, the learners can understand the properties and tastes of this medicine by associating it with its natural properties.

One may further use the associating way to findsome other functions of cicada slough. It may clear the ocular nebula. Nebula is often the cause of blurred vision of the elderly people. In some cases of nebula, based on syndrome differentiation, cicada slough is often added to achieve good result. Such curing process is like peeling off a layer of nebula from eyes, just as a cicada molting from its outer skin.

Cicada slough may also be used to treat skin diseases, surely based on syndrome differentiation. Usually in the middle or later stage of treatment, cicada slough could be added to the formula, aiming at "molting off" the affected skin.

It sounds absurd in such a strange way of talking, but sometimes the complicated nature might be easily comprehended in such a "poetic" way.

In addition, cicadas produce high pitched sound in summer, so cicada slough can be also used to treat hoarseness. In the formulas for singers and teachers, cicada slough might be used to help them produce ringing and clear voices. To treat husky voices, cicada slough in the formula usually will have a good effect, of course it should be used based on the right syndrome differentiation.

Some babies cry noisily at night. Does this remind you of cicadas? To treat this, first of all, it is important to clearly define the root causes, such as, due to cold or heat, or food retention, or scare etc. Cicada slough may be used for such cases.

In the case of husky voices, cicada slough could be used tomake the voice sonorous; while in the case of night crying of small babies, cicada slough could be used to suppress the voice. This tells us that one attribute could lead to functions of two different sides, all of which were tried and summarized in the past generations based on observation of the cicada slough. The functions may sound weird, but actually they have been practiced and verified continuously by many doctors in the history. Otherwise, many doctors would have raised objection to such efficacies.

The Way That Cinnabar Tranquilizes the Mind

Cinnabar is another example. It appears red or rubrical, quite eye-catching. It is often used to make top grade red ink paste for seal use. From TCM perspective, the red color goes to the heart meridian. Cinnabar also feels heavy, so if one purchases half kilo cinnabar, visually he finds it quite little in volume. Heaviness implies that it can press down. Entering the heart and functioning downwards, these two combined properties indicate that it can tranquilize and calm down the mind. Therefore, cinnabar can be used for curing insomnia and many other more serious mental disorders.

For the insomnia that is not so serious, just use magnet or lodestone instead of cinnabar. Lodestone or magnet also has the repressing function and can be used to allay excitement so as to calm down the mind, just as magnet attracting iron material. For the obstinate and chronic insomnia, a little bit of cinnabar, like cinnabar-coated Fuling (poria cocos) or Fushen (poria cum ligno hospite) , could be used, but cinnabar must not be used directly.

Mania, as one of the mental disorders, can be treated by adding a little bit of cinnabar to tranquilize (sedate) the patient. In addition, cinnabar is used to protect houses, i. e. , to exorcise the evil spirits from a house, which is also to take the advantage of its "repressing" function.

Some children may suffer from nightmares. In such cases, putting a little cinnabar in their pillows will help them to have sound sleep. Cinnabar functions well even without being swallowed. **Shennong Bencao Jing (Shen Nong's Herbal Classic)** says cinnabar "if taking for long, one can keep young. " Here, "taking" does not just mean to swallow, but also means to wear.

Cinnabar enters the heart meridian, and has the repressing function, but it is not good to take it excessively. Otherwise, it may suppress the Heart-Yang (the function of the Heart), which will cause the cinnabar users to appear feeble-minded or look foolish, as described in some folk saying "cinnabar-fooled". Taking too much cinnabar, one could become less intelligent, and very stubborn when losing temper.

Once before, when I talked about the principle of cinnabar use, I was challenged bya person, "according to your logic, may I cure mental disorders by taking a piece of heavy iron fried with hot peppers? These are also red, heavy and repressing! " My answer was "as it is your proposal, please verify it by yourself. "

Such ways of thinking like association and analogy are often the starting points for some people to question TCM. In fact, the key problem of such people is that they are indulged in empty talks, far away from real practices. Without repeated verification in clinical practice, neither scientific arguments nor the whimsical ideas of poets are worthy of anything. Chinese medical principles are profound learning rooted in the long practices, and verified through practices day by day. While imagination and analogy are just ways to explain something.

Understanding the Principles and Applications through Image Thinking

According to TCM theory, everything has its properties that enable the corresponding functions. Medication, in fact, is to experience and observe all things, and utilize the natural properties of things as well.

The way that Chinese are talking about "physics" is a quite different from that adopted by the westerners. In Chinese way, physics (literally means "the principles of things") covers a wide range of studies, which is more profound and flexible. It would be too elementary to just know a medicine according to its properties, taste, functions, compatibility, and diseases to treat. Such knowledge lacks of the macro view of looking up and down, making a thorough inquiry into the sense of physics of things. To learn TCM well, one must begin with an attitude toward depth and broadness of studying things.

In the above section, I took three examples to illustrate the functions of a medicine. Actually, that is a poetic, image-based way of comprehension, which intends to help the learners to understand a full range of properties of a medicine through associations. On the contrary, if one just makes a dull list that cicada slough can cure baby's night cry, remedy hoarse voice, remove eruptions, remove the nebula in the eyes, treat skin diseases and so on, it would be too difficult to understand and memorize the efficacies. Therefore, I try to illustrate them one by one to help the learners understand them all by associations, and avoid rote memorization. Such associations can help learners to forge their personalities and become more lively, cute, inclusive, open, and close to nature.

Movement of Medicines

It is not enough to know of the functions and properties of a medicine since the direction of its movement in the body is also important. In physics, there is a concept of "vector". For example, a force has magnitude and direction. Similarly, an herbal medicine is like a vector. It also has magnitude which refers to its property, and direction which refers to how and where the medicine goes after it enters the human body. This will involve its ascending, descending and channel tropism.

Most people attach great importance to the properties of medicines, but not to moving directions of the medicines, or tend to forget the movement while in the clinical practice, which will weaken the effects of medication.

Ascending or Descending

Different medicines move towards the different directions in the human body. Some medicines go upwards; some go downwards; some go into the five internal organs (heart, liver, spleen, bladder and kidneys); some go to the four limbs; some go to the Upper Jiao; some go to the Middle Jiao and some go to the Lower Jiao.... Therefore, medicines should be chosen based on the disease location, and the moving direction of the pathogens.

How can we grasp the moving directions of the medicines, i. e. , the ascending or descending? Definitely, rote memorization is not a proper way. My teacher never asks me to recite anything like *Yaoxing Fu* (*Medicine Properties in Verse*), rhyme or verses of formulas, which traditionally were required to learn by heart. I am encouraged to understand the real principles implied, by which I can know and learn a lot of things naturally. Without understanding the *Tao* or principle in the medicines, it is useless even I can memorize all the things.

In fact, the name of many medicines shows the moving directions. For example, Shengma (rhizoma cimicifugae), it definitely goes upwards, as the character "升" (Sheng) in Chinese literally means "rising". Another example, Chenxiang (agilawood), it definitely goes downwards as the character "沉" (Chen) in Chinese literally means "sinking". Generally speaking, wood usually floats on water, however, agalwood is an exception, and it sinks into water. So, when it is used as a medicine, it also goes downwards in the human body, and helps to depress Qi.

The TCM learners must pay much attention to the names/descriptions of herbs, formulas, or acupoints etc. in which many plant passwords need deciphering. For an herbal medicine, its properties and moving directions could be inferred from the position where it grows out of the plant.

Flowers and Leaves——Ascending; Seeds——Descending

Flowers and leaves have ascending and dissipating functions, as they are the most exterior parts of plants. Flowers send out fragrance and leaves evaporate water, which tells us they all dissipate or diffuse something. Therefore, they can function the similar way in the body when used as medicines. Those who have ever taken Chinese medicine for a cold should have such an experience that they will bring back a pack of herbs with only a few herbs in the prescription in which most of the herbs are flowers and leaves because of their ascending and dissipating functions. They are used for the purpose of getting rid of the pathogens from the body surface. Of course, there are some exceptions, for example, Xuanfuhua (inula flower) does not ascend or dissipate, but it descends instead.

All seeds have a descending effect. The mature seeds of plants will fall to the ground to take root and sprout, such as Laifuzi (radish seed), Wuweizi (fructus schisandrae chinensis), Baijiezi (semen brassicae), Cheqianzi (semen plantaginis), and Chuanlianzi (szechwan Chinaberry fruit). Therefore, they function the same way in human body. Some other seeds, such as Taoren (peach kernel), Xingren (apricot kernel), Baiziren (platycladi seed), Suanzaoren (wild jujube seed), are obviously oily. So, they can moisten the intestines and relax bowel. In addition, such sorts of seeds also tend to be warm. Otherwise, how can they have the power to sprout? There are also exceptions, too. For example, Manjingzi (fructus viticis), it is ascending, and it is also cold and light in properties, so it can be used to dispel the wind on the face and head.

Twigs Go to Limbs; Stems Go up and down

Twigs of plants go to the four limbs of the human body. It can be taken that it is following the principle of "like drawing to like", such as Guizhi (cassia twig), Sangzhi (mulberry twig), Zisuzhi (purple perilla twig), such herbs all go to the limbs. In case of pain in the arms and numbness at the finger tips, Sangzhi can be used as the guiding medicine. If such a case is serious due to the cold, Guizhi can be added. If it is only a little acute pain due to the cold for a short time, Zisuzhi and Sangzhi will work well.

Stems, as the mainstalks of plants, are the major trunk through which nutrition is transported from the roots to the upper branches, and the energy produced through photosynthesis at the leaves is transported to the roots for preservation. So, stems are considered to have the function of both ascending and descending. The herbs like Zisugeng (purple perilla stem) and Huoxianggeng (ageratum stem) can regulate Qi circulation inside the human body through ascending and descending process.

Roots Are Divided into Three Parts

It is a little more complicated when the roots of plants are used as medicines. The upper part of a root tends to go upwards because it is mainly functioning to supply nutrition to the upper part of the plant. The lower part of the root hair tends to go downwards since it always needs to grow deeper in the ground, so, it can cure the disease in the Lower Jiao. The middle part of the root tends to "stay in the center", so, it is often used to treat the diseases in the Middle Jiao. For instance, Danggui (angelica sinensis), it can be cut into three parts: Danggui Tou (angelica head), going upwards and invigorating the circulation of blood; Danggui Shen (angelica body), going to the middle part of the body to nourish blood; and Danggui Wei (angelica tail), going downwards to break blood stasis. However, roots are often used as a whole now without such a division. Of course, for some roots to be used as herbs, doctors have to differentiate the heads and root hairs, for instance, Lugen (rhizoma phragmitis).

At the top of the root of the reed is the head, which is the interconnection part between the root and the stem. The head part definitely goes upward, as this is the part where nutrition from the root goes up to the entire plant. When it is used as medicine, it has a very strong ascending effect, and even may cause vomiting. Therefore, when Lugen is used as a medicine, the head part is generally removed. Again, ginseng is a very valuable medicine, whose head, of course, should not be thrown away. Meanwhile, because of its special function, ginseng head is usually kept separately and will come in handy when those who are weak in physique suffer from the pathogens in the Upper Jiao. In that case, the doctor may need the ginseng head to promote the patient to vomit a little for curing their illness.

The lowest parts of roots are the root hairs that are always trying to go downwards deeper into the ground. So, they have the function of breaking through. For example, Gancao (licorice), when it is used to harmonize herbs in a formula, but the doctor may not want it stay in the Middle Jiao, and in that case, Gancaoshao (licorice root tips) can be used since it moves downwards faster. Cancaoshao can be also used in treating the painful urination with blood since it has the function of clearing the urethra.

Other Methods of Determining the Moving Directions

In addition to what has been discussed above, there are some other methods to make the judgment of moving directions of medicines, such as, the joints of a plant go to the joints of human body; the barks of a plant go to the skin of body; the core of a plant go to the heart; the fiber of a plant can go to the meridians and collaterals in the body; the vines go upwards; and thorns can prick something.... Therefore, the TCM learners must study the nature of things and properties of herbs.

Medicines such as metals, minerals, fossils, and shells are all very heavy. In fact, all the heavy medicines are endowed with the similar properties, that is, their basic moving direction is to go downwards.

Besides, there are some medicines taken from animals, which are usually called "medicines of flesh and blood". Based on the theory that like draws to like in the human body, such medicines will have tonifying effects to the human body, and can eliminate the chronic pathogens. Those who are physically weak can be nourished with such strong medicines as Lurong (pilos antler), which is able to tonify the kidney Yang, and Guiban (tortoise plastron), which is able to tonify the kidneys. Besides, there are medicines like Lujin (deer's sinew), Lubian (deer's testis and penis), Gejie (gecko), etc., and these are all strong tonics. However, such tonics could be used only when the patients are really in need. Otherwise, the strong tonics may function as bad as too little.

To deal with chronic pathogenic Qi in the body, when the common herbal medicines could not take effect, medicines processed from animal products, especially the insect medicines, are to be used for searching and scraping off (driving out) the pathogens. For instance, a piece of bone with some residual meat on the ground can attract many ants to quickly nibble off all the residual meat. This is called searching and scraping process. Similarly, the efficacies of the insect medicines are able to penetrate into the muscles and bones of the human body to dispel the wind-cold damp pathogens out of the fine gaps, which is like searching and scraping off the residual meat. However, it is not suggested to use the insect medicines unlimitedly at wills. Doctors are supposed to save lives, not just people's life. It is not proper to kill many lives of the other species for saving a person's life only. The insect medicines may be used only when they become a must for the treatment of certain diseases. In any case, try to avoid abuse of insect medicines.

Functioning on Qi System or Blood System

When insect medicines are to be used, some differences also exist between their functions on the Qi system or the blood system. Ye Tianshi, who was adept at using insect medicines, concluded that "(of insects) those that have blood can enter the blood system of the human body, and those that have no blood can enter Qi system". From the perspective of TCM concept, some insects have blood, and some don't. For instance, the ant, biologically, we cannot see the red blood in its body, and it may have blood of the other color rather than red color. Similarly, cicada does not have blood in its dead body, either. Therefore, in TCM, ant and cicada are considered as bloodless insects. Therefore, cicada slough will go to the Qi system. Snakes have blood, so, the snake slough will go to the blood system of the human body.

Similarly, herbs with red color enterthe blood system, and those with cyan color enter the Qi system. Suye (perilla leaf) is red on one side and green on the other side, and even, some are green in spring and summer, and will turn red in fall, which means Suye can communicate between Qi and blood. Therefore, it can be picked and used to function mainly on the Qi system while it is green, and can be picked and used to function mainly on the blood system while it is red.

Rules and Exceptions

Of course, where there is a rule, there is an exception. For example, Honghua (safflower carthamus) is red, going to the blood system, which is consistent with the rule. However, Jinyinhua (honeysuckle flower) is not red, going to the Qi system, which is also consistent with the rule. But Jinyinhua also goes to the blood system, which is an exception.

Again, Sanqi (notoginseng) is an herb that can go to the blood system to promote blood circulation to remove blood stasis. However, it is not red but appears gray white or yellow outside and dark green inside with very hard texture.

Moving Speed of Medicines

Medicines move in the human body at different speed. Some move faster; some move slower; some just move without any pause; and some stay (as if to guard there) without moving. For example, Dahuang (rheum officinale), it moves very fast in the human body, and never stays at certain position for a moment with an action style like General Guanyu, a famous warrior in the Three Kingdoms Period, who overcame all the difficulties to win glory in battle and never stayed at any pass to defend at the place. Once Dahuang is taken inside, it will also go all its way downwards in a very quick speed and forceful manner.

Some medicines move very slowly, or even tend to stay at a place as if they were guarding against something there. Many sweet-tasted herbs work in that way, for instance, Gancao (licorice) usually stays for a while at certain position, and especially, a small dose of Gancao will move extremely slow in the human body. Many bitter herbs usually move relatively faster. Of course, there are some exceptions, for example, Huanglian (coptis chinensis) always stays somewhere in the human body.

What the doctors should do is to carefully consider the interactions, i. e., the compatibility of such herbs? Dahuang and Mangxiao (mirabilite) used together will take effect almost immediately to cause bowel movement. Analogously, it is like two impatient persons who work together, they often lash out at each other. If another down-going medicines like Houpo (mangnolia officinalis) and Zhishi (fructus aurantii immaturus) are to be added and used together with Dahuang and Mangxiao, which make a formula of **Dachengqi Tang** (Dachengqi Decoction), they would go even much faster. However, if they are not expected to go too fast in order to avoid severe diarrhea, Gancao may be added to make another formula called **Tiaowei Chengqi Tang** to hold back the force of Dahuang and Mangxiao, and slow down their movement for a better effect of clearing the turbid things along the way.

Timely Collection of Genuine Medicinal Materials

Growing environment is also part of the natural attributes of herbal medicines. People growing up in different regions are endowed with different cultures. Similarly, herbs growing in different areas will have different properties. Wherever the herbs are growing, it is very particular about the time to pick or collect the herbal medicines, which tells us to follow their natural attributes.

Examples of Authentic Medical Herbs

Chinaberry trees, for example, grow in many areas, but the best Kulianzi (chinaberry seed) is that produced in Sichuan province, China, so, Kulianzi is also named as Chuanlianzi (szechwan chinaberry fruit), which are bigger in size than those produced in Anhui province, China. The seeds of the chinaberry trees in Anhui province are very small and cannot be used as medicine.

Another example is about Aiye (folium artemisiae argyi). Mugwort can grow all around China, but the best Aiye is from Qichun, Hubei Province, China. I heard that the mugwort leaf in Qichun is different from those produced elsewhere. It is different in shape of leaves and fragrance. It is said that just across one mountain, the mugwort leaf would be different in the next county.

And also, lycium is a very small bush along the Huaihe River, However, it is able to grow into a big tree in Ningxia autonomous region, China. So, Ningxia is considered to produce the best Gouqizi (fructus lycii) and Digupi (cortex lycii radices, or the root-bark of Chinese wolfberry). Similarly, Anqing of Anhui Province produces the best Jiegeng (platycodon grandiflorum). Xinhui of Guangdong Province produces the best Chenpi (pericarpium citri reticulatae, or tangerine peel) that is called Xinhuipi (Xinhui tangerine peel).

Korean ginseng should bethe ginseng produced in Korea (including the North Korea and the South Korea). American ginseng should be the ginseng produced in certain areas of USA and Canada. They were initially used as substitution for Jilin ginseng. But gradually their unique properties are discovered in clinical practices, so, the places of origin are specified for special uses.

Similarly, the place of origin is also important about the animal medicines. For instance, Qichun has a kind of snake called Qishe (long-noded pit viper, or agkistrodon) in addition to the mugwort leaf. And also, the best E-jiao (donkeyhide gelatin) is produced in Dong'e, Shandong Province, China.

The quality of mineral medicines depends upon the places of origin, too. For example, the best Zhusha (cinnabar) is from Chenzhou, Hunan province, China, so, it is named as Chensha (Chen-cinnabar).

There could be many reasons. As the saying goes, "Each place has its streams in from all over the country. " Therefore, we may induce that certain kind of water and soil raises special type of people. So, we may draw a similar conclusion that each place has its streams and soil for producing medicines.

Medical Herbs Produced in Specific Areas

Nowadays, we may see many so-called "Local Medicines", such as Qi Muxiang (Qi-radices saussureae), Bo Baishao (Bo-radix paeoniae alba), Bo Sanqi (Bo-notoginseng radix), which are produced respectively in areas around the few major herbal medicine trade centers like Anguo of Hebei Province, Zhangshu of Jiangxi Province, and Bozhou of Anhui Province, China, etc. .

Harvesting According to the Natural Attributes

It is best to collect the herbal medicines according to their natural attributes.

Roots, as medicines, should be collected before the plant sprouts, or after the plant is withered. In autumn, when plants get withered, all the life essence will be flooded and stored in the roots. So, the roots in autumn will be the most substantial of the life essence. Similarly, at the time of sprouting, the accumulated energy in the roots is also the most substantial. However, in summer, when the plants are luxuriant, the roots are usually getting thin and least powerful as medicines since the plant is viewed from two aspects, i. e. , the exterior part that refers to the section above the ground and the interior part that refers to the root. In spring and summer, Yang Qi goes to the exterior, which means the life essence lies outside and the root becomes empty. As such, it is not a good time to collect the root for medicinal purpose.

The same is true to the stems and leaves that should be collected when they are in the utmost luxuriance. By the season of autumn, the life essence has been exhausted, and the medicinal effect becomes much weaker.

Flowers, as medicines, should be collected when they are still in buds, or just about to blossom. Never try to pick the flowers till they are withering or falling since by that moment the medicinal effects have almost run out.

However, fruits, as medicines, should be collected when they are ripe. Of course, there exist some exceptions, such as Qingpi (the green tangerine peel) and Chenpi (pericarpium citri reticulatae) . Qingpi refers to the peel of the unripe small orange, which is like a teenager full of energy, with a bursting disposition or temper, so its peel can be used to relieve the stagnant Qi, while the ripe orange is like a grown-up person, quite experienced with personalities of calmness, so its peel becomes Chenpi after being processed or stored for a long period of time, which can be used to regulate the circulation of Qi (that is to regulate the circulation of vital energy and remove obstruction) . Similarly, Zhishi (fructus aurantii immaturus) and Zhike (fructus aurantii) are actually the same fruit, just because they are collected at the different time. Zhishi is picked when it is not ripe, which is to take advantage of its natural properties in terms of time.

Artificial Properties of Herbs

All that are discussed above are about the natural properties of herbs, because of which Chinese medicines can treat diseases. What shall the TCM doctors do when some of the natural properties are insufficient or inadequate? They can then apply some processing techniques to improve or enhance those natural properties, which are called "artificial properties" that can be illustrated in two aspects, i. e. , processing and compatibility of medicines.

Processing of Herbs

The southern Chinese usually say that "Herbs will not take effects without passing through Zhangshu (a city in Jiangxi province, China, the so-called southern capital of herbs)"; while the northern Chinese say that "Herbs only start to smell right after passing through Qizhou (the antient name of Anguo city in Hebei Province, China, the so-called northern capital of herbs)". They are the two major trading centers of the herbal medicines, where many of the herbs are processed into final medicines. Without processing, a lot of herbs won't be as effective as they should be.

Herbal processing involves complicatedtechniques. Even now, lots of processing methods and techniques are still being passed down orally, or even regarded as business secrets that are not to be passed on without the right candidates as apprentice. As the renowned maxim by Beijing Tongrentang (a well-known Chinese medicine store and processing factory, with a very long history) says, "Nobody really knows how you process; your intention is witnessed only by gods". Chinese herbal medicine processing is indeed a solemn task with many traditional rules and disciplines.

I have learnt some processing skills from a senior and experienced pharmaceutical worker in Tongrentang. Although complicated, the basic principles and rules could be illustrated with some examples.

Processing of Fuzi (Radix Aconiti Carmichaeli)

Fuzi, for instance, is an excellent herb, which is hot in its natural property. It can be used to tonify the primordial Yang, but it is also toxic to some extent. In order to remove its natural toxicity while its function of tonifying Yang is to be preserved, it must be processed. One of the processing methods is to use Gancao-soaked water with very complex procedures. Gancao can detoxify lots of herbal toxins, for example, Fuzi to be processed with Gancao-soaked water.

In many antient formulas, when a large dose of Fuzi is used, a large amount of Gancaowould be used, too, which is following the same principle as herbal processing with Gancao-soaked water. After all, detoxification cannot be thoroughly done with Gancao in the course of processing.

In recent days, it is claimed to use Danba water (calcium chloride water), also known as well-salt water, to process Fuzi. Since Fuzi is very hot in property, and well-salt is very cold, they may offset each other about their natural properties to some extent. This may explain why some practitioners are bold enough to use a large dose of Fuzi.

Processing of Banxia (Pinellia Ternate)

Another example is Banxia, which can be used to reduce phlegm and calm the adverse-rising energy. However, it is also toxic, causing numbness in the mouth and throat, or even inducing vomiting. Toxins in Banxi is restricted most by Shengjiang (fresh ginger). Therefore, for processing Banxia, the fresh ginger water is a must, and it is a complicated procedure that will take long hours for soaking.

The so-called Fa Banxia (rhizoma pinellinae praeparata) is processed by following a particular method unknown to the public ("Fa" literally means "method"). Besides, there is Jiang Banxia (ginger pinellia ternate) that is prepared by soaking Banxia even more thoroughly in ginger water. And also, Qing Banxia (purified pinellia ternate) is prepared by soaking Banxia in a water solution containing Sheng Jiang, Baifan (alum) and Gancao for very long hours, after which the toxins will be removed almost completely. Generally, Sheng Banxia (raw pinellia ternate) should not be used casually, but Fa Banxia or Qing Banxia should be used instead.

Processing of Dihuang (Rehmannia)

Processing could alter the medicinal properties holistically as well. For instance, Dihuang, if driedonly without other processing, is called Shengdi (radix rehmanniae recen), which has the function of cooling blood with a slightly greasy feature. If it is steamed, it will become Shudi (radix rehmanniae praeparata), and it will also turn from coolness into warmth in property with an increasing greasy property. Strictly speaking, the greasy property of Shudi could be removed, but it will need further complicated processing involving nine repeated steaming and sun drying, and thorough soaking with Chenpi-soaked water and Sharen (fructus amomi) -soaked water.

Turning from coolness to warmth, from blood cooling to Yin-nourishing, from greasiness to non-greasiness, it can be seen that great changes of its properties have taken place in the processing.

General Principles of Parching Herbs with Additional Ingredients

One may often read from books of formulas that claim some herbs need frying with alcohol, some need frying with ginger juice, some need frying with salt, and some need stirring and mixing with vinegar, etc.

For those soaked or fried with alcohol, the purpose is to use the ascending property of alcohol. As it is known to all that more drink of alcohol will make a drinker feel dizzy or giddy, which shows that alcohol has the ascending effect and goes upwards. Therefore, if it is needed to uplift the ascending property of an herb, it can be processed with alcohol. For example, Dahuang (rheum officinale) essentially goes downwards. If it is required to go up first, and then go down, it can be processed with yellow rice wine to make it into Jiu Dahuang (wine-treated rheum officinale).

Many herbs are processed with ginger juice in the way of frying or soaking. Fresh ginger is pungent and warm in property, so, it is used for its detoxifying and dissipating effects. For example, Houpo is a descending herb that is used to eliminate dampness and descend the turbid. If soaked with ginger juice, it will become Jiang Houpo (ginger mangnolia officinalis), so, it can not only descend the turbid, but also remove and dissipate dampness. Ginger, as the "killer" of Banxia, can eliminate the toxin, and also intensify the power of Banxia on reducing phlegm. However, the dosage of ginger must be moderate, which means it can neither be used too much nor too little.

Someherbs are processed with salt for the purpose of guiding the medicinal effect to the kidneys since salt has a function of entering the kidneys, which can help to guide the medicine to the Lower Jiao.

Some herbs are processed with vinegar for the purpose of guiding the medicinal effect to the liver to play an astringing function, for example, the vinegar-processed Xiangfu (rhizoma cyperi). Xiangfu is an herb that not only has the function of regulating the circulation of the liver Qi, but also has a stronger dissipating effect. In order to prevent it from being too strong in dissipating, it is processed with vinegar. Xiangfu targets to regulate the circulation of the liver Qi, so, vinegar is used to guide the effect of Xiangfu to the liver to intensify its effect of regulating the liver Qi.

Some herbs are processed with child's urine with the primary purpose of down-bearing the endogenous fire or clearing fire. Urine is cold and descending in property, so, it can descend the fire or reduce the endogenous heat without impairing the primordial Yang.

Some herbs are processed with rice-rinsed water since the rice-rinsed water has moist property that can nourish the stomach, moisten dryness and harmonize the Middle Jiao. For example, Cangzhu and Baizhu are usually prepared by soaking in rice-rinsed water for tonifying the spleen and eliminating dampness without impairing the vital Yin of the spleen and stomach. In southern China where people are relatively weak in the spleen and stomach, so, Cangzhu and Baizhu are usually processed with rice-rinsed water when they are used.

Some herbs are processed with human milk for the purpose of intensifying the function of blood hematogenesis. Some medicines are processed with honey for honey is sweet in taste, which can alleviate the medicinal function or slow down the movement of medicines. Meanwhile, sweet taste enters the spleen, so, honey can guide the effect of medicines to the Middle Jiao.

Some herbs are fried with some very particular soil. In the past, terra flavausta, i. e., the dirt in the core of the traditional stove is usually used since it has the function of tonifying the spleen and stomach and goes to the Middle Jiao. Sometimes, "old wall dirt" is used since it has been exposed to the weather for a long time, and fully mixed with Qi from the earth and human, therefore, it is the best thing for harmonizing the Middle Jiao. And especially, the "east wall dirt", i. e., the dirt taken from the wall in the east side, would be the best choice.

Some herbs are parched with wheat bran or rice bran. Bran is the outer skin of wheat that is left after wheat is processed into flour. Wheat grain is warm inside and cool outside, so, flour is warm and wheat bran is cool. Rice is just the opposite. Rice grain is cool inside and warm outside, so, the rice bran is hot-natured. If fried with rice bran, a cool or cold medicine could be turned partially warm; if fried with wheat bran, a warm medicine will become cooler. Therefore, to fry with wheat bran or rice bran, it is actually to make the necessary adjustment of coldness, hotness, warmth and coolness of medicines in their properties. In any case, regardless of using wheat or rice bran, they all have the function of tonifying the spleen and stomach.

To sum up, processing is to use proper methods toeliminate the natural properties that are useless or toxic, while the useful medicinal properties are preserved. Some people may think that toxicity is of the medicinal property, which is not so accurate. Some toxicity is directly related to its medicinal property, but some are not so directly related. They cannot be mixed.

Compatibility of Medicines

Processing is done by the pharmaceuticalworkers, while compatibility of medicines should be done by TCM doctors.

One medicine always has limited functions, but it will become more powerful when it is used together with some other medicines. This is the process of writing formulas. It is the same principle of $1 + 1 > 2$, like a team can be much more powerful than one individual.

A single medicine is the product of the nature, for example, Shidi (persimmon calyx) has the function of calming the adverse-rising Qi and checking the hiccup, which is the natural property of this medicine. However, in case of hiccup, only Shidi may be or may not be effective. Suppose it is not effective, the root cause of the hiccup must be found out, and an effective prescription is then made accordingly. For the cold hiccup, Dingxiang (clove) can be added; for the hot hiccup, Zhuru (bamboo shavings) can be added; if the patient is in bad mood, the medicines for soothing the liver can be added; if phlegm arises, medicines for reducing phlegm can be added. If a patient suffering from chronic or serious diseases suddenly starts to have hiccup, it could be a sign of dying, and more attention should be paid.

When many herbs are made into a formula, they will cover a large scope of curative treatment, which reveals the wisdom of doctors. This process is called compatibility of medicines.

Next, let us come to the formulas in details, that is, the relations between formulas and medicines. Formulas are composed of herbs, but are more powerful than individual herb. Therefore, the TCM leaners have to learn in the both ways of learning medicines through formulas and learning formulas through medicines. Medicines are all available in the drug store, but the way of using the medicines depends on the doctors' competence of formulating them correctly.

How to Mobilize the Power of Nature

The essential reason of the Chinese medicines to cure diseases is that all the medicines are the natural produces that reserve the unlimited power of nature. Of course, how to make full use of such inexhaustible power of nature depends upon the wisdom of our human beings. The more one knows about the nature, the more he could mobilize the natural power, and the more easily he is able to cure diseases. Otherwise, he may fail to mobilize the natural power and even feel helpless for the treatment of certain diseases.

Intuitive Comprehension about the Nature

How to understand the nature world and mobilize the power of nature depends upon the intuitive power of understanding. As part of the nature world, human beings can feel and respond to the call of the nature.

Some animals know what grasses to eat when they are ill, which is one of their natural instincts. I have heard about a story that the pregnant elephant would travel long distances to eat a specific plant that generally would not be to its liking. When it is back, it gives birth to a baby elephant. And, such plant is helpful for parturition. How could the elephant know about the medicinal function of the plant? From its instinct, it is a natural interaction to the nature. Human beings have that kind of instinct, too. Take a simple example, a pregnant woman might like to eat something sour, or something in particular, or enjoy the smell of certain flower or grass. Why is that? Because her body is telling her what she needs, and then, she would like to look for those things. Similarly, she would also reject certain taste or smell. That's a natural response.

I remember once my grandfather was seriously ill, and he suddenly asked for bamboo leaf-boiled water. After drinking such water, he felt a little relief. When he was dying, he asked for water boiled with roots of day lily. And he felt a little comfortable after my father gave him such water. He did not know much about herbal medicine, but why could he ask for those drinks made of bamboo leaves and day lily roots. It must be from his intuition. Now I understand that bamboo leaf has a function of clearing the heart fire, so my grandfather would feel better when bamboo leaves helped to clear the vigorous phlegm-fire inside the pericardium. And the day lily roots are very much like Maidong (radix ophiopogonis), which can enrich Yin, clear fire and promote the secretion of saliva or body fluid. That he wanted such drink indicated that his major problem was about Yin essence deficiency and vigorous heat. Root is the underground part of a plant, which means the pathogenic Qi was already in the kidneys. However, I did not have such knowledge at that time, which is a pity.

In the well-known story of Shennong tasting hundreds of herbs (Shennong, one of the cultural ancestors of Chinese people, is considered to be the legendary founder of Chinese herbal medicine. It is said that he tasted hundreds of herbs every day to discover medicinal herbs, and he taught people how to cure diseases with the help of those herbs. His knowledge has been passed down and captured in the first classic book about herbal medicine: **Shen Nong's Herbal Classic)**, he was not just simply tasting. He also observed carefully, thinking over and feeling about the herbs with all his perceptions. He is regarded as a sage, not because he was sacred, or he was powerful or rich, but because he was closer to the nature. He had a much more abundant sensing about the nature. Therefore, he could acquire more profound knowledge about herbs.

Nowadays, some learners are following Shennong's way to taste and feel the medicines by the way of drinking the herb decoction. Actually, that is far from enough. Real tasting is about thorough comprehension about the nature, which is involved with the natural intuitive talent.

Intuitive talent is not intelligence only. Some people might have petty shrewdness in many trivial matters, but has no talent. As Zhuangzi, a famous Taoist, put it, "the more thinking with brain, the less knowing about nature's mystery", or to say, "the more playing with tricks, the less understanding about nature's tricks". Thinking with brain is about human intelligence. Knowing about nature's mystery is about natural talent. The more talented one is, the closer one might be to the nature. The closer one gets to the nature, the more talented one might be. The talent is in people and in Nature, which is plain, flexible and delicate without any deliberately polishing.

It isoften said that learning TCM needs power of understanding that is dependent on one's talents to observe the nature and think over deeply. That is to integrate the principles in TCM with those in nature, and to make analogies and have dialogues with the nature. Otherwise, one may be entangled in a book only, which then wears down his power of understanding. Therefore, he who wants to cultivate his power of understanding must go to the natural world.

Learning from Books and Experts

Another way to mobilize the nature's power is by learning. The ancients were quite diligent to do observation and investigation into the nature, and recorded their findings into books, but not all. Why?

There are many reasons. First, it might be that the bamboo slips were expensive. In Chinese, bamboo slips are called "Jian", which literally means "simple". It might be a reminder to keep the written words as simple as possible. Otherwise, too many slips would become too heavy to carry. Second, the writer might think that it was unnecessary to record every detail, as everyone was considered to know the same as well. Third, the writer might not be willing to record everything, and leave something for the people to think over. Additionally, there might be a group of disciples learning from the master, who might think it unnecessary to write those familiar stuff. Instead, he might make simple records about a case study or a theory with quick notes. TCM is usually learnt from books and oral teaching that inspires true understanding in the learners' mind. So, it is impossible for learners to acquire the complete knowledge from books only.

Books record only part of things, and the other part needs the learners to understand by themselves.

Furthermore, knowledge can also be acquired from life. For example, reading the formulas made by some experts, one may feel that the formulas are quite simple. But when he further talks with the experts and gets to know them well, he may find their seriousness in the treatment of diseases. Such learnings about the seriousness in curing diseases may not be noted in books but will be followed in life. So, following an expert not only means acquiring knowledge, but also learning from his moral quality.

Walking on Two Legs

Now we know that learning about the natural world depends upon talent and knowledge. Talent arises from the power of understanding, while knowledge is acquired by learning from experts. Therefore, one should never take the attitude of pros of one side and cons of the other side.

There are always many angles and methods for learning about the natural world and understanding things. The more angles and methods we take, the more clearly we may learn about the nature and understand things. So, one should never just observe and investigate into the nature from one perspective and ignore it from the other perspective. It is normal that one has two arms. There are indeed some rare one-armed heroes who are also successful. However, I always encourage those who plan to learn TCM in both ways: by talents and by following experts, i. e., try to walk on two legs.

第二章　中药为什么能治病

不要割裂中药的整体性

何谓"中药"

认识中药为什么能治病，首先我们要排除一个错误的观念：就是认为中药里含有某种物质，某种物质对某种病有什么作用，某种物质对某种病菌有什么抑制作用，或者说能够给人补什么东西。

如果有这种观念，那么你就不是在讲中药，或者说就不是在用中药，你就是在用西药的观点来看待中药了。何谓中药？在中医思想的指导下所开的药，谓之中药。黄连、杜仲、石膏、龟板，从物质形态上讲，只不过是树皮草根、土石枯骨而已，中医思想发现它们的作用，赋予它们"灵魂"，它们才成为中药。

不要用分析的方法割裂中药的整体性

一说药里面含有某种物质，那你就把这个药给割裂了。比如说黄连，有人研究说黄连之所以有清火的作用，就是因为它含有黄连素。于是大家把黄连素提取出来，用来治疗这个病，还真的有用，但用久了，人体产生抗药性，没有用了。回过头来用黄连，却依然有用。

青蒿也是一样。青蒿截疟。治疗很多疟疾，青蒿是必不可少的一味药。后来屠呦呦老师发现青蒿中有青蒿素，青蒿素对疟疾有很好的抑制作用，于是把它提取出来，刚用也还是有效，但是用久了，没效了。屠老在诺奖获得者新闻发布会上也表示，她最关心的是疟疾可能对青蒿素产生耐药性的问题。怎么办？继续用青蒿，依然有效。可见青蒿跟青蒿素还不完全一样。当然，我们不能否认青蒿素在抗击疟疾中的巨大功劳，这是一个实至名归的诺奖成果。

这就好比一个人家兴旺发达，你不能说这是因为他家某一个人的功劳。其实，功劳是大家齐心协力取得的，全家人都在发挥作用，各有其功劳，不要割裂地看。某一个人哪怕再有本事，你把他从这个家里独立出来，他就什么都不是了。

从物质分析的角度看，一味中药里含有许许多多种物质，它们就像一家人，永远在一起，共同发挥作用，不可割裂。黄连就是整个黄连在发挥作用，青蒿就是整个青蒿在发挥作用，而不是其中含有的某种物质。这个作用是怎么发挥的呢？咱们如果用微观理论分析其物质组成、化学性质，将永远分析不到尽头。所以，我们用中国传统学问独有的分析方法，首先讲四气五味。

中药的四气五味

中药，是天地所生的。我们中国的传统学问，视野非常辽阔，看任何一个东西，首先都要想到天、地、人。中药生在天地之间，天生四气，地生五味。四气，就是一年四季、寒热温凉，这是天赋予的；五味，就是酸苦甘辛咸，这是地赋予的。每一味药的禀赋都不一样。

人得天地之全，药得天地之偏

你说天地偏不偏心？天地是非常偏心的，它在四气五味上给每一种动物、植物、矿物，都只给一部分。比如说，给了石膏、黄连寒性，给了附子、干姜热性，给了山萸肉温性，给了白芍酸味，给了黄连苦味……

有人要说，五味子不是酸苦甘辛咸都有吗？但这种情形较少。而且，五味都具备了，它在四气上必有所偏，五味子是温性的。

很多药，比如很多植物药，它是春天生，秋天就枯了；还有的药冬至时发芽，到夏至的时候就枯死了，一年四季它都没有走完；有的药只能生在南方，有的药只能长在北方，东西南北都没有走遍。其性之偏，显而易见。

只有人，是天地之灵，得天地赋予之大全。人的寿命是很长的，他要历经许多个春夏秋冬；人的适应性也强，可以东南西北到处跑，所以人身上是四气五味都有，禀赋很全。正因为如此，人才能成为人，跟动物有着本质的区别。咱们千万不要说，人也是动物。人有动物的属性，但人绝不是动物。佛家讲，人在人道，动物是在畜生道，畜生道属于三恶道，人道比畜生道的层次要高得多。人身难得啊！人是天地的骄子，自然的宠儿，天地对人是很眷顾的，所以，天地会生出很多的物来养人。人生病了，身体里四气五味的平衡状态被打破，有所偏了，这时，就可以用中药的四气五味来给人体补偏救弊。这是四气五味的第一重含义。

四气五味各有作用

第二重含义，四气五味都有各自的作用：

如果人体过于寒，就要用温药或者热药来温暖它；如果身体过于热，那么就要用凉药来凉它，甚至要用寒药去它的大热。这就叫"寒则热之，热者寒之"。

五味作用，主要是：辛散，咸软，酸收，甘缓，苦燥。

气味也有厚薄之分，我们可以概括为："气薄则发泄，气厚则发热，味薄则通，味厚则泄。"

这是一些基本的原则，就像数学里的定理、公理一样。我先不做过多解释，大家先记住。以后我们在具体讲解每一个药的时候会经常用到这些原则，并加深对他们的认识。

中药的其他自然属性

四气五味是理解药物的主要途径，也是大家非常重视的。中药不仅仅是四气五味，还有许许多多的自然属性需要我们去观察，古人说"仰观俯察"，仰观是在观天，俯察是在察地，如此去体悟自然万物的性质，再在实际运用去反复验证。这是非常宏阔的视野，也是非常有趣的过程。

下面以几味中药为例，来说明不同药的自然属性。

麻黄与葱管的异同

比如麻黄，从四气五味上讲，它是一味辛温的药。气温味辛。辛，就能开散邪；温，就能散寒。这就具备发汗的作用了。但辛温的药有很多，为什么麻黄发汗的作用比较大？这是因为麻黄又有它其他的特征，我们看它的形状：麻黄是一种草，绿色的，细管状，中间是空的，有节。中间空，就能通气，能通毛孔。很细，它就能开细孔，也就是开毛孔。

我们再想，气味辛温，同时又中空的还有什么？还有葱啊。但葱管比麻黄要粗一些。这意味着葱也能发汗，但葱发汗的力度比麻黄要弱一些。因为它粗，所以它对毛孔的作用比较小，而对鼻孔的作用相对大一些。因为葱管的粗细更接近鼻孔。

粗管通粗孔，细管通细孔。这是不是异想天开呢？很可能是，所以，还需验证。比如，风寒感冒的鼻塞，我们经常用葱豉汤，喝下去后，微微出点汗，鼻子马上就通了。葱豉汤的组成非常简单，而且是厨房常备——小葱和豆豉，都不用跑药店了。

还有很多情况，我们都会用麻黄和青葱，都是有效果的，这就一遍一遍地证明了这些异想天开的假设。所以，我们姑且承认其中的因果联系。

观鸣蝉则知蝉蜕妙用

再比如，蝉蜕，就是知了蜕下来的那层皮。书中讲，它气味甘寒，能散风热。它为什么甘寒？因为长在土里。我们看过法布尔的《昆虫记》，其中讲蝉，"四年地下的苦功，换来四个月枝头上的歌唱。"蝉的幼虫，至少要在土里生存四年。土里，冬天不会太冷，夏天也不会太热，温度比较均衡，土是平性的，能容纳万物。火性再大的东西，到了土里，时间久了，火性就去掉了。很多用火制过的药，如炒白术，炒苍术，炒完以后，要把它摊在地上，至少要摊一个晚上。因为你炒过了，有火性了，如果不经处理，直接使用，火热之性就能伤人。摊在地上，就是用土来收掉火性。蝉生存在土里时间长，也就被收掉了火性，所以它是偏凉的，从这里我们可以知道，它是一味甘寒的药。

为什么会甘呢？也是因为它在土里，土味就是甘的，它与土同气相求，也跟着味甘。为什么它又能散呢？因为它是动物的皮，皮在表，在表就主透散人体在表之邪。它能散风热，还能透疹，疹子也是邪在体表啊。所以从这些自然属性上，我们就可以联想出这味药的气味、作用，不用去死记硬背。

我们继续联想，蝉蜕还能干吗？它还能退翳障，人年龄大了，会感觉眼睛模糊了，这往往是有翳障。常在辨证论治的基础上，方中再加一味蝉蜕，效果会非常好。为什么呢？蝉是蜕皮的，蝉蜕下来的皮又能使人体眼睛上的那一层翳障，像蝉蜕皮那样蜕掉，重新拥有闪亮的眼睛。

蝉蜕还可以治疗皮肤病。皮肤病当然也要辨证论治，在疗程的中后期，往往方中加一味蝉蜕，其意也就是使身上这一层皮肤病能够像蝉蜕皮一样蜕掉，甩开。

咱们这里用的是一种诗意的说法，似乎很荒谬，但自然界的微妙往往要通过这种诗意的思维去把握。

— 46 —

还有，蝉在夏天叫得很欢，声音很大，所以，嗓子哑了可以用蝉蜕，它能亮嗓子。在给很多歌唱家、教师开方子的时候，可以加一味蝉蜕，他说话的声音会特别脆，特别亮。如果嗓子沙哑了，咱们在辨证论治的基础上，加蝉蜕，效果也会非常好。

小孩子晚上老哭，声音还非常大，吵得四邻不安，这不也跟知了似的吗？要治这个，当然也要弄清原因，是寒还是热，是有食积还是受过惊吓，方中也常加蝉蜕。

嗓子哑了的，蝉蜕可以使其洪亮；小儿夜啼，嗓子很洪亮，蝉蜕又可以来抑制。一种事物往往有不同的两方面作用。这些都是古人在观察蝉蜕的性质的基础上慢慢摸索出来的。听起来似乎有点悬乎，但实际上历代的医家都在这么用，在实践中不断得到验证。屡用屡效，大家才津津乐道；如果屡用无效，早就有人提出异议了。

朱砂何以镇心安神

再举一个例子：朱砂。朱砂是红色的，红得非常好看，历来最高档的印泥，就是用天然朱砂做的。色红入心。同时，它又非常重，我们要是买一斤朱砂，会发现只有一点点，但拿到手里沉甸甸的。重，就能往下镇压。入心且能重镇，所以它镇静安神，小到失眠，大到精神病，都可以用到它。

当然，如果不是非常难治的失眠，请不要用朱砂，一般用磁石就行了。磁石就是吸铁石，也是重镇的，而且磁石吸铁，能收敛人失散的元神。如果是那种久治不愈的失眠，咱们可以用一点朱砂，当然仍不要直接用朱砂，用朱茯神或朱茯苓就行了，也就是用朱砂染过的茯苓或茯神，红色的。

精神病中的狂症，在辨证用药中，可以加一点朱砂来使之镇静。此外，朱砂还能镇宅、辟邪，也是通过它的重镇的作用。

有的小孩晚上梦多，甚至做恶梦，总是从梦中吓醒，咱们可以用一些朱砂放到枕头里，虽然没有吃下去，但仍有用。《神农本草经》说，朱砂"久服通神明，不老"，服，并非内服，它有佩戴之义。

当然朱砂入心且能重镇，吃多了肯定不好，心阳被它镇压下去了，人就容易傻傻呆呆的，用我们当地方言说就是犯了"朱砂孬"。孬，就是有点傻。吃多了朱砂，人会变得有点傻，发起脾气又会很倔很犟。

— 47 —

以前我在讲这些的时候，有人抬杠说："按你的逻辑，我用红辣椒炒秤砣，就能治疗精神病了？因为它也是红色、重镇的啊。"我只答复了一句话："这是你提出来的，还得请你亲自验证一下。"

这种联想、类比的思维方式，往往成为某些人质疑中医的突破口。其实，这些人脱离了实践。脱离了实践的检验，无论是科学的高头讲章，还是诗人的异想天开，都同样一钱不值。而中医，是源于实践，并且天天在实践中验证的学问，联想、类比只不过是其说理的方式。

以形象思维穷究物理，明其实用

物有其性，性有其用。用药其实就是在体察万物，在利用万物的自然属性。

中国人讲的物理，跟西方的物理是不一样的，中国的物理范围很广，也更深奥，更灵动，中医的用药必须上升到这个高度。仅仅知道某味药的性味归经，功效，跟什么配伍，治什么病，这也未免太初级了，没有上升到仰观俯察、穷究物理的高度。我们学中医，一开始就要站在这样的高度，方能势如破竹。

上面我们举了三个例子，来看一味药的功效。其实这是一个很诗意、很生动形象的理解，它是通过联想，让你把这些药的性质全部掌握。如果是干巴巴地讲蝉蜕能止小儿夜啼，能够亮嗓子，还能够退疹，还能够退眼睛上的那一层翳障，还能治皮肤病，一个一个地去背，这就太难了。现在我根据知了的特点，一层一层地讲，就比较容易记住，它还能激发人的联想，帮助人记住这些药的性质，而不是去死记硬背。这种生动活泼的联想可以陶冶人的性情，可以铸就我们生动、活泼、宽容、豁达、自然的人格。所以说，学中医会让人成为一个很有诗意、很灵动的人。

药物的行走

光知道一个药物的作用和性质还不够，还得明白它的走向。西方的物理学里有一个概念叫"向量"，比如力，有大小、有方向。中药也与此类似。大小就相当于药物的性质，而方向则意味着这味药物到人体后会怎么走、到哪里去。这就涉及升降浮沉和归经的问题。

药性，大家都很重视；但药的走向大家都不是太重视，或是一到运用的时候就忘了，这大大影响了用药的效果。

升降浮沉

不同的药走向不同。有的药往上升，有的药往下降；有的药走五脏，有的药走四肢；有的走上焦，有的走中焦，有的走下焦……都不同。所以你要根据病位，根据邪气的出入来选择用药。

怎么把握药的升降浮沉呢？靠死记硬背当然不行。我们师门从来不要求背任何东西。过去要求背的《药性赋》，什么方歌、歌诀，我们从来没有背过。咱们要去体会。明白了它的道理，这些东西自然就记住了。不明白其中的道理，死记硬背是没有用的。

很多药，药名本身就体现了升降浮沉。比如升麻，肯定是往上升的；沉香它肯定是往下沉的。沉香就是沉香木，一般的木头都浮于水，唯独沉香木，扔到水里会下沉，用于人体它也会往下沉，它能降气。

我们必须非常注意中医里的药名、方名、穴位名称，其中都含有很多密码，可以去破解。植物类药，我们可以看它长在植物哪个部位，以确定其性质和走向。

花叶升散，凡子必降

花和叶是升散的，它们在植物的最表层。花散发出清香，它是散的；叶子上每天蒸发出大量的水分，这也是在散。用于人体也有升散的作用。抓过感冒药的人应该都知道，一个方子，药味不多，药量也不大，但是抓回来却是一大包，以花和叶居多，质地都是非常轻的，因为要取它的升散之性，来发散掉我们体表的邪气。花叶升散，但也有例外，比如旋覆花，它不升不散，而是降的。

凡子必降。植物的种子，比如莱菔子、五味子、白芥子、车前子、川楝子等，种子在枝头成熟了以后，都要掉到地上，才能生根发芽，这就是在往下降。作用于人体，它也有下降的作用。还有比如桃仁、杏仁、柏子仁、酸枣仁，他们不但是种子而且还有很明显的油性，所以能润下，润肠通便。这些种子药还有一个特点，就是偏温。没有温热，它哪有力量发芽呢？但也有例外的，比如蔓荆子就是往上升的，而且性凉，它质地轻，可以用于升散头面之风。

枝走四肢，梗通上下

植物的枝丫就会走人体的四肢。我们可以说，它们同气相求。比如桂

— 49 —

枝、桑枝、紫苏旁枝，都是走四肢的。像胳膊痛，手指发麻，引经药可用桑枝，如果因为受寒较深，也可以加桂枝；如果只是因为临时受了一点寒，用紫苏旁枝和桑枝就可以了。

梗，就是植物的中间的梗子，也叫主茎。养料要通过茎从根部往上输送；叶子通过光合作用合成的能量，输送到根部去储藏，也要通过茎。所以说，茎是能升能降的。我们经常说的紫苏梗、藿香梗，在人体内，能通气、调气，能升能降，调气就在这升降之中完成。

根分三部

根部入药要复杂一点。靠上部的根，主要往上面的植株输送养料，它偏往上走；靠下部的根须，是要往下扎的，它的性质偏往下走，治下焦的病；至于中间的那一截根，就是守中的，治中焦的病。比如当归，按上中下的部位，可分为当归头、当归身、当归尾三部分，当归头上行而活血，当归身守中而养血，当归尾下行而破血。现在大家用根都不是太分明了，整个根都放在一块用了。当然，现在用芦和用须还是有讲究的。

芦在根的最上方，是植物根和茎的交会处，比如说人参有一个参芦。芦是一心向上升的，因为根的养料在芦这里往整个植物上输送，芦也就具有了很强的上升的作用，甚至能够引发呕吐。我们在用根部的药的时候，一般都把芦去掉。像人参这样比较珍贵的药材，我们舍不得扔掉它的芦，又因为它有很特殊的作用，所以我们就留下来，遇到体质比较虚的人，上焦有邪，你想让他吐一下，又不敢用那些峻烈的催吐药，就用参芦。

根须在根的最下方，它使劲往下走，往土里钻，所以又有攻破作用。比如甘草，你要是用它来调和诸药，又不想让他过于固守中焦，就可以用甘草梢，他会往下走得快一点；再比如小便带血，小便刺痛，一般也会用甘草梢。甘草梢能走阴茎，走尿道，有清利的作用。

药物走向的其他判定方法

此外，植物的节则走人体的关节，皮则走人体体表，心则入心，络则通络，藤则上行，刺则刺破……这都需要我们格物致知，观察这个药的本身。

金石、介类药，即金属、矿物、化石、贝壳之类。这些药都很重，药只要重就会往下走，这是它们的基本走向。

还有动物药，被称为"血肉有情之品"，它跟人体血肉同气相求，对人体的作用就会非常明显，它能峻补不足，搜剔顽邪。人体有虚，用它可以很峻猛地给你补一下。比如说鹿茸，是峻补真阳的；龟板，是大补真阴的。还有鹿筋，药店里卖的蛤蚧、鹿鞭等，都是用来峻补人体的。当你需要补的时候可以补，不需要补的时候用了反而会过犹不及。

人体有非常顽固的邪气时，一般的药攻不下来，可以用动物药，尤其是虫类药来搜剔。一块骨头，啃完了，上面还剩一些碎肉，咱们怎么啃也啃不下来，有的在缝隙里，剔也剔不下来，扔在地上，很多蚂蚁爬上去了，开始吃骨头上面的肉，很快骨头就被啃得光溜溜了，这就是虫类的搜剔功能。虫类的药也会钻到人体筋骨的缝隙里，把一些顽固的风寒湿邪，像从骨头上搜剔筋肉一样剔除，从而达到很好的祛邪的效果。但是，咱们不要轻易用虫类的药。医者是救人的，是拯救众生生命的，不能因为救一个人而杀害更多的众生。当用则用，不必用时，就千万别滥用。

入气入血解

虫类药也是有入气分入血分之区别。叶天士比较善于用虫类的药，他总结说："有血者入血，无血者入气。"有的虫子有血，有的虫子没有血。比如说一只蚂蚁，你把它掐死，就没有红色的血。当然从生物学意义上你可以说它有血，它的血可以是其他颜色，但是它没有红色，在中医里面就叫无血，这样的虫子入药就往往走气分。知了死了以后，你把它剥开，看不到红色的，知了没有血，蛇则肯定有血。所以蝉蜕就走气分，蛇蜕就走血分。

其他的药也是如此。红色的入血分，青色的以入气分为主。紫苏叶一面是红的一面是绿色，还有的叶子春天夏天是绿的，到了秋天的时候成红的了。这说明它一定能沟通气血。或者说当它青的时候采就入气分为主，红的时候采就以入血分为主。

有规律就有例外

当然，有规矩就有特权，有规律就有例外。比如红花是红色的，入血分，这是规律；金银花不是红的，所以入气分，这也是规律；但金银花也入血分，这又另当别论。

再比如，三七是一味活血化瘀的药，它肯定要入血分。三七是什么颜色？它外表是灰白色或是黄色的，里面则是墨绿色的，而且很坚硬。没听说它是红色的，但是依然走血分。

药的行走速度

药的行走也有速度。有的药走得快，有的药走得慢；有的药是走而不守，有的药是守而不走。比如大黄，它在人体内走得非常快，从来不停留，就像关公过五关斩六将那样，那就叫做走而不守，从东岭关到黄河渡口，他不会占领了哪个关就守在那儿不走了，这味药下肚会迅速从上往下通，夺关斩将而出。

有的药则是守而不走，喝下去了以后走得特别慢，甚至会在某个地方守一阵子。比如甘草。其实很多甘甜的药都喜欢守；而很多苦药，它都走得相对快一些。当然也有例外，比如黄连走得就慢。黄连、甘草都是守而不走的。尤其是小剂量的甘草，它走得尤其慢。

这些药怎么配伍呢？要相互牵引。就好比两个人，如果他们都是急性子，会互相催促着赶紧走，大黄和芒硝在一起就是这样，喝下去了马上就要大便了。如果在此基础上再加厚朴、枳实这两个下行的药，它们就走得更快了，这就是大承气汤。有时候我们并不想让他们走得那么快，拉肚子拉的太厉害了，人会受不了。这时候可以配点甘草，它走得就慢了，走得慢了，它们就会在路上把涤荡污浊的工作做得更细。这就是调胃承气汤，用甘草来牵制大黄和芒硝。

地道药材与顺时采摘

生长环境也是药材的一个自然属性。不同地方生长的人不一样，生长的药材也不一样，那么哪里产的最好、最适用呢？于是就有地道药材的说法。不管是不是地道药材，采收的时间也要有讲究，要符合它的天性。

地道药材举例

比如苦楝树，很多地方都有，但四川的苦楝子是最好的，叫川楝子，个头比安徽的大，安徽的苦楝树子是不入药的。

再比如艾叶，全国各地都有，最好的是湖北蕲春的，叫"蕲艾"。我在蕲春的时候听人说过，蕲艾跟其他地方的艾叶不一样，叶子的形状不一样，香气也有所区别。有人曾经翻过一道山梁，到了武穴地界，就发现武穴的艾跟蕲春的艾有所不同了。

再比如枸杞，在淮河沿岸是非常小的灌木，到了宁夏就能长成大树，宁夏的枸杞子、地骨皮是最好的。桔梗，以安徽安庆的最好；陈皮，以广东新会产的为好，叫新会皮。

高丽参就要出自高丽，也就是朝鲜和韩国。西洋参产于美国和加拿大的某些地区。他们虽然最初都是作为吉林人参的替代品而出现的，但久而久之，在应用中也体现了它们的独特性，所以慢慢地也有了产地要求了。

动物也是这样的，蕲春除了蕲艾还有蕲蛇，阿胶以山东东阿的为好。

矿物也看产地，比如说朱砂以辰州的最好，叫辰砂。

至于这是为什么，解释可以有多种。说到底，俗话说"一方水土养一方人"，我们也可以说"一方水土养一方药"吧。

地产药材

现在有很多"地产药材"，就是在河北安国、江西樟树、安徽亳州等几大药材市场所在地种植的药材，如祁木香、亳白芍、亳三七等。

药材须顺其自然属性而采摘

采摘药物，也要顺随它的自然属性。

根，要在植物还没有萌芽的时候，或在植物已经枯萎的时候采。植物到秋天枯萎时，会把全身的精华全部灌注到根里，这时的根是最充实的。快要萌芽的时候，根部积聚了很大的能量，所含精气或者说药力是最足的。要是在植物长得最茂盛的时候，比如说夏天，它的根就可能比较枯瘦，药力也薄。为什么呢？植物也有表里之分，它的表就是在地上的部分，它的里就是根。春天夏天，阳气走表，它的精气全部在外面，根是很空虚的，这时候你去挖它的根做药，效果必然不好。只要动动脑筋就能想到这一层。

茎和叶就得在它们最茂盛的时候采，秋天采枯叶，药力就薄了，它的精气已经耗尽。

花一般都是在含苞待放的时候采，或者在刚刚开放的时候采，不要等花快开败了再采，因为这时它的精气已经泄掉，效果就不大了。

果实要在成熟的时候采，这是众所周知的。当然也有例外，比如青皮和陈皮。青皮就是还没有成熟的小青橘子的皮。当橘子还没成熟的时候，它的皮就像小年轻，浑身是劲，脾气暴烈，可以用来破气；成熟了的橘子的皮经过炮制或者经过长期的保存就成了陈皮，就像一个成熟了的人，经历了很多风雨，办事更加沉稳了，所以用来理气。还有枳实和枳壳，也是同一个实物，只是采收的时间不一样。采摘枳实，也得趁枳还没成熟的时候采。这也是在利用其不同时期的自然属性。

药物的人工属性

上面所讲的，都是中药的自然属性，正因为有了这么多自然属性，中药才能够治病。那么，当自然属性不够或者不足的时候，怎么办呢？我们可以稍加人工，去改善这些自然属性，或者加强这些自然属性，这就叫人工属性了，也就是人为加给这些药物的属性。这主要体现在两个方面：炮制和配伍。

炮制

南方人讲："药不过樟树不灵。"北方人讲："药过祁州始生香。"南方的"药都"是在江西的樟树，北方的"药都"是河北的安国，古称祁州，这是中药材的集散地，很多药材的炮制就在这里进行。不经过炮制加工，很多药都不灵。

药物炮制，工艺比较复杂，现在很多炮制的技术，仍是师徒之间口耳相传的，而且有很多是行业的机密，非其人不传。"修合无人见，存心有天知。"中药炮制是一件很严肃的工作，现在这个行业里的规矩还是非常多。

我是在同仁堂的一位老药工那里学习中药的炮制的。炮制工艺虽然复杂，但其基本的原则和道理我们还是必须讲一讲的，我们通过具体举例来讲。

附子的炮制

比如，附子是味非常好的药，性热，能壮元阳，但它也有毒，这些都是附子的自然属性。要把附子有毒的自然属性去掉，把扶阳的自然属性留着，就必须炮制。怎么炮制呢？有一种方法就是用甘草水，具体操作比较复杂。甘草是能解百药之毒的，附子中毒，也要用甘草水来解。

在很多古方里，如果附子用的量比较大的话，后面必然跟着大量的甘草，这跟炮制用甘草水是同一个道理，毕竟炮制的时候甘草用得还不彻底。

现在有种说法，说附子用胆巴水，即井盐水来炮制。附子大热，而井盐大寒，一寒一热就会抵消一些，有人敢把附子的剂量用到那么大，跟这种炮制方法也有很大关系。

半夏的炮制

再比如半夏，也是非常好的药，化痰、降逆，但它也有毒，让嘴、喉咙发麻，喉咙一发麻甚至就会吐。半夏的毒最怕生姜，所以炮制半夏就要用生姜水，炮制过程工艺也非常复杂，要浸泡很长时间。

我们现在看到的法半夏，就是如法炮制的半夏，至于这个法是什么样的，他不告诉你。还有姜半夏，用姜汁浸泡得更透。还有清半夏，是用生姜、白矾、甘草水浸泡的，浸泡的时间相当长，基本上没有毒性了。生半夏，不要轻易用，平时尽量用法半夏或清半夏。

地黄的炮制

炮制还可能从整体上改变一味药的性质。比如地黄，地黄不经其他工艺，仅仅是晾干，就是生地。生地凉血，滋腻性小。如果你把它蒸熟，就成了熟地。生地本是凉药，到熟地它性就温了，且有滋腻性。严格地讲，熟地也是可以没有滋腻性的，炮制也就更复杂了，得九蒸九晒，还得用陈皮水、砂仁水充分浸泡。

从一个凉药变成了温药，从一个凉血的药变成了滋阴的药，从一个滋腻的药变成一个不滋腻的药，这对它的改变就比较大了。

加料炒拌的一般原则

我们在方书里会经常看到，某药要用酒炒，或姜汁炒，或盐炒，或醋拌。

凡是酒泡、酒炒，都是取酒的升提之性。我们知道酒喝多了就会上脸、上头，说明酒是往上走的，具有升提的性质。你如果想把一味药往上升提，就可以用酒制。比如，大黄本来是往下走的，如果我想把它先提上来，再往下走，就要用酒来炮制了，叫"酒大黄"。炮制用酒，都是黄酒。

很多药用姜汁来炒或浸泡。一是取它解毒的作用，二是取它发散的作用，因为生姜是一味辛温发散的药。比如厚朴，是一味往下降的药，燥湿降浊，现在我们用姜汁一浸泡，就成了姜厚朴，能够降浊化湿，还能够散湿，这样作用就更健全了！姜是半夏的克星，能解半夏的毒，其温散之性还能加强半夏化痰的力度。但用姜必须有一个度，不能太过，也不能不及，如何把握，这就是炮制工艺的不传之秘了。

有的药要用盐制，目的是将其往肾里面引，因为咸入肾，能引药入下焦。

有的药是用醋来制的，目的是让它走肝，让它收敛，比如醋制的香附。香附是一味理气的药，它发散的作用也比较强，为了防止它发散的力度过强，所以用醋来制。香附是理肝气的，为了加强理肝气的性能，所以用醋的酸引药入肝。

有的药用童便制，主要是取其降火、清火的功能。小便寒凉，是往下走的，能降火、去火，但又不伤元阳。

有的药需要是用淘米水来制，淘米水也叫米泔水，有润性，能养胃、润燥、和中。比如苍术、白术往往都用淘米水来浸泡，这样，它们在健脾燥湿的前提下，又不伤害脾胃的真阴。南方人脾胃较弱，用到苍白术就经常用米泔水来制。

有的药用人的乳汁来制，这是为了加强它生血的作用；还有的药用蜂蜜来制的，因为蜜是甜的，甘则能缓，用它来缓解药性，或者减缓药物行走的速度；同时甘还能入脾，能引药入中焦。

有的药用土炒，所用的土也是有讲究的。过去炒药，一般都用"伏龙肝"，就是灶心土，取它能"健脾胃，走中焦"。有时还用"陈壁土"，取其久耐风吹日晒，且接地气、人气，和中最妙。"东壁土"，就是东边老墙上的土，尤其好。

还有的药用麦麸或米糠炒。麦麸是什么东西？麦子碾成面粉，外面的麦皮就成了麦麸。麦子里边温，外边凉，面粉是温性的，麦麸是凉性的。稻子正好相反，稻米是凉性的，而外面稻壳（碾碎以后叫作"糠"）则是热性的。如果一味药用糠来炒，本来的寒凉性就会变得偏温；如果用麦麸来炒，本来是温药，温性就会稍微降低一些，或变得偏凉。所以用麸炒，用糠炒，是在寒热温凉上对药进行必要调节。同时，糠也好，麸也好，都是谷物的外壳，它们都有健脾胃的作用。

总而言之，炮制就是用合适的方法来去掉药物没有用的自然属性，保留它有用的自然属性，去掉它的毒性，保存它的药性。有的人认为毒性就是药性，这个是不一定的。毒性是毒性，药性是药性，有的毒性就是药性，有的毒性不是药性，这是不能混为一谈的。

配伍

炮制，由药工来完成；配伍，则由医生来完成。

一味药的作用是有限的，当它跟别的药物团结起来的时候，作用会更大，这就成了一个方子。"1＋1"是大于2的，好比一个人的力量是有限的，一个团体的力量远远比几个人的力量加起来要大得多。

单个的药物是自然的东西，比如一味柿蒂，能够"降逆止呃"，这就是它的自然属性。遇到呃逆，你光用这一味药，可能有效，也可能没效，如果没效怎么办呢？就要对它进行配伍，进一步找出呃逆的原因，是寒呃还是热呃，如果是寒呃，可以配丁香，如果是热呃，可以配竹茹。如果跟心情不好有关，可以配上疏肝的药，如果有痰，可以配上化痰的药，如果久病重病，忽然呃逆，那就得注意了，很可能是临终的征兆。

当很多药配成一个方子的时候，它治病的范围就会更广，这就体现了人的智慧，这就是配伍。

我们接下来会仔细谈到方剂，就是方和药的关系。方是方，药是药。方是由药组成，但是方剂的作用比药的作用要大得多。我们既要学方，也要学药，要通过方来学药，也要通过药来学方。可以说治世间百病的药都在药店里，看你会不会抓、会不会配。

如何调动自然的力量

中药为什么会治病呢？因为它是自然的产物，蕴藏着自然的力量。自然的力量是无穷无尽的。当然，要调动这无穷无尽的自然力量，还要靠人的智慧。有人认识得多，他就能更多地调动自然的力量，很多病对于他来说就很简单；有人认识得比较少，他就没法调动自然的力量了，遇到某些病就会觉得非常的无助。

灵气与自然

怎么去认识自然，怎么去调用自然的力量呢？第一要靠灵气，靠人的悟性。人也是自然的一部分，人能够跟自然相感应。

有的动物生病时知道去选择该吃什么草，这是它的一种本能。我听说过这样的故事：一只大象生小象之前，跑很远的路，去吃某种平常并不爱吃的植物，回来后，就生下小象了。而这个植物，恰好有催产的作用。大象怎么也知道药性呢？靠的是本能，靠的是跟自然的那种感应。人也有这个本能，最简单的例子，怀孕的时候喜欢吃酸，或者喜欢吃某种特殊的东西，或者喜欢闻某一种特殊的气息，如某一种花草的气息。为什么会这样呢？因为她的身体需要什么，她就会喜欢什么，也就会本能地想去寻取。当然她还可能排斥另外一种气味，道理也是一样。这是人的自然本能。

　　记得我的祖父病重期间，忽然想喝竹叶水，喝了以后，病情缓解了。他在临终前，想喝黄花菜根熬的水，我父亲也给他弄来了，他喝了以后，也感觉舒服一些。这是为什么呢？平时他也不懂药理，但他忽然会想到这个。大自然中可以用来熬水喝的东西太多了，他为什么会想到竹叶，为什么会想到黄花菜的根？这是一种本能。现在我想，竹叶是清心火的，老人家心包络中痰火非常的旺，所以用竹叶来清利一下，人就会舒服一些；黄花菜的根非常像麦冬，能滋阴、清热、生津，忽然想喝这个，也说明最后是精亏热盛。根在下部，这就说明这个时候邪气已经入肾了。可惜我当年还并不明白这些，现在想来就非常遗憾。

　　所以神农尝百草，并不是仅仅品尝一下百草的味道而已，他是在仰观俯察，在思考，在感受。他是圣人，他跟自然更接近。什么是圣人？并不是他神圣不可侵犯，或者有很大的权力、有很多钱。而是他跟自然更接近，他对自然的感受比常人更丰富，所以他能对本草认识得更深。

　　我们现在有些人听说学中医要尝百草，就拿一些药来自己熬着喝看看什么味道，喝下去有什么反应，他以为这就是在学神农尝百草了，其实这是远远不够的。真正的神农尝百草是对自然进行全面的体察，而这种体察要靠人的灵气。

　　什么是灵气？灵气不是看你聪明与否，有人小聪明很多，但灵气全无。庄子说："心机深者天机浅。"心机是人的小聪明，天机才是人的灵气。灵气越足的人跟自然越接近，跟自然越接近的人灵气越足。灵在心里，也在自然，它是朴素的灵动与精致，没有刻意的雕琢。

　　我们常讲："学中医要有悟性。"靠什么来悟呢，靠我们的灵气，到自然中去观察，去思考，就会有所悟。或者说，把中医的道理和自然界的东西结合起来，能够用自然界的现象比喻中医里的道理，跟自然有对话，你就有所悟，跟自然没对话，你就永远困在书本里出不来，你就没有悟性。所以悟，从根本上讲，你是在悟自然，因为世界上最博大的也就是自然，力量最大的也是自然。人心要获得悟性，要获得能量，也只能到大自然中去。

学识与师承

调动自然的力量，第二要靠学识。

古人非常努力，他们仰观俯察，把自己的成果写在书里，但又不全写在书里。为什么呢？

原因有很多：第一，可能因为当时竹简比较贵，竹简之所以叫"简"，也是提示人们在上面书写要尽可能简洁，否则搬不动；第二，他可能觉得没有必要写那么详细，他以为别人也跟他一样懂了；第三，可能他不愿意全写出来，他要写一半留一半，剩下一半让大家去想。第四，可能当时有一批弟子，天天耳濡目染，大家耳熟能详的东西，他就不写在书里边了，大家看到一句话想起一个病例，看到一个方子就能想起很多理论，所以他在书里只用做一个简单的记录。如今，斯人已去，我们无缘在他门下聆教，光看他记在竹简上干巴巴的一句话，当然不明白是什么意思。中国传统学问的传授，尤其是中医的传授，往往是书本传授和口传心授的一个结合体，书并不能承载所有的学问。

书中只能写一半，还有一半没有写出来，需要我们去领悟，去破解，好比坚果，首先要剥掉壳才能吃。这就需要一位师父带着你，为你点拨，你会事半功倍。

更何况，学问有的是在书里，有的是在平常生活中。比如说，有的中医，我们看他病历，老是用那几个方剂，粗浅一看，觉得这个人也就那么回事。你进一步接触他，会发现其实不然，这个人说话行事，包括看病，都是非常细致严谨。他看病当然也会非常地认真。这些严谨与认真，他不会写在书里边，但在日常生活中，他会做出来。你只有通过跟他交流，甚至跟他共同生活，才能学来他的严谨。所以，跟师不仅是学习知识，还要学习师父更多的品性。

不做独臂侠

认识自然，一靠灵气，二靠学识。灵气产生悟性，学识来自师承。我们千万不可以站在一端，来否定另一端。

认识自然，认识事物，永远有很多的角度和方式，角度和方式越多，我们就能看得越清楚。千万不要轻易否定哪一个角度，轻易放弃哪一种方式。就好比人有两只胳膊才是常态，独臂大侠固然也能行走江湖，但毕竟是少数，而且都是迫不得已的，他们要比别人付出更多的辛劳。认识自然，一靠灵气，二靠学识；学习中医，一要靠悟性，二要靠师承。单靠悟性，或者仅凭家传，不否认也有学得不错的，但只是少数，是独臂侠。

Chapter 3   Relationship between Formulas and Medicines

Monarch-Minister-Assistant-Envoy Theory

Based on understanding of the medical principles, doctors can compose a formula containing many different herbs. Then, what is the relationship between the formulas and the medicines?

One medicine does have its specific functions on certain diseases, as clearly stated in **Shennong Bencao Jing.** However, when facing a disease on a real person, one may find a single medicine alone may be helpless, as the Chinese proverb says one single hand cannot clap (which means it is difficult to achieve anything without support). This is because human beings are complicated, so are the diseases. Treatment of diseases needs ideas or concept that arises in the mind of human beings. Medicines reflect the natural properties, while formulas reflect the ideas of doctors.

A single medicine is like an individual who may have certain capabilities and some personalities, or certain strengths and weaknesses. But in any case, one's own capabilities, strong or weak, are limited, so, the unity of a team will be quite necessary. Medication for curing diseases definitely needs the power of a team, especially for curing the serious and complex diseases.

A big project usually needs many people, while a small task may just take one person. For some simple vulnus, for example, a little hurt of scraped skin may be treated with a little Sanqi powder (notoginseng powder). However, a complex disease will have to be treated with a combination of many medicines. Of course, it cannot be denied that on some occasions, single medicine can work well to cure a serious disease, which is so-called "single herb formula shocks the experts". After all, such occasions are very rare.

Roles and Responsibilities in the Monarch-Minister-Assistant-Envoy Team

In the light of the common practice, even a slightly complicated disease will require a formula with many medicines. This can be compared to a working team, in which there must be a leader to make decisions. This leader in a formula is named as the **monarch medicine,** which needs several helpers who are capable and experienced, i. e., the **minister medicines**. Besides, the **monarch medicine** also needs some members who not only could help to do something, but also provide some constructive opinions, and play a function of counterbalance to restrict the other members. Such members are named as the **assistant medicines**. In addition, some members who are functioning like envoys or guides are then named as the **envoy medicines**. A working team often needs to divide its work and responsibilities to its members, so does a formula.

In *Huangdi Neijing*, there is discussion about the medium-sized formulas and large-sized formulas. "The formulas composed of one monarch herb, three minister herbs and five assistant herbs are taken as medium-sized formulas. The formula composed of one monarch herb, three minister herbs and nine assistant herbs are taken as large-sized formulas. " In fact, we have to understand such descriptions with flexibility. "One monarch herb", it can be regarded as one herb, or can be understood as one solution. If such a solution needs to be represented by many herbs, then such a group of herbs can be regarded as "one monarch herb". Similarly, the "three minister herbs" can be either 3 kinds of herbs, or three groups of herbs representing three ideas, all supporting the monarch herb from different perspectives. The same is true for the five or nine assistant herbs. Moreover, sometimes one herb may serve multiple roles. Therefore, the composition principle of monarch-minister-assistant-envoy is obvious in some formulas, but not so obviously stated in the others.

Monarch Herb: to Cure or to Dominate

Once I was explaining the monarch-minister-assistant-envoy theory, I got one question like this: "the monarch-minister thing is from the old dynasty time, and now we are already out of the feudal society. That is true, but this theory is still alive in talking about TCM formulas. "

The truth is, in modern times, although we do not have emperors any more, in all walks of life we do have leaders, who are actually the "monarch" in the corresponding group or team, such as a chief, a head, or a director in an office, a section or a department and so on. Otherwise, a team without a leader may become "sheep without a shepherd". A monarch means a core, or a direction. Where there is a monarch, there will be ministers who are playing supporting roles.

It is often said that the monarch medicine is to cure diseases. But I think the monarch is like a sovereign who governs by doing nothing that goes against the nature. So, the monarch medicine is not used to cure diseases, but used for body conditioning/regulating. Maybe, neither of these two ideas are fully correct. Therefore, we should take an attitude that in the formula for a minor illness, the monarch medicine is for the purpose of curing the illness; while in the formula for a serious illness or body regulating, the monarch medicine is playing a role of controlling the overall situation.

To treat a minor illness is like to do a trifle thing. For example, now I am taking two or three people to go with me for shopping. I am the "monarch" and decide what to buy. I have helpers but I may carry more stuff in my hands than they do. This shows that in treating the minor illness, a monarch medicine is playing a major role.

To treat a serious illness is like to accomplish a big task. The leader cannot do everything personally, but he/she should control the overall situation. So, the monarch medicine in such a case is to take a control of the overall situation, i. e. , to deal with the body regulating for the minister medicines to play their functions of curing the illness.

For example, one patient has been suffering from the liver stagnation with enclosed masses in the breasts, which are diagnosed as hyperplasia of mammary glands by a western medicine doctor. For her problem, a formula may be prescribed with the following process: **Xiaoyao San** is used as the monarch medicine to disperse stagnated liver Qi to relieve depression, which is to control the overall situation, but **Xiaoyao San** itself does not cure the hyperplasia. However, it is not enough to control the overall situation only, as the real problem is still there without being solved. Therefore, the minister medicines also need to be added to remove the hard lump, like Xiakucao (spica prunellae), or Zhe beimu (thunberg fritillary bulb) etc. If it is serious hyperplasia, more medicines can be added such as Haigeqiao (concha meretricis seu cyclinae), and Fuhaishi (costazia bone/pumice) etc., which are specially for the treatment of the hyperplasia of mammary glands. Next, the addition of the assistant and envoy medicines should also be considered. Considering that **Xiaoyao San** is dry and strong and those medicines for removing hard lumps also consumes the body fluid, some assistant medicines can also be added, like Lugen and Tianhua Fen (radices trichosanthis), to make up the body fluid. Since the breasts lie at the upper part of the body, Jiegeng can be used to guide the medicinal effect upwards; By the way, the mammary glands are usually related to the collaterals, so the herbs such as the envoy medicines of Sigualuo (loofah sponge) or Juluo (tangerine pith) and the like can be used to guide the medicinal effect into the collateral channels so as to dredge the collaterals. Such a formula is made for the hyperplasia of mammary glands that is not a real serious illness. Still, the monarch medicine is used for controlling the overall situation in this formula rather than for curing the illness directly.

Therefore, the formula to be used for the minor illness is different from that for the serious illness.

It may be asked that why the body conditioning is put together with the treatment of the serious illness rather than with the minor illness. As a matter of fact, the body conditioning is more difficult than curing the minor illness. A minor illness can be cured easily and quickly, but the body conditioning might be a huge project, just like governing a state. One may have nothing wrong with his physical health, but he requests a doctor for his body conditioning. For such a "simple" request, the doctor may have to spend a lot more time on it than treating a serious illness. It is equally difficult to cure a serious illness and to nurse one's health.

There is such a saying among those veteran doctors of TCM in Beijing as:

they are not worried about the patients who are carried into the hospital, but they are afraid to see those patients who walk into the hospital, especially those who walk in with a smiling face. For the patients who are carried in, their problems are already serious, which are easy to identify with half an eye. The doctors may just give treatment to their illness accordingly, or at least explain clearly to them if their illness could not be cured. For those patients who walk into the hospital, their symptoms might not be obvious, and sometimes they may just tell half of the truth about their illness, or they may even intentionally test the doctors. So, it is difficult to handle such cases. For those patients who walk in with smiling face, they may just come to see whether the doctors could help to nurse their health. In such cases, it is hard to see any obvious symptoms, or even harder to define their physique, cold or warm. The doctors have to ask them in details or even guess what illness they are suffering.

Assistant Herbs: Help and Not to Help

What does it mean by "assistant"? What are the differences between "ministers" and "assistants"? Once I asked a student from a TCM university about the implication of monarch-minister- assistant-envoy, he could explain very well about the monarch medicines, and said that both the minister and assistant medicines refer to those medicines to support the monarch medicine. I further asked, if they both are medicines to support the monarch medicine, what is the difference between the two?

The Chinese character "佐" (Zuo in Pinyin) in antient Chinese was written as "左"(Zuo, which means "to assist"). In the annotation book "*Shuowen Jiezi*" (*Origin of Chinese Characters*) (The first Chinese dictionary, compiled by Xu Shen, 121 A. D), the writer put that "佐", the antient form is "左", which means the left hand. The character implies the meaning of the left assistant hand. " However, it also implies the meaning of "not to assist". In the antient history book *Zuo Zhuan (The Commentary of Zuo)* (the first chronological history book in China, compiled by Zuo Qiuming during 403BC- 386BC, recording the history of 722 BC to 468 B. C.), there is wording like this: "If the emperor gives his right hand, I will also give my right hand. If he gives his left hand, I will also give my left hand". The note says that: "a person has a right hand and a left hand. Usually, the right hand is convenient and the left hand is inconvenient. So, the right hand means to help; the left hand means not to help".

So, the character "佐" (assistant) means both "to assist" and "not to assist". Then, is the assistant helpful or helpless? The truth is that to assist implies the meaning of "no assistance", and no assistance implies the meaning of assistance. Both "to assist" and "not to assist" refer to a real assistant. For example, if I always assist one person, he may become more dependent on me and less capable. The result of my assistance is not assisting him at all. If I do not assist him, he may become independent and successful by using his own full potential. So "not to assist" turns to be "the best assistance". This shows a distinct feature about the Chinese wisdom, which never tells something absolute.

Now we know that the best assistants are those who will give assistance when necessary and will not give assistance in some cases. What the monarch needs is such kind of assistants. In Chinese, we often use the phrase "辅佐" (fu zuo) that is composed of two characters, i. e., "辅" (fu) and "佐" (zuo), of which "辅" is partial to the meaning of "assistance", and "佐" means "using corrigent", which is more partial to the implication of "no assistance". Of course, no assistance does not mean to make troubles deliberately, but to propose some good opinions when the monarch has faults, which is very important (as we often say the phrase "having different opinions"). So, in the past, one with great vision and mind was said to have "the capabilities of a prime minister". It should not be assumed that the monarch has the supreme power and he could do whatever he wants. In fact, the more power he possesses, the more assistants he will need, and the more check and supervision he will be imposed. Only when he enjoys more assistance and more restrictions, could the monarch then keep his balance and stay long in his throne. The same is true to the medication in life. The assistant medicines undertake the functions of assistance or none to the monarch medicine.

Take the example of **Zuojin Pill**. It is only composed of two ingredients: Wuzhuyu (fructus evodiae) and Huanglian (coptis chinensis). The formula, just as its name implies, is for "assisting metal (referring to the lung and large intestine) and soothing the wood (referring to the liver and gallbladder)", which is to purge the liver fire. However, instead of directly purging the liver fire, it uses Huanglian to discharge the heart fire in order to purge the liver fire indirectly, which is following the principle of "treating an excess syndrome by removing the pathogenic factors from its sub-organ". As to the liver, this formula does not purge the liver fire, but uses a small dose of Wuzhuyu to warm the liver, which is to play cat and mouse, that is, let the cat go first in order to catch it at the end. Similarly, in order to clear the liver fire, let it warm up first. Wuzhuyu is warm in property while Huanglian is cold, so they hold each other up to make a mutual containment so as to achieve a balance in this formula. According to the books of formulas, the standard dosage of Huanglian and Wuzhuyu is 6: 1. In clinical practices, the proportion of these two medicines may be adjusted according to the actual cold-heat situation of the patient.

Another example is **Yinqiao San**, which is essentially a pungent-cool formula, containing Jinyinhua (honeysuckle flower), Lianqiao (fructus forsythiae), Jiegeng (platycodon grandiflorum), Bohe (mint), Zhuye (bamboo leaf), Jingjiesui (schizonepeta spike), Douchi (fermented soya beans), Niubangzi (fructus arctii), and raw Gancao (licorice). In the formula, Douchi is warm in property. In the traditional way of processing Douchi, soybeans are cooked first with Suye (perilla leaf), then fermented. In modern times, since we are not sure about the real processing method of Douchi, we often use Suye to substitute for Douchi, for Suye is also pungent and warm in property. Suye, added in the cold-pungent formula, can help to induce perspiration on the one hand, and also gives a restraining factor to the formula to prevent it from being too cold.

Use of Assistant Herbs: the True Level of Clinical Competence

Medicines usually have partial properties, but a formula should not be too off-balance. So, TCM doctors are required to have qualified skills in order to achieve balance in formulas. All TCM practitioners are aware of the basic medicinal functions of herbs, such as Shudi nourishing Yin, Fuzi warming Yang, Ginseng reinforcing the primordial Qi, and Fuling removing dampness etc. However, in clinical practices, under the guidance of the same principles of writing prescriptions according to syndrome differentiation, why are some prescriptions functioning well, and some not? Generally speaking, all practitioners use monarch and minister medicines, or even envoy medicines in the similar way, but great differences may arise in using the assistant medicines. A common problem is off-balance existing in prescriptions. At the beginning, the formula might be effective since it focuses directly on the illness. Then in the later stage, with the counteraction of the pathogenic factors, the formula fails to react to the changes and gets stuck. That could have been avoided if the assistant medicines were better used to give considerations to more perspectives. We have known that between the medium-sized formula (one monarch herb, three minister ones, five assistant ones), and the large-sized formula (one monarch herb, three minister herbs and nine assistant herbs) as stated in **Huangdi Neijing,** the difference is all about using the assistant herbs. This is like performing an opera on the stage, where the leading performers are the same four roles: one monarch and three ministers; it makes a lot of differences by adding five or nine supporting actors, who will make the stage effect grand and wide. However, it is much more difficult to arrange nine supporting actors than five supporting actors on the stage.

Therefore, to evaluate the ability of a practitioner to write prescriptions in clinical practices, one of the most important criteria is to see whether he can make the monarch, minister, assistant and envoy medicines in his formulas woven together in balance. To achieve such a balance, the assistant medicines should be well used so that they could supervise and restrain the monarch medicine but not inhibit its curative effect, and also could help to tackle some accompanying symptoms. Therefore, the most critical points of using medicines are on the assistant medicines; and the key of writing a prescription is to keep a balance of all herbs in a formula.

As to the envoy medicines, they are the envoys or messengers, leading the way or guiding the medicines to the target locations.

Proficiency in Using Herbs and Formulas

Rational Use of Medicines based on Understanding of Herbal Properties

Different tasks need accomplishing accordingly in different ways. The same is true for composing formulas. A doctor should know the medicinal properties very well in order to use the medicines properly. It is like deploying troops, for which the general should know the characters and capability of his soldiers and the inter-relation among them as well, so that he can deploy all his troops rationally.

In the stories about the Three Kingdoms in the history of China, many people have read so many good examples, for instance, for the great warrior Guan Yu, his son Guan Ping and his loyal follower Zhou Cang were assigned to support him, so they made a great team. In another example, it is said that the marshal Liu Bocheng tackled each and every problem in a very serious manner, while Deng Xiaoping tackled the complicated problems in a very easy manner. So, they could bring out the best in each other, restrained and promoted each other. Therefore, they could cooperate very closely in the liberation cause of China, which created mild and peaceful situations.

The same is true to the use of medicines. For example, Cangzhu is a good medicine for drying dampness and strengthening the spleen, but it has a very dry property that must be removed in the way of soaking it in rice-rinsed water so that it not only can maintain its functions of drying dampness and strengthening the spleen on the one hand, but also will not hurt the stomach Yin due to its dry property. One can also use Yin-nourishing and body liquid generating medicines like Lugen and Xuanshen (radix scrophulariae) to counteract it. Such processing and compatibility with other ingredients are the rational uses of medicines.

Therefore, it is critical and important for a TCM doctor to get familiar with the medicinal properties, the principles of medical science and the diagnostic methods before he starts to write prescriptions.

Using Formulas like Deploying Battle Array

An old Chinese saying goes like "use of medicines is like deploying troops",

I would also say, "use of formulas is like organizing a defense. " Troops are usually deployed in certain tactical ways to serve military purpose. There are many legendary stories about various patterns of tactical deployment of troops in antient times. Those can be regarded as the formulas applied in battle fields. In study of formulas, the notion of tactical deployment of troops was also borrowed for the purpose of analysis, for instance, the medical encyclopedia *Jingyue's Complete Works*, written by Zhang Jingyue (distinguished medical scientist in Ming Dynasty) described the "eight arrays of ancient formulas" and "eight arrays of new formulas" in order to do researches on the formulas in an analogical way of troop deployment.

The great *Tao* (Way) can be applied in many different fields. In military science, there is tactical deployment of troops. Similarly, in TCM science, there are formulas. However, these tactical deployment of troops and medical formulas cannot be copied directly, and they must be modified according to the practical situations.

The emperors in the Song Dynasty were especially afraid of their military generals to become overwhelmingly powerful. So, they often send deployment charts to guide those generals to organize and fight battles, of which the intention is to issue a guideline on the one hand and to bridle those generals on the other hand in order to guard against the potential threat to the central government by the generals due to their military power expansion. Later, Yue Fei, a well-known general of that time, expressed his feeling in his famous remark: "the magic of deployment only lies in the heart", which has become a well-known quotation in TCM field though it was originated for the military battle. That is to say, the military strategy and tactics cannot be indiscriminately imitated, but should adapt to the changing circumstances like the weather, favorable geographical position, human power, landform, and soldiers' potential etc. Similarly, the formulas should also be modified according to syndrome differentiation.

Let us take **Maxing Shigan Tang** as an example. Its formula is composed of Mahuang (ephedra), Xingren (apricot kernel), Shigao (gypsum) and Gancao (liqorice), as introduced in *Shanghan Lun* (**Treatise on Cold Pathogenic Diseases**) *written by Zhang Zhongjing, the medical sage in Han dynasty. This is a* *drastic formula, pungent and cool in properties, targeting at opening the exterior pores and clearing the endogenous heat. It represents a concept regarding the treatment of the diseases in lungs. The pores on the skin are considered as the orifices of the lungs, so, Mahuang is used in the formula for it moves towards the exterior and opens the pores. Xingren is used to descend the lung Qi since, in the normal state, the lung dislikes adverse rising of Qi. The obstruction of the lung orifices may result in the failure of the lung Qi descending, which can incur heat in the lungs. Of course, the lung heat may also arise from the external pathogenic factors (exogenous pathogens). So, Shigao is used to clear the heat in the lungs. The vigorous heat in the lungs may easily result in short breath of the lungs due to the failure of Qi descending. Therefore, Gancao is used to relieve such symptom in the lungs. It may be concluded that in the formula of* **Maxing Shigan Tang**, Mahuang functions to open the orifice of the lungs; Xingren functions to descend the lung Qi; Shigao functions to clear away the lung heat; and Gancao functions to relieve the short breath. When the damp pathogen is present but without heat in the lungs, Shigao can be substituted by Yiyiren (coix seed), which can eliminate the pathogenic Qi and the damp from the lungs.

Do Not Mechanically Follow the Existing Formulas

Today, many TCM learners talk about using a specific formula to treat a specific disease or symptom, which is basically focusing on formulas without considering the medicines. Some even claim that they belong to "the school of classic formulas". Excellent as the classic formulas are, they should not be applied mechanically for all symptoms. What needs to do is to learn the underlying principles in the classic formulas. In the preface of **Shennong Bencao Jing**, Tao Hongjing mentioned that some quack doctors "feel shameful to study the herbs", and "solely depend on the established formulas", which would impede the others and themselves.

In the Three Kingdoms Period, a powerful troop of 800,000 soldiers were defeated by Zhuge Liang and Zhou Yu, who successfully applied the strategy of fire attack. Does this mean such a troop can be always defeated by a fire attack? Definitely not. Different tactics should be applied under different situations, the same is true to the treatment of the same disease on different patients.

Fire attack is like a formula. It can be applied to different enemies. In each fight, details of fire attack might also be different based on different situation. So, when using formulas, TCM doctors could use different medicines for the same purpose, or use the same formula to treat different illness, or treat the same illness with different formulas.

Do not simply take the existing formulas to treat diseases mechanically. If a doctor believes that such a formula is specially for treating such a disease, it would be the same as the belief that a troop can always be defeated with fire attack. Furthermore, do not label a general as a "school of fire attack" just because he is good at using fire attack.

Spend 90% of Time on Studying Herbs

For learning TCM, three key points should be kept in mind. The first point is about the principles of medical science, which exercise control of the overall situation; the second is about the properties of medicines, which can help a doctor to know how to use a medicine properly; and the last but not least is about diagnosis, which helps a doctor to identify and recognize an illness. Formulas should be made based on the above three points.

In learning medicines and formulas, the principle is to apply 90% of the time to studying medicines, and 10% of the time to formulas. This has been emphasized by my respected teacher Mr. Hu Youheng. Getting familiar with the medicinal properties should be the key point among focuses.

The purpose of learning formulas is to understand the ideas and concepts about formulating the medicines. The classic formulas were developed by the ancients through continuous groping experiences, which include a lot of valuable insights. So, to learn the classic formulas is actually to learn the underlying principles and the methods of creating the formulas, which needs thorough comprehension of principles of medical science and properties of medicines. Hence, the best way to learn the formulas is to learn the methods of creating a formula but not limited to the classic formulas themselves.

Methods Embedded in the Formulas

Many books just record formulas with methods being embedded, especially the books before and in Tang Dynasty, such as *Waitai Miyao (Medical Secrets of an Official), Qianjin Yaofang (Thousand Golden Prescriptions), Zhouhou Fang (Handbook of Formulas for Emergencies), Shanghan Zabing Lun (Treatise on Cold Pathogenic and Miscellaneous Diseases)*, all of which mainly contain formulas with little discussion of the principles of medical science. All the medical principles were actually learnt through oral teaching that inspires the learners to have true understanding by themselves, instead. So, those who learn TCM from the same teacher are able to understand the medical principles once they see the formulas, while the laymen could only apply the existing formulas mechanically at the best.

In TCM, thereare sorts of prescriptions called "forbidden formulas". "Forbidden" actually in Chinese implies two meanings. One is that they are kept secret, and the other one is that they are forbidden to be used randomly by the laymen because nothing is described about how to use such formulas. Only those who have been learning TCM under the direct guidance of a medical expert can understand the secret of how to use such forbidden formulas. In the past, royal court or other places always had some forbidden formulas. There is a book available, named *Lufu Forbidden Formulas* compiled by Gong Tingxian in Ming Dynasty, in which a lot of formulas are recorded.

As to the "classic formulas", it is known that they are from *Shanghan Lun (Treatise on Cold Pathogenic Diseases) and Jingui Yaolue (Synopsis of Golden Chamber)*. It is said that the ancient saints, after fully understanding the universe, the earth and the supernatural beings, created the classic formulas, the best of which could not be comprehended by the people of today. Therefore, nothing in these classic formulas should be modified. I cannot agree with such a biased idea. People today should and also can reach the level of wisdom of the ancient sages by learning, exploring and thinking deeply, and then, will be able to make effective formulas after deeply understanding the medical principles and medicinal properties.

The purpose of learning the formulas is to gain the experience from the ancients on how to create formulas. For example, in **Shanghan Lun, and Jingui Yaolue,** only formulas are listed with very little explanation of medical principles in most cases. With time passing by, now there is no way to figure out how Zhang Zhongjing taught his followers at that time, but only read the book that was edited by the others later on. So, all the scholars who are elaborating on **Shanghan Lun** are actually trying utmost to conjecture the underlying meaning of those formulas.

Another example is **Furen Liangfang (Effective Formulas for Women)** written by Chen Ziming in the Song Dynasty, which also takes formulas as the core. Each formula he created reflects his thought in some way. It is a great pity that his concepts or ideas about those formulas were gone although his formulas stay with us today.

Integrity of Theories, Methods, Formulas and Medicines

In the process of TCM development, only by the time of theJin-Yuan Dynasty, the Four Great Medical Masters (They are Liu Wuansu, the representative of fire-heat theory; Zhang Congzheng, the representative of attacking pathogen theory; Li Dongyuan, the representative of spleen-stomach theory; and Zhu Zhenheng, the representative of Yin nourishing theory in Jin-Yuan dynasty), to be more specific, that is, Zhang Yuansu, a Chinese medical expert before the Four Great Medical Masters, who was the teacher of Li Dongyuan, one of the "Four Great Masters, gradually put medical theories and the formulas together to explain TCM more thoroughly. To a large extent, they are called the "Four Great Medical Masters"since they established a theory along the line of integrity of medical principles and formulas, and enlightened the later TCM learners. The train of their medical thoughts have been being followed till the Dynasties of Ming and Qing, and even up to now. Since then, medical experts are no longer trying to explain medical theories via formulas only.

In the early Qing dynasty, a TCM doctor named Chen Shiduo wrote many TCM books, such as, **Shishi Milu (Secret Records of the Stone Chamber), Bianzheng Qiwen (Legends of Syndrome Differentiation)** , all of which integrated the medical theories, methods, formulas and medicines into one. For example, **Shishi Milu** takes the methods of disease treatment as the core, like the methods of "direct treatment", "indirect treatment" etc. The writer brought out the facts and causes first, and then gave the formulas that are very effective in most cases. Such books are very valuable since they can satisfy the needs of doctors at various levels. Those doctors who are not so experienced can use the listed formulas directly, while those medical experts would do some research on the methods and principles embedded.

"Theories, methods, formulas and medicines" are considered as the four pillars of TCM. After the Four Great Masters of Jin and Yuan Dynasties, many TCM experts took the four pillars as a foundation to establish new TCM theories, which received much criticism like the comments of "reddish violet and obscene music" (means "just various attractive colors and disturbance to the orthodox principles and nothing else) described in *Yixue Sanzi Jing (Three-Character Medical Verses)* compiled by Chen Xiuyuan (Medical scientist of the Qing Dynasty).

In fact, all the medical books, if they could be handed down from the past, will definitely contain some valuable things that are worth learning. Therefore, the learners should try to absorb what is best in them.

第三章　方和药的关系

君臣佐使

一个方剂要用很多味药，我们必须在熟悉药理的情况下组织一个方剂，那方和药之间的关系是什么呢？

药固然有它的作用，就像《神农本草经》上就说某味药治什么病，都写得很清楚。但真正面对一个病，面对一个人，单味药依然可能是孤掌难鸣的。因为人是复杂的，病也是复杂的，治病是要有思想的，思想是人的思想。药体现的主要是自然属性，而方体现的是人的思想。

一味药就好比一个人，有它的本领，它的性格；有长处，也有短处。它的本领再大，都是有限的，所以就要依靠团队的力量。用药治病往往也需要依靠团队的力量，尤其是在面对大病、重病的时候。

办大事通常需要好几个人，办小事有时候一个人就行。有一些简单的小病，用一味药就行，比如蹭破皮出血了，涂点三七粉就行。当然有时候一个人也能做大事，一味药也能治大病，这就是"单方一味，气死名医"，但这种情况毕竟不常见。

君臣佐使的团队分工

按照常规，对于稍微复杂一些的病，就需要好几味药了。好比一个工作组，其中，肯定就有一个为首的，能说了算，这就是君药；还应该有几个帮忙的，他们有能力，有经验，这好比臣药；还有人，既能帮忙，又能提出一些建设性的意见，还能对其他人起到制衡作用，这相当于佐药；还有人纯粹是跑腿的，带路的，这相当于使药。一个团队的人员往往会形成这种分工，一个方子也如此。

《黄帝内经》里有中方"君一臣三佐五"，大方"君一臣三佐九"之说，我们要灵活地看，君一，可以说是一味药，也可以说是一种思路，如果这个思路要用很多药来体现，那么这几味药在一起也叫"君一"。臣三，可以认为是三味药，也可以认为是三种思路，三组药，从多个方面去辅助君药，佐五、佐九也是同样的道理。而且，同一个药，有时候还要身兼数职。因此，在一个方子里，君臣佐使，有时候很明显，有时候又不是很明晰的。

君药：治病还是控局

一次我在另外一个场合给大家讲君臣佐使，有个同学就说："君臣是封建社会的东西，我们现在已经不用了，方剂依然讲这个，是不是过时了呢？"

实则，虽然现在没有皇帝，但"君"依然是存在的，他就是为首的，就是领导，这个长，那个主任，都是他对应的团体里的君。否则，"无帅之兵，谓之乌合"，团队没有主帅，就成了乌合之众。君，是核心，是方向。有君就有臣，臣是辅助君的。

人们常说，君药是用来治病的；但前几天我在微博上说："君药好比君主，君主无为而治。君药是不治病的，它是用来调整体质的。"这就是两种说法了，哪个对呢？都对，但都不全面，二者合在一起讲就完整了：治小病的方，君药是用来治病的；治大病的方或者说调整身体的方，君药是用来控局的。控局就是控制整个局面。

治小病相当于做一件小事情。比如说，我现在去采购，带两三个人去，买什么我说了算，我是君；虽然他们几个帮我的忙，可我也没法闲着，可能我手上拎的东西比他们还多呢。这是治小病的方，君药是治病的主力。

治大病好比做一件大事，为首的没法事必躬亲，但他要能够把控大局。君药控局，也就是调整体质，然后让臣药来治病。

比如说，某人长期肝郁，乳房中出现很多包块，一检查，西医说是乳腺增生。咱们给她开的方子，逍遥散为君，用来疏肝解郁，这是调整大局的，它本身并不治疗乳腺增生。现在有的医生遇到乳腺增生就开一些加味逍遥丸之类的中成药，这是不管用的，光调整大局，不干实事，问题会始终存在。所以我们还得加上臣药，也就是软坚散结的药，比如夏枯草啊、浙贝之类，如果严重还得加海蛤壳、浮海石之类的，这就是针对乳腺增生的啦。再加佐药、使药。因为逍遥散比较燥烈，软坚散结的药也要消耗津液，咱们可以加上芦根、花粉之类的东西来补充津液，这是佐药。乳房偏人体上部，可以加点桔梗把药往上带；乳腺增生跟络脉有关系，咱们还要通络，可以用丝瓜络、橘络之类的，把药力引入络脉，这都是使药。这是一个方子。虽然乳腺增生不是什么大病，但是咱们在组方的时候依然把君药拿来控局，而不直接把君药拿来治病。

所以说，治小病的方跟治大病的方是不一样的。

有人会说，调理身体为什么要跟治大病放在一起，而不是跟治小病放在一起呢？其实啊，调理身体比治小病要难，小病可能很快就治好了，调理身体却是一个庞大的工程，好比治理一个国家。可能这个人什么病都没有，他说大夫你给我调一调，他说得轻巧，可你花的精力不亚于治一个大病。所以说，治大病难，调理体质也难。

北京过去的老中医经常讲这么一句话："不怕抬着进来的，就怕走着进来的，最怕的是笑呵呵走着进来的。"抬着进来，说明这个病已经很严重了，哪儿出了问题，一目了然，我们该怎么治就怎么治，实在治不好也可以说明，这个不用怕。走着进来的，他的症状不明显，可能还想考考你，你问他的病情，他说一半瞒一半，这就有点不好对付了，现在很多这种病人呢。笑呵呵走着进来的，可能也就没什么病，就是想叫你给他调理调理身体，这时候症状不明显，寒热也不明显，甚至体质都不明显，你得问，还得猜。

佐药：既帮助又不帮助

佐是什么呢？臣和佐有什么区别呢？以前我问过一位中医药大学的学生："君臣佐使是什么意思？"君药他解释得很好，臣药是辅佐君药的，佐药也是辅佐君药的，我问："既然都是辅佐君药的，那他们之间有什么区别？"

佐，古字写作"左"，有"帮助"的意思。《说文解字》段注云："左者，今之佐字。……左手也。谓左助之手也。以手助手，是曰左。"但同时，它又有"不帮助"的意思。《左传·襄公十年》："天子所右，寡君亦右之；所左，亦佐之。"疏曰："人有左右，右便而左不便，所以所助者为右，所不助者为左。"

有人也许要问，既有"帮助"的意思，又有"不帮助"的意思，那么到底是帮助还是不帮助呢？其实，帮助就是不帮助，不帮助就是帮助，既帮助又不帮助，才是真正的帮助。比如，我一味帮助你，使你产生了依赖，变得无能了，效果就适得其反，帮助成了不帮助，这就是我们经常说的"帮倒忙";不帮助呢？或许会使人独立自主，发挥潜能，最后自己成功，这样，不帮助成了最好的帮助。中国的学问，永远不是绝对的。

所以，最善于帮助别人的人，是既帮助又不帮助的。君王就需要这样的帮助。我们经常把"辅佐"二字连用。辅是辅助，更偏重于"帮助"；佐是反佐，更偏于"不帮助"。不帮助，当然不是故意捣乱，而是在君王有过失的时候能够提出不同意见（我们经常说"意见相左"），这往往是非常重要的。所以，过去我们经常把具有雄才大略的人叫"王佐之才"。我们不要以为君王的权力至高无上，可以为所欲为，其实，你权力越大，帮助你的人越多，制约你的人也就越多。有帮助有不帮助，有生有克，君王才能保持一个平衡的状态，才能当得长久。处方用药也是如此。佐药作为帮助君药的药，也是既帮助又不帮助的，或者说，是通过不帮助来帮助。

比如，左金丸中，只有吴茱萸和黄连两味药，这个方子，顾名思义，是用来"佐金平木"，泻肝火的。它不直接泻肝火，而是采取"实则泻其子"的方法，通过黄连泻心火来间接泻肝火。对于肝，它不但不泄其火，反而用少量的吴茱萸来温它一下。这叫欲清先温，欲擒故纵。吴茱萸性温，黄连性寒凉。一寒一温，互相牵制，达成了这个方子的平衡。方书上的标准计量是黄连六份，吴茱萸一份，但在临床中，我们还可以根据寒热的多少来重新调配剂量比例。

再比如，银翘散本是辛凉方剂，其组成是：银花、连翘、桔梗、薄荷、竹叶、荆芥穗、豆豉、牛蒡子、生甘草。其中豆豉性温。古法制豆豉，是用苏叶煮豆，然后发酵而成。现在的豆豉，因为不知其制作过程，所以临床上一般用苏叶代替豆豉，苏叶也是辛温之品。在辛凉剂中加一味辛温之品，其作用，既是帮助辛凉剂发汗，也是为了给方子中的凉药一个反佐，使其不过于寒凉。

佐药的运用体现临床的功夫

药性是有偏的，但方子的性质却不能过偏。这一点要做到是需要很深的功夫的。所有的中医都知道熟地滋阴、附子温阳、人参大补元气、茯苓淡渗水湿……但在具体运用中，在辨证立法都一样的情况下，为什么有的有疗效有的没有疗效呢？君药、臣药，甚至使药，大家用得都会差不多，但佐药怎么用，却有很大差别。往往很多方子开出来，有欠平衡：先是高歌猛进，直达病所，初服有效，但孤军深入，马上陷入困境，病邪反攻，变证蜂起。如果佐药用得好，兼顾面较多，绝不致如此。《黄帝内经》中，中方"君一臣三佐五"，大方"君一臣三佐九"，差别全在佐药的运用上。这好比唱戏，主要演员就是"君一臣三"这四个人，再来五个配角，场面就不小了，如果来九个配角，舞台效果会更加宏阔，但安排九个配角要比安排五个配角难得多。

所以，我们看一个中医开处方的水平，很重要的一个标准就是看这个方子的君臣佐使诸药之间是否丝丝入扣，达成平衡。要达到平衡，就要善于使用佐药，这个佐药既要对君药有监制作用，又不能影响君药发挥疗效，还得对治疗一些兼证有辅助作用。所以，用药不难，难在用佐药；组方不难，难在平衡。

还有一个使药。使药就是信使，就是我们前面讲的它能够把药带到该去的地方，是带路的或送信的。

用药如用兵，用方如用阵

知药善用好比知人善任

工作有大小之分，工作的方法就不一样，用方的思路也是如此。医者得非常熟悉药性，才能很好地调遣这些药，好比是分兵派将，你得熟悉这些人的性格，还有他们之间的关系。

关羽是主将，是君，派谁跟着他呢？必然是周仓、关平，为什么？上阵父子兵，关平跟着关羽，肯定没错；周仓最服关羽，会配合得非常好。据说，邓小平和刘伯承，是一对很好的搭档。刘伯承举轻若重，非常的谨慎，一点小事，他会看得非常的大，严肃认真；邓小平相反，他举重若轻，再大的事情，他都能够以一种很轻松的姿态去完成，这两人在一起就能够相得益彰，又互相约束，互相促进，这样就平和。

用药也如此，我们使用苍术，这是一个燥湿健脾的好药，但它也非常燥烈，要减掉它燥烈的性质，就放在淘米水里浸泡一下，使之既不失燥湿健脾的作用，又不会过于燥烈伤了胃阴。还可以用芦根、玄参等养阴生津的药来反佐它。我们这么炮制和配伍苍术，是"知药善用"。

所以熟悉药性是最重要的。熟悉了药性，再熟悉了医理和诊断，你就能开处方了。

用方如用阵

"用药如用兵"，这是古人常讲的一句话，我在后面加一句，"用方如用阵"。阵是作战的方法，排兵布阵。张景岳在他的《景岳全书》里就有古方八阵、新方八阵的说法，用排兵布阵的思想来研究这些方剂。

大道相通，中医里有方子，军事上也有方子，有一些固定的排兵布阵的方法，但是你能照搬吗？不能。你还得根据具体的情况来对这个阵图进行相应的变化。

宋朝的皇帝特别害怕在外作战的将军势力过大，就常常派人送阵图过去，教这些将军怎么打仗。意图就是一方面对你进行指导，另一方面是要掌控你，防止你军事势力扩张太大，对中央造成威胁。后来岳飞说了一句很有名的话："运用之妙，存乎一心。"这话现在中医经常讲，其实它源于军事，意思是说，兵法不能照搬死的方子，不能照搬死阵图。要根据天时、地利、人事，根据地形、兵势，随机应变。方子也是这样的，我们经常讲"方法"，一个方子只是意味着一个法，一种思想，你要变通来用。

比如麻杏石甘汤，由这几味药组成：麻黄、杏仁、石膏、甘草。这是《伤寒论》的方子，辛凉重剂，能够开表，也能够清里热，这个方子体现了一个治肺的思想。我们知道肺开窍于皮毛，麻黄能够走表，开肺窍；杏仁降肺气，肺苦气上逆，所以用杏仁来降；在肺窍闭住，肺气不降的情况下，容易产生肺热，在外邪犯肺的情况下，也很容易产生肺热，我们用石膏来清肺热；在肺窍闭、肺热盛、肺气不降的情况下，肺容易急，所以用甘草缓肺急。这就是麻杏石甘汤的方义："麻黄开肺窍，杏仁降肺气，石膏清肺热，甘草缓肺急。"如果肺没有热而有湿邪，石膏就不要用了，可以改用薏苡仁，这要求我们对薏苡仁非常熟悉，知道它能够降肺里的邪气，利肺中的水湿。

不可死守成方

现在有很多人抛开治疗思想谈某病用某方，某症用某方，往往就只讲方不讲药了。有人还以此自诩"经方派"。经方虽好，但也不能生搬硬套，我们仍要学习其中的思想。陶弘景在《神农本草经》序言里就提到过有的庸医"耻看本草"、"倚约旧方"，结果误人误己。

诸葛亮和周瑜面对曹操八十万大军，都开出了"大破曹兵，要用火攻"的方子，果然火烧赤壁，大败曹军。那么是否意味着下次再遇到曹军依旧用火攻呢？当然不行。在不同的情况下遇到曹军，打法不一样，在不同人身上遇到同一个病，治法也不一样。

一个火攻就好比一个方子，不仅可以对付曹丞相，还可以对付藤甲兵，对付司马懿，陆逊拿它来对付刘备。但是他们每次用火的情形都不一样，每次发动火攻，用的人也不一样。这就好比一个法，比如说，同样是一个疏肝的方法，用的药不一样；同样一个养阴的方法，用的药也不一样，都是依据具体的情况而定的。因此一个方子可以对付很多病。同一种病呢，也会用到很多的方。

千万不要拿方和病去相对应，对应不上的。如果你认为某某病就用某某方，那么你会很机械，就像遇到曹操就用火攻，你是打不过曹操的。而且，也不要因为诸葛亮善用火攻，就觉得他是"火攻派"。

九分药一分方

学习中医的重点，有三个。首先是医理，接着是药性和诊断。医理是最重要的，是一个统摄。药性让你知道怎么用药。诊断这是让你认识这个病。方剂是以前面三点为根据拟出的。

学习方药，我们有一个原则：九分药一分方。这是我的恩师胡有衡先生跟我一贯强调的。熟悉药理药性，应该成为重点中的重点。

那为什么还要一分方呢？不是说熟悉了医理药理就行了吗？这是为了学习组方用药的思想。方剂都是古人慢慢摸索出来的，其中有很多真知灼见。学方，其实是在学方中之理及组方之法，这需要通晓医理，熟知药性。因此，学方的最佳状态是"师其法而不泥其方"。

"以方说理"时期

有很多书就是以方说理。尤其是唐朝及以前的一些医书，如《外台秘要》、《千金方》、《肘后方》、《伤寒杂病论》，里面主要是方子，医理没有完全写出来，而是靠口传心授。师门内部的人，看到这个方子就知道这个方子是什么道理，这叫"见方知理"。门外人见方茫然，只有照搬。

中医里有一种方叫"禁方"。禁，有两重含义：一是秘方；二是禁止使用，一些方子在那里，并不说明治什么病，禁止外行人乱用。怎么用？只有这个师门里面的人才知道。你得入了师门，经过口传心授，才能慢慢知道这些禁方的使用方法。过去宫廷里，还有一些其他地方，都会有禁方，我们现在还能找到一本书叫《鲁府禁方》。里面也是列了一些方剂。

而"经方"，我们都知道，是出自《伤寒论》和《金匮要略》里的方，有一种说法：经方是古圣先贤参天地、通鬼神，用无上智慧得出来的，今人愚钝，参不透其中的妙处，也不能改它。我觉得这种说法太过偏颇，古人有的智能今人也应该去达到，去学习、去探索和思考。千万不要这样，我们要通过深究医理，深究药理，自己来拟方。

学习方剂，目的是为了学习古人拟方的经验。我们看《伤寒论》《金匮要略》，其中讲"理"极少，主要是列举方子。随着时光的流逝，张仲景师门当时讲习的是什么东西我们现在已经不得而知了，留下的就是一本《伤寒论》，还是经过整理的，所以大家就茫然无措。后面注解《伤寒论》的人，都是在揣测这些方子背后的含义。

宋朝有一本书，叫《妇人良方》，也是以方为核心，用一个方剂体现一个思想，可能方剂写出来了，思想没有写出来。

"理法方药俱全"时期

一直到金元四大家的时代，确切地说是从张元素开始，大家才逐渐把医理和方剂结合起来讲，这也是为了把中医讲得更加透彻。金元四大家，他们之所以能够成为"大家"，在很大程度上讲，是因为他们著书立说，变换了一种表述方式，启迪了更多的后学。一直到明、清，大家都是沿着这个思路下来，就没有人仅仅用方剂来讲医理了。

清初有一位医家叫陈士铎，他写了很多书，比如《石室秘录》《辨证奇闻》，都是很注重理法方药的。比如说《石室秘录》，它以治法为核心，什么"正治法""反治法"，列举了非常多的治法，先讲道理，接着再把方给出来，而且都是非常管用的方子。像这样的书非常好，它适合不同层次的人。如果是非常笨的人，翻这书，会觉得这书里有很多有效的方剂可以用，可以去套，这也是允许的；如果是有一些聪明劲儿的人，就不会拘泥于这些方子，那就会去看它的法、看它的理。所以说它适合不同的人。

"理、法、方、药"，这也是中医的四大支柱。金元四大家以后，各家著述往往理法方药兼备，也正是如此，此后的医家才招致许多非议，如陈修园就在《医学三字经》中说这些人是"红紫色，郑卫音"，这也不是陈修园一个人的观点，当时人们喜欢对这些著书立说，详言理法方药的医家指指点点。

其实，无论什么样的著作，只要能流传到今天，其间都有值得我们学习的地方，我们要跟它们对话，取其精华。

Chapter 4　Understanding of Medicinal Quality

Three Levels of "Moral Quality" in Medicines

Shennong Bencao Jing lists 360 kinds of medicines that are classified into three categories: top grade, medium grade, and low grade, according to the properties ("characters", or "moral qualities") of the medicines. Moral quality is very important for selection and recruitment of human power. Similarly, the quality of a medicine is important for curing illness. Tao Hongjing (medical scientist in the Southern Dynasties) described the medicine properties about the three categories in the preface to *Shennong Bencao Jing*.

Top-Grade Medicines Follow the Nature Way

"A top-grade medicine can cure diseases; however, its effect is mild and slow in properties. So, if in a rush, it may not take immediate effect as expected but it will last long for the treatment of diseases. However, if it is used for a long period of time, it will definitely benefit the patients a lot. It not only can cure illness, but also nourish the health for longevity. The medicines in this category are in conformity with the *Tao* of Heaven, i. e. , "Heaven takes pleasure in the welfare of living things. " Therefore, one can say that the top-grade medicines follow the natural way.

Those who seek quick success and instant benefits may not be interested in such top-grade medicinessince they are slow for treatment. They may prefer the quick-effect medicines, which, however, may maintain their effects for merely a short period of time.

Here's a story in the Southern Dynasties(420-589) . The emperor was going to promote one of his officials named Fan Yun. However, just before the ceremony was about to be held, Fan Yun fell ill. He invited a famous doctor of the time named Xu Wenbo, who told Fan Yun that he needed a gradual treatment for complete cure. But Fan Yun asked for a quick cure, due to which he might die within two years. Fan Yun insisted on a quick cure with a quotation of Confucius "if in the morning one could comprehend the Way to Morality, in the evening he would die contented" to persuade Doctor Xu, who made a fire to bake the ground to a burning hot condition, and then covered the ground with peach leaves, after which Fan Yun was asked to lay down on the leaves, and he sweated immediately. On the next day, Fan Yun recovered happily and surely received his accolade. However, what Doctor Xu had said was finally proved to be true that Fan Yun died two years later.

Using the top-grade medicines is like following the **Nature Way** or the so-called **King Way**. The effect might be slower, but the patient will get healthy after he recovers from his illness, which tells us that the top-grade medicines focus on the long-term benefits.

Medium-Grade Medicines Follow the Human Way

"Medium-grade medicines are discussed more about their curing effects, but less about their functions on maintenance of health. They can cure illness quickly, but have limited effects for longevity. They are like human beings, born with certain temperament. Therefore, it is said that such medicines follow the **Human Way**."

In **Shennong Bencao Jing,** when the medium-grade medicines are discussed, there are more words about what illness they can cure, but much fewer words like "long-time use of such medicines make people feel light and stay young", which are frequently repeated for describing the top-grade medicines. The so-called "feel light" means one feels light-footed and lively, not so much about real body weight lost. When one feels heavier, he or she is becoming weaker physically. When one feels lighter, he or she is definitely becoming stronger physically. The medium-grade medicines may cure illness quickly, but such medicines have very little effect on longevity.

Low-Grade Medicines Follow the Tyranny Way

"Thelower-grade medicines specifically target at diseases. They are intensely strong, which may damage the balance and harmony. So, such medicines cannot

be taken for long, and should be immediately stopped once they strike the diseases. They are like the earth, which will bury everything. Therefore, it is said
that such medicines are corresponding to the earth", or to be more frankly, they
are corresponding to the Tartarean road.

The lower-grade medicines cannot be used for the purpose of health maintenance, and they follow the **Tyranny Way** only for curing illness specifically.
So, stop using such medicines once the illness is cured.

The ancient administrators usually took a policy by force yet with tolerance
in governance, i. e. , combination of harshness with mercy. For the unruly people
and mobs, force would have to be used, after which some lenient policies would
be taken to pacify the society.

Staying Close to the Virtuous Men and Keeping Away from the Mean Men

Zhuge Liang, the famous Prime Ministerof the State Shu in the Three Kingdoms Period, followed the principles of "staying close to the virtuous talents, and
keeping away from the mean persons" for choosing a person for a vacancy, for example, Zhuge Liang left an important position to Jiang Wei who was noble and
capable. The virtuous men are those with excellent moral quality, like the top-
grade medicine. The mean men are also needed for some jobs, for example, Wei
Yan, who was low in his moral quality, just like the low-grade medicine, so,
Zhuge Liang only used him to fight against the enemies, and took some measures
to control him when necessary.

Again, many people frequently use Fuzi (radix aconiti carmichaeli), or e-
ven use it for healthcare, which is quite unsuitable. According to the **Shennong
Bencao Jing,** Fuzi is of a low-grade medicine, i. e. , "a mean person" that is
very capable in respect of saving lives in case of severe cold syndrome, like the
declining kidney Yang in the body. But normally, it cannot be used at wills or in
a long run. Zhu Liangchun, a famous TCM expert, said that "Fuzi should be rationally used, but never abused. "

In an institution or organization, one may be appointed at an important position just because he or she is very capable, but his or her moral quality is not se-

riously taken into consideration, which will finally result in some bad consequences. However, TCM strongly advocates the principles of staying close to "the virtuous talents" (the top-grade medicines), and keeping away from "the mean persons" (the low-grade medicines).

Seven Emotions of the Medicines

Medicines, like humans, have "seven emotions", too, i. e. , joy, anger, worry, pensiveness, sadness, fear, and shock. The seven emotions of the medicines refer to the interconnection between medicines. Some medicines function individually; some are mutually needed; some are mutually intensified; some are mutually restrained; some are mutually inhibitive; some are mutually incompatible; and some are mutually detoxicating. Emotions define the relations. To choose a medicine is just like choosing a person.

Explanation of the "Seven Emotions"

The medicines that function individually means that only one single herb will have a specific effect for curing illness without necessity of combining with other herbs.

Some medicines are mutually needed, which means that it is necessary to use two medicines together since both of them need each other in the process of curing illness, for example, mulberry leaf and chrysanthemum are often mutually needed.

Some medicines can intensify each other, which means that each of the two medicines used together can function more effectively with mutual assistance than individually used.

Some are mutually restrained, which means the two medicines "fear" each other, therefore, they should not be used together.

Some are mutually incompatible means the two medicines are against each other, which will result in negative effects.

Traditionally, there are totally three sets of eighteen incompatible medicines, called the **"Eighteen Incompatibilities"**; and eight pairs and one trio of medicines that are restrained mutually, called **"Nineteen Restraints"**. Such medicines should be used with special caution.

The **Eighteen Incompatibilities** refer that the various forms of Wutou (aconite) is incompatible with Banxia (pinellia ternate), Gualou (trichosanthes kirilowii maxim), Beimu (fritillaria), Bailian (radix ampelopsis), and Baiji (bletilla).

Gancao (liquorice) is incompatible with Haizao (seaweed), Daji (euphorbia pekinensis), Gansui (euphorbia kansui), Yuanhua (lilac daphne flower bud).

"Lilu (Veratrum nigrum) is incompatible with Renshen (ginseng), Danshen (radix salviae miltiorrhizae), Shashen (radix adenophorae), Xuanshen (radix scrophulariae), Xixin (asarum), Chishao (radix paeoniae rubra) and Baishao (radix paeoniae alba).

The **Nineteen Restraints refer to the following** eight pairs and one trio of medicines that are restrained mutually: Liuhuang (sulfur) vs Poxiao (mirabilite); Shuiyin (hydrargyrum) vs Pishuang (arsenic); Langdu (radix euphorbiae lantu) vs Mituoseng (lithargite); Badou (croton) vs Qianniu (amomum cardamomum); Yujin (radix curcumae) vs Dingxiang (clove); Yaxiao (saltpeter) vs Sanleng (rhizoma sparganii); Guangui (cassia bark) vs Shizhi (halloysit); Renshen (ginseng) vs Wulingzhi (trogopterus dung); Chuanwu (aconite root), Caowu (radix aconiti agrestis) vs Xijiao (rhinoceros horn). If these pairs of medicines are used together, they may become toxic. Therefore, they should be used with extreme caution.

As is known, where there is regularity, there will be exceptions. In some formulas, incompatible medicines are indeed used together. For instance, in the formula of **Haizao Yuhu Tang** recorded in *Yizong Jinjian (Golden Mirror of Medicine)*, Haizao and Gancao are used together for a specific effect. So, the regularity might be broken sometimes under some specific circumstances.

The mutual inhibitive medicines in TCM refer that some medicines dislike the others. So, if they are used together, they may interact mutually. For example, tortoise plastron dislikes Dangshen (codonopsis pilosula), Renshen, Shashen, and so on. However, in the formula of **Guilu Erxian Jiao**, ginseng is intentionally used together with the tortoise plastron, the purpose of which is for them to take precautions against each other. Just like in a working team, it is not good for all the members to be too close-bonded since it may be more likely for them to form a clique to pursue selfish interests. Having a few members to keep watch on each other, the team is more likely to work at its best strength.

The mutually detoxicating medicines can also be used together in some cases. They are quite similar to those mutually inhibitive medicines but with more severe interaction. For example, ginger can restrain or detoxify Banxia. Just for such an effect, the normally used Jiang Banxia actually refers to Banxia processed with ginger. Another example, Fa Banxia (rhizoma pinellinae praeparata) also refers to Banxia processed by ginger. So, the seven "emotions" of medicines in TCM tell us to make best use of the advantages and avoid the disadvantages.

The Weird Way vs the Balance Mechanism

Now some doctors like to use raw Banxia to reduce phlegm. It may function effectively and quickly, but the toxicity of raw Banxia will make the patients feel numb or sore in the throat. The side effect might be less serious in the case of excessive phlegm. However, this is not following the **King Way**, or even not the **Tyranny Way**. That's a **Wired Way**.

The **Wired Way** is a shortcut sometimes, but it may bring about disastrous consequences later. Banxia is a low-grade medicine, which can be used, but must be restrained in some way in order to find a mechanism of balance among different medicines.

Medicines in Five Categories

Various Medicines Categorized by Properties Based on the *Wuxing Doctrine*

In this book, five categories of medicines will be discussed, which are corresponding to the Five Elements (wood, fire, metal, water, and earth) (**Note:** these five elements, to some extent, do not really refer to the five physical substances, but the five symbols. According to **Wuxing Doctrine**, or the Five-element theory, all things in this word based on their properties and attributes are classified into five categories that are represented by the five symbols/elements respectively: wood, fire, metal, water, and earth) and the five directions (east, south, west, north, and middle), representing the five properties of medicines. It is like a company consisting of five departments with over 360 employees in total. What the leader needs to do in that company is to guide the managers in the five department, not necessarily manage every employee. So, what the TCM beginners should do is to concentrate on the main points on the herbal medicines.

The first category is about Mulberry of Genera——Wood-categorized Formulas and Medicines, in which mulberry is taken as a representative mainly used for the treatment of the wind related-diseases. The second category is Cassia of Genera — Fire-categorized Formulas and Medicines, in which cassia is taken as a representative mainly used for the treatment of the febrile diseases. The third is Gypsum of Genera — Metal-categorized Formulas and Medicines, in which gypsum is taken as a representative to explain the cold and cool medicines. The fourth is Rehmannia of Genera - Water-associated Formulas and Medicines, in which rehmannia is taken as a representative to explain the cold and cool tonifying or nourishing medicines. The fifth is Atractylodes of Genera - Earth-associated Formulas and Medicines, which will focus on the medicines for transportation and transformation (T&T) purposes. All the commonly used medicines in TCM will be discussed in line with these five categories.

Learning from Books vs Learning from Experts

In the bookstores, one may find many books on herbal medicines, some of which categorize the medicines by plant herbs, metal and stone herbs, and animal herbs, for instance, **Bencao Gangmu (Compendium of Materia Medica)**. The advantage is that medicines can be explained in details. For example, when mulberry is discussed, all the herbs related the mulberry, like leaves, bark, and fruits will be illustrated clearly. The disadvantage is that it is impossible to discuss the medicines with similar functions in the category.

Some other books, like **Bencao Qiuzhen (Seeking Truth in Materia Medica)**, categorize the medicines by their respective functions, such as the medicines for the exterior dissipation, the internal treatment, warm tonification, the cold and cool medicines, etc. , which is usually categorized in too much details.

The traditional way of learningTCM is to follow an expert to acquire the knowledge in a free and flexible way without any dogmatic constraints, which is also a way I am trying to follow in this book.

第四章　如何把握药性

药分三品

《神农本草经》把三百六十味药分成了上、中、下三品。为什么要分品呢？用人要讲人品，用药也要讲药品。用药也是如此。陶弘景在《神农本草经》的序言中对药的上中下三品做了一个说明。

上品药应天，行王道

"上品药性，亦皆能遣疾，但其势力和厚，不为仓卒之效，然而岁月常服必获大益，病既愈矣，命亦兼申。天道仁育，故云应天。"上品的药也能治病，但是力量比较缓和，可能仓促之际没有什么效果，或者效果要来得慢一些，但是服用这个药的时间一长，它对你的身心必然有很大的益处。等你病好了以后，寿命也会延长。它治病不伤人，而且还养人，这些药它符合"天有好生之德"的天道，所以应天。

那些急功近利的人对此必然不感兴趣了，他们可能更喜欢"霸道"。你用霸道，成功可能很快就来了，但维持的时间往往比较短。用王道，成功来得慢一些，但持续的时间会很长很长。

南朝陈武帝属下有位官员叫范云，武帝打算给他加"九锡"，也就是给他加封一个很高的爵位。加九锡的仪式快要举行的时候，范云病了。他请来当时的名医徐文伯。徐文伯说："您这病得慢慢治，一时半会儿好不了。"范云说："有什么办法可以很快就好么？"文伯说："有，但是用了这个方法后，再过两年你就会死。"范云这时候开始引经据典了，说："朝闻道，夕死可矣！何况两年呢？"于是徐文伯用火把地烧得滚烫，然后铺上桃叶，让范云躺上去，范云马上出了一身的汗，第二天病就好了。范云非常高兴，拜官受爵去了。徐文伯却说："没什么值得高兴的。"果然，两年后，范云就死了。

用上品的药相当于用王道，可能效果来得稍微慢一点，但当病好了以后，人的身体也好了。所以，用上品药，有长远的效果。

中品药应人，行人道

"中品药性，疗病之辞渐深，轻身之说稍薄，于服之者，祛患当速，而延龄为缓。人怀性情，故云应人。"

《神农本草经》谈到中品药的时候，说它治什么病的言辞多了，而说它"久服轻身不老"之类的话就少了。要知道，《神农本草经》在解释上品药的时候，动不动就在最后来一句"久服轻身不老"。所谓"轻身"，就是觉得自己的身体变得轻快了，而不是身体的重量真的变轻了。当一个人觉得自己的身体变重的时候，就是说他的气力变衰了，觉得自己的身体越来越轻快的时候，肯定就是身体变好了。服中品药，病好得快，但可能它没有什么令人长寿的作用了。

下品药应地，行霸道

"下品药性，专主攻疾，毒烈之气，倾损中和，不可恒服，疾愈即止，地体收杀，故云应地。"下品药是专攻疾病的，它有毒烈之气，能够很快地伤害人的中和之气，不能经常服用，病好了就得停下来。它对应的是地道，说白了，就是通地狱的。

用下品药没法养生，我们只能利用它的能力，把事情做完就行了，不可重用它，不可跟它深交，否则它会害你，可以用于一时而不能长久，它行的是霸道。

古人讲，治理百姓应该宽猛相济，王道和霸道相结合，有时候应该宽厚，有时候应该严厉一些，交替着用。真的有这种刁民、暴民，我们可以用武力镇压，但是镇压完了马上就要实行仁政，进行宽抚。

亲贤臣，远小人

用药如用人。诸葛亮讲，用人的原则是：亲贤臣，远小人。贤臣是上品的人，好比上品药；小人好比下品的药。但是小人也可以用，用他的能力。像姜维这样的人，人品、武功都是上品的，所以诸葛亮会重用；像魏延这样的人，诸葛亮一直以为他人品不好，所以只用他的能力，不亲近他，防备他，有必要时打压他。

比如，现在很多人用附子，有人甚至靠大量的附子来养生，这样做是否合适呢？当然不合适。我们查《神农本草经》，可以知道附子在下品。它就是一个小人，但这个小人很有能力，如果我们遇到大寒证，遇到人体真阳衰微，可以用它，但千万不要轻易用它，更不要长时间地用它。朱良春老先生说："附子要善用，不要滥用。"

当今社会上，某些机构也会出现这种情况：看到某一个人能力很强，就不问他的人品，委以重任，最后造成的祸害就很大。中医用药中提倡亲贤臣，远小人。

药有七情

人有七情，药也有七情。人有七情是喜、怒、忧、思、悲、恐、惊。药的七情则用来表达药和药之间的感情：有单行者，有相须者，有相使者，有相畏者，有相恶者，有相反者，有相杀者。感情决定关系，用人如此，用药也如此。

"七情"解

单行就是一味药，不需配伍就有某种作用。

相须，就是你需要我，我需要你，就像我们接着要讲到的桑叶和菊花，它们就是相须的。

相使，就是我有你会作用更大，你有我作用也会更大。

相畏，就是这两味药在一起，你怕我，我怕你，在一起不和。

相反，就是两个药在一起会对着干，产生坏的影响。

中药里有十八反，十九畏，这个药就要慎用了。

这些都是有歌诀的。十八反的歌诀："本草明言十八反，半蒌贝蔹芨攻乌，藻戟芫遂具战草，诸参辛芍叛藜芦。"半夏、瓜蒌、贝母、白蔹、白芨与乌头相反，海藻、大戟、甘遂、芫花与甘草相反，人参、丹参、沙参、玄参等所有的参，细辛、赤芍、白芍与藜芦相反。

十九畏是："硫黄原是火中精，朴硝一见便相争。水银莫与砒霜见，狼毒最怕密陀僧。巴豆性烈最为上，偏与牵牛不顺情。丁香莫与郁金见，牙硝难合京三棱。川乌草乌不顺犀，人参最怕五灵脂。官桂善能调冷气，若逢石脂便相欺。大凡修合看顺逆，炮爁炙煿莫相依。"硫黄畏朴硝，水银畏砒霜，狼毒畏密陀僧，巴豆畏牵牛，丁香畏郁金，川乌、草乌畏犀角，牙硝畏三棱，官桂畏石脂，人参畏五灵脂。尤其是相反的，用了可能就会有毒，相畏稍微要好一些，但是最好慎用。

当然，有规律就有例外，在有的方子里，比如《医宗金鉴》里的海藻玉壶汤，偏偏要把海藻和甘草同用，以达到某种效果。你不能死守规律，不敢越雷池一步，更不能拿例外来否定规律。

相恶，就是你讨厌我，我讨厌你，但在一起的时候可以相互制约。比如龟版恶参，与党参、人参、沙参什么的都相恶。但是龟鹿二仙胶里，偏偏要把人参跟龟版放在一起，其用意就是相互提防着。一个团队里大家太团结了也不好，容易结党营私，如果其中有几个人相互提防，反倒可以用彼之长，防彼之短。

相杀的药也是可以同用的，它跟相恶有点相似，只不过是更明显，作用的力度更大。比如生姜和半夏，生姜可以杀半夏毒，它们是相杀的，但现在我们偏偏要用它这个相杀的，用生姜来制半夏，所以配药的时候经常讲姜半夏，姜半夏就是用姜制了的半夏，法半夏其实也是用姜制的。这就是利用他们之间的七情来互相制约扬长避短。

诡道与平衡机制

现在医界还有些人喜欢用生半夏化痰，的确化得快，但生半夏有毒，吃了会让人喉咙麻、肿痛，当然如果痰多的话，它去化痰了，副作用会小一些。这些人敢用生半夏，取快于一时，痰化掉了，他就觉得自己本事很大，其实这不是王道，这连霸道都称不上，这是诡道。

诡道有时是一种快捷方式，其实大祸就在后面。半夏也是下品药，可以用，但应该得到应有的抑制，即寻找药品之间的一种平衡机制。

药分五部

中药众多，五行统括

我们的整个"方药之道"，只讲五个药。它们对应的是五行（木、火、金、水、土）、五方（东、南、西、北、中）。代表药的五种属性。就好比做领导的，这个公司有五个部门，一共三百六十多个人，他只需管好这五个部门的经理就行了，没必要每个人都管。咱们掌握中药，也要提纲挈领地来。

第一类是"桑之属"，木部方药，以桑为核心，主要是治风的；第二类是"桂之属"，桂枝、肉桂什么的，火部方药，主要是温热类的；第三类是"石膏之属"，金部方药，在这一部里面我们主要讲一些寒凉药；第四类是"地黄之属"，生地、熟地之类，为水部方药，主要是滋补类的。

第五种是"术之属"，土部方药，为运化类的。我们常用的方药，都将围绕着五种药来展开。

书上的讲法与师门的传授

市面上的中药书籍，有的是按草木、金石、动物药来分类的，如《本草纲目》，这种分类的优点是可以把某一个药讲透，比如讲到桑，可以把桑叶、桑皮、桑葚放在一起讲清楚；缺点是难以将同类功效的药全部放在一起讲。有的是按发表之药、攻里之药、温补之药、寒凉之药等等来分类，如《本草求真》，这样分类太细。

传统的讲法是师门传授，没有条条框框，往往想到哪里讲到哪里，这样讲才灵动，我们也争取这样讲。

Volume 2
Mulberry of Genera—Wood-categorized Formulas and Medicines

Chapter 1   Introduction of Wood-categorized Formulas and Medicines

Analyses of Wood Properties

Let us start with the wood-categorized formulas of mulberry of genera. *Huangdi Neijing (The Inner Classic of Huangdi)* says, "The east generates wind, and the wind then produces wood. ...... In the air it is wind, and in the earth it grows woods; in the body it refers to anadesma, and among the internal vital organs it refers to the liver. " The spring, east, wind, liver and anadesma, all of these appear to be unrelated, but they all have a common feature, that is, all of them are subsumed to wood of genera from the perspective of Wuxing (the five elements referring to metal, wood, water, fire and earth). That is called "like drawing to like", which means the objects of the same function like to be together.

In the four seasons of a year, the spring always comes the first. Whenever talking about a year, one always starts from the season of the spring. In the spring, it is always windy. After Lichun (the first of the 24 solar terms in a year, on the day of February 3 to 5), cold as it is of the wind, one can feel the different in some way since the cold draught is getting less and less, and the fragrance of the earth is getting more and more, which signifies that Yang-qi (the healthy energy) is growing from under the earth, and together with the wind from the horizon, it sends us the spring smell of great strength and vigor. The spring starts with the wind, and wind indicates the beginning of a season, and it also is the source of diseases. "Wind is the primary pathogen", as such, when talking about the traditional Chinese medicine (TCM) , one will have to start with the category of wood - the prescribed herbs that are used to cure the diseases caused by the wind.

What is the feature of wood in Wuxing? Regarding this question, one must experience and comprehend it from the wood in the nature.

The wood is growing in between the sky and earth, from where it links up Yin-qi and Yang-qi. Water produces wood and wood then produces fire. The wood lying in between water and fire can links up water and fire. The wood grows and withers following the changes of the four seasons, and it has a quite sensible response to Qi from the nature, earth and the dynamic changes of seasons. The wood and grass had already been there in the nature before the animals and human came into being. Where there is abundant vegetation, there will be a better environment and less dust, and smaller temperature difference round the clock as well, so the wood has a much stronger regulating function.

The Book of History says, "Wood is characterized by growing freely and peripherally". Wood, having the characteristics of flexibility and pliability, may be bended or straightened. In spring, wood becomes vigorous. Under the influence of the rising energy, the grass and wood will grow most rapidly. Wood is easily subject to wind in that it grows rapidly in the wind. That is why it is said that **Spring Wind Blows the Growth of All Things on Earth** in a verse. Such a poetic line does have its grounded support. "The strong wind always destroy the wood that stands high in the forest. " Such a saying tells us that the woods can guard against the wind, however, if any of the wood grows exceptionally high out of the woods, it will be definitely destroyed. This is called hurting of pathogenic wind, which gives us a reminder that the liver-qi (the energy in the liver) in the human body must not get too strong, but keep mild instead.

Trees cannot survive or grow without water. According to TCM theory, water is subsumed to the kidney, and the liver and kidney are closely related, which is called "Yi-Gui Homology" in TCM. Wood has the nature of liveness, so the liver-Yin must be strong enough, but liver-Yin originates from kidney-Yin because water produces wood. If the liver shows deficiency of Yin, it would be like wood getting withered easily for the shortage of water. Once wood withers, it will lose its flexibility, and be blown off, or even it may catch fire easily. Therefore, if the liver is in deficiency of Yin, the human body will lose its toughness, and all muscles, bones and blood vessels will become vulnerable, and even appear to get inflamed in various way. Well, no doubt, if there is too much water, wood will get rotten, so will be the liver. That is why liver is terribly unbearable to the hot and humid conditions.

Out of earth grows wood, which, with liveness, is able to loosen the earth and conserve water and soil. "Wood restricts earth", which in fact manifests a lot. Again, sand storm and haze are also subsumed to earth. If land is covered with dense woods, air will be purified and the sand wind will quiet down.

All in all, where there is wood, there will be clear and beautiful environment, so will be the human body. Of great importance is the wood-caterigorized-formulas for curing diseases and keeping human being in good health.

Therefore, the wood-categorized formulas will be explained and analyzed with all these natures of wood encompassed.

Analyses of Mulberry Properties

Mulberry is a token of the spring. In Chinese language, there are two characters making a phrase called "sāngzǐ" (which means "one's native place"), of which "sāng" refers to mulberry tree and "zǐ" refers to catalpa tree. When these too types of trees are put together, they refer to "one's native place". Why is it so? Mulberry tree is the leading actor in spring, whose green color is quite eye-catching in this season, and people climb up the tree to pick mulberry leaves (folium mori) and fruit, so one's memories about spring may not go on if without the images of mulberry. The catalpa tree is a little more eye-catching in autumn. It has strong branches and red leaves, bearing white seeds, which is a picturesque scenery in autumn. As seasons are changing from spring to autumn, mulberry tree and catalpa tree not only represent the two special trees in one's hometown, they also mean something of the years and time in one's childhood. And for me, only by now when I think of my hometown, I am aware of the implication of these two Chinese characters.

The spring is a reproducing season, and mulberry tree is a most vigorous plant, so there are a lot of herbal medicines related to mulberry like mulberry leaf (folium mori), Sangzhi (mulberry twig), Sangbaipi (cortex mori), mulberry fruits, Sangjisheng (parasitic loranthus) (parasitic plantlets on the mulberry trees), and Sangpiaoxiao (mantis egg-case) (eggs spawned by mantis on mulberry trees). The mulberry leaves can be used as food for silkworms. The dead silkworms can also be used for medicine called Baijiangcan (silkworm larva), and even Cansha (silkworm faeces or silkworm excrement), too. All these will be discussed in the following parts. There are series of medicines related to mulberry trees, which just answer the questions about vitality of life and growth in the mulberry trees.

第二卷　桑之属－木部方药

第一章　木部方药概论

木性解

我们今天先讲桑之属，木部方药。《黄帝内经》说："东方生风，风生木。……在天为风，在地为木，在体为筋，在藏为肝。"春天、东方、木、风、肝、筋，这一系列看似风马牛不相及的东西都有一个共同的属性，就是在五行上属木，它们同气相求。

四季春为首。论及一年，必然从春天说起。春季多风，立春过后，风虽仍然很冷，但我们已经能从其中感觉到有些不一样了，其中少了寒气，多了一些泥土的芳香，这告诉我们，地下的阳气在往外透了，它和天际吹来的风一起，让我们感受到浩浩荡荡的春的气息。春，又是从风开始的。风为季节的开端，又是疾病的源头。"风为百病之长。"所以在讲药的时候，我们也从木部，这些治风的方药讲起。

五行中的木，有何特征呢？我们要联系到大自然中的木来体会和理解。

木在天地之间，它沟通天地阴阳。水生木，木生火，木在水火之间，能沟通水火。木随着四季的交替而枯荣，它对天地之气、季节律动的反应非常敏感。自然界在有动物之前就有了草木，然后才有了动物、人类。哪里植被丰富，哪里的环境就会好一些，灰尘就会少，昼夜温差也不至于太大，所以木有很强的调节作用。

《尚书·洪范》讲："木曰曲直。"木有活性、柔韧性，能曲能直。木旺于春，升发最速，在春天的升发之气下，生长得最快的就是草木。木喜风，草木见风而长，所以人们常说是春风吹生了万物，这种诗意的表达并非毫无依据。然而"木秀于林，风必摧之"，森林可以防风，但如果这片森林中哪棵树长得格外高，高出整个树林，就会被风吹坏，这又是风邪伤木。也提示人体肝气不能过旺，要以平为期。

树木的生长离不开水，水属肾，故肝肾关系密切，中医里称"乙癸同源"。木有活性，所以肝阴要旺，肝阴源自肾阴，水生木。如果肝阴虚，就好比木头缺水就容易枯萎，木头一枯萎就失去了柔韧性，容易被风吹断，甚至容易着火。肝阴虚，人体也会失去柔韧性，筋骨、血管都会变脆，甚至出现各种火症。当然，如果水太多了，木头也会腐烂，肝也是如此，最怕湿热。

木生在土上，能让土壤松软、有活性，又能保持水土，所谓"木克土"，其表现也是非常丰富的。再比如，风沙、雾霾也属土，如果树木多，空气就会净化，风沙就会平息。

总而言之，有木方有美丽明净的大自然，人体之自然也是如此。木部方药，对于治病养生也非常重要。

我们的木部方药，将围绕着肝木的这些属性逐步展开。

桑性解

桑树是春天的象征。

有一个词叫"桑梓"。桑就是桑树，梓就是木梓树，这两种树放在一起为什么可以用来指代故乡呢？桑树是春天的主角，其绿色在春天非常显眼，大家在上面采桑叶、摘桑葚，关于春天的回忆，都可能有桑树。木梓树在秋天比较显眼，枝干苍劲，叶红白籽，是秋天的一番风景。于是，春去秋来，秋去春回，桑梓既是故乡的两种树，又意味着故乡的岁月，春秋轮转。直到现在，我想起故乡，才体会到这两个字的内涵。

春天是一个生发的季节，桑树是最有"有生之气"的，所以围绕桑树的药也就非常多。桑树的叶子就是桑叶，桑树枝叫桑枝，桑树的根皮叫桑白皮，桑树的果实叫桑葚，桑树上还有一种寄生的小植物叫桑寄生，螳螂在桑树上排的卵叫桑螵蛸。桑叶可以喂蚕，蚕死了也可以入药的，叫白僵蚕，蚕的粪便又是蚕沙。这些我们都会讲到。围绕桑树的药非常多，我们这个系列的药也会非常多。这也正好应了桑的生生之气。

Chapter 2   Mulberry Leaves and
Dispelling Medicines

Mulberry Leaves Dispelling the Wind

As can be seen in the nature, the mulberry trees are big with luxuriant foliage, striking their roots deeply into the earth. The mulberry branches and twigs sprout in spring and grow through the whole summer and autumn. When it is cold and the frost falls, part of the leaves will fall, but the remaining leaves will hang on the tree until the winter set in. Without doubt, after experiencing the weathering in the heat of the sun and the strike of the wind blow of the whole year, the mulberry leaves will be in a disastrous state with scars and holes in them by the season of winter. In spring, mulberry leaves are picked from trees for feeding silkworms, but the mulberry trees never stop growing new leaves over and again in an endless succession. But as medicine, mulberry leaves can only be picked after being stricken by the frost. When doctors make a prescription, the mulberry leaf is often written as "frosted mulberry leaf" or "winter mulberry leaf". As said in **Wuxing Doctrine** (theory of the Five Elements) about "metal restricting wood", the mulberry leaf takes in the life essence of "metal" in autumn (according to Wuxing theory, autumn is corresponding to "metal", so "life essence of metal" in fact refers to "the life essence of autumn") , so the leaves picked in winter can soothe the liver. The mulberry leaves hang on the branches and twigs of trees and do not fall to the ground even after wind blow, indicating they would have a strong force to quiet down the air flow and wind blow, therefore, mulberry leaf used as medicine should not be picked until winter is come. When leaves are picked and collected, they must dry in air in such a way of hanging on thread in order to further absorb the energy of air. The hanging leaves hit against each other and make sounds like metal and stone impacting upon each other, which implies that the dried mulberry leaves would have the properties of metal and stone.

Shennong Bencao Jing mentions that mulberry leaves are bitter cold. But actually, it also has a little sweet taste under the cover of bitter cold, so it is sweet, bitter and cold in properties. Regarding the efficacy of mulberry leaves, in the book of **Bencao Biandu (Chinese Herbes Reading)** , there is a nice poetic couplet describing it as under:

Collecting vita llife essence from the *Jī* star,

Searching liver collaterals for diseases due to wind;

Holding the balance weight of the Lord *Qingdi*,

It can purge the fire from *Shaoyang* Channel.

Collecting vital life essence from the Jī star, Searching the Liver Meridian for Wind Pathogens

The twenty eight stars (in ancient time, the Chinese ancesteral astronomers grouped the sidereal stars in the south meridian passage into twenty eight constellations in order to facilitate the observation of running of the sun, the moon and the Five Planets) cover seven constellations in each direction of the east, the south, the west and the north. The seven constellations in the east called *Qinglong* (Green Dragon) Seven Constellations include the stars of *Jiǎo, Kàng, Dī, Fáng, Xīn, Wěi, Jī*. After observing the celestial phenomena, the Chinese ancestors found when the *Jī* star becomes very bright in the sky, then wind will rise on the earth, so it was concluded "the *Jī* star likes wind. " Now it is a little harder to observe the celestial phenomena in cities due to the air pollution. All the things on the earth including the five internal solid organs (heart, spleen, liver, lung and kidney) and the six hollow organs (stomach, large intestine, small intestine, bladder, gallbladder, Tri-jiao) of the human body may be linked up with the twenty eight stars. The liver Qi is linked with the seven constellations in the east, while wind is linked up with the *Jī* star and so is the mulberry. Therefore, mulberry leaves are linked up with the Jī star and will collect the vital life essence from the star. That is why mulberry leaves can enter the liver meridian to cure wind pathogens.

It may be asked: "wind can be divided into endogenous wind and exogenous wind, so, which one can the mulberry leaves cure? As a matter of fact, it can cure both, but it depends on how one will use it. The ancients said "the *Jī* star likes wind", but they did not mention the *Jī* star likes the endogenous wind or exogenous wind. Furthermore, the wind has diversities of forms.

If one holds a piece of mulberry leaf in the hand, he or she can clearly see the veins in the leaf, which are dense and clear. As veins in the leaf can be useful for collaterals in human body, one can use mulberry leaves to search the liver collaterals for the wind pathogens. The liver governs wind in human body, so, when the liver shows *Yin* deficiency, the liver wind will be easy to move; and when the wind enters collaterals, it will become chronic, as such, mulberry leaves can be used to "search liver collaterals for wind pathogens".

Holding the balance weight of the Lord Qingdi, Purging the fire from Shaoyang Channel

Qingdi is the God of the East, i. e. *Qinglong* (Green Dragon) [one of the four images, representing the four holy beasts of *Qinglong* (green dragon), *Baihu* (white tiger), *Zhuque* (rosefinch) and *Xuanwu* (turtles) in Chinese traditional culture]. *Shaoyang* Channel is of gallbladder meridian. The liver and the gallbladder meridians cooperate with each other to function like the exterior and the interior mutually. Therefore, **"holding the balance weight of the Lord *Qingdi*, it can purge the fire from *Shaoyang* Channel"**, which means the mulberry leaves (folium mori) can reconcile the liver and gallbladder.

The liver is an organ that generates wind and governs the fire of *Shaoyang* meridian. Each person has liver wind, but for the healthy person, the liver wind is just a gentle breeze, which can blow all things to grow. And all the energetic and vital Qi in human body will rise under the blow of such gentle breeze. By the senior ages, the ascending and rising functions in human body become weak, while the liver keeps on generating wind. Under such a circumstance, the wind will become "pathogenic wind". In that case, it is necessary to nourish Yin in order to prevent the pathogenic wind and minimize the adverse effect of sucn immoderate wind. Try to transform the wind generated into gentle breeze or make a proper room for the liver wind.

The gallbladder is subsumed to the *Shaoyang* meridian, which governs the slight fire. **Huangdi Neijing** says, "*Shaohuo* (the slight fire) generates Qi (here referring to the healthy Qi) while *Zhuanghuo* (the sthenic fire) consumes Qi".

The slight fire is soft and mild, which is also the most energetic and vital, so it can generate healthy Qi. If the fire is too strong and sthenic, it may burn out all things and leave nothing energetic, so the gallbladder fire should be soft and slow in order to let the healthy Qi rise. Otherwise, it will become pathogenic fire.

Once the liver generates pathogenic wind and the gallbladder generates pathogenic fire, the wind and fire may help to encourage each other and get stronger gradually. In the nature, the wind and fire fan up each other and become higher and stronger. The fire itself is featured with burning hot, and the wind fans and blows up the fire. They together will whirl upwards. The wind and the fire inside the human body follow the similar way and whirl upwards. In such cases, the diseases always occur in the head and eyes.

For instance, one feels light in the head (or dizzy and giddy) or feels bloodshot in the eyes. That must be connected with wind and fire, so mulberry leaves may be used to reconcile liver and gallbladder in order to quiet down the pathogenic wind and downbear the endogenic fire since mulberry leaf has the effect of clearing the dizziness and giddiness in the head and eyes. By the way, mulberry leaf may also be used for washing eyes, hairs and pinkeyes. If pinkeyes arise from the exogenous wind, mulberry leaf decoction can be used to wash eyes directly. Mulberry leaf may also be used for washing hair. The scalp is likely to be itchy, which is often due to cold or exposure to wind-pathogens on the top. In that case, one may decoct mulberry leaf and chrysanthemum together, or mulberry leaf only to wash hair with the decoction, which has proved quite effective.

Sangma Pill

Hair loss is somewhat related to the wind-pathogens. My teacher frequently mentioned before that hair can be compared to leaves on the trees. The leaves, if healthily growing on trees, will not fall in wind until they get withered and dried-up. In order to solve the problem of hair loss, one should nourish both Yin and blood, and dispel the pathogenic wind at the same time. For this purpose, a medicine named **Sangma Pill** has been developed, which is mainly made out of mulberry leaf and black sesame. As for the dosage of these two ingredients, it depends on the degree of seriousness. If the pathogenic wind symptom is more serious, more mulberry leaf may be used, or if Yin deficiency is more serious, more black sesame may be used. Both of these ingredients should be made into fine grinding, and then into pills with whitish honey. Take the pills with salt water in the morning and with liquor in the evening on the long-term basis. In this way, it can help to nourish Yin and dispel the wind, which will bring about a very good effect for curing hair loss. **Sangma Pill** must be taken with salt water since in the early morning stomach is empty and salt can get into the kidney to nourish Yin, while liquor in the evening can help to send the medical effect up to the head to dispel the wind. As such, the effect of the pills on the one hand is sent upwards for dispelling wind and on the other hand is sent downwards for nourishing Yin. Of course, **Sangma Pill** is primarily used for curing hair loss due to deficiency of Yin plus pathogenic wind disturbance. However, it is effective for some eye diseases due to deficiency of liver-Yin, vigorous liver wind, and hot gallbladder fire, too.

Common Medicine With Uncommon Effects

As to high blood pressure (hypertension) stemming from the liver and gall-bladder, mulberry leaf is also used since mulberry leaf can search liver collaterals for wind-pathogens. The high blood pressure in most cases arises from liver wind disturbance and hyperactivity of liver-Yang. Whenever there exists hyperactivity of liver-Yang, **Zhengan Xifeng Tang** (decotion for suppressing liver and quieting wind) will spring to the mind of most of people, but few will think of mulberry leaf since it is too common and unimpressive.

TCM is not to uphold any novelty or newness. If common medicine can cure diseases, there will be no necessity to seek for using new or unfamilar medicines, or large dosage of medicines, or even toxicant medicines. Medication follows the similar principles to the use of human power. Seeing strangers and passers-by, one always feels they are quite common and never see them better than any others, but the deeper he/she makes friends with them, the more competence he/she may find in them, and the more he/she may benefit from them to accomplish a lot of tasks. So it is the real ace in the hole to use the common medicines to a-chieve the desired effects.

It is quite sure that reasonable combination of medicines is very important likethe compilibility with the medicines for nourishing liver and Yin, reducing phlegm or removing blood stasis.

Mulberry Leaf Restrains Sweating

Mulberry leaf has another effect of restraining sweating.

Yijian Zhi (a note-style classical novels collection, featured with ghost stories, weird and supernatural things written by Hong Mai in Song dynasty) described such a story that a travelling Buddhist Monk, quite thin physically and with poor appetite, suffered from night sweating every day, and always became wet all over himself, even his sleepwear and quilt. For over twenty years, he tried every possible means and prescription, but failed. Finally, he gave up further treatment and waited for death to come. Later on, he came to Tangshan Temple in Yanzhou, Zhejiang province, where a monk told him a very effective formula, that is, to dry up some mulberry leaf and grind into powder, and then wash down two *qian* of the powder (*"qian"* is a Chinese unit of weight in the ancient time) with cooked rice soup at the moment of empty stomach. At that time, it was just in between the seasons of autumn and winter, the right moment of collecting mulberry leaf. Three days later after he took the powder of mulbrry leaf, his chronical disease of night sweating was surprisingly cured.

I fully believe this story. The reason why the treatment of his night sweating was not effective and the illness was not cured in the previous twenty years was that his illness had penetrated into meridians. Generally, the disease at its early stage just stays in the main channels, and as time goes on, the chronic diseases will penetrate into meridians. That can be compared to the invasion of enemies. At the very beginning when the enemies start to invade, they may walk on the highroad and concentrate on certain spots. If the victims of aggression stand to defend against them, it would be much easier. But if the enemies carry on their aggression for long, they may then run all over into each and every village. By that stage, it would not be easy to defend against them since they scatter around and may become concealed. The collaterals inside the human body are equivalent to the blood capillaries. When the pathogenic factors (or pathogens) get into capillaries, it would be difficult to drive them out. When the above-mentioned Buddhist monk travelled around for begging for alms or kobo activities, he might not have continued to get his illness properly treated. Later, when mulberry leaf was used to penetrate into collaterals and drive out pathogenic wind, sweating was then restrained naturally.

Mulberry leaf is essentially a sudorific herb in that herbal leaves always induce perspiration through the exterior, but here mulberry leaf functions to restrain sweating. To induce perspiration is nothing but to drive out the pathogenic factors. Therefore, when the leaf drives all the pathogens out of the collaterals, sweating will not take place any more.

Mulberry Leaves Tonify Life Essence

Newly Compiled Chinese Materia Medica, an excellent book written by Chen Shiduo, a medical expert in Qing dynasty, introduces that mulberry leaf has the medical effects of "tonifying life essence and filling up bone marrow", which means mulberry leaf can nourish Yin.

In the past, I always thought this is its second effect, of which the precondition is to dispel wind because when the wind-pathogen inside human body is too vigorous, the pith or marrow could not be filled up even it wants to since the pathogenic wind always causes impairment of Yin. The wet clothes, hanging outdoor, will dry up very quickly when the wind starts to blow, which shows that wind can win over wetness and dry up dampness. The primodial Yin in human body refers to fluid in fact. When the pathogenic wind inside becomes comparatively much stronger, Yin will be easily dried up, and the life essence and blood will get lost easily. When the wind is driven out, the life essence and blood will naturally restore to a good condition, as such, the bone marrow will definitely be filled up under the help of the inborn self-cure function of human body.

But later on, my idea in this respect has some changes. In an early winter, after the severe frost, a few pieces of leaves were still hanging on mulberry trees in my living blocks. I reached out to pick a leaf and chewed it in mouth. I felt pleasantly sweet and sticky. That tells me that mulberry leaf can also nourish Yin. From that experience, I am sure that mulberry leaf can directly supplement life essence and blood and fill up the bone marrow in addition to the effect of its dispelling wind, but it must be the winter mulberry leaf. Many things will become sweet after expericing frost, so does mulberry leaf. The winer mulberry leaf can nourish Yin and dispel wind, which tells us the importance of right time for collecting herbs in TCM.

"Nothing can be comprehended profoundly unless it is done in practice." Nothing can be described in all aspects with great details in books, either. Therefore, one must find chances to the greatest extent to carry out practices personally with "the courage of Shennong tasting hundreds of herbs", try to approach each and every herb for observation and learning through his own personal experience, and finally may find many unexpected gain.

Sangju Yin

Mulberry leaf enters into the liver, gallbladder and lung meridians.

The meridian tropism of a medical herb may be memorized through imagination or comprehension: mulberry leaf, green in color and collecting vital life essence from the Jī star, is sure to enter the liver meridian. At the same time, it can also purge the gallbladder fire, and enter into the gallbladder meridian, too. It is pungent in taste and cool in property. It can relieve the exterior syndromes, and enter into the lung meridian. Again, because of its fine and close leaf veins, it can enter both the liver and lung meridians.

Mulberry leaf is often used for curinga cold due to exogenous pathogenic factors. For that symtom, there is a typical formula called **Sangju Yin** (Mulberry leaf and chrysanthemum decoction).

The formula of **Sangju Yin** contains Sangye (mulberry leaf) 2. 5 *qian*, Juhua (chrysanthemum) 1 *qian*, Xingren (apricot kernel) 2 *qian*, Lianqiao (fructus forsythia) 1.5 *qian*, Bohe (mint) 8 *fen*, Jiegeng (platycodon grandiflorum) 2 *qian*, Lugen (rhizoma phragmitis) 8 *fen*, Gancao (liquorice) 8 *fen*.

The dosage of all the herbs mentioned in the above formula refers to the dosage recorded in the ancient books. For the dosage to be used today, some changes may be necessary. For example, Lugen 8 *fen* is too small in quantity, and it is now used with a dosage around 1 *liang*. So I hereby give a regular dosage for reference: Sangye (mulberry leaf) 3 *qian*, Juhua (chrysanthemum) 4 *qian*, Xingren (apricot kernel) 3 *qian*, Lianqiao (fructus forsythia) 3 *qian*, Bohe (mint) 1 *qian*, Jiegeng (platycodon grandiflorum) 3 *qian*, Lugen (rhizoma phragmitis) 1 *liang*, Gancao (liquorice) 2 *qian*. The dosage of the herbs usually changes according to the herbal quality fluctuation, the changing decocting method or the dosage form since the ancient time.

When shall **Sangju Yin** be used? In accordance with ***Wenbing Tiaobian*** (***Treatise on Differentiation and Treatment of Epidemic Febrile Diseases***) written by Wu Tang in Qing dynasty: "The patient who suffers from the wind-warm syndromes arising in the foot-taiyang bladder meridian, slight coughing, without too much fever, can just use the pungent-cool **Sangju Yin**", which tells that just a little fever and slight coughing indicates a slight cold. The symptom of coughing mentioned here refers to that caused by heat impairment of the lung meridian. But why just a little pathogenic influence can cause fever? The book of ***Shanghan Lun (Treatise on Cold Pathogenic Diseases)*** recorded few such cases, but by the time of Qing dynasty, many such cases were recorded in ***Wenbing Tiaobian***. This shows that such a symptom of coughing is related to the physiques and habitus of different people. By the time of Qing dynasty, people were much easier to get excessive endogenic heat. ***Shanghan Lun*** aims at the cold-pathogens, so many diseases can be cured with the concepts reflected in this book. But the formulas in ***Shanghan Lun*** target at the people living in Han dynasty. That is to say the people in Han dynasty could normally bear the herbs of Mahuang (ephedra) and Guizhi (cassia twig), but by the time of Qing dynasty, people could not bear such herbs too much. TCM is developing with the change of time. Although the doctrine or principles are not changed, yet the methods, formulas and herbs all keep on developing ceaselessly.

Mulberry and Chrysanthemum as Monarch Medicines

Easily occurring endogenic heat is always closely related to the liver and gallbladder. If the liver-heat occurs frequently, the wood-fire (the liver fire) will impair the metal (the lung), i. e. the liver-fire attacking lungs. That is why the liver-heat will impair the lung meridians, which echoes the exogenous pathogens and causes symptoms of coughing and fever. And so, the mulberry leaf and chrysanthemum are used to relieve gallbladder-fire and clear the liver and gall-bladder.

Still, people in the modern time frequently use **Sangju Yin**. For the dizziness in the head at the time of a cold, **Sangju Yin** can work well to clear the head and eyesight. By the way, it also can dispel wind and clear heat. Especially, the mulberry leaf is particularly good for dispelling wind, and chrysanthemum is good for clearing heat. So, when they are used together, they may bring out the best in each other.

In this formula, chrysanthemum is used instead of peach flower because chrysanthemum blossoms in autumn, obtaining the "metal" (corresponding the autumn) Qi. The "metal" governs the cool and refreshing, and sternness, and it also restricts "wood". Peach flower blossoms in spring with ascending and rising Qi; and it is red in color, and able to enter the blood system. The pathogenic factors mainly lie in Qi system, so herbs for blood system cannot be used, otherwise, it may guide the pathogens to go deeper into the Qi system.

Mint: Pungent-cool to Relieve the Exterior Syndromes

Sangju Yin contains another herb of Bohe (mint), which is a very important herb, pungent in taste and cool in property for relieving the exterior syndromes. However, it was not mentioned in **Shennong Bencao Jing** (**Shen Nong's Herbal Classic**), and it is discovered by the medical experts in the later generations. mulberry leaf and chrysanthemum are pungent in taste and cool in property for relieving the exterior syndromes, but they are not strong enough, so Bohe is added to reinforce the effect. The pungent and fragrant taste of Bohe is quite distinct and clear, and it is strong enough for relieving the exterior symptoms. As a matter of fact, this herb is only used by the later generations for inducing perspiration. However, in the case of heat presence, the warm and pungent herbs cannot be used for inducing perspiration. At the time of Zhang Zhongjing, the pungent and warm Mahuang and Guizhi could be used for inducing perspiration. But now, people in the modern time have much stronger liver-fire, and suffer from fire frequently, so the pungent and cool herbs are preferred instead of the pungent and warm herbs. Pungent herbs can relieve the exterior and induce perspiration, and cool herbs can clear heat, as such, Bohe is the best choice here.

The patient who suffers from the cold-pathogen may use the pungent and warm herbs for relieving the exterior symptoms, but due to the excessive sudorific effect, Mahuang and Guizhi are not suitable. In that case, Suye (perilla leaf) may be used instead since Suye can enter into both Qi and blood systems. Hence, learning Chinese medicines, the learners should never be constrained by *Shennong Bencao Jing* only, but keep open-minded.

Lianqiao (Fructus Forsythiae): Bitter-cold to Clear the Endogenic Heat

Lianqiao goes through the Middle Jiao, and it can clear stomach heat and eliminate heart-fire as well. "The pathogenic heat always affects the lung first, and then the pericardium", therefore, Lianqiao can be used to prevent the pathogenic factors from transmitting to pericardium.

It may be asked why Huanglian is not used now that it also has the function of clearing stomach heat and eliminating heart-fire. As for this point, there are two reasons.

First and foremost is that Huanglian can defend but not move since it is a little lazy and moves comparatively slow. However, when getting a cold, the patients always need quick effect of treatment since pathogenic factors must be driven out of the body. The pathogenic factors on the body surface may be driven away by way of inducing perspiration with Bohe. While the pathogenic factors inside the body should be induced down the large intestine with Xingren. Huanglian is effective, but it works too slow.

Second, doctors often in prescriptions write "Lianqiao Yi" (fructus forsythia coat), i. e. the hull of lianqiao since the hull always goes on the surface, and Lianqiao with permeability has the effects of opening orifices with its fragrance. While Huanglian, as a root herb, does not go on the surface. Also, it has neither fragrance nor permeability.

All the herbs used in **Sangju Yin** are quite permeable, and they will neither stay at certain points without moving, nor induce the pathogenic factors into deeper points. In the well-known formulas passed down from the ancients, each herb used is worth researching carefully.

Xingren (Apricot Kernel) and Jiegeng (Platycodon Grandiflorum): Ascending and Descending

A good formula for treatment of influenza not only has to take account of the exterior and interior, but also gives consideration to ascending and descending. **Sangju Yin** contains Xingren and Jiegeng for ascending and descending purposes respectively in order to reguate Qi function of the lung, even of the whole system of human body.

Xingren is an herb for soothing the lungs, but it also goes to the large intestine and clear the hollow viscera and discharge heat. As a matter of fact, all nuts contain oils and fats that can lubricate the intestines and relax bowels. Xingren can soothe the lungs to lower the lung Qi and lubricate the large intestine with the oil and fat contained, so it is very effective for clearing the hollow viscera and discharging heat. The lung and large intestine are interior-exteriorly related, so the lung heat may be excreted with faeces through the large intestine. By the way, Taoren and Xingren look almost the same, but they are different in fact since Xingren goes into Qi system, while Taoren goes into blood system. In spring, it can be seen the apricot blossom and the peach blossom. The former is white with slightly reddish color, while the latter is red in color, so Taoren goes into the blood system. Hence, Taoren and Xingren should not be misused, otherwise, the pathogenic factors could be induced into deeper points.

Jiegeng is an herb for "Kai Ti" of the lung Qi ("Kai" here means "open"; "Ti" here means "uplift", so "Platycodon grandiflorum is an herb for opening and uplifting the lung Qi).

When in opening, it will become permeable. So opening the lung Qi means the hair pores will open, and then the medicines like Bohe for inducing perspiration can be more effective.

When a medicine has the effect for lifting up, it will not fall down. When getting a cold, a patient may have been suffering from a lot of pathogenic factors that must be guarded against their falling down. Otherwise, if the pathoges fall down to the intestines and stomach in the Middle Jiao, it will cause diarrhea; if falling down into the kidneys, it will cause nephritis and the like. The acute nephritis is cured in many cases with modified **Sangju Yin**, which is usually effective.

Lugen (Rhizoma Phragmitis) and Gancao (Liquorice): Nourishing the Middle Jiao

Considering the pathogenic factors may be transformed into heat very fast, causing impairment to body fluid, which, if impaired, must be made up, so Lugen is added. Lugen is the root of reed growing in water, and it is quite moistening, nourishing and permeable in properties. As a medicine, it can generate body fluid. The body fluid generated by Lugen will not be inclined to change into phlegm. Meanwhile, Lugen can also clear the unnecessary dampness and make up the necessary fluid.

As is known, learning requires thinking. If a learner frequently asks questions himself and tries to find answers as well, he will make progress gradually. Lugen has the effect of generating body fluid, so does Tianhua Fen (radices trichosanthis). But why is Lugen used here instead of Tianhua Fen? Tianhua Fen is the root of Gualou (trichosanthes kirilowii maxim), and its permeability is not as good as that of Lugen. When a prescription is written for influenza, permeability of herbs is very important and should be attended all the time, which can ensure the pathogenic influences to be eliminated timely.

Furthermore, Gancao added in the formula on the one hand can reconcile all the other herbs, and on the other hand harmonize the stomach Qi. Generally speaking, for the purpose of reconciling different herbs, 3 to 5g Gancao is used. But if for more additional purposes like relieving endogenous heat or fever, 10g or even 20g Gancao may be used.

Both Lugen and Gancao enter into the Middle Jiao with the effects of consolidating and protecting the stomach Qi and generating body fluids. Moreover, "protecting the stomach Qi" and "storing body fluids" are the more important principles according to **Shanghan Lun**.

Evaluating Medicinesls like Evaluating Persons

When talking about a prescription, one must concentrate on each and every herb in it. At the same time, he also has to compare each herb with the other herbs over and again, and then he can understand the properties of all herbs profoundly.

Just like doing something, one must start with comparing different people and then discovering the capable persons and put them at suitable posts. In the same way, one must discover the properties of herbs and put them in the right formulas. To know an herb is like knowing of a person. For instance, one is going to get to know a man named Tom today, so he must print out his curriculum vitae and hand it out to the concerning people and let everyone of them get a primary impression. As to the moral quality and working style of Tom, his curriculum vitae may not reflect all information. For knowing one person, it is so complicated. Suppose one receives the curriculum vitaes from 356 persons, he may then become blurred up.

So, in order to know a person well, it would be much better to meet him repeatedly and observe him about his response at different occasions and compare him with the other people simultaneously. Only in such a way can that person be known. Such a way is also the right way to learn about medical herbs.

Therefore, it is necessary to introduce different herbs for discussing formulas. The first time when one reads my introduction about Bohe or Xingren, he may feel a little more unfamiliar, but later on, the same herbs will be frequently mentioned in many other formulas. Much frequence of reading these two herbs, even bored with reading about them, will help the readers get familiar with them.

Three Pungent-Cool Medicaments

Sangju Yin is named as "pungent-cool light medicament" in the book of **Wenbing Tiaobian**. Now that there is a light medicament, there must be a heavy medicament too, and a mild medicament as well in between. That is to say, there are three pungent-cool medicaments, or even four: The pungent-cool light medicament refers to **Sangju Yin**; The pungent-cool mild medicament refers to **Yin Qiao San**; The pungent-cool heavy medicament refers to **Maxing Shigan Tang** and one more is **Baihu Tang**. The last two Formulas are from the book of **Shanghan Lun**, and the other two are from the book of **Wenbing Tiaobian**.

Some learners often ignore the knowledge regarding epidemic febrile diseases, which is not the right and proper learning attitude. One should learn all the useful and helpful things. Even the featherwit is not always free from gain, and much less, Wu Jutong, the writer of the book of **Wenbing Tiaobian**, was not a featherwit in any aspect. So, all those who want to learn TCM well must have a broad mind and take down all the strengths of different medical schools.

Yinqiao San

The pungent-cool mild medicament of **Yinqiao San** (or Yinqiao powder) contains the herbal ingredients:

Jinyinhua (Honeysuckle flower) 1 *liang*, Lianqiao (fructus forsythia) 1 *liang*, Bohe (mint) 6 *qian*, Jingjiesui (schizonepeta spike) 4 *qian*, Douchi (fermented soya beans) 5 *qian*, Zhuye (bamboo leaf) 4 *qian*, Niu Bangzi (fructus arctii) 6 *qian*, Jiegeng (platycodon grandiflorum) 6 *qian*, and Lugen (rhizoma phragmitis) decocted for drinks.

Powder and Decoction

San(means powder) refers that the herbs should be ground into powder, which has the meanings of divergency and dispersion. For instance, **Yinqiao San** is to disperse the pathogenic factors, **Xiaoyao San** is to disperse the pent-up symptoms. "Tang" (means decoction) is to boil herbs into decoction for drinking, which is relatively more common form in use. "Tang" also means "Dàng" in Chinese, which means to wash away, and it can wash away all the pathogenic factors swiftly.

The book of **Wenbing Tiaobian** prescribes to process **Yinqiao San** into powder form, but in modern times, it is often made into decoction form. When there are changes of dosage forms, there will also be some changes of dose and decoction method accordingly. Generally speaking, present dosages of ingredients for **Yinqiao San** contain Jinyinhua (honeysuckle flower) 30g, Lianqiao (fructus forsythia) 10g, Bohe (mint) 6 to 10g, Jingjiesui (schizonepeta spike) 10 to 12g,

Douchi (fermented soya beans) 10g (to be discussed later on), Suye (perilla leaf) 8 to 12g, Niu Bangzi (fructus arctii) 10g, Jiegeng (platycodon grandiflorum) 10g, and Lugen (rhizoma phragmitis) 30g. Here are the common clinical dosages, which are a little different from the dosages listed in the book of **Wenbing Tiaobian**.

Jinyinhua (Honeysuckle Flower) - Lianqiao (Fructus Forsythiae)

This formula takes Jinyinhua and Lianqiao as the monarch medicines. Jinyinhua should be picked before it blossoms since it is more effective to soothe the liver, dissolve the turbid with delicate fragrance and relieve the endogenous heat or fever while it is green in color. There is no such a thing as channel tropism of Jinyinhua, but it can go through the whole body, not only to clear the heat in Qi system, but also to relieve endogenous heat of the blood system. When Jinyinhua and Lianqiao are used together, they will be more effective in relieving endogenous heat. Furthermore, Lianqiao can be classified into the green one and the yellow one. The green Lianqiao enters into the liver and tends to relieve endogenous heat, while the yellow Lianqiao in most cases enters the Middle Jiao and tends to clear heat. So choices can be made according to the specific clinical cases.

As previously discussed, people in modern times often suffer from more serious liver stagnation and gallbladder fire. Once encountering the exogenous pathogens, they will suffer from the collaboration from endogenous heat with the exogenous pathogens, which will then cause quick heat transformation, so mulberry leaf and Juhua are contained in **Juhua Yin**, on the one hand for pungent-cool dispersion of the pathogenic factors, and on the other hand for relieving the liver and gallbladder heat. **Yinqiao San** still follows this concept, that is, the liver is to detoxicate, but if the liver heat is not fully dispersed, the liver will not be able to detoxicate completely. The toxic factors will continue to accumulate inside the body and cause long liver stagnation, which will then lead to heat transformation. As such, the heat may be stagnated over and again and transformed into toxic factors. The liver is essentially able to relieve the endogenous heat, but now due to its limited power, it becomes unable to relieve the toxic factors, so Jinyinhua and

Lianqiao have to be used to help the liver for detoxication.

In fact, Jinyinhua and Lianqiao not only relieve the toxic factors related to a cold, but also relieve the toxic factors or influences related to skin diseases and the miscellaneous diseases involving the internal medicine department. Now it is often heard about the viral cold (influenza), which, though, is a name given in the western medicine, TCM approves it regarding virus, but the toxic influences and factors referred in TCM involve a more extensive scope.

Medicines inYinqiao San for Relieving Exterior Syndromes

Though Jinyinhua and Lianqiao can also go to the body surface, yet they are not powerful enough, so Bohe must be added in order to relieve the exterior syndromes with some pungent cool medicines in order to disperse the exterior pathogens.

In addition, Jingjiesui (schizonepeta spike) is added. Jingjie (schizonepeta) is pungent in taste and warm in property, but in most books of Chinese materia medica, it is classified into the group of pungent-cool medicines for relieving the exterior syndromes. In essence, it is slightly warm. But because of its properties of pungency and dispersion, in the process of dispersion of toxic factors, the properties of slight warmth cannot be felt any more; and on the contrary, it can give the patients a cool feeling. Hence, it is taken as a medicine that is warm in property and cool in effect. Jingjiesui is just the tassel of Jingjie with a very powerful effect of dispersion. The tassel of Jingjie smells aromatic and very comfortable at the first smelling, but long smelling can make people feel dizzy and giddy.

Douzhi contained in **Yinqiao San** is actually processed from the soya beans soaked in Suye soaked water and then fermented. The fermentation itself is a process of ascending and effusion, in which the hardened things can become loose and permeable. So the fermenting property of Douzhi is able to loosen the hardened stale odour inside human body and disperse the pathogenic factors in the Upper Jiao. Having soaked in the Suye soaked water, Douzhi will have another effect of inducing perspiration. Surely, Suye soaked water plays a very important role therein. Presently, Douzhi in most cases is not processed in such a traditional way, so Suye may be used straightforward instead.

Generally, the dosage of Suye is 6 to 10g, which is of pungent-warm herb for relieving the exterior syndromes. By the way, so many pungent-cool medicines have been used already, why is a pungent-warm herb used hereby? Actually, the cold is often included in the warm-pathogen, and sometimes, the human body it-self also suffers from the cold. Therefore, Suye is added to disperse the cold patho-gens. But even if without the cold, Suye used with the pungent-cool medicines is nothing too much since the pathogenic factors in any case will be diverged to the outside. Under such a condition, a little warm herb is helpful for dispersion.

In the *Compendium of Materia Medica*, it is recorded that Suye, pungent and warm in properties, can enter the liver, lungs and stomach meridians; it can induce perspiration, disperse the cold, promote the circulation of Qi, and harmo-nize the blood. It not only enters the system of Qi but also the system of blood.

From the profile of Suye, its upper side is green while the back side is red. The geen color goes to the system of Qi and the red color signifies that it can go to the system of blood. So it is a medicine for treatment of the diseases lying in be-tween the system of Qi and the system of blood. While Mahuang enters the system of Qi, it is light in property and dark green in color, so it cannot enter the system of blood. Mahuang is used with Guizhi since Guizhi is red in color going to the system of blood and the system of Ying (nutrient Qi that lies in between the sys-tem of Qi and the system of blood). With the help of Guizhi, Mahuang can then concurrently enter the system of Qi and the system of blood, the role of which can be played by Suye concurrently in this aspect. So, to some extent, Suye is equiv-alent to Mahuang plus Guizhi but simply its effect is much weaker than Mahuang plus Guizhi. Meanwhile, Suye can enter the Middle Jiao to get rid of the stale and bring forth the fresh. By the way, Suye goes on the body surface and Sugeng (caulis perllae) can get through up and down and regulate the flow of vital energy and remove obstruction. So Zisu (purple perilla) can play the same role as Douzhi for getting rid of the stale and bringing forth the fresh.

Medicines Contained in Yinqiao San for Clearing Endogenous Heat

Some of the heat pathogens will be dispersed from the exterior, but some other heat pathogens will be diverged from the interior, that is, discharged with faeces and urine, for which Zhuye and Niubangzi are used here.

Zhuye has the effect of clearing the heart fire, going to the small intestine, inducing urination and discharging heat with urination. Lianqiao contained in **Sangju Yin** can clear both the fire in the Middle Jiao and heart in order to guard against pathogenic Qi reversing to pericardium, while **Yinqiao San** contains Zhuye in addition to Lianqiao, enhancing the dimension for guarding against pathogens reversing to pericardium.

Niubangzi is pungent and bitter in taste and cool in property. In the formula, this herb must be noted to be crushed. It not only can dispel wind and discharge heat, but also lubricate bowel movement and clear the hollow viscera to release heat. For such a purpose, **Sangju Yin** uses Xingren, while **Yinqiao San** uses Niubangzi. Xingren has a slight effect of relieving the exterior symptoms and lubricating bowel movement. Niubangzi has some similarities to apricot kernel, but it is much stronger comparing with Xingren. So Niubangzi is used instead of Xingren. Meanwhile, Niubangzi can open and discharge the lung Qi. When used together with some other exterior sysdrome relieving medicines, Niubangzi can open the hair pores to dispel wind and discharge heat and detoxicate for dermexanthesis as well. At the same time, one must know it is a medicine with cold and cool nature. Niubangzi, as seeds of a special plant, always goes downward to relax the large intestine and lubricate bowel movement because of oil lubricity so as to discharge endogenous heat and toxic things quickly with faeces.

Besides, Niubangzi has another important effect of curing sore throat.

The throat is a very important channel, as a Chinese idiom says "throat thoroughfare", which refers to the extremely important and narrow passageway where one man can hold out against ten thousand enemy soldiers, so is the throat. Whenever there is an infringement of the lung heat due to a cold, the throat will be the first to be affected and become sore. Niubangzi can get through the lung Qi, lower and clear away the lung heat, so it is very effective for curing sore throat.

Most Common Process of Wind-Heat Type Cold

The wind-heat type cold is often accompanied by sore throat. In many cases, the patients have sore throat in the previous evening, and then the next morning, he would have some symptoms like feeling uncomfortable, dizzy and giddy, and nose stuffed-up. By this moment, they realize that they catch a coat.

The pulse is beating fast and the body temperature is basically normal or almost the same as usual. But though there is no fever in the morning, yet there will be high temperature in the afternoon definitely, and "the heat symptom of Yangming meridian is always flourishing at the time of Shenyou", i. e. in the period from 15:00 to 19:00 p. m. (In the ancient time, the people divided a whole duration of a day and night into 12 periods in total, i. e. Zi, Chou, Yin, Mao, Chen, Si, Wu, Wei, Shen, You, Xu, Hai. Each of these 12 periods equals to two hours of the modern time, so Shen refers to 15:00 to 17:00 p. m. , and You refers to 17:00 to 19:00p. m.). In the period of Shen-You, the patients will have fever most probably.

Why does the fever take place in this period? As is known, in the morning, Yang in the human body is flourishing and vigorous, and it becomes strong enough to resist the pathogens, which do not break out but is pent-up inside the body. This can be proved by the number of pulse beats. In normal case, the pulse beats around 80 times per minute. However, those who have strong endogenous fire will have 90 or even over 100 times per minute but they may have no fever. In the afternoon, Yang restrains itself inside the body and fights hand-in-hand against the interior endogenous pathogens, so the body temperature will rise quickly; or in another aspect, after Yang restrains itself, the exogenous heat pathogens will run riot unscrupulously, which can also result in fever. If no action is to be taken to control such heat, the fever will last till the midnight, that is, by the time of Zi period (23:00p. m. to 1:00 a. m.) when Yang restarts to rise, the fever will come down gradually.

The process of wind-heat type cold is now very common. In case of a sore throat in the previous evening when the patient uses **Yinqiao San**, such a cold may be wiped out in the bud. But if **Yinqiao San** is to be taken by the next day when there is a fever, Shigao (gypsum) has to be added since it can clear away the heat from the system of Qi.

Yinqiao San is pungent-cool, and it can relieve the exterior symptoms, and clear away endogenous heat or fever. If a patient do not like to decoct medical herbs, he may take **Yinqiao Jiedu Pill** (lonicerae and forsythiae pills) or **Yinqiao Jiedu Granule** (lonicerae and forsythiae granules) instead for relieving endogenous heat or fever. But when the cold and fever become very serious, the patent medicines like pills or granule appear to be less effective because of insufficient dosage or the fixed ingredients without any other necessary addition or subtraction of herbs to/from the fixed formula. In fact, it would be much better if Shigao is added in **Yinqiao San** when the fever becomes very serious. Just like a stuffy room, the easy way to cool it down is to open the window. However, if there are more ways to be adopted simultaneously, that would be more effective. That is, when opening the windows of the stuffy room, one may also put some ice blocks in the room at the same time. **Yinqiao San** used here is like opening the windows for the patient, and Shigao added is like the ice blocks, which takes both the interior and the exterior factors into consideration at the same time, and help to bring down the fever much quicker.

For the warm-heat type cold (influenza), one or two doses of modified **Yinqiao San** will work to bring down the fever, after which the patient will feel much light-footed, but he often has more phlegm and cough by that time. In that case, please do not try to relieve the cough with medicines at that stage, and just let the phlegm come out through coughing since it is in this process that human body is trying to clear the lungs and wipe out all the wastes arising from the cold by itself, after which the lung will become refreshing. Some people, after having caught a cold, would clear away a lot of phlegm through coughing, and especially those who are chain smokers would cough out, if properly treated, a lot of grey phlegm, i. e. the smoking phlegm. This is called "ailment keeping in good health" .

Of course, the patient should not be kept to cough and spit. If the coughing could not stop after a certain period of time, medicines then should be taken to tonify the spleen and clear the lungs in order to relieve cough and reduce phlegm. While doing the treatment of a common cold, the doctor cannot just give treatment to the lungs, but also give consideration to both the spleen and lungs since the spleen is the source of producing phlegm. When the spleen is tonified and strengthened, it would no longer produce so much phlegm.

In the whole process, fever, the sputum excretion and clearing would consume the body fluid, which must be made up timely by adding Lugen into **Yinqiao San**. Undoubtedly, more sweet cold and moistening medicines like Lugen, Zhuye, Maidong should be added to nourish and build up the body fluid. This is a whole process for curing a cold.

Generally, thecommon cold taking place in spring and autumn, especially the spring warm type cold, usually follows the above principle. However, for the cold in the other seasons, some differential treatments should be given depending upon the specific cases. In brief, the treatment of a common cold needs relieving the exterior syndromes, clearing endogenous heat or fever, clearing the lungs, relieving cough and reducing phlegm and nourishing Yin for inducing the body fluid. Many people ignore such a process and deal with the cold casually, which may cure the cold for the time being but will bring an endless flow of disastrous aftermath, such as allergy, chronic rhinitis, acute nephritis, and meningitis etc. .

Maxing Shigan Tang

Dosage of Maxing Shigan Tang

Maxing Shigan Tang is a kind of heavy pungent-cool dosage, containing Mahuang (ephedra) 4 *liang*, Xingren (apricot kernel) 50 Pcs, Shigao (gypsum) 0. 5 *jin* and Gancao (liquorice) 2 *liang*.

The dosage of these herbs are that recorded in the book of **Shanghan Lun** for **Maxing Shigan Tang**, which should not be copied today in any case, because of the different weights and measures adopted in the different times and the different quality of herbs, even changing physiques of people. The different era needs different formulas with different dosages that even cannot be converted proportionally, either. For instance, the book of **Wenbing Tiaobian** in Qing dynasty gives the formula as: 3 *qian* for Mahuang, Xingren and Shigao respectively, and Gancao 2 *qian*, while the textbook of **Formulas of Chinese Medicine** published in 1964 gives the dosage for the same formula as: 1 *qian* for Mahuang and Gancao respectively, Xingren 2 *qian* and Shigao 3 *qian*.

In modern times, the dosage in **Maxing Shigan Tang** is again different.

For the Chinese southerners, only 3 to 5 *fen* (1 to 2g) Mahuang will be enough, but for the northerners, especially the northwesten Chinese, more Mahuang may be used. Xingren 3 to 4 *qian* (10 to 12g), Shigao around 1 *liang* (30g) and Gancao 2 to 3 *qian* (5 to 10g) may be used respectively.

Shanghan Lun says **Maxing Shixan Tang** mainly focuses on the sweating and panting symptoms. Sweating means the exterior superface is open, and panting means the lung Qi is impassable and obstructed or stagnated. The lung Qi, if obstructed, will produce heat and then cause lung Qi upward reversal, resulting in panting. Mahuang used here is not to induce perspiration but to open the lung Qi, so it is unnecessary to use a large dosage. Regarding **Maxing Shigan Tang**, four points can be concluded as: "Mahuang opens the lung Qi; Xingren descends the adverse rising of lung Qi; Shigao clears the lung heat; and Gancao relieves the lung heat. " Therefore, this formula not only can relieve the exterior symptoms but also clear away the endogenous heat or fever. This formula is quite similar to **Yinqiao San**, of which the dosage of the four herbs should be decided primarily in line with their due effects on the specific patients rather than on the records in the books.

Mahuang (Ephedra)

To discuss **Maxing Shigan Tang**, the major target is on the herb of Mahuang. In the traditional chinese pharmacology, Mahuang always comes on the top. It grows in the northwest of China, receiving the lucid Yang and the strong Qi from the sky and earth.

I have seen the wild Mahuang: green and thin tubulous grass without much special taste or smell. Many people dare not believe that it is so strong for sweating (diaphoresis) use. In fact, it feels very light in taste, smell and weight. Three grams of such herb may give you a surprise in its size. So, light in weight means it is able to float up and go to the superficies and send up Yang-Qi as well. Mahuang can enter the Ying system [human body can be analyzed from the four levels of "Wei (defensive system), Qi, Ying (nutrient system), and Blood". "Wei" is on the skin layer of the body and it is like a defence shield, which can be taken as bodyguard. Under "Wei" is Qi, and then comes "Ying".

As to "Ying", we can compare it to "military camp" located inside the body. "Blood" is the innermost part] for inducing perspiration only when it is used together with Guizhi. For inducing perspiration purpose, Mahuang may be used individually, but it was primarily used by the ancients in this way since the ancients had very densified skin and strong lung Qi, and Mahuang is comparatively suitable for such characterized people. For the modern people, some changes about the physique have taken place, therefore, attention must be paid to the clinical use of Mahuang. Now, doctors generally use the processed Mahuang, the old Mahuang or the processed Mahuang tomentum. The processed Mahuang refers to that processed with honey; the old Mahuang refers to that having been stored on shelf for a logn time. In fact, the longer Mahuang is stored, the better it would be in property, and it would not be so fierce and would become mild but without losing its efficacy; the processed Mahuang tomentum refers to that pounded with a pestle, after which the pounded Mahuang is made into tomentum like the fibre of Airong (mugwort) with a very mild property.

Mahuang is generally used at a dosage of 1 to 2g. Based upon its characteristics of "being light in weight and able to float up", a small dosage of Mahuang will do well. Quite similarly, in **Buzhong Yiqi Tang**, only 5 to 6g of Shengma (rhizoma cimicifugae) is used. Though it is used at a small dosage, it is more powerful for upbearing the clear. The same is true for Mahuang, which can upbear the clear and relieve the exterior symptoms with a small dosage, but too much of it will consume and dissipate the promordial Qi (archaeus), for which Renshen may have to be used for remediation. Renshen can be used for remedying the malpractice due to excessive use of Mahuang since Renshen can "restore the promordial Qi from nowhere", retrieve the consumed and dissipated promordial Qi, and promote the secretion of saliva or body fluid at the same time.

A few years ago, I met a TCM doctor from the northwest of China, who told me that his home land grows Mahuang. The local people, whenever catching a cold, go to pick some Mahuang straightforward, more or less, and after drinking the decocted water of Mahuang, they would recover. I asked him whether the decoction would induce perspiration or not. He told me there would be no perspiration after drinking generally but anyway the cold was cured. He said that was a very strange phenomenon. As a matter of fact, it is not strange at all. The reason why Mahuang can induce perspiration is that it can open the lung orifice. People in the northwest of China usually have fine and densified skin similar to that of the people at the time of Zhang Zhongjing, therefore, after drinking Mahuang decocted water, they would not have perspiration, but in fact their lung orifice is indeed opened and Qi function would also be in work. As such, the exogenous pathogens would pass through and be dispersed naturally. In spite of no perspiration, the hair pores are open indeed, which are invisible.

Compatibility of Mahuang and Shigao (Gypsum)

Chen Shiduo, a famous Chinese doctor in Ming dynasy, once said Mahuang essentially is a cool medicine; And however, when used together with Guizhi, it would become a warm medicine. Chen Shiduo, having given such a comment, mainly stressed the significance of Mahuang – Guizhi combination, which is helpful for understanding the concept implied in **Maxing Shigan Tang**.

Guizhi, as a pungent-warm medicine, if used together with Mahuang, can induce perspiration. While Shigao, as a pungent-cool medicine, if used together with Mahuang, will become pungent-cool. Some people claim that Shigao is a severe cold medicine, but in fact, it is not that horrible. The book of **Shanghan Lun** records that Mahuang 4 *liang* and Shigao 0.5 *jin* were used, which doubles the dosage of Mahuang (in the ancient time, 0.5 *jin* equals to 8 *liang* according to the ancient unit of weight in China). Later on, this dosage ratio has been changed, but the dosage of Shigao is never smaller than that of Mahuang. In such a case, Mahuang will almost lose its warm property. So, when Mahuang is used together with Shigao, it may induce less perspiration than it is used individually.

People in the northwest of China may not have perspiration after taking Mahuang, while the southerners on the contrary may perspire with sweat streaming down their backs since the southerners have less densified grain of skin and the texture of the subcutaneous flesh comparing with the people in the northwest of China. The book of **Shanghan Lun** indeed has profound implication concerning the dosage of each and every herb in formulas. Mahuang is still used under the condition of sweating in that Shigao is used as a corrigent medicine in the formula, and the dosage of Shigao doubles that of Mahuang, which guarantees the medicines to reach the maximum effects from the perspective of compatibility. So, in reading the medical classic, the most critical point is to work out the principles implied rather than copy the fromulas since the person who wrote that formula is gone and the era has greatly changed for the recorded fromulas, too. It is true that time is changing, but the principles followed in TCM remains the same and runs through all the time, under which the specific formulas and methods always keep on changing.

TCM keeping pace with the times, that means the formulas and medical skills must change and be improved with the time and people. Formulas and specific treatment are necessary to be renovated in allusion to the physique of the modern people, but simply all the renovation should be concentrated upon the methods and techniques rather than on the principles, which in fact are impossible to be renovated since the medical principle of TCM has already been in a state of harmony, and what it needs now is to aim at absolute perfection.

Sequence of Apricot Kernel in Decocting

The function of Xingren is to lower the lung Qi. *Huangdi Neijing* says, "the lungs dislike Qi upward reversal. " Xingren has the effect of slightly opening the exterior, and it can clear the lung, moisten and lubricate the large intestine. The two effects of moistening the large intestine and lowering the lung Qi can bring out the best in each other.

Inthe formula of **Maxing Shigan Tang**, Mahuang plays the function of opening the exterior. Although Xingren has an effect of slightly opening the exterior, in this formula, it is not for the purpose of opening the exterior. Therefore, it can be decocted with all the other herbs simultaneously.

Now, many drugstores in Beijing require that Xingren be put in for decoction later, which is not advisable. But only when Xingren is used for the purpose of relieving the exterior syndromes and inducing perspiration, it needs putting in later. Otherwise, it is not advisable or necessary when it is used for the purpose of moistening the large intestine.

As for **Maxing Shigan Tang**, there is requirement for the sequence of putting in herbs, i. e. decoct Mahuang in advance for 20 to 30 minutes and remove the white froth or foam. Shigao should be decocted 15 minutes in advance prior to decocting the remaining herbs.

As for the formula of **Yinqiao San** mentioned previously, the decoction also needs particular attention. When a doctor writes a prescription, he usually puts a remark beside, like Suye to be put in later for decocting 5 minutes only, Niuban-gzi to be crushed, Bohe to be put in later for decocting 2 minutes only, i. e. put Bohe in 2 minutes before the first decoction is over, because the fragrance of mint can be easily dispersed and it should not be decocted for over 2 minutes. Two-mi-nute decocting can assure the fragrance of herbs staying in the decoction and the pungent-cool herbal property remaining in it as well.

Xiangru Yin

The cold in summer in most cases is not due to suffering from heat but from cold because most people in summer like cold food and cool wind. Those who stay in the cold place for a long time, may easily catch a cold with the hair pores being closed up. Summer essentially causes sweating. But those who catch a cold will not sweat at all and have no appetite either, even feel dizzy and giddy all o-ver, which are the general syndromes of summer cold. Sometimes there is a fe-ver, but sometimes there is not. So, in that case, **Xiangru Yin** may be helpful and useful.

Xiangru Yin contains three herbs: Xiangru (elsholtzia ciliate), Houpo (mangnolia officinalis) and Bai Biandou (white lentils) .

Xiangru (Elsholtzia Ciliate)

Xiangru, pungent-warm in property, can open the exterior. When the hair pores are closed up, they have to be opened by the way of relieving the exterior syndroms and inducing perspiration.

Mahuang is not used here for such a case since summer is a season when people will be sweating and Yang will go to the exterior surface. If Mahuang is used in this season, it will cause sweat streaming down and even result in Yang depletion. So, Xiangru is used instead of Mahuang. Xiangru used in summer is equivalent to Mahuang used in winter with equal effect of inducing perspiration for different seasons respectively.

Xiangru, having white flower, smells fragrant and goes to the system of Qi. As is known, the white flower usually goes to the system of Qi and the red flower usually goes to the system of blood. It can play both ascending and descending roles, and it always functions to ascend to relieve the exterior symptoms and induce perspiration first, and then functions to descent to lower Qi and remove dampness. Hence, it is extremely good for use in the hot summer.

There are many pungent-warm herbs like Mahuang, Guizhi, Cong (scallion), Huoxiang (ageratum), Suye etc. , but Xiangru is used here instead of Suye since Suye does not have the effect of removing dampness and lowering Qi comparing with Xiangru. In hot summer days, once the hair pores are closed up, sweat cannot penetrate out and the Middle Jiao of the spleen and stomach will hold dampness easily. In that case, Xiangru will be the best choice to relieve the exterior symptoms and induce perspiration on the one hand, and lower Qi and eliminate dampness on the other hand.

Analyses of Xiangru Yin Formula

Xiangru, pungent and warm in properties, mainly functions to open the exterior, though it can lower Qi and remove dampness. Therefore, some other herbs are added to help Xiangru to further lower Qi and eliminate dampness.

Houpo goes to the spleen and stomach in the Middle Jiao to soothe the stomach and eliminate dampness and purge the large intestine as well. In summer, the spleen and stomach often suffer from dampness, so Houpo is used here for further eliminating dampness through the large intestine.

Bai Biandou is tasteless, and it can excrete dampness, so Biandou is used instead of Gancao to harmonize the spleen and stomach.

In brief, **Xiangru Yin** can relieve the exterior symptoms and regulate the spleen and stomach in the Middle Jiao. In summer, many people suffer from poor appetite because of the dampness trapping the spleen and stomach, which can be treated with **Xiangru Yin**.

Xin Jia Xiangru Yin

Wu Jutong, a well-knownChinese medical expert on febrile diseases in Qing dynasty, developed **Xiangru Yin** into **Xin Jia Xiangru Yin** (newly developed Xiangru decoction) that contains the ingredient herbs of Jinyinhua (honeysuckle flower), Lianqiao (fructus forsythiae), Xiangru (elsholtzia ciliate), Houpo (mangnolia officinalis), Xian Biandouhua (fresh lentils flower).

He added two more herbs ofJinyinhua and Lianqiao based on the formula of **Xiangru Yin**. When the pathogenic Qi is enclosed or trapped inside the body, it will cause stagnation that will be transformed into heat. If the pathogenic heat is not timely dispersed, it will then be transformed into heat toxin. Jinyinhua and Lianqiao have the effects of clearing heat and removing toxicity. Meanwhile, in **Xin Jia Xiangru Yin**, Bai Biandou is substituted by the fresh lentils flower that not only can harmonize the spleen and stomach, but also play the function of dispersion. But sometimes the fresh lentils flower is not so easy to find that Bai Biandou may still be used instead. In fact, they have the similar effects.

For treatment of a common cold in summer with the symptoms of fever and poor appetite but without sweating, **Xin Jia Xiangru Yin** can be more effective.

Huoxiang Zhengqi San

In case of failure of **Xiangru Yin** in curing a cold in summer, there is another typical formula for curing summer heat symptom, that is, **Huoxiang Zhengqi San** (ageratum Zhengqi powder). It is also commonly used medicine in summer, which now has been processed into a patent medicine, containing the ingredient herbs of Huoxiang (ageratum), Zisu (purple perilla), Baizhi (radix angelicae), Fuling (poria cocos), Banxia (pinellia ternate), Baizhu (white atractylodes rhizome), Jiang Houpo (gingered magnolia officinalis), Ku Jiegeng (bitter platycodon grandiflorum), Dafupi (pericarpium arecae), Chenpi (pericarpium citri reticulatae), Gancao (liquorice).

Huoxiang (Ageratum)

Huoxiang, pungent, warm, aromatic and hydrophilous in properties, is generally growing in the wet land. In most cases, the hydrophilous plants can eliminate dampness. Huoxiang not only relieves the exterior symptoms but also reconciles the Middle Jiao, eliminates dampness and enters the spleen and stomach, which are different in properties from those of the other pungent-warm medicines for relieving the exterior symptoms.

Huoxiangis also different from Xiangru whose aromat can consume Qi more easily though Xiangru can eliminate dampness, yet it is too much powerful for inducinig perspiration. The summer-heat pathogen can impair Qi, and people are always sweating in summer. Therefore, Xiangru should be used with much care in summer. By contrast, Huoxiang is much milder in preoperty.

Huoxiang in prescriptions is often written as Guang Huoxiang, which refers to the Huoxiang produced in Guangdong and Guangxi provinces of China, especially that produced in Guangdong province. Besides, Zhejiang province also produces Huoxiang called Zhe Huoxiang. Guang Huoxiang has more powerful effect for going inside and into the Middle Jiao, while Zhe Huoxiang is inclined to go on the exterior. By the way, the peduncle of Guang Huoxiang is square-shaped, and that of the ageratum produced in other areas is round-shaped. Therefore, they can be distinguished quite easily. In practice, Huoxiang, when used, has to be considered from the perspective of the leaf and peduncle respectively. Its leaf is partial to disperse the pathogen, while its peduncle is inclined to protect the stomach and regulate the circulation of Qi, but sometimes they are used together.

Analyses of Huoxiang Zhengqi San Fromula

Huoxiang, pungent and warm in properties, can relieve the exterior symptoms and reconcile the spleen and stomach in the Middle Jiao. Zisu (purple perilla) includes Suye (perilla leaf) and Sugeng (caulis perllae). Suye is primarily used to disperse the exterior while Sugeng is primarily used to regulate the circulation of Qi, so Zisu not only disperses the exterior but also regulates flow of Qi. Baizhi (radix angelicae), pungent and warm in property, goes to Yangming meridians. So when these three herbs are used together, they can open the exterior.

Besides, Jiegeng is added to open and uplift the lung Qi. "Open" means to open the pores for discharging the pathogenic Qi; "uplift" means to let the lung Qi rise up, which is much better for discharging the pathogenic Qi out of human body.

Houpo, Dafupi, Banxia, Fuling, Chenpi, and Gancao are all medicines to go to the Middle Jiao. The cold in summer is always related to both the exterior and the interior. The interior is mainly reflected in the spleen and stomach. In summer, Yang going to the exterior, the Middle Jiao is in deficiency-cold that can easily contain dampness, resulting in people suffering from poor appetite and weakness all over. Hence, the medicines for the Middle Jiao are to be used for removing dampness in the Middle Jiao.

Huoxiang Zhengqi San is quite similar to **Xiangru Yin** in the ingredients. **Xiangru Yin** uses Xiangru, while **Huoxiang Zhengqi San** uses Huoxiang, Zisu, Baizhi, and Jiegeng. The former uses Houpo and Bai Biandou, while the latter uses Houpo, Dafupi, Banxia, Fuling, Chepi, and Gancao. It can be seen that a lot of herbs have been substituted, therefore, the effects become more complicated and more comprehensive accordingly. Dafupi is actually the shell of areca nut. Just as its Chinese name implies that it can eliminate the abdominal distension. If any patient feels abnormal distension in abdomen, he or she can use Dafupi to regulate the flow of Qi and elimintate the distension. The herbs of Banxia, Fuling, Chenpi, and Gancao are the ingredients of the formula of **Erchen Tang** for reducing phlegm. Much more cold-dampness staying in the spleen and stomach too long will turn into phlegm, which can be removed with **Erchen Tang**. All in all, **Huoxiang Zhengqi San** is more comprehensive and more complicated than **Xiangru Yin** in all aspects.

Jiuwei QianghuoTang

It is relatively wet and damp in south China. Once a person in those areas catches a cold, he or she may feel pain in all joints, especially the back side of head down along the back, even further down, and also feels heavy all over. Such a cold keeps lingering for long, which always makes the patient feel rotten. In that case, **Yinqiao San** may become ineffective, but **Jiuwei Qianghuo Tang** can then be very helpful and effective.

Jiuwei Qianghuo Tang was created by Zhang Yuansu, a Chinese medical expert before the Four Great Medical Masters (Liu Wuansu, Zhang Congzheng, Li

Dongyuan, and Zhu Zhenheng in Jin-Yuan dynasty), in which his medical thought is fully reflected. Zhang Yuansu was the teacher of Li Dongyuan, and he also once gave medical treatment for Liu Wuansu, one of the above Four Great Medical Masters. Therefore, from this point, there are Five Great Medical Masters in Jin-Yuan dynasty. Zhang Yuansu was actually the greatest Medical Master before the Four Great Medical Masters in Jin-Yuan dynasty.

Jiuwei QianghuoTang contains Qianghuo (notopterygium root), Fangfeng (radix sileris), Baizhi (radix angelicae), Chuanxiong (ligusticum wallichii), Xixin (as arum), Cangzhu (rhizoma atractylodis), Huangqin (scutellaria baicalensis), Shengdi (radix rehmanniae recen), Gancao (liquorice), Shengjiang (fresh ginger), Congbai (fistular onion stalk).

When a common cold is mingled with the damp pathogens, Mahuang will not be suitable since Mahuang is too powerful for inducing perspiration. The damp pathogen is a sort of greasy and obstinate pathogenic factor, which can only be driven out and cleared away gradually but not instantly, as it is always said "more haste, less speed". If anyone wants to expel damp pathogens in a snap by instantly inducing perspiration, he may achieve nothing but impairment of body fluid only.

Qianghuo (Notopterygium Root)

Qianghuo is mainly produced in the northwest of China with a very strong and intense smell. It can open the exterior and disperse the pathogens. By the way, it is inclined to search for wind and excrete dampness, so it is very effective for curing the cold mingled with damp pathogens.

Qianghuo goes to Taiyang channel. When wind-dampness pathogens trap Taiyang channel, the patients will feel heavy all over and pain in joints. The treatment with Qianghuo is different from the way of using Mahuang and Guizhi for dispersing the cold pathogens due to cold impairment of Taiyang channel at the time of Zhang Zhongjing in East Han dynasty. The pathogenic factors in the case referred here is of wind and dampness. Therefore, Qianghuo is used to go to Taiyang channel to search for wind and excrete dampness.

In particular, for the pain in the upper limbs, Qianghuo is more effective.

In the following sections, Sangzhi (mulberry twig or ramulus mori) will be discussed, and it also goes to the upper limbs, too. Duhuo (radix angelicae pubescentis) goes to the lower limbs to Shaoyin channel for driving out the wind-cold pathogenic influence, and it is very effective for curing the pain in lower limbs.

Analyses of Jiuwei Qianghuo Tang Formula

So far, a number of pungent-warm medicines have been discussed for opening the exterior like Qianghuo, Fangfeng, Baizhi, and Xixin.

A lot more southerners in China suffer deficiency of kidneys, and the pathogenic wind can take advantage of such deficiency to enter into Shaoyin channel, so Xixin is used for inducing perspiration from Shaoyin channel.

Cangzhu is essentially used to eliminate dampness, but it can also induce perspiration through the Middle Jiao. Its peculiar effect is to restrain from sweating, or to induce perspiration. Scientifically speaking, Cangzhu has two-way regulation effects of the sweat gland, and it can regulate human body to the most comfortable state.

Congbai can also induce perspiration. It is green in color, going to Jueyin liver meridian.

Fangfeng can dispel wind and excrete dampness, but it is moister than Qianghuo in property. When it is used together with Qianghuo, it not only strengthens the dispersion intensity of Qianghuo, but also guards against its dryness intensity.

Baizhi, pungent and warm in property, is white in color with moistening effect. Its white color means it goes to Yangming meridian. As a guiding medicine, it is able to cure the Yangming-meridian headache. The cold in the south of China is often accompanied with ache at forehead and superciliary ridge and head heaviness as well. Such a cold is resulted from the wind-dampness pathogen entering into Yangming meridian. Therefore, Baizhi is used for dispelling the wind and dampness.

Chuanxiong is a lubricant in the wind. As a guiding medicine for Shaoyang meridian, it can harmonize the blood and soothe the liver. Chuanxiong has a strong and intense smell and penetrating effect as well, so it can search for the wind-cold in the blood system, eliminating stagnation and curing the headache.

All these medicines can go to the different channels and meridians: Qianghuo and Fangfeng go to Taiyang channel; Baizhi to yangming meridian; Chuanxiong to shaoyang channel; Xixin and Shengdi to Shaoyin channel; Cangzhu to foot Taiyin meridian of spleen, and Huangqin to hand Taiyin meridian of lungs. When the wind-dampness pathogen traps the body surface, there is often heat or fever inside, so Huangqin and Shengdi are used to clear the heat on the one hand and nourish Yin on the other hand.

Because of the strong and heavy wind and dampness in the south of China, this formula is often used for curing the cold. Meanwhile, it is much hotter in the south normally, Yang usually goes out of human body more than collecting Yang from outside. Moreover, in the hot and wet environment, the vital life essence inside body is always weaker, i. e. "When pathogens gather, the healthy Qi will definitely be in deficiency." When the healthy Qi is weak, the wind-dampness pathogen will take advantage of the weakness. While the base is weak and the exogenous wind-dampness is so heavy, it then needs to dispel the pathogenic factors, clear away the endogenous heat and re-nourish Yin as well.

Yupingfeng San

Reasons of Frequently Catching a Cold

Many formulas have been discussed for curing a cold, but a question will arise: is there any effective precaution against a cold?

Surely, there is, but nothing is absolute in the world. In fact, catching a cold is one of the physiological reactions against the exogenous pathogens. The defensive Qi of human body can guard against exogenous pathogens, but sometimes it can win, and sometimes it may fail. Once in failure, the pathogenic factors will begin to invade, resulting in a cold. As the Chinese saying goes, "Victory and defeat are both common in battles", so occasional failure or defeat in battles does not matter too much. But if frequent cold takes place, that is, frequent failure or defeat taking place, that will need a special attention.

Many people may have such an experience as: after a cold, there will not be any cold again for certain period of time, but after which there will be another cold. This is called "antibodies" in the western medicine. In reality, the TCM takes it in another way that the previous cold has cleared away the pathogenic factors and the fouling things out of the lungs, which means that the lungs have experienced an exercise and strengthened their ability against the pathogenic influences. From this point of view, catching a cold is not a bad thing completely.

However, this is not a good or proper case for those who frequently catch a cold. Some people always have a cold continually at intervals, and some other people catch a cold continuously for a long time without worsening or alleviating, both of which are resulted from the spleen-lung Qi deficiency and weakness of the defensive Qi. As it is known that the lungs dominate the skin and hair, so the lung deficiency will result in weak defense ability of skin against exogenous pathogens that may invade at any time they want to, and the lung itself fails to eliminate the pathogens, either. As such, some people always have a cold continually or continuously. Though a cold is a minor ailment, yet it will consume some primordial Qi to repair the impairment arising from a cold when the body mobilizes to guard against the pathogenic factors. The continual or continuous cold, if not treated and cured timely or delayed over and again, the primordial Qi of body will get further consumed and impaired, and then result in some other diseases.

The spleen-lung Qi deficiency will not only result in frequently catching a cold, but also result in some symptoms like sensation of chill and wind and more sweating etc. Besides, another disease like chronic rhinitis and allergy may also arise. Once in cold air blast, the patient will sneeze continuously. All of these are due to the malfunction of "lungs dominating skin and hair" arising from primordial Qi deficiency, causing the pathogenic factors to enter into human body easily. This case is just like a weak country without strong army at frontier will be suffering from assaults frequently.

Analyses of Yupingfeng San Formula

All the above-mentioned seems horrible, but in fact, if treated with proper medicines, the problems may be solved quite easily. Now let us see the Chinese medicine **Yupingfeng San** (or Jade Screen Powder).

Yupingfeng San, as its Chinese name implies, is like a jade screen for human body, which is specifically prepared for our human body to keep out pathogenic wind. It contains three ingredient herbs: Fangfeng (radix sileris), Huangqi (radix astragali), and Baizhu (white atractylodes rhizome).

It is always said that "grass falls with the wind", which means grasses always swing to the direction where the wind blows toward, but only Fangfeng is an exception since it always stands still in the wind. The ancient people adopted the theory of "comparative states" (the thinking of classification according to manifestation), and took Fangfeng as a medicine with very peculiar effects for guarding against various wind pathogens. It not only guards against the exogenous wind invasion, but also drives the wind pathogens out of the human body. Huangqi not only reinforces the vital energy, but also provides Fangfeng with power and impetus. Furthermore, Fangfeng, while it is eliminating and defending the pathogens, will also consume some of the primordial Qi of human body, and Huangqi by lucky coincidence can make up the lost primordial Qi. As such, the side-effect of Fangfeng will be cleared up. Baizhu is to tonify the spleen, which means to support Qi in the Middle Jiao. If Huangqi and Fangfeng are taken as the fighting soldiers at frontier juncture to guard against and dispel the pathogenic factors on the skin of human body, Baizhu can be regarded as support crew at the rear area to prepare the strong and substantial backup force for the frontier warriors to assure them a strong Qi in the Middle Jiao.

Chinese Patent Medicine and Home-made Yupingfeng San

The formula of **Yupingfeng San**, because of its effectiveness and common use, has been processed into a Chinese patent medicine, i. e. **Yupingfeng San**, **Yupingfeng granule** and **Yupingfeng capsule**, which can be taken respectively according to the dosage specified in the introduction.

Yupingfen San has a very simple formula and involves no quite special processing workmanship, so it can be made at home by oneself. Of course, there are a lot of different ways: it can be made with the crushed powder of Fangfeng, Sheng Huangqi (raw radix astragali), Chao Baizhu (parched white atractylodes rhizome) mixed at a proportion of 1 : 2 : 2. Then take it twice a day in the morning and evening respectively, and 10g for each time to be washed down with warm water. Or in another way, take the three herbs mentioned above as tea, i.

e. put Fangfeng 2g, Huangqi 4g, Baizhu 4g in a glass and pour in boiling water and cover up for soaking half an hour and drink. Boiling water may be added continually as needed until the soaked water is very thin. This can be done twice a day.

第二章　桑叶与发散类方药

桑叶祛风

桑树我们应该都见过，树大根深，枝繁叶茂。桑叶春天发芽，一直经过夏天秋天。寒霜之中，它会掉一小部分，入冬以后，才慢慢掉光。当然，到了冬天这些叶子会千疮百孔，毕竟它经历了近一年的日晒风吹。春天的桑叶被人采来喂蚕，但是采了又长，生生不息。但桑叶入药，要等到下霜以后再采。我们开方子的时候通常把桑叶写作"霜桑叶"或者"冬桑叶"。金克木，桑叶在秋天得金气则能平肝，在枝头经风不凋，则平风的力量强，所以要冬天采。把冬桑叶采来后，要穿在在线晾干，这也是为了使它继续得风气，晾着的桑叶之间相碰撞，能发出金石之声，就像金属箔相碰撞，这个意味着，桑叶有金石之性。

《神农本草经》说，桑叶是苦寒的。其实在苦寒里面还有一丝甜味，所以我们说它的性味是甘苦寒。桑叶的作用，《本草便读》用一副对联来形容，非常美：

得箕星之精气，能搜肝络风邪；

秉青帝之权衡，善泄少阳气火。

得箕星之精，搜肝络风邪

二十八宿，东南西北各七宿，东方青龙七宿：角、亢、氐、房、心、尾、箕。古人仰观天象，发现天上的箕星非常明亮，地上就会起风，所以总结说"箕星好风"。现在大气污染了，在城里仰观天象就显得比较困难。大地上的一切，包括人体的五脏六腑，跟天上的二十八星宿都有着信息的沟通和往来。肝气通于东方七宿，风通于箕星，桑也与箕星相通，得箕星精气，故能入肝治风。

有人要问："风，有内风，有外风。那桑主要治内风还是外风呢？"其实，它内风外风都治，看你怎么用。古人讲箕星喜风，但并没讲它喜内风还是外风。何况，风的形态也是多样的。

我们拿一片桑叶在手上看，会发现桑叶的脉络，致密而清晰，以络入络，所以桑叶可以入络，搜肝络的风邪。肝主风，当肝阴虚的时候，肝风就容易动，当风入络脉的时候，就比较顽固了，可以考虑用桑叶来"搜肝络的风邪"。

秉青帝之权衡，善泄少阳气火

青帝就是东方之神：青龙，少阳是胆经，肝胆两经相表里，"秉青帝之权衡，善泄少阳气火"，就是说桑叶能调和肝胆。

肝是生风的，主生发。肝风，每个人都有，在健康的人那里，肝风是和风，吹生万物，人体的一切生生之气都靠这和风。到了老年，身体的升发机能已经很弱了，肝依然在生风，那么这个风就成了"邪风"，是一种不和的风。怎么办呢？养阴息风，把风带来的不利影响减轻到最低。要让肝生的风变成和风，或者说给肝生的风一个合理的安置。

胆为少阳，主少火，《黄帝内经》讲"少火生气，壮火食气"，少火小小的，温温的，最有生机，所以能生气。火太过了，什么都烧掉了，就没有生机了。所以胆火应该慢慢地让气生起来，如果过旺，就是邪火了。

肝生出邪风，胆生出邪火，风火相煽，风助火势，火助风威，慢慢地越来越大。自然界有风火相煽，越旋越高。火性本身就是炎上的，风又把火往上吹，大家一起往上旋。我们在火灾现场就会看到这种景象。人体的风火相煽也一样会往上旋，所以病往往在头、在眼睛。

比方说，头晕、眼睛发昏或者发红，都跟风火有关，都可以考虑用桑叶，调和肝胆，息风降火。所以，桑叶有一个作用，就是清利头目。桑叶可以用来洗眼睛、洗头发。红眼病，如果是因为外风的话，可以直接用桑叶熬水来洗。桑叶也可以洗头发：头皮容易痒，往往是风邪客居巅顶，你抓一把桑叶和菊花，一块熬汤来洗，效果会很好，单用桑叶也可以。

桑麻丸

头发老掉，跟风邪也有关系。

我师父以前经常说，头发好比树叶，好好长在树上的叶子不会掉，得干枯了，再刮一阵风，才会掉。所以，治疗脱发，要一边养阴养血，一边祛风，这就有了一个药，叫桑麻丸：桑叶和芝麻做丸。剂量看具体情况：如果风象比较重，桑叶可以多用一些；如果是阴虚比较重，芝麻可以多用一些。把两者碾成细末，用白蜜做成丸，早晨用盐汤服，晚上用酒服，这可以养阴祛风，对于脱发有很好效果，但要长期坚持服用。为什么早晨用盐汤呢？因为早晨肚子是空的，盐是咸的，能入肾，能很快进入肾里，养阴；晚上用酒是把它往上带，带到头上来祛风。一上一下，往下养阴，往上祛风，都兼顾了。桑麻丸主要用来治疗阴虚兼风的脱发，对于因肝阴虚、肝风盛、胆火旺导致的眼睛疾病，也会有效。

深交便觉不寻常

针对肝胆性的高血压，桑叶也很常用。因为它搜肝络的风邪，而高血压多因肝风内动，肝阳上亢。见到肝阳上亢，大家马上想起镇肝息风汤，很少有人能够想到桑叶，因为它太平常了。

中医不尚奇，能用平常药解决的问题，就没有必要用新奇药、冷僻药、大剂量药、毒药。用药往往像用人，若是路人，我们一眼看过去，会觉得这些人都很平常，看不到任何过人之处，你跟某个人相交越深，越会发现他的能耐，觉得他很得力，能够完成很多事情。用平常的药达到不平常的效果，才叫出奇制胜。

当然它还得跟养肝、养阴、化痰或者化瘀的药合理配伍，单打独斗是不行的。

桑叶收汗

桑叶还有一个作用就是收汗。

《夷坚志》里面有这样一个故事：有一位游僧，非常瘦，吃得又少，每天晚上就盗汗，到了早晨，身子、衣被全都湿透了。二十多年，各种方法、方药都用了，就是治不好。他也就不治了，等死。后来到了严州山寺，寺里的和尚说，他有一个方子，非常有效，就是单用一味桑叶，烘干，碾成碎末，每次用两钱，空腹用米汤来调服。当时正好是秋冬季节，可以采桑叶，于是采了很多。吃了三天以后，这个二十多年的病就好了。

这个故事我是相信的。前面为什么百医无效啊？因为病已经入络了。通常，疾病都是这样，初病在经，久病入络。好比敌人刚刚来侵犯你的时候，都是走大路。此时比较集中，你要说打他，也会很利索。入侵时间长了，他们会遍布每一个山村、每一条田间小路。这就坏了，不好打，因为太分散、太隐蔽了。人体的络脉相当于毛细血管，当邪气进入毛细血管的时候，你想把它赶走，就不那么容易。这位游僧到处化缘弘法，可能也没有坚持去治。用桑叶入络，把风祛出去，汗自然就收了。

本来桑叶是一个发汗的东西，因为它是叶子，叶子就会走表而发汗，但在这里它是收汗。发汗只不过是为了驱邪，当它把络脉中的邪全部驱走了以后，络脉里面就没有风邪扰动，汗也就不会出来了。桑叶的收汗作用就是这样实现的。

桑叶补精髓

陈士铎有一本很有名的书叫《本草新编》，其中讲桑叶还有"补精髓、填骨髓"的作用，意思就是说它能养阴。

过去，我一直认为这是它的第二重功效，前提仍是祛风。当体内风邪太盛的时候，精髓、骨髓想满也满不了，因为风是一个伤阴的东西。湿透了的衣服晾在外边，只要起风，它会干得更快。这就是"风能胜湿"，风能够把水吹干。人体的真阴也是水啊，当体内的邪风比较旺的时候，它就容易干，精血就容易亏耗。当你把风驱走了以后，精血自然恢复得好，骨髓自然充满，这项功能是借助人体的自愈机能实现的。

后来，我的这一认识又有所改变：那一年初冬，严霜过后，我们小区的桑树上还残存着几片叶子，我摘下来，放在嘴里细细咀嚼，甜丝丝，黏乎乎的，分明能养阴嘛。我这才发现，桑叶，于祛风之外，仍有直接补精血、填骨髓的作用。但必须是冬桑叶。很多东西都是经霜则甘甜，桑叶也是，冬桑叶能养阴祛风。可见药材的采摘时间是多么重要！

"纸上得来终觉浅，绝知此事要躬行。"书本不可能把一切都讲得面面俱到，我们要尽量创造条件，亲身实践，拿出神农尝百草的精神，亲近每一味药材，去观察它、体验它，这样会有很多意想不到的收获。

桑菊饮

桑叶入肝、胆、肺三经。

一味药的归经，我们可以通过想象，或者在理解中记忆：桑叶是绿的，而且作为箕星之精，肯定入肝经；它还能泻胆火，所以必定入胆经；它辛凉解表，所以入肺经；又因为它的叶脉非常致密，所以它还能够入肝络、肺络。

治疗外感会经常用到桑叶。有一个典型的方剂，就是桑菊饮。

— 143 —

桑菊饮

桑叶二钱五，菊花一钱，杏仁二钱，连翘钱半，薄荷八分，桔梗二钱，芦根八分，甘草八分。

这是古书中的剂量，我们现在用的时候，还会有所改变，比如说芦根用八分就太少啦，我们一般会用到一两左右。我可以给出我常用的一个常规剂量，供大家参考：桑叶三钱，菊花四钱，杏仁三钱，连翘三钱，薄荷一钱，桔梗三钱，芦根一两，甘草二钱。为什么剂量会有变化呢？可能是药材的质量变了，也可能是煎法、剂型上古今有差异。

什么时候用到桑菊饮呢？《温病条辨》是这么讲的："太阳风温，但咳，身不甚热，微咳者，辛凉轻剂，桑菊饮主之。"病人略微有点发热，略微有点咳嗽，这是感冒很轻微的证状。这里的咳嗽，是因为热伤了肺络，为什么只受了那么一丁点邪，他就会有热？在《伤寒论》中，这种情况是比较少的，但是到了《温病条辨》的时代，也就是清朝，这种情况就比较多了，这跟人的体质有关。这时候，人们比张仲景时代更加容易动火。《伤寒论》主要针对寒邪，我们用它的思想可以通治百病。但是它的方剂主要是针对那个时代的人。老用麻黄桂枝，汉朝人受得了。到了清朝，大家就有点受不了啦。中医也是随着时代的变化而变化的。道不变，但是它的法、方、药，都是在变的。

桑菊为君

容易动火，跟肝胆有关。动辄肝热，木火刑金，所以肝热会伤肺络，与外邪呼应，造成咳嗽、身热。所以，用桑叶菊花，去胆火、清肝胆。

我们现在的人依然是这样的，所以桑菊饮仍经常用到。感冒的时候会出现头脑昏沉，正好桑菊来清利头目。何况它都能疏风清热，桑叶更擅长疏风，菊花更擅长清热，他们配在一起就能够相得益彰了。

那我们想，为什么在这里用到菊花，而不用桃花呢？桃花不也是花吗？不也有宣发的作用吗？但是，菊花是秋天开的，得金气，而金是主清凉、肃杀的，而且金克木。桃花是春天开的，有生发之气，它是红色的，入血分，现在邪气主要在气分，当然不能用入血分的药。邪还没到血分，你却用了入血分的药，就可能会引邪深入。

薄荷：辛凉解表

桑菊饮里还有一味薄荷，是一味非常重要的辛凉发表药，《神农本草经》中没有，是后世医家发现的。桑菊辛凉发表，但是它发表的力度不够，还需要加大，所以用了薄荷。薄荷的辛香之气味非常明显，开表的力度很大。这个药到后世才用，也是因时制宜。为什么呢？因为有邪，要发汗，但同时又因为有热，不能辛温发汗。在张仲景时代，发汗都用辛温的麻黄、桂枝，但是现在时代不同了，这个时代的人肝火更大，动不动就是火，不敢用辛温，只好用辛凉。辛能开表发汗，凉又能清热，于是大家就找到了薄荷。

即使是受了寒邪，可以用辛温发表，但由于麻黄桂枝发汗的力度太大了，也不适合。那就用苏叶。一味苏叶，就能替代麻黄加桂枝，因为苏叶既入气分又入血分。我们学本草，千万不要拘泥于《神农本草经》，而要有一种开放的心态。

连翘：苦寒清里

连翘是走中焦的，能清胃热，又清心火。"温邪上受，首先犯肺，逆传心包"，温热之邪传到心包就会成为重症，所以用连翘防止邪气逆传心包。

有人要问了：既能清胃热，又能清心火，黄连不也有这个作用吗？为什么不用呢？有两个原因：

第一，黄连是守而不走的药，它比较懒惰，走得比较慢，而我们感冒是需要速战速决的，邪气在这里，必须赶紧把它赶走，排出体外。体表的邪气用薄荷以发汗的方式把它赶走，在里的则用杏仁把它从大肠往下引。黄连虽然有用，但速度不行，耽误事儿。

第二，我们在开方子的时候写"连翘衣"，就是连翘外面的一层壳，外壳往往走表，而且连翘有幽香开窍之功有通透性。黄连是根，不走表；也无幽香，没有通透性可言。

桑菊饮里面的药都比较通透，没有赖在那里不走的药，也没有引邪深入的药。古人流传下来的名方，其中每一味药都是很值得我们研究的。

杏仁桔梗，升降之机

一个治疗感冒的好方子，不但要兼顾表里，还要考虑升降之机。桑菊饮中用杏仁、桔梗，一升一降，在升降之间调整肺的气机，乃至整个人体气机。

杏仁是一味开肺的药，又走大肠，通腑泄热。所有的仁都含有油脂，能润肠通便，杏仁开肺，降肺气，又有油脂通润大肠，所以它通腑泄热的功效尤其好。肺与大肠相表里，肺热可以通过大便从大肠泻下去。那么，这里为什么不用桃仁呢？桃仁跟杏仁不挺相似吗？因为杏仁走气分，桃仁走血分，它们不一样。怎么区分呢，我们不需要死记硬背，春天的时候我们出去看看杏花和桃花。杏花是白的，可能微微有那么一丁点红；桃花则是红的，所以桃仁走血分，邪在气分你用走血分的药可能又是引邪深入了。

桔梗是一味开提肺气的药。开就是打开，提就是往上提。

开就能透，肺气一开也就意味着毛孔开，毛孔一开，薄荷之类发汗的药，就会发得更快。

能够往上提，它就不会下陷。感冒受了很多邪气，要防止它下陷。邪气如果下陷，陷到中焦肠胃，那就是拉肚子；陷到肾里，那就是肾炎之类的。急性肾炎，很多就用桑菊饮的加减来治，效果非常好。

芦根甘草养中焦

考虑到人体受邪，很快会化热，一化热就会伤津，津液伤了要赶紧补上，所以这里用了一味芦根。芦根就是芦苇的根，长在水里，是一味生津液的药，它很滋润，同时又很通透。这味药生津液而不易成为痰。它还能把不好的水利出去，把好的水给你补上。

我们这里又要问了——学东西要学会思考，多问自己，学问需要自己设问题问自己，等自己把问题给解决了，就是不知不觉地在进步——芦根有生津的作用，那花粉不也有生津的作用吗？这里为什么不用花粉而非要用芦根呢？因为花粉是瓜蒌的根，通透性不如芦根。感冒用药始终要注意通透，要能够让邪气及时透出去。所以，在这里用芦根而没有用花粉。

方中的甘草一是调和上面各种药的，同时还能和胃气。我们一般用十克。甘草是调和诸药的，我们经常用三五克；如果用到十克或者二十克，那它是具有清的作用，能清热还能解毒。在这里，甘草有解毒的作用。

芦根、甘草都是入中焦的，能固护胃气，生津液。而"保胃气""存津液"是《伤寒论》中重要的原则。

识药如识人

我们在讲方子的时候，每味药都要认真地讲一讲，同时，我们要把这味药跟别的药反复比较，这样才能深入地认识药性。

就像做一件事的时候，把人和人反复比较一样，达到知人善任。我们要知药善用。认一味药就好比认一个人，比如说今天我们要认识张三同志，把他的简历打出来，发给大家。大家就有了一个初步的印象，至于这个人的人品、办事的风格，简历上还不能完全体现。一个人尚且如此，如果是三百六十五个人的简历都发给我们，我们就迷糊了。

我们最好是在不同的场合反复见到这个人，观察他在不同场合有什么反应。同时，又跟别人做比较，这样我们就能很快熟悉他。这也是学药的正路。

所以我们现在讲方子的时候要介绍药，第一次听我介绍薄荷或者杏仁的时候，你可能会比较生疏，但是以后大家还会常常听，因为杏仁、薄荷的药在很多方子里都会有。在不同的场合反复地遇到，甚至听腻了，你就熟悉它了。

辛凉三剂

桑菊饮在《温病条辨》里被称为"辛凉轻剂"。既然有轻剂，那么肯定就有重剂，还有介于轻重之间的平剂。所以，辛凉有三个方子，或者说有四个方子。辛凉轻剂是桑菊饮，辛凉平剂是银翘散，辛凉重剂一是麻杏石甘汤，还有一个是白虎汤。后两个方子都出自《伤寒论》，而银翘散和桑菊饮这两个方剂都出自《温病条辨》。

有的同学一看到讲的是温病的东西就走了，不听了，这种心态不好。只要有用的东西我们都要学。愚者千虑，必有一得。何况吴鞠通并非愚者。学中医必须有开阔的胸襟，能纳百家之长为我所用。

银翘散

辛凉平剂银翘散

银花一两，连翘一两，薄荷六钱，荆芥穗四钱，豆豉五钱，竹叶四钱，牛蒡子六钱，桔梗六钱，芦根煎汤代水。

散剂与汤剂

散，是把药打成粉服用的，且有发散、疏散的意思。比如，银翘散是发散邪气的，逍遥散是疏散郁结的。汤，就是把药煮成汤来喝，比较常用。汤者荡也，用于涤荡邪气，速度较快。

《温病条辨》把银翘散做成散剂，而我们现在是把它作为汤剂。剂型变了，药量及煎法都会有一些差别。一般来说，我们现在银花要用三十克左右，连翘十克，薄荷用六到十克，荆芥穗十到十二克，豆豉十克（我们到后面还要讲），苏叶八到十二克，牛蒡子用十克，芦根三十克，桔梗十克，这是临床常用的剂量，跟《温病条辨》列出来的不太一样。

银花连翘

这个方子是以金银花和连翘为君药的。金银花在它没有开的时候就得采，它绿色通肝，清香化浊，解毒的功能非常好。金银花没有归经之说，它能通行全身。既能清气分的热，也能解血分的毒。银花连翘一起用，解毒的作用更大。如果要细致地讲，连翘还分青连翘和黄连翘，青连翘入肝，作用偏于解毒，黄连翘更多的入中焦，偏于清热。临床上还可以根据具体情况来选择。

前面我们讲过，近世之人，肝郁、胆火比较重，一旦遇到外邪，往往里应外合，迅速化热，所以桑菊饮里面用了桑叶菊花，一面辛凉散邪，一面解肝胆之热。银翘散依然遵循这个思想。肝是解毒的，但如果肝热未能充分散掉，那么肝解毒也就不彻底，毒存在我们体内，郁久化热，热再郁久而成毒。本来肝是应该解掉这个毒的，现在它能力有限，不能完全解掉，我们就用银花连翘来协助它解。

其实，银花连翘并不仅仅只是解感冒的毒。一些皮肤病、内科杂症的毒，也可以用银花连翘来解。我们现在讲病毒性感冒，虽是西医的说法，但中医也认同有病毒，只不过中医里毒的范围更为广泛。

银翘散中的解表药

虽然银花连翘也能走表，但力度还远远不够，所以必须加薄荷，辛凉发表，透散在表的邪气。

再加荆芥穗。荆芥，味辛微温，但一般的本草书都把它归为辛凉发表，它本质上是微温的，但因为它辛、散，在散的过程中，微温就感觉不到了，它反而能够给人一种凉的感觉。我们可以说它是体温而用凉的一味药。荆芥穗就是荆芥的穗子，发散的力量更强。荆芥穗很香，刚闻上去非常舒服，但若闻太久，可能会头晕。

银翘散里的豆豉，是用苏叶水浸泡豆子，再让它发酵。发酵，也是一个升发的过程，它还能使板结的东西变得松透。豆豉的发酵性，能松动体内板结的陈气，宣散上焦之邪；经过苏叶水的浸泡，它又有了发汗的作用。苏叶水在其中起了重要的作用。现在很多豆豉不是按这个方法做的，所以我们干脆不用，用苏叶来代替。

苏叶的用量一般是六到十克，它辛温发表。前面用了那么多辛凉的药，这里为何忽然用了一味辛温的呢？因为温邪往往夹杂着寒，有时候人体本来是受了寒，入里才化热，所以可以加苏叶来散寒邪。即使没有寒，苏叶跟前面这些辛凉的药在一起也不为过，因为邪气要往外发，稍微用一些温有助于发散。

本草里讲，苏叶是入肝经入肺胃经的，它辛温，能够发汗、散寒，能够行气、和血，既走气分又走血分。

我们来看看苏叶的外形特点，它的叶子正面（向上的一面）是绿的，背面是红的。绿的它就走气分，红色意味着它能走血分。它是介于气分和血分之间的一味药。麻黄是走气分的，很轻而且很绿，它不会走到血分去。麻黄为什么要加桂枝呢？桂枝色红入血分、入营分。麻黄得到了桂枝，所以就能兼走气分和血分。现在苏叶一味药就能同时走气分和血分，从某种程度上讲，它就等同于麻黄加上桂枝，只不过力度要轻得多。而且苏叶还入中焦，能推陈致新。苏叶走表，苏梗通上下，能够理气。所以紫苏也有类似于豆豉的推陈致新的作用。

银翘散中的清里药

一部份热邪从表发散掉了，还有一部份热邪要从里走，也就是通过大小便泻下去。这便是竹叶和牛蒡子两味药。

竹叶清心火、走小肠、利小便，能让热从小便中排出来。桑菊饮中用连翘能清中焦的火还能清心火，防止邪气逆传心包，银翘散里除了连翘还有竹叶，加大了防止邪气逆传心包的力度。

牛蒡子味辛、苦，性凉。开方的时候，一定注明要打碎。它既能够散风泄热，又能够润大便，通腑泄热。为了达到这些目的，桑菊饮用了杏

— 149 —

仁，银翘散则用牛蒡子。杏仁也微微有一些透表的作用，还能润大便，牛蒡子跟杏仁有相似之处，但它的力度比杏仁要大得多。所以这里就不用杏仁而用牛蒡子。牛蒡子能开泄肺气，配上其他解表的药，就能打开毛孔，散风泄热，解毒发疹。同时我们还要知道，它是一味寒凉药，又是植物种子，种子是往下走的，能通大肠，带有油润性，又能润大便，把大便迅速通下去，体内的火和毒也会跟着大便一块往外走。

牛蒡子还有一个最重要的作用就是治疗咽喉痛。

咽喉是人体重要的通道。有一个成语叫"咽喉要道"，指那种非常重要，同时又比较狭窄的通道，一夫当关，万夫莫开。咽喉也是如此。感冒肺热上犯，咽喉首当其冲，所以咽喉痛；牛蒡子宣通肺气，肃降肺热，所以对咽痛有很好的疗效。

最常见的风热感冒过程

风热感冒往往伴随咽喉痛。很多人往往是头天晚上咽喉有点痛，第二天上午就不舒服，有点头晕，还可能有点鼻塞之类的证状，这才感觉可能感冒了。

脉是数的，体温还算正常，或者比平时高不到哪去。这时要非常注意，上午虽不发热，但到下午就会发热了，而且"阳明之热，旺在申酉"，申时酉时就是下午三到七点，最容易发热。

为什么热要到这时才发呢？因为上午人体阳气旺盛，阳气抗邪的能力很足，邪气不便发作，郁在体内，脉数就是证据，一般都有每分钟八十次以上，如果内火重的人能够达到九十多一百多，但是不发热。到了下午，阳气往里收敛，与体内热邪短兵相接，打起来了，所以体温迅速升高；或者说，阳气收敛了，在表的邪热无所顾忌，也能够导致发热。这个热如果不采取措施的话会一直热到半夜，等到子时一阳生的时候，发热又会有所减轻。

这个感冒的过程，现在很常见。如果在头天晚上嗓子有点疼的时候就开始用银翘散，这个感冒就很有可能被你消灭在萌芽状态。等到第二天发热的时候，再用银翘散就要考虑加石膏了。石膏清气分的热。

银翘散辛凉开表，清热解毒。有时我们感冒了懒得熬药，可以直接用银翘解毒丸、银翘解毒颗粒。但是到了感冒、发热比较严重的时候，成药作用就会弱一些，因为剂量可能不够，还因为它的药味无法加减。发热严

— 150 —

重，用银翘散加一味石膏多好呢！好比一间房子里面很热，怎么才能凉下来？开窗子。但是如果多种方法同时使用那不更好吗？我们在开窗子的同时，在房子里放很多冰块。用银翘散相当于开窗子，再加石膏就相当于放冰块。里外都考虑到，退热也会更快。

温热性的感冒，用银翘散加减，往往一两剂就能把热退下去。热退后，人就轻快多了，但往往痰比较多，还有一些零星咳嗽。这时候，不要急于止咳，要让痰通过咳嗽排出来。这也是人体在自动清理肺部，把感冒产生的垃圾清出来，这样肺里就更清爽了。有人通过感冒，一次咳了很多痰。尤其抽烟的人，通过感冒，治疗的比较得当，咳出很多灰色的痰，这是烟痰，排出来总是好的。这就是"小病养生"。

当然，也不能一直这样咳嗽吐痰，如果咳嗽到一定的时候还不见好，那就应该用药，健脾清肺，止咳化痰了。不能光治肺，一定要脾肺兼顾，扶土生金。脾为生痰之源，健脾之后，就不再产生那么多痰了。

在整个过程中，发热要消耗津液，生痰、排痰又要消耗津液。消耗的津液需要及时补充，所以，虽然银翘散里面有一味芦根，但到了善后的时候，我们还要用更多甘寒滋润的药来补养津液，如芦根、竹叶、麦冬之类，才算最后扫尾。这是治热性感冒的一个完整的过程。

通常，发生在冬春两季的感冒，尤其是春温感冒，采取的是这个思路，其他季节还是要区别对待。那种最常见的感冒就是刚才这个步骤，要开表，要清里，要清肺，要止咳化痰，到最后还要养阴生津。现在很多人都无视这个过程了，感冒了就胡乱对付，当时好了，但后患无穷，所以现在有这么多过敏的，有这么多慢性鼻炎，往往是感冒的邪气没有排出来，留在了肺里。还有很多其他的病，也是由感冒导致的，说出来大家都不信，急性肾炎多是由感冒导致的，脑膜炎也是由感冒导致的……

麻杏石甘汤

麻杏石甘汤的剂量
辛凉重剂麻杏石甘汤
麻黄四两，杏仁五十个，石膏半斤，甘草二两。

这个剂量是《伤寒论》中麻杏石甘汤的剂量，今天不能照搬。因为不同时代的度量衡不同，药材质量不同，人也不同。不同的时代，方子会给出不同的剂量，而且往往不是按比例换算的。比如，清朝《温病条辨》给出的剂量是：麻黄、杏仁、石膏各三钱，甘草二钱；而 1964 年版《方剂学》教材给出的剂量是：麻黄、甘草各一钱，杏仁二钱，石膏三钱。

我们现在用麻杏石甘汤，剂量又不一样。如果是南方人，麻黄一般用三五分（1－2 克）就可以了，如果是北方人，尤其是西北人，可以多用一点。杏仁可以用三四钱（10－12 克），石膏一两（30 克）左右，甘草则两三钱（5－10 克）。

《伤寒论》说麻杏石甘汤的主证是"汗出而喘"，出汗意味表是开的。喘意味着肺气不通，肺气遏郁。肺气被遏就生热，且使肺气上逆，致喘。麻黄用在此并不是发汗，而是开肺气的，所以不需要用那么多。麻杏石甘汤方义可以概括为这四句话："麻黄开肺气，杏仁降肺逆，石膏清肺热，甘草缓肺急。"这个方子，既解表又清里，它的结构跟银翘散有很相似的地方。其中四个药的剂量如何确定，首先是要看能不能在特定的人身上起到它们应有的作用，而不是看是否跟书本记载的一致。

麻黄

讲麻杏石甘汤，主要是为了仔细讲讲麻黄这味药。麻黄在《中药学》中往往是第一个讲，它生在我国西北，秉天地清阳刚烈之气以生。

我见过麻黄自然生长的样子：绿色的管状草，细细的。摘一根尝尝，也没有明显的味道和气味，很多人都不敢相信这个药发汗那么厉害。它气味俱薄，质地很轻，三克能有不少。质地轻，就能够轻清上浮而走表，还可以升发阳气。麻黄必须跟桂枝配伍才能入营分以发汗，单用也能发汗，古人用的比较多，因为古人肌肤比较致密，肺气刚强，用它非常适宜。现在的人，体质发生了变化，临床使用就要注意。现在我们用麻黄，一般用制麻黄、陈麻黄或制麻绒。制麻黄，就是把麻黄用蜜制过；陈麻黄，就是把麻黄存放得时间越长越好，这样它的性质就不那么刚烈，会平和一点，同时仍不失其作用；制麻绒，就是把麻黄捣过之后留下的绒，就像艾绒一样，性质也很平和。

麻黄一般用 1－2 克就足够了，少用是取其"轻清上浮"之意。就像升麻，在补中益气汤中一般用 5－6 克就行了，用得少，它升清的力度反而比较大。麻黄用得少，能够升清、散表，用多了，它就耗散真气了，这时要用人参来补救。人参可救过用麻黄之弊，因为人参能够"回元气于无何有之乡"，及时挽回耗散的真气，同时还能够生津。

前几年我遇到一位西北的中医，他说他们当地就产麻黄，当地人感冒，直接采一些麻黄回来，不拘多少，煎水喝完就好了。我问这么喝可以发汗吗？他说不，一般喝了也不出汗，但感冒就会好。他说这个现象有点奇怪。其实并不奇怪，麻黄之所以发汗，是因为它开肺窍。西北人肌肤比较致密，这一点跟张仲景时期的人更加接近，所以喝下麻黄之后，不会出汗，但肺窍已开，气机也开了，外邪自然透散，虽然没有出汗，但是毛孔已开，这是用肉眼看不到的。

麻黄石膏之配伍

陈士铎曾说：麻黄本不是温药，而是凉药，跟桂枝在一起，才成为温药。陈士铎这么说，主要还是强调麻黄和桂枝配伍的意义，也有助于我们理解麻杏石甘汤。

桂枝是辛温药，麻黄配桂枝，是辛温发汗的。石膏是辛凉药，麻黄配石膏，就是辛凉的了。有人说石膏是大寒的药，其实它并没有那么可怕。《伤寒论》里，麻黄用的是四两，石膏用的是半斤，石膏的用量正好是麻黄的两倍（古代的半斤是八两）。后来这个比例又有所改变，石膏的剂量永远不会比麻黄小。这时麻黄的温性基本上就没有了。麻黄配伍石膏，比单用麻黄出汗更少。

西北人喝麻黄可能不会出汗，而南方人喝麻黄可能就会汗出不止了，南方人肌肤腠理没有西北人那么致密。《伤寒论》里面的方子，在剂量上很见功夫。敢在有汗的情况下依然用麻黄，是因为有石膏来反佐它，而且，石膏的量是麻黄的两倍，在配伍上能够使药尽其性。我们要弄懂它的道理而不要照搬它的方剂，因为用这个方剂的人已经不在了，用这个方剂的时代也已经有变迁了。随着时代的变迁，道是不会变迁的，它一以贯之，但具体的方和法，要变迁。

我们讲中医要与时俱进，意思是，医方、医术要随着时代和人的变化而变化，针对现代人的体质，是有必要在方药和具体疗法上翻新的。只能在术的层面创新，在道的层面是创不了新的。因为，中医的医道已经圆融了，它要止于至善。

杏仁与上几方的先煎后下问题

杏仁是降肺气的。《黄帝内经》说"肺苦气上逆"。杏仁略微有开表作用，它能肃肺、通润大肠，通过润大肠又可以降肺气，两个功能相得益彰。

麻杏石甘汤有麻黄开表，杏仁虽然有微微解表的作用，但是我们可以不靠它来解表，因此，杏仁在这里与其他药一块煎就行了，不需要后下。

现在北京有很多药店，要求杏仁后下，并不可取。如果你要用杏仁来解表发汗，你就后下；如果你用杏仁润大肠，那就不需要后下了。

麻杏石甘汤是有先煎后下的：麻黄应该先煎，先煎二十分钟到半个小时，把表面泛起的白沫去掉。石膏先煎十五分钟就行了。

前面讲的银翘散方，煎药同样有讲究，我们在开方子时要标注在旁边。苏叶要后下，只能煮五分钟；牛蒡子要打碎；薄荷后下，煮两分钟就行了，也就是头煎的最后两分钟下薄荷，因为薄荷的香味非常容易发散，只能熬两分钟。熬两分钟，香气已经在药里边了，辛凉的性质已经在药里边了，再煎香气便会散失。

香薷饮

夏天的感冒，很多不是因为受了热，而是受了凉。因为夏天人们喜欢吃凉的，喜欢吹风乘凉。待在凉的地方久了，人就容易受凉，把毛孔闭住了。夏天本来应该出汗，但这种感冒反而不出汗，不想吃东西，头晕，昏沉，身体非常重。这是夏天感冒常有的一些证状。可能发热，也可能不发热，这时候我们就要用到香薷饮。

香薷饮由三味药组成：香薷　厚朴　白扁豆。

香薷

香薷辛温开表。毛孔被寒邪闭住了，就要试图打开，需要解表发汗。

为什么不用麻黄呢？因为夏天本身就是出汗的季节，阳气走表，如果再用麻黄就特别容易导致汗出不止，甚至大汗亡阳。所以我们用香薷来代替麻黄。夏天用了香薷，也就相当于冬天用了麻黄，发汗的作用就有这么强。

香薷气息芳香，走气分。它开白花，开白花也往往走气分，开红花往往走血分。而且，它能升能降，先往上升，解表发汗；然后它还能往下降，所以又能下气、利湿。所以暑天用它会非常好。

辛温的药有很多，麻黄、桂枝、葱、藿香、苏叶都是辛温的。此处为何用香薷不用苏叶？因为与香薷相比，苏叶少了利湿和下气的作用。暑天，毛孔一旦闭住，汗出不来，中焦脾胃就容易停湿，所以用香薷，一方面解表发汗，一方面下气利湿。这是最佳的选择。

香薷饮方义

香薷虽然能够下气利湿，但它主要的作用依然是辛温开表。所以我们要加几味药来帮助香薷进一步下气利湿。

厚朴是走中焦脾胃，能平胃燥湿，也能通大肠。夏天脾胃多湿，用厚朴进一步来化湿、燥湿，再让湿从大肠走掉。

白扁豆味淡，淡以渗湿，故用白扁豆来调和脾胃，而不用甘草。

这就是香薷饮的作用：解表、和中。夏天很多感冒，人都不想吃饭，只是因为湿困中焦脾胃，这也正是香薷饮所善治的。

新加香薷饮

后来，吴鞠通在香薷饮的基础上做了一些发挥，创造出新加香薷饮：银花 连翘 香薷 厚朴 鲜扁豆花。

他加了两味药，银花和连翘。邪气闭在体内，郁而化热，邪热不散就成了毒，银花、连翘清热解毒。新加香薷饮把白扁豆换成了鲜扁豆花，鲜扁豆花不但能够调和脾胃，还有发散作用。鲜扁豆花我们现在就不好找，咱们依然可以用白扁豆，效果差不多。

新加香薷饮，针对夏天受凉的感冒，发热无汗，食欲减退，效果较好。

藿香正气散

如果香薷饮解决不了问题，还有一个治阴暑典型的方剂，藿香正气散。这也是夏天经常用的方剂，而且做成了成药：

藿香、紫苏、白芷、茯苓、半夏、白术、姜厚朴、苦桔梗、大腹皮、陈皮、甘草。

藿香

藿香辛温芳香，但它一般生在水湿之地。它喜欢水，而喜欢水的植物药多能利湿，所以藿香不但能够解表，还能和中化湿，能入中焦脾胃，这

— 155 —

是藿香跟其他辛温解表药不一样的地方。

它跟香薷也不一样，香薷虽然能够利湿，但是它的芳香更容易耗气，而且发汗的力度太强。暑邪本来就伤气，夏天人本来就容易出汗，所以往往要慎用香薷，相比之下，藿香要平和得多。

藿香，我们开方子的时候一般写广藿香，就是两广（广东广西）产的藿香，一般以广东为主。还有浙江也有藿香，叫浙藿香。广藿香入里入中焦的作用要强一些，浙藿香更倾向于走表。广藿香的梗是方的，其他地方藿香的梗是圆的，很容易区分。藿香分藿香叶和藿香梗，藿香叶偏于散邪，藿香梗偏于宽中理气，有时候我们就一块用了。

藿香正气散方义

藿香辛温，解表和中；紫苏包括苏梗和苏叶，苏叶主要是散表的，苏梗能理气，紫苏既散表又理气；白芷辛温走阳明。这三味药合用，辛温开表。

再加桔梗，开提肺气，开就是打开门户排出邪气，提就是让肺气往上升，肺气上升则更有利于把邪气透出体外。

厚朴、大腹皮、半夏、茯苓、陈皮、甘草，都是走中焦的药。因为夏天的感冒跟表有关，跟里也有关。里，主要体现在脾胃上。夏天阳气走表，中焦虚寒，容易停湿，一停湿人就食欲减退，浑身乏力，所以咱们要用走中焦的药来健脾助运，化中焦的湿。

藿香正气散跟香薷饮在结构上非常相似。香薷饮用了一味香薷，藿香正气散则用藿香、紫苏、白芷、桔梗。前者用厚朴、白扁豆，后者用的是厚朴、大腹皮、半夏、茯苓、陈皮、甘草，药味变得更多了，作用变得更复杂也更全面了。大腹皮就是槟榔的皮，顾名思义，它能够消胀，有人感觉到肚子很胀，可以用大腹皮理气、消胀。半夏、茯苓、陈皮、甘草则是二陈汤，化痰的。脾胃的寒湿停留太多太久就变成了痰，咱们就用二陈汤来化。

所以，藿香正气散比香薷饮更加全面和复杂一些。

九味羌活汤

南方湿气比较重，一旦感冒常会骨节疼，尤其是后脑勺连着背疼，甚至还有腰痛、身体沉重。那种感冒非常缠绵，人很难受。这时候用银翘散可能就不管用了，九味羌活汤可以派上用场。

九味羌活汤是金元四大家之前的医家张元素所创立，这个方剂体现了他的学问。张元素是金元四大家中李东垣的老师，他还给四大家中的刘完素看过病，因此，与其说是金元四大家，还不如说是五大家，张元素是排在金元四大家前的一大家。

九味羌活汤

羌活、防风、白芷、川芎、细辛、苍术、黄芩、生地、甘草、生姜、葱白。

感冒夹湿邪，不宜用麻黄，因为麻黄发汗力度太大了。湿邪是一种粘腻的邪气，你要慢慢地把它赶出去，不能太快，欲速则不达。湿邪是很顽固的，要慢慢赶才能够赶得清。通过迅速发汗的方式驱逐湿邪，只是白白伤害津液而已。

羌活

羌活产自西北，气味雄烈、辛温发表、散邪。它的作用偏于搜风渗湿，所以感冒夹杂湿，用羌活非常好。

羌活走太阳经，风湿之邪困太阳经，人就会觉得身体沉重，骨节痛。这跟张仲景时代的寒伤太阳，用麻黄桂枝来散寒邪不一样，这里是风湿之邪，不能乱用麻黄和桂枝，而要用羌活走太阳经搜风渗湿。

尤其是它走上肢的痛，用羌活效果好。后面我们还要讲桑枝，也走上肢。走下肢用独活，独活走少阴经的，祛少阴经的风寒邪气，治下肢的疼痛效果非常好。

九味羌活汤的方义

通过九味羌活汤这个方，我们又认识了一系列辛温发表的药。羌活、防风、白芷、细辛。

南方人肾虚的比较多，虚邪贼风乘虚而入少阴经，所以用细辛来发少阴经的汗。

苍术本来是燥湿的，但也能发汗，它是通过走中焦来发汗的，而且它有汗就收汗，没汗就能发汗，用科学的话讲就是它能够对汗腺进行双向调节。能把人体调节到最舒服的状态。

葱白也是发汗的，它是绿色的，所以能走厥阴肝经。

防风祛风渗湿，但它的性质比羌活润，跟羌活同用，既能够加大羌活发散的力度，又能防止羌活过于燥烈。

白芷色白，辛温，也能润泽。色白则走阳明，是阳明经的引经药，所以治阳明头痛。南方的感冒往往伴随着前额及眉棱骨疼，头重，这种感冒是风湿邪气已经入阳明经了，所以用白芷来散。

川芎是风中润剂，是少阳经的引经药，能够和血通肝；香气浓烈，有走窜的作用，能够搜血分的风寒，还能够解郁，治头痛。

这些药，走六经的都有了：羌活、防风走太阳经，白芷走阳明经，川芎走少阳经，细辛、生地走少阴经，苍术走足太阴经脾，黄芩走手太阴经肺。当风湿之邪困在体表的时候，体内往往是热的，所以黄芩和生地，一方面清里热，一方面养阴。

在南方，风湿比较重，人们感冒经常要用到本方。南方比较热，体内的阳气往外走的多，往里收的少。而且在比较湿热的环境中，体内的精气就要稍微弱一些。"邪之所凑，其气必虚"，正气一弱，风湿邪气趁虚而入，那就坏了。底子很弱，外面的风湿邪气又那么重，所以要一边散邪，一边清里热，一边再养阴。

玉屏风散

频繁感冒的原因

讲了这么多治疗感冒的方子，大家自然就会想到：预防感冒有什么方法么？

当然是有的，但凡事也不能绝对。感冒是人体对外邪的生理反应之一，人体的卫气抵御外邪，有时候能抵御，有时候也会打败仗，卫气战败，邪气入侵，人就感冒了。胜败乃兵家常事，偶尔打一次败仗也不要紧。但如果经常感冒，那就是经常打败仗了，那就需要注意。

很多人有过这样的体验：每当感冒一次之后，近期就不会感冒了，要隔很长一段时间才有可能再次感冒。西医把这种现象叫"产生了抗体"。其实，从中医的角度来讲，这是因为上一次感冒肃清了肺里的邪气和污浊，使肺经历了一次锻炼，抵抗邪气的能力增强了。从这个意义上讲，感冒也不完全是坏事。

然而，经常感冒的人则不然。有人隔三差五就感冒了，有人的感冒则绵绵不断，很长时间既不恶化也不减轻，这都是因为脾肺气虚、卫外不固。肺主皮毛，肺虚则肌肤没有很好的抵抗外邪的能力，邪气何时何地想进来就进来了，肺本身也不能迅速排出邪气，所以，感冒要么隔三差五，要么缠绵不断。感冒虽是小病，但人体抵抗感冒的病邪，修复感冒带来的损伤确实需要消耗不少元气的。感冒反复发作或缠绵不断，如果不能及时治疗，拖延下去，人体的元气将会进一步耗伤，变生出各种各样的疾病。

脾肺气虚不仅会导致经常性的感冒，而且还会导致怕冷、怕风、汗多等症状，还有一种慢性鼻炎过敏，一遇到冷风就不断打喷嚏。这些，都是因为元气虚亏使"肺主皮毛"的功能失常，导致邪气容易进入人体为患。就好比一个国家国力不足，边境上没有精兵强将，所以不断遭受敌人袭击。

玉屏风散的方义

这些，看似可怕，其实，只要用对了药，治疗起来还是很容易的，玉屏风散即可。

玉屏风散，顾名思义，它是人体的一道玉屏风，专门为我们遮风挡邪。它的组成药物相当简单，只有三味药：防风、黄芪、白术。

人们都说"风随草偃"，风朝哪个方向吹，草就朝哪个方向偏，可唯独防风这种植物不同，风吹不动他，在风中能静止不动，古人取象比类，用它来做为抵御各种风邪的药，效果非常奇特。它会防止外界的风侵入，又会把已经侵入人体的风邪驱赶出去。黄芪既为人体大补元气，又给防风提供动力。而且，防风在祛邪和御邪的过程中会耗散人体的一部分元气，而黄芪恰好可以把这部分元气补足，这样，就消解了防风的副作用。白术是健脾的，健脾就是养人体的中气。如果说黄芪和防风在人体肌表抵御和驱逐邪气像是在边关作战，那么，白术这是在大后方，为边关的勇士们提供强大的物质后盾，使他们中气十足。

中成药与自制玉屏风散

玉屏风散这个方子，由于很有效、很常用，被做成了中成药，就是现在市场上玉屏风散、玉屏风散颗粒、玉屏风胶囊等，我们按照说明书上的用法用量服用即可。

由于玉屏风散组成药物简单，没有什么特殊的加工工艺，我们也可以自己制作玉屏风散。方法是多种多样的：可以按照 1∶2∶2 的比例，从药店买来防风、生黄芪、炒白术这三味药，打碎成粉，混合在一起，每天早晚各一次，每次 10 克，温开水冲服。还可以用这三味药泡水当茶喝，每次取防风 2 克，黄芪 4 克，白术 4 克。放在水杯里，倒进去滚开的开水，密封浸泡半小时后服用，喝完还可以继续加水，一直泡到淡了为止。每天可以这样泡两次。

Chapter 3　Sangzhi (mulberry twig) and Medicines for Dispelling Wind and Dredging Collaterals

Sangzhi (Mulberry Twig)

Wind is the leading factor in causing various diseases, and many diseases arise from a common cold, which can be generally named as the exogenous wind. In addition, many other diseases arisedue to senior age, which can be generally named as the endogenous wind. In the previous part, a lot of formulas involving Sangye (mulberry leaves) for treatment of the exogenous wind have been discussed. When wind- pathogen goes deeper further, it will enter into in between the blood vessels and bones, for which other medicines represented by Sangzhi (mulberry twig) will be needed.

Characteristics of Sangzhi (Mulberry Twig)

Sangzhi refers to the little branches of mulberry trees. A normal mulberry tree is always flourishing with luxuriant foliage with twigs on branches interlaced. In spring, mulberry trees shoot out new twigs that grow very quickly and will become rough and long by the time of summer. It shows a strong vitality, and therefore, Bao Pozi (i. e. Ge Hong, a medical expert and well-known alchemist in East Jin dynasty) said, "No medicine of panacea should be taken unless it is decocted over the mulberry wood fire". Many panacea or health maintenance formulas of Taoists were decocted over the mulberry wood fire because of its vitality. In fact, wood charcoal fire is vital, but the mulberry charcoal fire is the best.

The best season for picking Sangzhi is at the end of spring and the beginning of summer, and the newly sprouted twigs every year should be collected and cut into slices, which will become yellow in color after being dried up.

The mulberry twig is sweet in taste with slight bitterness and mild in nature. Compared to the whole mulberry tree, new twigs are far smaller, and they are like the collaterals, indicating that the mulberry twig can function to dredge collaterals. Generally, the twigs of plants can dredge the limbs of human body, so the mulberry twig is also corresponding to limbs, especially the upper limbs. Combined with the previous analyses about the mulberry tree that collects the vital life essence from the Jī star, it is able to dispel wind. Therefore, Sangzhi can go through the limbs, dispel wind and activate collaterals.

Common Medicines for Limbs and Neck and Shoulder

By the way, the mulberry twig is often used as Yaoyinzi (an ingredient herb added to enhance the effect of a dose of medicine), which can guide the effect of the prescribed medicines to limbs and collaterals. Meanwhile, it is characterized with vitality to go upwards, so its most important efficacy is on the upper limbs of human body, especially on fingers. All ailments related to limbs, especially those related to the upper limbs are often treated with mulberry twigs.

The book *Benshi Fang* (*Effective Formulas for Universal Relief*) by Xu Shuwei in Song dynasty records an empirical formula: "to cure arm pain, take one small *Sheng* (a unit of dry measure for grain in ancient time of China) of Sangzhi and cut it into fine slices and parch it, then decoct it with 3 litres of water till 2 litres of decoction is left, and then drink it up now and then within a day." To be exactly, one *Sheng* roughly equals to the present 60g, and add 4 to 5 times of water for decocting. The mulberry twig is able to guide its vitality to the arms, and the pathogens will then find nowhere to hide inside. This formula can be used for the acute arm pain, but for the chronic arm pain, it has to be treated based on syndrome differentiation, or with Pianjianghuang (zedoary) and the like to be added. Pianjianghuang also goes to the upper limbs and has very good effect for driving out pathogens and relieving pains.

If there is a pain in the lower limbs, Niuxi (radix achyranthis bidentatae), Mugua (pawpaw), Wujiapi (cortex acanthopanacis) and Duhuo and so on can be added to guide the effect of Sangzhi down to the lower limbs.

The medicines are always interactive, and Sangzhi is inclined to go to the upper limbs, so it can be used as a guiding medicine to lead the efficacy of the other medicines to arms; but for the lower limbs, one use other medicines to guide the efficacy of medicines to play the guiding functions.

Sangzhi can also go to shoulder to relax the cervical vertebra. Many people keep on bending over their desk excessively, resulting in cervical spondylopathy, so some Sangzhi may be added in the prescription; if the cervical spondylopathy is going serious, add some Gegen (radix puerariae) for relaxing the muscle, shoulder and neck; if the cervical spondylopathy is getting more serious, or even there appears some wind-phlegm, Tianma (gastrodia elata) may also be added. So aiming at the uncomfortable cervical vertebra, Sangzhi around 30g, Gegen 10 to 15g, and Tianma 10 to 12g are often used together.

Sangzhi Jian (Decoction) and Treatment of Vitiligo

Sangzhi can dredge collaterals, while the vitiligo is related to the obstruction of collaterals. Can Sangzhi be used to cure the vitiligo? The book of *Taiping Shenghui Fang* (*The Peaceful Holy Benevolence Formulas)* records a formula called **Sangzhi Jian** (Mulberry Twig Decoction).

Take Sangzhi 10 *jin* and Yimucao (motherwort) 3 *jin* to boil into a paste, and then take it after mixing with warm liquor (referring to yellow rice wine) before sleep for treating purpura wind and vitiligo until they are healed up.

Take Sangzhi 10 *jin* and Yimu 3 *jin*, and add enough water to boil for decoction, then filtrate away the dregs. Boil the filtrated decoction with soft fire slowly into paste. Of course, a little honey may be added or some other ingredients to extract the paste. As for the paste preparing, in fact, only very small amount can be extracted, but the finally prepared paste has a very high medical concentration, which then is to be taken before sleep after mixing it with liquor.

Yimucao is a medicine for cooling and dispersing blood stasis, and it can nourish blood without causing phlegm-dampness. Generally, medicines for nourishing blood, like Shengdi, is able to cause phlegm-dampness, and Shudi (radix rehmanniae praeparata) is even worse in this respect, but only Yimucao will not. When used together with Sangzhi, Yimucao can dispel wind, and so, it can cure purpura wind and vitiligo. The said warm liquor in the past generally referred to yellow rice wine that is perfectly heated to a proper temperature for mixing with the paste and drinking before sleep. "Wine travelling to the four limbs" tells us that it is able to extend to the whole body to warm up all collaterals. Sangzhi has the function to dredge collaterals, and with the promotion of liquor, it obtains much stronger power to get through collaterals.

In addition, what I want to call attention to "the extent of using the paste" is to the degree that the disease is cured, that is to say, the patient can take the paste until his disease is completely cured. Definitely, it may take much longer time since vitiligo itself is a kind of chronic disease that is difficult to be cured.

The disease of vitiligo, to a great extent, results from collaterals being blocked up, due to which blood cannot extend to the obstructed points where white spots arise. The ancients left behind this formula, but whether it is effective or not, I dare not make a comment since I have not practiced it fully, however, the learners may borrow the ideas in it. Sangzhi is a medicine with great vitality and efficacy for dredging collaterals, and Yimucao is a medicine for cooling blood and eliminating blood stasis and nourishing blood as well, both of which give a reminder that one should try to get through collaterals, nourish blood, eliminate blood stasis, try to avoid using the medicines that may constitute phlegm-dampness and attend to dispel wind while he/she is trying to give treatment of vitiligo. This is the idea for vitiligo treatment drawn from the ancient formula.

Regarding treatment of vitiligo, there are now many formulas, for instance, **Siwu Tang Jiajian** (Decoction of four medicines plus and minus), with some medicines added mainly for dispelling wind and dredging collaterals. Surely, Sangzhi and Yimucao may also be added. The specific addition and subtraction of medicines will be determined according to the specific conditions of individual patients. In the case of deficiency Yin, the medicines for nourishing Yin should be added, while in the case of phlegm condition, the medicines for reducing phlegm may be added, or even the carminative medicines like Wugong (centipede) or Jiangcan (stiff silkworm) etc. may be added, but these additives are only made in due time and cannot be used on long-term basis.

Sangzhi and Guizhi

When it comes to Sangzhi, it always brings up with Guizhi. Both of them are branches of plants that, as medical herbs, can go to the arms and legs. However, Guizhi is more often used than Sangzhi. Both Sangzhi and Guizhi can enter the upper limbs, but Sangzhi is mild in nature and it can be used for both chills and fever, while Guizhi is hot in nature. So, if the diseases in arms and legs arise from chills, Sangzhi should be used with a little Guizi added. The hot Guizi can warmly remove all the wind-cold damp pathogens.

Regarding Guizi, there will be a detailed description and discussion in the next volume. Here the focus will be put on the functions of Guizi in the treatment of various rheumatoid arthritis, arm and leg pains. Guizi can induce perspiration and relax muscle, and warmly dredge collaterals. Whenever there arise any symptoms of chills, Sangzhi and Guizhi may be used together. They can function very smoothly, and at the same time, the warm nature of Guizi can help Sangzhi to dredge collaterals.

Qianghuo (Notopterygium Root) and Duhuo (Radix Angelicae Pubescentis)

In relation to Sangzhi, a series of medicines will be discussed for treatment of wind-pathogens in between blood vessels and bones. In the commonest case, when suffering from the wind pathogens, a patient will have some obvious symptoms of a common cold. There is another case that the exogenous pathogenic factors may imperceptibly infringe upon the human body, stay in between skin, bones, meridian and collateral channels, "pitch a camp" there, do some destruction furtively, and collaborate from within with the exogenous pathogenic factors from outside as like draws to like. Under such conditions, the patients will feel sore, or ache, or swelling, which are the troubles caused by the wind, chills, dampness and heat in between skin, meridian and collateral channels, muscles and bones. All of these symptoms will then result in many related diseases like arthritis, rheumatosis, and other chronic pains in body.

Especially in the south of China, it is warm, and the hot season always lasts long. Generally, the human body Yang is inclined to go to the superficies. So, in most of the time, the skin pores on human body are inclined to be in an open state, combined with the wind and heavy dampness, rheumatism may easily launch intrusion through the pores. As such, a lot of people suffer from rheumatism and rheumatoid disease. Also, air conditioners may blow the neck directly, which may also easily result in the troublesome cervical spondylosis that is rooted deeply. Such a disease also arises unconsciously from exogenous pathogenic factors. However, the exogenous pathogenic influence is always a slow process in which the pathogens will first "pitch a camp" inside and then run its small groups to develop its own bases. But after it is rooted deeply, it would be much more troublesome than a common cold to cure.

Functions of Qianghuo and Duhuo

Qianghuo goes to upper limbs while Duhuo goes to the lower limbs. Qianghuo has a very strong medical efficacy, running extremely rapidly, going to Taiyang channel and running wildly across arms. It is good at curing urticaria, i. e. the faintly discernible and penetrating wind-pathogen running here and there like the roving bandits who are quite difficult to catch if without some special techniques to be used. By the way, Qianghuo is often used together with Fangfeng.

Duhuo is slightly slow in its curing effect. It goes through chest, abdomen, waist and knee, going to Shaoyin channel, and being good at driving away the concealed wind. The so-called concealed wind refers to the wind lurking deep inside the human body. Duhuo is slow in nature, but it can search out the pathogenic wind even if it is lurking tightly deep inside.

The urticaria is inclined to go to the upper side or to the superficies, while the lurking wind is inclined to go to the lower side or inside. Qianghuo is good at driving away the drifting wind, going to arms; and Duhuo is good at driving away the lurking wind, going to lower limbs. According to the medication experience, Qianghuo is for curing the arm pains and Duhuo is for curing pains in the lower limbs. When the pathogenic factor is shallow at the superficies, Qianghuo can work well, which has a strong and rapid effect so as to quickly drive out away the superficial pathogenic factors. When the pathogenic factor is deep inside, Duhuo may have to be used, which is slow in nature but it is able to search out the pathogenic factors one by one in no hurry.

Much Ado About Strengthening Healthy Factors over Unhealthy Ones

Both Qianghuo and Duhuo are pungent, warm and penetrating in properties, and they usually disperse pathogenic wind at the cost of consuming Qi and blood, to which attention must be paid when they are used. In the treatment of various rheumatic diseases, try to use less tonic medicine if the pathogenic influence is strong. When the pathogenic influence becomes weaker, try to follow up with Danggui, Shengdi and Jixueteng (caulis spatholobi) in time. All of these medicines are to nourish Yin and blood in order to revitalize blood sufficiently. Otherwise, too much consumption of blood will cause that the loss outweights the gain. "When the pathogens gather, the healthy Qi will definitely be in deficiency. " Too much consumption of blood will result in failure of defense of body against exogenous intrusion. So, at the time of medication, one has to consider to fix the adverse factors caused by medicines at the same time. And that "nourishing blood should always comes first in order to dispel wind. When blood circulates smoothly, wind will extinguish itself". So, nourishing blood is another way of dispelling wind.

Arthralgia refers to the wind-cold damp pathogen stagnated in between skin, bone marrow, meridians and collaterals, especially in the joints. The dampness always stays or prefers to stay in the joints. However, joints are the blood vessel intersections where there are a lot of blood vessels. Besides, the liver dominates anadesma, and attracts the wind as like drawing to like. So the pathogenic wind will easily remain in the joints. When wind and dampness pathogens fall together, they will become chronical. Combined with the complex architecture and fine aperture inside the joints, the pathogenic factors will stay in the aperture and become quite difficult to penetrate out. For all these diseases, rheumatism or rheumatoid diseases, the most important thing is to give priority to driving away the pathogen while it is vigorous. As soon as the pathogen is getting weaker, try to drive out the pathogen on the one hand, and strengthen healthy factors on the other hand.

It sounds simple, but in fact, it indeed takes time and difficulties in nursing and treating arthralgia to a normal healthy condition. In clinical treatment, medication needs adjusting in accordance with specific circumstances concerning what percentage of dosage is for nourishing the healthy factors and what percentage of dosage is for driving out the pathogenic factors. If the proportion for medication is not properly controlled, the fierce and strong medicines like Qianghuo and Duhuo will consume and impair the healthy factors once they are overused, or mild medicines like Danggui, Dihuang, and Jixueteng etc. will invigorate the pathogenic factors once they are overused. So, of all these medicines, their respective dosage proportion must be adjusted timely and accordingly, which is a basic principle for treatment of arthralgia.

Wujiapi (Cortex Acanthopanacis)

For treatment of arthralgia or rheumatism, there is another good medicine, i. e. Wujiapi (cortex acanthopanacis).

Wujiapi is pungent, warm and aromatic in properties, which can dispel wind, eliminate dampness, induce diuresis to alleviate edema and strengthen muscles and bones. The water-dampness often lies in the lower part, so Wujiapi combined with Mugua (pawpaw) will go downwards to the lower limbs to induce diuresis.

From the perspective of divination, five signifies the earth. The plant of Wujiapi contains five elements with its leaves, flowers, joints, roots, stem respectively in five different colors of blue, red, yellow, white and black, and its flower with five petals, and its twigs with five leaves. It is the quintessence of the five stars, which is a constellation in the sky. The slender acanthopanax grows from the five stars constellation nutrients. Besides, there are a lot of medicines related to "Five" according to their Chinese names, like Wuweizi (fructus schisandrae chinensis), Wulingzhi (trogopterus dung), Wujiapi (cortex acanthopanacis), which are all related to the earth in the five elements (metal, wood, water, fire and earth).

Fairy Medicine for Health Maintenance

Many books say Wujiapi is a fairy medicine for health maintenance. In fact, its main function is to drive out the wind-cold damp pathogens.

I guess, probably because most of those who take some pills of immortality and try to cultivate themselves to become immortals dwelling at certain places in the famous mountains and along the great waters, or even directly in some cases, where the environment is heavily moist and damp, so they used Wujiapi to drive out the wind-cold damp pathogens, but it does not mean it is effective for all people.

One may say he or she has met with such-and-such a Laojun (originated from the holy title given by Taoists to Lao Tzu, founder of Taoism, a philosopher in the Spring and Autumn Period, here referring to those who are cultivating themselves with wish to become an immortal) and he takes Wujiapi every day. However, one may fail to know that the so-called Laojun dwells in the cave throughout the year and has to drive out the wind-cold damp pathogens in order to treat his wind-cold-dampness type of arthralgia that can make him feel comfortable. The modern people who live in the high-rise building and take fat meat and fine grain in fact need not take Wujiapi as Laojun did.

Functions of Wujiapi

If a child is not able to take a step to walk by five years old, that would indicate that his postnatal somatic function cannot support him to collect and store the refined nutritious substances from water and grains in his kidneys because of his congenital deficiency, which then causes the phlegm-damp to be accumulated in the body and retards the vitality. In this case, Wujiapi can be used to aromatically refresh the spleen, remove the cold-dampness, and dredge meridians and collaterals, after which he will be revitalized gradually. Of course, such a case seldom takes place.

Wujiapi is often used with Nuzhenzi (fructus ligustri lucidi) as Nuzhenzi can nourish Yin, and it can astringe the vital life essence inwardly. However, Wujiapi is pungent-warm in nature, and it can disperse from inside to outside. So the two medicines can make the best of them and complement each other when used together.

But now in Beijing, one may fail to find Wujiapi in the drugstore since such a medicine is rarely used in the north of China where is dry. Therefore, many people in the north feel uncomfortable after taking Wujiapi. However, in the south of China, this medicine is quite often used, especially those people along the Yangtze River, they take this medicine directly to soak in liquor for drinking every day. Those who suffer from arm or leg pains, after drinking, will feel very comfortable since it can eliminate dampness, dispel wind, induce diuresis to alleviate edema, and strengthen muscles and bones.

Why is it able to strengthen muscles and bones? In fact, it cannot nourish muscles and bones directly, but it can drive the wind, coldness, dampness and pathogens out of muscles and bones. Without disturbance from pathogenic factors, the muscles and bones will naturally become strong, so Wujiapi just plays an indirect role in building up strength of muscles and bones.

Qinjiao (Gentiana Macrophylla) and Weilingxian (Radix Clematidis)

The best Qinjiao (gentiana macrophylla) grows in places of high altitude in the north of China, so in the prescription, this medicine is often written as "northern Qinjiao". It can dispel wind, eliminate dampness, relax muscles and activate collaterals, clear heat and relieve pain.

Analyses of the Cool Nature of Qinjiao

Qinjiao always reminds of the formula "**Qinjiao Biejia San**", which is for curing hectic fever. it is used only when there is a fever. The ancients described it as: pungent, bitter and mild in properties. Mildness in nature means that it is neither cold, nor hot, nor warm, nor cool, but now it is generally used as a cool medicine. Why is it so? For any medicine, if it is pungent in taste, it will have the property of dispersion; if it is pungent but not warm, it may be inclined to be cold. And if it is bitter additionally, bitterness plus mildness will then make it tend to be cold. Many medicines take such properties, and the medicines themselves are mild in nature, but because they are pungent and bitter in taste, their medical properties are influenced and then have the cooling function. So, it is mild in nature but it is used for cooling effect, and that is why it is now used as a cool medicine. For general arthralgia with hot symptoms, Qinjiao should be used; but for arthralgia with cold symptoms, never use Qinjiao.

Regarding the four properties of medicines, those medicines which are mild in nature are inclined to be cold if they are pungent and bitter in tastes. Otherwise, they will be inclined to be warm if they are pungent and sweet in tastes since the medicines that are pungent and sweet in tastes always have dispersing effect.

Uses of Qinjiao and its Compatibility

Qinjiao has a very good effect for relieving pains, especially the heat pain. When a joint is red, sore and swollen, Qinjiao will be very effective, and it always goes to the lower limbs to dispel wind and eliminate dampness in legs. It is commonly used with the herbs of Duhuo, Mugua, Niuxi and Shenjincao (lycopodium clavatum) etc. Generally, 3 to 5 *qian*, i. e. 10 to 15g of Qinjiao will do. Meanwhile, it is also a common medicine for treatment of rheumatic diseases.

There is a saying: so long as one feels uncomfortable when making a move, neither sore nor painful, or either sore or painful, that is, feel rotten anyway, two herbs are added right away in the medical formula: Qinjiao and Weilingxian (radix clematidis). The dosage of Qinjiao about 10 to 15g and Weilingxian around 12g will do. Is it really so? Definitely! But I do not advise it. It is better to give treatment based upon syndrome differentiation since the patient feels comfortable after taking the two medicines, it is often just a temporary solution.

Qinjiao, after all, is a dispersing medicine, which will consume Qi and blood, so it should not be used too long. How about Weilingxian then? For this medicine, just use its root, which is very thin and hard like a steel wire with a core in it. It is often called "steel foot Weilingxian", whose medical property is strong, fierce and acute, moving but without holding. It can go through 12 meridians and collaterals. Generally speaking, doctors do not talk about what meridian the medicine of Weilingxian is subsumed to since it does not go to any specific meridian and also it goes very rapidly. It can dispel wind, and especially for those swelling and pain, numb, and uncomfortable scleromere arising from meridian obstruction due to wind cold, Weilingxian may be used for getting it through. By the way, Weilingxian should never be used long since it is too fierce and acute, and it can cause too much consumption of energy of human body.

Meanwhile, when it is used, many other adjuvant medicines must be used as well. However, under no circumstancess should it be used for long since lasting use of such a medicine will impair the bones.

Weilingxian: "Bone-Resolving Holy Pill"

Weilingxian (radix clematidis) has a Chinese name "Huagu Shendan" (bone-resolving holy pill) or "Huagu Dan" (bone-resolving pill), which means it can resolve bones. Now that it can resolve the bones of human body, of course, it is able to resolve fish bones as well. Those who are accidentally caught by fish-bone at throat can simply soften the fishbone by drinking Weilingxian-boiled water, or drinking decoction of Weilingxian boiled with yellow rice wine or liquor mixed with white sugar, which will have a good effect.

Can Weilingxian really resolve a bony spur? It certainly can. Many people have lumbar disc herniation or bone spurs, which can be treated based upon syndrome differentiation with Weilingxian around 10g added, and the bone spurs will then be resolved easily. It may be asked whether Weilingxian will impair the bone. In fact, when the patients suffer from the bone spurs, Weilingxian will only resolve the spurs without causing impairment to the good bones. But, stop using Weilingxian when the spurs are almost resolved. Otherwise, the good bones will get hurt indeed.

In fact, there are some other cases related to bones. When lying-in women deliver babies, the maternal bone (pubis) must be open, as such the cunnus will become bigger, which will give a sufficient channel for the birth of a baby. In case the maternal bone does not open, it will result in dystocia. The opening and closing are related to Qi and blood. The failure of maternal bone opening arises from either Qi or blood deficiency, which can also be treated with Weilingxian. Generally, it is used together with Danggui, Chuanxiong and Guiban (turtle plastron), which can open the maternal bone with an amazing speed. If it is not strong enough for descending downwards, Chuan Niuxi (radix cyathulae) can be added in order to guide the medical efficacy to go down quickly. In case of Qi deficiency at the same time, add some Renshen. In addition, Zuomuzhi (xylosma twig) may also be used, but it is a medicine of rarity, special for oxytocic use.

Zuomuzhi actually are the branches of oak trees, growing in the south of China.

Weilingxian tastes bitter and also descends downwards. It goes through the whole body, and then downwards finally, so it has a very good effect for curing the swelling of the lower part of body. Of course, it is effective for curing upper limb swelling as well.

Lulu Tong and Shenjincao (Lycopodium Clavatum)

Many different medicines are available for treatment of rheumatic diseases, and hereunder are a few commonly used and more effective medicines.

Modified Siwu Tang Used for Arthralgia

Generally, for treatment of arthralgia, **Siwu Tang** (decoction of four medical herbs) is taken as monarch medicines in a formula.

Siwu Tang contains four ingredient herbs: Danggui (angelica sinensis), Shaoyao (paeonia lactiflora), Dihuang (rehmannia), Chuanxiong (ligusticum wallichii).

These four medicines are very special: if there is serious blood stasis, the tail part of Danggui should be used since the tail part is inclined to break and disperse the blood stasis; if deficiency of blood arises, the main stem part or simply the whole of Danggui should be used.

Shaoyao is divided into Chishao (radix paeoniae rubra or red peony root) and Baishao (radix paeoniae alba or white peony root). If the pathogenic Qi is vigorous with blood stasis, use Chishao; when blood is needed to cool down, use Chishao with Danpi (cortex moutan radices) added. In case that the pathogenic Qi is not so vigorous and the blood vessels are not so flexible, use Baishao to nourish the liver and soften the blood vessels. By the way, if ankylosis arises, use more Baishao about 30g to 60g, or even up to 90g.

Dihuang (rehmannia) is classified into Shengdi (radix rehmanniae recen) and Shudi (radix rehmanniae praeparata). In case that Yin deficiency arises and the pathogenic Qi is not so vigorous, use Shudi; in case that blood-heat is very serious, use Shengdi.

When a lady is in the period of menstruation, remove Chuanxiong from the prescription since it is a breaking medicine that may easily result in excessive volume of menses, so it requires specific handling in clinical practices.

"Nourishing blood should always comes first in order to dispel wind. When the blood circulates smoothly, the pathogenic wind will extinguish itself". Hence, take **Siwu Tang** as monarch medicine in a formula, and make some proper modification as necessary based upon the symptoms of chills and fever. Generally speaking, the chill-oriented arthralgia is easier to cure, while the fever-oriented is harder to cure. As the old saying goes that "thousands of chills are easier to be dispersed, but one fever is harder to be eliminated!" The cold-pathogen can be dispersed just through warming treatment. Like the cold weather, it is just a piece of cake, and switching on the heater will make the house warm up. Just think of it, no matter how cold it is, the food and vegetables that is left in the house will not go stale easily. However, the heat is very terrible. In the burning hot summer, the food one forgets to put into refrigerator will go stale easily, or even one puts the food into refrigerator, it still goes stale. In the cold season, the food one puts into refrigerator may go frozen, but it does not matter, after he heats it up, it is still delicious. Anyway, this is just a comparison that may not be quite appropriate, but one can take it for reference.

Regardless of wind- or cold- or damp-pathogen, if it is long trapped in joints, it will be definitely transformed into pathogenic heat, which is like an enemy staying in a place for a long time, he would make some troubles of fire and sword. Such a heat is usually more difficult to get rid of, so sometimes a little Shigao may even need to be used.

And then, deficiency and excess symptoms also have to be taken into consideration. That is, in case that deficiency arises, the nourishing method should be adopted, or otherwise, in case that the excess symptom arises, the discharging method should be adopted instead. The deficiency here refers to deficiency of healthy Qi, which should be nourished, while the excess symptom here refers to the vitality of the pathogenic Qi, which then should be discharged mainly. The medicines like Qinjiao, Weilingxian, Wujiapi, Qianghuo, Duhuo, Sangzhi etc. are all for driving out the pathogens.

Sangzhi can drive out the pathogens but also dredge collaterals. It is vital somehow with a slight nourishing effect, but its nourishing will not cause any phlegm-dampness. Based upon deficiency and excess symptoms, and the disease location as well, if the pathogenic factor is in the upper part of body, use Sangzhi and Pianjianghuang (zedoary) to guide the medical efficacy to go upwards; if the pathogenic factor is in the lower part of body, use Mugua, Chuan Niuxi, Duhuo and the like to guide the medical efficacy to go downwards.

Again, try to give the treatment according to the extent of seriousness of pathogenic wind, coldness, dampness and heat: in the case of more serious wind-pathogen, the first priority should be given to dispeling the pathogenic wind; in the case of more serious cold-pathogen, the first priority should be given to warming and dredging; in the case of more serious damp-pathogen, the first priority should be given to removing dampness; in the case of more serious heat-pathogen, the first priority should be given to clearing heat, but make clear where the heat exactly comes from: the Qi system or the blood system.

So, based upon all the above discussed, adjustable medication and clinical practices should be controlled flexibly based on the syndrome differentiation.

When the pathogen is vigorous, stop nourishing; when the pathogen becomes weakened 70 to 80%, start to increase nourishing. All in all, while dispelling the wind-pathogen is being carried on, nourishing blood should be carried out as well. In that way, diseases will then be eliminated. Generally, the deeper the pathogenic influence goes, the longer time it will take to get rid of it, and vice versa; the shallower the pathogenic influence goes, the easier it will be to get rid of the diseases, and probably, only a few doses of medicines will do. Hence, it depends on the specific circumstances, including the treatment for many gouty diseases.

In the process of treatment, more rattan-type medicines can be used, for instance, Jixueteng mentioned previously in which there exists much gum looking like chicken blood when it is cut apart. Rattan-type medicines can be used frequently since rattan or vine is much like meridians and collaterals, or blood vessels in human body. They can play a dredging function. Besides, the medicines for dispelling wind include Luoshiteng (Chinese starjasmine stem), Qingfengteng (sabia japonica) etc, both of which follow the above principles in medical functions.

Lulu Tong to Vitalize the Whole Body

In case that wind-cold-damp pathogens spread all over the body, or when one finds the medical effect fails to function quickly, Lulu Tong (in Chinese, it means "all channels are clear and through") can be used. Lulu Tong, just as its Chinese name implies, it can travel here and there in each and every channel in the body without any obstruction.

Lulu Tong here refers to the maple fruit like chestnuts with small thorns on its surface. The maple tree has a much longer fruiting season, starting at the end of spring and beginning of summer to bear fruits that keep hanging high on the branches by the time of later autumn when all maple leaves drop completely, or even in the long-lasting severe winter while snowflakes are whirling in the roaring north wind, the fruits will still not fall down until the next spring when the maple tree starts to sprout again. Such a feature of its withstanding wind signifies that the fruit is good for the treatment of the wind pathogens. Falling down by the time of spring shows that it reacts to the vitality of this season and then falls down. However, if used as a medicine, it should be picked in winter timely before it is about to fall. Otherwise, when it becomes withered, its medical efficacy would become weaker.

Lulu Tong can go through the whole body with the effects of dispelling wind, activating collaterals, alleviating fluid/water retention and smoothening menstruation etc. Of course, if a medicine can smoothen menstruation, the female should not take it in the menstrual period, otherwise, it may result in excessive volume of menses, and then consume the normal blood in body. If a lady suffers from metrorrhagia or metrostaxis (uterine bleeding) occurs, she must take great caution against the use of this medicine since it can go through the whole body and has greater promoting effect. In addition, for some skin diseases, Lulu Tong may also be used to guide the medical efficacy to the whole body.

Many Medicines Are Available for Rheumatic Diseases

Many different medicines are available for treatment of rheumatism. Why is it so? Generally, rheumatism is hard to cure, and in the process of treatment, some physicians throw doubt upon some medicines and then look for some other medicines. That process definitely would take a lot of work, but also give an index to another problem: a lot of people would lose patience and back down when they find one medicine ineffective, and they would prefer to look for another medicine.

The patient is often like a drowning man who will clutch at a straw, and doctors sometimes may also try to look for medicines one after another when they find it difficult in treatment of complicated diseases. Occasionally, they may run across a few medicines that are effective. And then, they would note the herb and reuse it next time for the similar cases. In such a way, they figure out a lot of medicines for treatment of rheumatism. Regarding medicines, it does not mean the more the better, but the key is the doctors' efforts for the proper utilization of medicines.

A few common medicines like Qingfengteng and Luoshiteng etc. for treatment of rheumatic diseases have been discussed, but for some major commonly used medicines, one should have confidence and patience in them since rheumatic diseases are really hard to cure within short time. The most important thing for medical workers to do is to spare no efforts on the study of the specific disease pathologically.

Shenjincao Used for Relaxing Muscles

Shenjincao, as its Chinese name implies, is able to outstretch blood vessels. Because of long lasting disturbance of the pathogenic wind, coldness, dampness and heat, the blood fails to nourish the vessels, causing that the patients fail to stretch out their arms or fingers, i. e. the blood vessel may shrink. As it is known that Baishao can relax the blood vessels, but in case that Baishao does not work well to relax the blood vessels, Shenjincao should be added, which would bring better effect. By the way, Shenjincao is also commonly used for treatment of rheumatism.

Of course, some rheumatism lasts a long time, even resulting in the bone joint deformation. In that case, it is necessary to use some animal medicines like Qishe (long-noded pit viper), Xiezi (scorpion), Wugong (centipede) and the like. But for animal medicines, try to use less as far as possible.

The treatment of rheumatism always takes exceptionally long time, and that is why some patients may lose confidence after a certain period of treatment. So both patients and doctors must proceed with firm confidence. Do not consider that the medicines having been used are not the right choices just because of no obvious effects within a short time, and then resort to some other medicines. In that case, one may fail to cure the disease for lack of a last effort.

Those who major in science of medicine sometimes should try to do some self-examination and find the reasons and solution by oneself. Sometimes, it is the doctor himself who does not make clear medical theories or make sure of the diseases, but he raises doubt on the efficacy of medicines: "Is this medicine not effective? Or is there anything wrong with that medicine? Or should I try to find some other medicines?" All these are to find reasons from the outside, which may only help to get half the result with twice effort.

第三章　桑枝与祛风通络类药

桑枝

风为百病之长，很多病是来源于伤风感冒，这可以很笼统地称为外风；还有很多病是来源于衰老，这可以笼统的称为内风。前面我们通过桑叶，讲了很多治外风的方药，当风邪继续深入，就会进入肢体筋骨之间，这就需要以桑枝为代表的另一类方药。

桑枝性状

桑枝就是桑树的枝条。一颗正常的桑树是枝繁叶茂的，枝上有枝，枝桠纵横交错。每到春天，桑树就抽出新的枝条，枝条长得非常快，长到夏天就很粗很长了。从这点可以看出它有很强的生发之性。所以抱朴子（即东晋的葛洪）说"一切仙药，不得桑煎则不服"，道家的很多奇方灵药、养生方药，都是用桑木火来熬的，因为桑木火有生生之气。其实木炭火就已经有生生之气了，桑木炭的火最好。

春夏之交时采摘桑枝最好，而且一定要采当年发出来的嫩枝，切片，晾干以后，颜色金黄。

桑枝甘平、微苦。相对于整个一棵大桑树来说，当年新发出来的桑枝就比较渺小了，它相当于络脉，所以桑枝有通络脉的作用。植物的枝能通人体的四肢。桑枝也对应人体的四肢，尤其是上肢。再结合上次讲的，桑树是箕星之精，它能够驱风。我们把这几条全部归纳起来，就可以知道，桑枝通行四肢而驱风活络。

走四肢肩颈的常用药

桑枝还经常用来做药引子，把方子的药力带到四肢、络脉中。由于它的性质是生发向上，所以更主要作用于人的上肢，尤其是手指；四肢的病痛，尤其是上肢的各种病症，往往都要用桑枝。

《本事方》记载了一个小验方："治臂痛，桑枝一小升，细切，炒香，以水三大升，煎取二升，一日服尽，无时。"一小升，我们现在大概要用60克的样子，加水的体积大概是桑枝的四五倍。桑枝能把它的生生之气带到胳膊里，胳膊里面的邪气自然就没有容身之所。一时半会儿的胳膊痛可以用这个方子，如果胳膊痛时间长，那就得辨证论治了，还可以加片姜黄之类的药。片姜黄也是走上肢的，有很好的驱邪止痛的效果。

如果是下肢疼，我们可以加牛膝、木瓜、五加皮、独活等，用这些药把桑枝的药力引到下肢。

药和药之间是互相牵引的。桑枝善于走上肢，所以可以作为引经药把别的药引到手臂上来；当要它走下肢的时候，我们又可以用另外一些药把它的药力往下肢引。

桑枝还能够走肩膀，能松颈椎。很多人伏案埋头过多，颈椎不太好，我们可以在方子里面加上一些桑枝；如果比较严重，还可以加葛根，葛根能解肌，使肩颈部放松；如果更严重，甚至有风痰之象，还可以加天麻。所以针对颈椎不舒服，桑枝、葛根、天麻这三味药经常是一起用的。一般桑枝30克左右，葛根用10到15克，天麻用10到12克。

桑枝煎与白癜风的治疗思想

桑枝能够通络，白癜风就跟络脉不通有关。那么用桑枝能不能治白癜风呢？《太平圣惠方》有一个方子叫桑枝煎。

桑枝煎

桑枝十斤，益母草三斤，熬膏，睡前温酒调服。治疗紫癜疯、白癜风，以愈为度。

用十斤桑枝、三斤益母草，先加很多水煮出汁，再把药渣滤掉，把熬出来的汁用小火慢慢煮，药汁就渐渐形成了膏状，当然还可以放一点蜜或者别的什么来收膏。熬膏，最后熬出来的很少，但是药的浓度却很高。熬成膏以后，睡觉前用酒来调服。

益母草是一味凉血化瘀的药，能养血但不滋腻。养血的药，像生地，就有些滋腻，熟地更滋腻了，唯独益母草不滋腻，配桑枝就可以驱风，所以它治疗紫癜风、白癜风。温酒，在过去一般都是黄酒，加热到适口的温度，睡前调服。"酒行四体"，行于全身，是温通的；桑枝是通络的，它得到了酒力的鼓动，透络的能力会更强。

"以愈为度"就是说这个膏你要一直用，用到好为止。时间会比较长，因为白癜风是一种很难治的病，需要时间。

白癜风很大程度上是因为络脉不通，络脉一旦不通，血到不了的地方，就会发白。古人留下的这个方子是否有用，我没有完全照此实践，不好说，但我们可以借鉴它的思想。桑枝是一味有生生之气、又能够通络的药，益母草是一味凉血化瘀又养血的药，这提示我们在治疗白癜风的时候，应该通络、养血、化瘀。少用滋腻的药，并注意驱风，这便是治疗思想。

治疗白癜风，现在方剂很多，比如说用四物汤加减，主要是加驱风通络的药，桑枝和益母草也可以加进去。具体加减法就要根据患者个体情况而定了，如果阴虚就要养阴，如果有痰就要化痰，甚至可以加进去蜈蚣、僵蚕等驱风的药，这是适时加进去的，不能长期用。

桑枝与桂枝

讲到桑枝我们就会想到桂枝，同样是树枝，同样是走四肢的，同样是很常用的药，桂枝比桑枝用得更多，如果说桑枝是走上肢，那么桂枝同样也是走上肢的。桑枝是平性的，寒热都可以用。但桂枝是热性的，如果说病在四肢，又是因为受了寒，那么在用桑枝的同时再加一点桂枝，桂枝是一味温药，风寒湿邪都能被桂枝温化掉。

关于桂枝，我们将在下一卷详细讲。这里我们主要讲桂枝在治疗各种风湿关节炎、胳膊疼、腿疼方面的作用。桂枝可以发汗解肌、温通经脉，我们主要取它温通经脉的作用，有寒象时可以桑枝桂枝一块用，它们会走得非常顺利，而且桂枝的温性也会加速桑枝通络的作用。

羌活和独活

围绕桑枝，我们要讲一系列治疗筋骨之间风邪的药。

人受了外邪，最常见也最明显的反应就是感冒。还有一种情况，就是外邪在不知不觉中侵犯了你的身体，病留在肌肤骨骼经络之间，偷偷地搞破坏，慢慢安营扎寨，而且跟外邪同气相求，里应外合。人在这种情况下，或者酸、或者痛、或者肿，这就是风、寒、湿、热在肌肤经络筋骨之间作祟。现在很多关节炎、风湿病、各种慢性身痛等，都与此有关。

尤其是在南方，气候温暖，炎热的时间较长，人体阳气偏于走表，毛孔张开的时候偏多，又加上风多、湿重，风湿更容易从毛孔侵入，很多人都得风湿、类风湿病。还有，空调对着人的脖子吹，也容易吹出颈椎病来，很难受，这也是受外邪而不觉，病根子就落下了。因为受邪有一个过程，邪气先在里面安营扎寨，再经营自己的小团体，发展自己的根据地，扎下了根，治疗起来就比感冒麻烦得多。

羌活、独活的作用

羌活走上肢，独活走下肢。

羌活的药力很峻猛，跑得也特别快，它走太阳经，且能横行于手臂。它善治游风，也就是若有若无、游走不定的风邪。就像那种流寇，今天在这里，明天在那里，没有点儿本事你还真的抓他不住。羌活经常跟防风相配。

独活的力量要稍微缓一些，它通行胸腹腰膝，走的是少阴经，善理伏风。所谓伏风，就是潜伏很深的风。独活，它的性质是慢悠悠的，风邪躲得再紧，都能够被它揪出来。

游风偏上、偏表，伏风偏下、偏里。羌活和独活一个善治游风，走手臂，一个善治伏风，走下肢。上肢痛用羌活，下肢痛用独活，这也是用药的经验。当邪气比较浅的时候用羌活，因为羌活的药力峻猛，速度快，能速战速决，把表浅的邪气及时地赶出去。当邪气很深的时候你就只能用独活了，因为它很缓和，能够慢悠悠地给你找，把一个一个的特务揪出来。

扶正去邪费拿捏

羌活和独活都是辛温走窜的，它们驱风，都要以消耗气血为代价，这点我们在用的时候要注意。在治疗各类风湿病时，邪气盛就少用补药，当邪气弱了，要及时用当归、生地、鸡血藤等来跟进。这些药都是滋阴养血的，要及时把血养足，不然，耗血耗得太多恐怕就得不偿失了。"邪之所凑，其气必虚"，血耗得太多，机体就没有抵御能力了。所以我们在用药的时候，还要同时考虑修复它们可能带来的一些不利因素。而且，"治风先治血，血行风自灭"，治血也是治风的另一途径。

痹症，是风寒湿邪阻遏在肌肤、骨髓、经络之间，尤其是在关节。我们可以去分析：首先，湿留关节，湿气就喜欢留在关节里面。此外，关节为筋之会，关节部位的筋都是很多的，而肝主筋，肝与风同气相求，所以风邪也容易留在关节里面。风湿之邪结合起来，缠绵不去，加上关节里面结构比较复杂，有很小的缝隙，这些邪气躲在小缝隙里面，更不容易透出去。对于所有这些病，风湿或者类风湿等，首先在邪气比较盛的情况下，以驱邪为主，当邪气驱得差不多了，一方面驱邪一方面要扶正。

这话听来简单，实际上，把痹症调理正常是需要一段时间的，这个颇费拿捏。在临床上根据具体情况，把握好用药，几分养正？几分驱邪？如果比例把握不准，羌活、独活这些比较峻猛的刚燥之药，用多了就耗伤了正气；而当归、地黄、鸡血藤等阴柔之药，用多了又会助长邪气。在这二者之间，应该时时注意调整它们的比例。这是治疗痹症的一个基本原则。

五加皮

治疗痹症，或者说风湿，还有一味比较好的药就是五加皮。

五加皮辛温芳香。它能够驱风除湿，利水消肿，强筋壮骨。水湿往往在下，所以五加皮跟木瓜一块用，就往下肢走，可行水利水。

从术数上讲，五为土。五加皮这种植物色备五行，它的叶、花、节、根、秆，分别具备青、红、黄、白、黑五种颜色，而且花有五瓣，枝分五叶，是五车星之精。五车星是天上的一个星宿，五加是得此星精气而生的。此外还有很多含"五"的药，比如五味子，五灵脂，五加皮，都与五行中的土有关。

仙家养生要药

很多书上都说五加皮是仙家养生的要药，其实它的主要功用还是驱风寒湿邪。

我猜想，可能是因为这些修仙之人大多居住在名山大川之间，甚至有些人就是直接居于洞穴之内，湿气比较重，就以此驱邪，并非所有人吃五加皮都管用的。

可能你在某某洞府中遇见某某老君，发现他怎么天天服用五加皮呀，殊不知他常年居住在那石洞中，必须以此来驱他的风寒湿邪，来治他的风寒湿痹，他吃得很舒服。而你住在高楼广厦之中，每天吃膏粱厚味，就没必要像他那样用五加皮了。

仙家养生的要药，不一定是我们这些凡夫俗子的养生要药。

五加皮的作用

小孩子如果到五岁以上还不能走路，那是因为先天不足，而后天水谷之精微不能收藏入肾，造成体内痰湿积聚，阻滞了气机，可以用五加皮，芳香醒脾，化寒湿，通经络，气机转过来就慢慢好了。当然这种情况现在很少见。

五加皮经常配女贞子。女贞子是一味养阴的药，能往里收敛精气；五加皮则辛温耗散，是从里往外通的。二者正好相互取长补短。

但现在在北京，如果你方子里开五加皮，在药店里通常是抓不到的，因为北方很少用这味药。北方本来就干燥，很多北方的人服用五加皮就会不舒服。而南方用得多，长江沿岸的人服用此药比较多，很多人就直接拿五加皮泡酒喝，一天喝一点，胳膊疼腿疼的人，喝得会很舒服，因为它能够利湿行水，驱风除湿，利水消肿，强筋壮骨。

它为什么能够强筋壮骨？并不是说它直接能补你的筋、补你的骨，而是它能够把风、寒、湿、邪从你的筋骨里驱逐出去，没有邪气的骚扰，你的筋骨就自然强壮，在这里它是起间接的作用。

秦艽与威灵仙

秦艽以北方海拔高处产的为好，开方子时往往写"北秦艽"。它能驱风除湿，舒筋活络，清热止痛。

秦艽性凉

说到秦艽，我们就会想起"秦艽鳖甲散"这个方子，它是治骨蒸痨热的，有热才用。古人是这样描述它的作用：辛苦平。平性，就是说它不寒不热不温不凉，但我们现在一般把它当做凉药来用，为什么呢？因为它味辛，辛就能散，一味药辛而不温，它可能就偏凉了。加上它又苦，苦而平则偏寒。很多药都是这样，本身是平的，但因为辛苦之味，影响了它的性，它就有凉的作用了。可以说，它是体平而用凉。我们现在都拿它当凉药来用。一般痹症有热象的会用到秦艽，如果寒象重就不用秦艽了。

在四气上，本质是平性的药如果味辛苦就会偏寒，如果味辛甘就会偏温，因为辛甘发散为阳。

秦艽的配伍及使用

秦艽止痛的效果也非常好，尤其止热痛，当关节又红又肿又痛的时候，秦艽是很常用的一味药，而且秦艽善于往下肢走，驱下肢的风湿，与独活、木瓜、牛膝、伸筋草等药一块用比较多。一般用三至五钱，也就是10到15克就够了，秦艽也是在治疗风湿性疾病经常用的一味药。

有一种说法：人只要身体的筋骨感觉不爽利，身体筋骨动起来，酸不是酸，疼不是疼，或者说要么是酸要么是疼，很难受，只要是身上难受，马上在方子里加上两味药：秦艽和威灵仙。秦艽可以用到十到十五克，威灵仙用十二克左右，用下去就舒服了。有没有这个作用呢？有！但是我不太主张这么用，还是得辨证论治，喝下去身体舒服了，往往只是一时的功劳。

毕竟秦艽它是一味往外耗散的药，它能耗人的气血，不宜久用。威灵仙呢？威灵仙这味药，用的是根。它的根很细很硬，跟铁丝似的，中间有心，所以我们也经常叫它"铁脚威灵仙"。威灵仙药性比较猛，比较急，走而不守，通行十二经络。我们一般不讲威灵仙归什么经，因为它每一经都去，而且跑得特别快。它能够驱风，尤其是风寒壅滞经络的一些肿痛，麻木，骨节不舒，都可以用它来通一通。威灵仙更不宜久用，因为它太猛太急，对人的消耗量太大了。在用的时候要用很多佐药来佐它。即使有佐药也不能久用，因为久用就会伤骨头。

化骨神丹威灵仙

威灵仙别名叫"化骨神丹"，又叫化骨丹。它能把骨头给化了。既然能化人的骨头，那么它同样能化鱼的骨头化肉骨头。如果吃鱼的时候不小心被鱼刺卡住了，很简单，用一丁点威灵仙熬水，喝下去鱼刺就软了；或者用威灵仙拌白糖，用黄酒或者白酒煎服，效果会更好。

威灵仙能不能化各种骨刺呢？也是可以的。很多人有腰椎间盘突出或者长骨刺，咱们在辨证论治的基础上加一些威灵仙，十克左右就可以了，它会化得很快。大家会问，威灵仙不是会伤骨头吗？当你有骨刺的时候，威灵仙就是化骨刺的，不伤骨头。当你把骨刺化得差不多了，再用它就伤骨头了。

还有什么问题是关于骨头的呢？产妇在生孩子的时候，交骨（耻骨）必须要开的，交骨一开，阴门就会变大，就会有足够的通道让孩子出来。

若交骨不开，就会导致难产。交骨的开合跟气血有关系，交骨不开，要么气虚要么血虚。治疗临产交骨不开，也会用到威灵仙。一般跟当归、川芎、龟版配伍，开交骨非常地神速。如果嫌它往下走的力度不够的话，还可以加川牛膝，迅速地把药力往下引。如果同时有气虚，还可以加人参。此外，柞木枝也可以用，它是一味比较冷僻的药，是催产的专药。柞木枝是柞树的枝，柞树生在南方。

威灵仙又是苦降的，通行全身，最后它会往下降，所以对于下身的肿，效果是非常好的。当然，上肢的肿用它也有用。

路路通与伸筋草

治风湿的药非常多，在此只列举几味常见常用而且效果比较好的。

痹症常用四物汤加减

治疗痹症一般以四物汤为君药。

四物汤

当归、芍药、地黄、川芎。

这四味药很有讲究：如果瘀血严重，那当归就用尾，因为当归尾偏于化瘀破血；如果血虚，就用当归身，或者索性用全当归。

芍药分赤芍和白芍。如果邪盛，有瘀血，可用赤芍；需要凉血的时候，赤芍又可以配丹皮。邪不盛，但筋不柔，可以用白芍来养肝柔筋。白芍的量可大一些，当关节僵硬的时候，白芍可以用30克到60克，甚至90克。

地黄分生地和熟地，当阴虚邪气又不盛的时候，可以用熟地，当血热比较严重的时候就用生地。

如果是女性来了月经，川芎可以去掉，因为川芎是一味走蹿的药，它一走蹿就容易让月经的经血变得特别多。这都需要在临床的时候灵活把握。

"治风先治血，血行风自灭"。所以要以四物汤为君，进行加减。加减的依据，首先是寒热。一般来说，痹症以寒为主的好治，以热为主的难治。"千寒易散，一火难除！"有寒邪，我一温就可以了。冷，咱们不怕，再冷，把暖气一开，屋里面很快就暖和了。哪怕屋子里边再冷，我放在屋子里边的菜啊什么东西不会坏。热就比较可怕了，炎热的夏天，剩菜没搁冰箱里，你回家会发现这些菜很多都馊了，你再把它放进冰箱，它依然腐臭。寒不要紧啊，菜放在冰箱里冻上了，你拿出来热热，还能吃。这是一个模拟，不一定确切，但可以借鉴。

不管是风邪、寒邪还是湿邪，在关节盘踞得久了，都要化热，好比敌人在这里久了就会杀人放火。这个热比较难以除掉，甚至可以用一些石膏。

然后，还得根据虚实，虚则补，实则泻。虚就是正气虚，可以补；实就是邪气旺，就要以驱邪为主了。秦艽、威灵仙、五加皮、羌活、独活、桑枝等，这些都是以驱邪为主的。

桑枝驱邪，也通络，但是它毕竟有生生之气，还是略微有那么一点补的作用。但它补而不滋腻。根据虚实，再根据病位，病在上，用桑枝、片姜黄来把药往上引。如果邪在下，那就木瓜、川牛膝、独活之类，把药力往下引。

再根据风、寒、湿、热这四大邪气的轻重施治：风邪重的以驱风为主，寒邪重的以温通为主，湿邪重的以化湿为主，热邪重的以清热为主，既要清气分的热，也要清血分的热，看这个热到底在哪。

根据这些，灵活用药，灵活把握。

当邪气盛的时候就不要补了，当邪气退去七八分了，你要开始加大补养的力度。总之，一边养血一边驱风驱邪，病就是这样慢慢磨下来的。邪气越深，磨的时间越久，邪气越浅，可能几剂药就给磨掉了，看情况而定。包括很多痛风的治疗，也是这个思路。

在这过程中，藤类的药物可以多用。比如上面我们略微提到了一下鸡血藤，鸡血藤里面有很多树胶，把它切开了挺像鸡血的。藤类药为什么可以经常用呢？藤很像经络，很像血脉，所以能通。驱风的药里面还有络石藤、清风藤等等，都是遵循这个大法。

路路通，通全身

如果风寒湿邪遍布全身，或者你嫌药力行得不够快，可以用路路通。路路通，顾名思义，它能够到处跑，每条路它都能通。

路路通是枫树结的果实，长着刺，跟小板栗似的。它的果实果期特别长，春夏之交结果，深秋季节枫叶落光了，它依然高挂着，漫长的寒冬，雪花飞舞，北风呼啸，它都不掉下来，一直到第二年春天，枫树要发芽了，它才落下来。它很耐风，可见善治风邪。它春天才掉，是感春生之气而落的。但不能等它掉下来再捡回家作药，此时它已经枯死，药力就小了，你必须去采。这味药一般是冬天趁它还在树上的时候采。

路路通通行全身，有驱风活络、利水、通月经等作用。当然，一味药既然可以通月经，那么当女子经期，就不要用它了，否则月经的量可能会变得特别大，从而损耗人体的正常血液。如果女子有崩漏之类的，这味药就更要慎用了。因为它通利的作用较大，它通行全身，是有一定力度的。此外，对于一些皮肤病，要把药力引向全身，都可以用路路通。

治风湿的药为何那么多

治疗风湿的药特别多。为什么有那么多呢？因为风湿难治，治疗过程中一些医家就会对药产生怀疑，于是转而寻找别的药。当然这也颇费了一番苦心，但同时也反映出另外一个问题：很多人没有耐心，用的药没有效果就会打退堂鼓，去找别的药。

病人往往病急乱投医。医生有时候也会犯这样的错，病难乱求药。试试这味药，试试那味药，偶尔会碰到一两味药，效果非常好，他就把这味药记下来，下次再用。慢慢地他们摸索出很多治疗风湿的药，但是药不在多，关键是在运用上下功夫。

所以治疗风湿的药，上面我讲了几味经常使用的，像清风藤、络石藤等，我们可以自己去观察、使用，但一些主要的、常用的药要用好，用的时候要有信心，也要有耐心，因为风湿病不是一时半会能治好的。最重要的是，一定要在病理上，在对疾病的具体把握上下功夫。

舒筋常用伸筋草

伸筋草，顾名思义，能够让筋伸展的一味草药。风寒湿热之邪长期搅扰，血不养筋，病人胳膊、手指伸不直，这就是筋收缩了。前面我讲了用白芍可以舒筋，如果白芍舒不动怎么办呢？配上伸筋草，效果会更好一些。伸筋草也是在治疗风湿时经常用的药。

当然，有的风湿病程实在是太长，骨节关节都变形了，那还是有必要用一些动物药，比如说蕲蛇、蝎子、蜈蚣之类的。只是，这些药能少用就要尽量少用。

风湿病治疗时间特别长，有人治疗了一段时间就没有信心了。所以无论病人还是医生一定要坚定信心。不要短期内效果不明显，就觉得以前用的药是不对的，然后去找其他的药，这样可能会功亏一篑。

学医很多时候要内求而不要外求。反思自己，从自己这边去寻找原因，寻找答案，这叫内求；明明是自己理论把握得不好，对疾病把握的不精，却去怀疑药：是不是路路通这味药不管用啊？是不是桑枝这味药有问题啊？我要不要再去找找别的什么藤啊？这就叫外求，这样反而事倍功半。

Chapter 4　Sangjisheng (Parasitic Loranthus) and Sangbaipi (Cortex Mori)

Sangjisheng(Parasitic Loranthus)

Rarity of Genuine Sangjisheng

In the south of China, in between branches of big mulberry trees accidentally grows a smaller plant, which is usually about 2 to 3 *chi* high with obviously different leaves from those of the mulberry trees. It is called Sangjisheng (parasitic loranthus). Its leaf is slightly round, but thicker than the mulberry leaf and soft. On its back grows a thinnish fluff, which will become light yellow when it is withered.

Sangjisheng is quite common in Sichuan, Guangdong and Guangxi provinces in China, but they only exist on the mulberry trees from which the mulberry leaves are seldom picked. If leaves are often picked, the vital life essence of the mulberry tree will become deficient, and therefore, Sangjisheng may not be easy to grow out. Some mulberry tree planters often pull out Sangjisheng whenever they see it for fear of its damaging the mulberry tree. Therefore, it is rare to find the genuine Sangjisheng right now.

Now Sangjisheng in use is actually miscellaneous parasitic with similar appearance to Sangjisheng. They grow out of some other trees rather than out of mulberry trees, or some similar plants parasitizing the other different trees, but their medical effect is far from that of Sangjisheng. The purely genuine Sangjisheng is quite hard to find. The miscellaneous parasitic anyway does have certain effect to some extent, but the worst thing is that some people substitute the ficus microcarpa twigs for Sangjisheng, which actually is not effective at all.

Dispelling Wind and Going Upwards

The twigs and leaves of Sangjisheng, sweet in taste and mild in nature, can be used as medicines, entering into the liver and kidney meridians, dispelling wind and removing dampness, and strengthening blood vessels and bones.

Sangjisheng can dispel pathogenic wind since it grows through sensing the vital life essence of mulberry trees, and it shares some similar properties and efficacies to the mulberry trees. But Sangzhi (mulberry twig) always goes to limbs, while Sangjisheng goes to the back to disperse the wind thereon. Therefore, AS (ankylosing spondylitis) is often treated with Sangjisheng. The genuine Sangjisheng is very effective for treatment.

As it is known that a plant is often rooted deep in the earth, but Sangjisheng is rooted in a tree, which is nourished by the wind dew in the air and by the vital life essence of the mulberry tree at the root without soaking any turbidity of the earth. It is a comparatively clean and pure plant, hence, the ancients said that it can "nourish blood vessels. "

Going up means it can dispel pathogenic wind and improve eyesight, and consolidate teeth, hair and grow beard and eyebrows as well. Hair is of the end of blood, and only when the blood is sufficient, hair and beard can then grow. Some patients, after chemotherapy or radiotherapy, would lose hair, eyebrows and beard because the blood is impaired. In that case, they can use Sangjisheng for treatment.

Chantui (cicada slough) can remove the ocular hide, but Sangjisheng cannot. Attention: Never use Sangjisheng when a patient suffers from ocular hide.

Miscarriage Prevention With Sangjisheng

Sangjisheng is taken as the top grade medicine in **Shennong Bencao Jing** (**Shen Nong 's Herbal Classic**). It is parasitic, representing an "image of child". When a woman is pregnant, the child is parasitizing the body of mother, which is like Sangjisheng parasitizes mulberry trees. Being parasitic, as "like attracts like", Sangjisheng can prevent miscarriage. Generally, Sangjisheng together with E-jiao, and Aiye will be very effective for curing threatened abortion.

Of course, there are many other medicines for miscarriage prevention like-Huangqin, Baizhu, and Sharen.

As for Huangqin, it is a medicine for clearing heat, but the roasted Huangqin should be used here. It is the common sense that it is appropriate to have a cool prenatal temperature and a warm postpartum temperature since the mother and her child huddle together before delivery and heat is easily produced, so Huangqin can be used for clearing up the heat.

Baizhu is a medicine for tonifying the spleen. That the baby can settle in the mother's womb peacefully depends upon the dominance of the spleen Qi, so roasted Baizhu is used.

Sharen is an aromatic medicine. Generally, an expectant mother should not try any aromatic medicine. But in case she has to, the first choice should be Sharen, which is aromatic, though, its fragrance will not impair the fetus. The medicines that may impair the fetus are Shexiang (musk) and Bingpian (borneol), especially Shexiang, since it has a very strong spurting power. Sharen is also characterized with aroma and spurting influence, but its spurting power is not so strong, and it also has ascending effect. The fetus is the most afraid of descending, when it is consolidated with Baizhu and slightly uplifted with Sharen, the expectant mother will feel quite comfortable and feel light of the falling weight.

Image Thinking in Medication

Regarding the efficacy of Sangjisheng for miscarriage prevention, it is determined from its image, and so are many other medicines, whose efficacies can be perceived from their respective profiles.

It is said that Shi Jinmo, a medical expert, once proposed another medicine for miscarriage prevention, i. e. Canjian (silkworm cocoon), in which there is a silkworm chrysalis. Is it like a baby staying in its mother's womb? When the silkworm moth pips out of the silkworm cocoon, it is a fetus to be born, and the silkworm cocoon is like a tuck net to pocket the cocoon. Shi Jinmo often said the fetus is afraid of falling out, so Canjian can be used to pocket it.

Later on, some followers of Shi Jinmo stop believing in this concept, or they even take it as a joke, which is a great pity. In truth, this tells us the unique features of TCM. It is nothing but that the scientized traditional Chinese pharmacology either ignores the unique features or disdains it or dare not mention it. As a matter of fact, all of these are quite natural. When different things are similar in images, they may share some similar effects, which are worth thinking deeply and practicing as well.

One should have a concept of resonance and understanding to look at some uniqueness of TCM rather than bring it down just because it is not proved scientifically. As a son must look like his father, but why is it so? It is the connection between images, or so to say it is because of gene. The silkworm cocoon looks like a placenta, or so to say the silkworm cocoon takes the image of a placenta. Sangjisheng is parasitic, which is similar to a fetus parasitizing its mother's womb. Therefore, they are similarly interlinked. From this perspective, it might be concluded that they share similar gene to certain extent.

Duzhong (Eucommia Ulmoides) and Parasitic Plant

When Duzhong (eucommia ulmoides) and parasitic plant are used together, they can dispel pathogenic wind and eliminate dampness, and tonify the liver and kidneys.

In Beijing Botanical Garden, there is a large tree, i. e. a tree of eucommia, around which a 3-meter-high tubular wire entanglement is set up. The bark of eucommia can be used as medicine. In order to keep off anyone to peel off bark of the eucommia tree, the lower section of the tree is shielded with wire entanglement. When the bark of an eucommia tree is peeled off, it can be seen that it is purple in color inside, and some very soft filament that needs to take some effort to pull it apart. The soft filament may let us connect it in mind to blood vessles in human bodies. The purple color means it can enter into the blood system; and the liver is known to dominate the anadesma. Therefore, Duzhong can enter the liver meridian and the blood system. It is sweet and warm in properties, and comparatively good at driving out the cold dampness in the Lower Jiao. Meanwhile, it is the rind of tree. Generally, the rind goes on the superficies, so it can drive away the cold dampness from the superficies. Duzhong, similar to parasitic plant, is inclined to dispel pathogenic wind and eliminate dampness, but their tonifying effect is not so powerful. Then, why are they always used for tonifying the liver and kidneys?

Huangdi Neijing says, "The accumulation of pathogens will definitely result in deficiency of Qi". Many people often have lumbago, backache and weak legs, which are all attributable to the deficiency of liver-Yin or kidney-Yin. The kidney deficiency is likely to have sprain of waist, and the liver deficiency is likely to have sprain of ankle, since the waist and the lower part of body are susceptible to the exogenous pathogens (the exogenous pathogenic factors). The pathogenic wind and dampness staying at the lower part of body will make the patients very uncomfortable. Meanwhile, the pathogenic wind and dampness staying continuously at the waist and knees will consume a lot of energy, which will then cause the liver and kidneys of the patients to become more deficient, so Duzhong and parasitic plant are used mainly to dispel and eliminate the lingering pathogenic wind and dampness. As such, the liver Qi can fully develop itself, and the kidney Qi will not lose itself pointlessly. Therefore, to use Duzhong and parasitic plant to tonify the liver and kidneys is, in essence, to accomplish the tonifying purpose by way of driving out the pathogens. Actually, Duzhong and parasitic plant themselves are not powerful enough for tonifying effect.

Duzhong (Eucommia Ulmoides) Guides Qi and Blood to Go Downwards

Duzhong can guide Qi and blood to go downwards. What about going upwards? Those who suffer from Qi and blood going upwards in parallel will then suffer high blood pressure. Duzhong can guide Qi and blood to go downwards. Is this just helpful to reduce blood pressure? Duzhong mainly reduce the high blood pressure arising from wind-cold pathogens Qi in the Lower Jiao. The lumbago and knee pain in those patients with the trouble of hypertension are generally resulted from deficiency of liver-Yin and kidney-Yin, exogenous pathogens intrusion, the liver and kidneys trapped in the above troubles, hyperactivity of liver-Yang, and failure of kidney Yang to store up. Hence, Qi and blood will go upwards in parallel. Duzhong can guide Qi and blood to go downwards and drive out the wind-cold-dampness pathogens.

Duzhong also has a function for miscarriage prevention. In the first place, its bark implies protection. Inside the bark, there is filament looking like blood vessels, which also has the implication of protection.

Contraindications of Duzhong (Eucommia Ulmoides)

Duzhong is a good medicine. In fact, no matter how effective a medicine is, it always has some contraindication.

Generally speaking, if deficiency fire exists in kidneys, try to avoid using Duzhong since it is warm after all and can boost the deficiency fire.

Never use Duzhong when one catches a cold since it always goes to the blood system first and then to the liver and kidneys till it goes to the innermost point of human body. When catching a cold, the patient always has the pathogenic influence on the superficies. At that moment, if Duzhong is used, it will pull and press the pathogens downwards to the interior, causing nephritis when it goes into the kidneys, or icterus when it goes into the liver.

In addition, in case the coating on the tongue is rather thick, caution should also be taken for using Duzhong. The thick coating on the tongue indicates existence of heat and dampness in the Middle Jiao, which has to be removed. In that case, if Duzhong is used, it may guide the heat and dampness to the Lower Jiao, which then will be harder to be eliminated.

Sangbaipi (Cortex Mori)

Collection of Sangbaipi (Cortex Mori)

In **Shennong Bencao Jing**, Sangbaipi (cortex mori) is named as Sanggen Baipi (the root bark of white mulberry).

Strictly speaking, when collecting the root bark of white mulberry, try to select over-10-year-old mulberry tree and collect the bark from the tender roots growing eastwards. But now, in most cases, a mulberry treeis simply cut down to collect the bark of all roots for medicine use.

The newly dug-up mulberry roots are usually bluish yellow or golden in color, but such yellow color is only a very thin cover, after which is removed, a thicker white bark is exposed. That is what should be used as medicine.

By the way, a copper knife should be used for scraping off the outer bluish yellowskin since the mulberry tree is contradictory to iron. The mulberry may be deactivated if it is cut with an iron scraper. While collecting the root bark of white mulberry, one can see much saliva and juice, which is the life quintessence of the mulberry tree and must not be removed.

Generally, the root bark of white mulberry should be soaked with rice-rinsed water (i. e. the left-over water of rice rinsing), because it is slightly pungent and dry in properties. After soaked with rice-rinsed water, it will become more moistening and nourishing.

What Is Meant by "Killing"

Also note that the mulberry root growing out of the earth is toxic, whose bark collected "may kill people" according to the ancient medical books. "Killing" here does not mean it can cause a person to die immediately, but means it could not be beneficial to the person.

The ancients said that many things could "kill" people, for example, Xingren (apricot kernel). In each apricot pit, basically there is only one kernel, but if there are two in a pit, that would be called twin-kernel apricot pit, which should never be eaten according to the ancients because it is "killing". Such a thing is called "loss of its essential state", which is harmful to the human body.

On one occasion, one of my friends visited Xinjiang Uygur Automonous Region of China and brought me a lot of apricot pits, of which I found some with twin-kernel. I ate them deliberately and wanted to prove whether I would be poisoned to death. At that moment, I was thinking that I could give some treatment myself in case I was poisoned, but after taking the twin-kernel of apricot, nothing happened and I was not "killed" anyway.

Did the ancients cheat us? So I made another try and ate the mulberry root exposed to the air. Nothing happened, either.

The humanbody actually has very powerful force of vitality. How can only a few pieces of apricot kernel or mulberry bark "kill" a person? What the ancients said "killing" does not mean to take a knife in the hand and cut off the head down to the ground, but "a soft knife" cuts off the head without any feeling, that is, consuming the life force soundlessly, which may cause some impairment to the body without any sensation.

Therefore, what the ancients said should not be ignored or misunderstood. Never try the things that have been warned against, or deny what the ancients concluded from experiences just because one is not poisoned to death after taking apricot twin-kernels.

Functions of Sangbaipi

Sangbaipi or so-called the root bark of white mulberry is cold from the perspective of the four properties of medicines (cold, hot, warm and cool) , and it is sweet from the perspective of the five tastes (sweet, sour, bitter, pungent and salty) with slight pungency and bitterness. It enters the lung because of its white color; it purges the fire of the lung because of its sweetness and coldness; it smoothens the blood and Qi circulation in the lung because of its slight pungency and bitterness. It enters the lung because of its pungency; and it enters the spleen because of its sweetness. Furthermore, as a root medicine with the property of coldness, it can enter the urinary bladder. Therefore, it can eliminate the dampness and pathogenic heat out of the urinary bladder through urination.

The lung, as a tender organ, is not cold-resistant, but sometimes there exists some deficiency heat in the lung. The deficiency-heat in kidneys goes upwards. As it is known that fire restricts metal, so the kidney fire enters the lung to play a restricting function. The deficiency fire in lung cannot be cleard within a short time. Sangbaipi is only used to clear the lingering and deep heat in the lung. As for the temporary pathogenic influence in the lung arising from a common cold due to wind-cold, it is not deep, and the obstinate deficiency- fire has not taken shape yet, therefore, never use Sangbaipi to clear it in such a case.

Sangbaipi is a medicine for the interior, and it can go deeper in the lung. The heat arising from the pathogenic factors due to a common cold usually lies in a relatively superficial location. In such a case, if Sangbaipi is used, it may guide the pathogens due to a common cold to the interior. In that case, it would be much harder to clear it out again.

In addition, Sangbaipi is also good for treating alopecia (loss of hair) , withering of hair, and kids' dribbling, which are all related the spleen and lung heat. Sangbaipi can purge the spleen and lung heat and give a thorough cure.

Toughness of Sangbaipi

"The mulberry bark paper" is still available in the market. In the ancient time, such paper was taken as the top grade paper, pure white and tough.

The mulberry bark was a necessity in the military supply since it can be rubbed into a thread for stitching incised wounds. The large wound cut with knife, ax, or bayonet had to be stitched with the mulberry bark thread, which is not only good for the wound, but also tough and strong with vitality.

Besides, the silk, related to the mulberry leaf, is also featured with toughness. In spring, the new Sangzhi (mulberry twig) is much tougher, and it cannot be broken easily in the strong wind, which shows the vitality of mulberry trees.

The vitality actually is a sort of toughness, showing its indomitable nature. What is the toughest thing in human body? It is the blood vessel. For sure, the bone is also tough since it obtains the liver Qi and vitality. Children are not susceptible to fracture in case of tumbling, but the old are when falling down since the bone of the old people become fragile.

Let us see the strokes of the Chinese character "脆" (cuì, means fragile): the component of the left side refers to bone and flesh, i. e. the character of "月" ("yuè", means "moon"), while the right side is a Chinese character "危" ("wēi", means danger), indicating that the body is in great danger of fragility.

With time passing by, the old people will become fragile, either the bone or the blood vessel. Once the blood vessel loses its toughness, it will become fracted and cracked, especially the blood capillary, whose fracture or crack will cause cerebral hemorrhage and stroke (apoplexia). Generally, the young people are energetic with vitality and their blood vessels are also flexible, so, few young people in their twenties suffer from apoplexia; The old people are not so energetic and vital because of their senior age, so their bones, blood vessels and hair become fragile. . . .

So are the characters and morals of people. Only those who have strong and tough characters can have vitality of life. Toughness is a quality of indomitability. Those who are indomitable with the ability to stand against temporary setbacks will definitely have a more promising future.

From the toughness of Sangbaipi and silk, it can be seen that the vitality of mulberry trees lies in its toughness. In order to keep healthy, one must keep tough physically and psychologically. Otherwise, the pathogenic wind will arise physiologically, which then results in various diseases. Surely, the pathogenic wind may also arise psychologically, which then results in irrationality, or even loss of control.

Xiebai San

Sangbaipi always reminds of a formula of **Xiebai San**.

Xiebai San contains the herbal ingredients: Sangbaipi (Cortex mori) 1 *liang*, Digupi (cortex lycii radicis) 1 *liang*, Zhigancao (honey-fried licorice root) 0.5 *liang*, Gengmi (polished round-grained rice) 100 grains, taken with warm water after meal.

1 *liang* is equivalent to 30g. **Xiebai San** is a sort of powder that is not required to orally take all once, but only a little each time. Both Sangbaipi, Digupi should be parched yellow, after which they are mixed with Zhigancao and Gengmi, and then crushed into powder.

The lung is corresponding to the white color. **Xiebai San** actually is a powder for purging the lung of the pathogenic fire. Digupi can enter the kidney to clear the deficiency fire and the endogenous heat due to Yin deficiency. A sort of heat seems to be emitted from the bone, which can make patients feel the endogenous heat due to Yin deficiency. The long lasting low-temperature fever arising from Yin deficiency should be cleared with Digupi. The lung is the upper source of fluid, from which the kidney receives fluid and obtains real life essence. The lung generates the life essence for the kidneys. The lung is the mother of the kidney, and the mother always gives the best to her son, while the son, on the contrary, often brings his mother troubles, so the deficiency fire in kidney is always transferred to the lung easily, but the deficiency fire in the lung in most cases stems from the kidney. When the kidney is in deficiency of Yin, the kidney Yang will not be able to be stored up, and the kidney fire will spurt upwards to the stomach or lung, which will then result in pathogenic fire. The kidney essence (or genuine fluid) coming from the lung is a physiological phenomenon, while the pathogenic fire in the lung stemming from the kidney is a pathological phenomenon. Therefore, some young people suffer from tuberculosis, and look very thin with deficiency fire in lung and coughing. Sangbaipi and Digupi can purge the pathogenic fire, but the former mainly purges the lung of the pathogenic fire, and the latter purges the kidney of the pathogenic fire.

Both Sangbaipi and Digupi are partial to the sweet-cold but not very bitter, otherwise, the bitter-cold may spoil appetite. The sweet-cold can purge fire but will not cause any side effect like spoiling appetite due to the bitter-cold. The excess fire can be cleared temporarily with the bitter-cold, but the deficiency fire is hard to be cleared within short time. Hence, only the sweet-cold can be used here.

Gancao used in the formula can also purge fire, but also relax the Middle Jiao. Gancao is sweet, and it goes to the spleen. Gancao, in case of a small dosage, can function as a blender for coordinating the medicine actions of a formula, but in case of a large dosage, it not only will purge but also clear the fire of the Middle Jiao. **Xiebai San** contains a larger dosage of Gancao, so it can purge fire as well. Meanwhile, The sweet taste has an effect of relaxing the spleen and stomach. Generally, in case there is fire in the lung and kidney, the spleen will become impatient since it lies in the middle with fire at both the upper and the lower sides.

Gengmi functions to clear the lung-heat, nourish the spleen and stomach, help the spleen to support the lung and nourish blood as well.

Those who sufferfrom deficiency fire in lung that, however, has no deficiency symptoms yet, can use **Xiebai San**. However, those who suffer from deficiency in the lung and a lot of urination should not use **Xiebai San**.

Analyses of Xiebai San Formula

Though **Xiebai San** only contains four herbs, it reflects three superpowers: universe, earth and human being. Sangbaipi goes to the lung, which is corresponding to the universe; Digupi is an herb that goes downwards to the kidney (corresponding to earth); Zhigancao and Gengmi go to the Middle Jiao, corresponding to the human being. This formula covers a vast train of thinking, so do many other ancient formulas.

The book *Ancient and Modern Famous Medical Prescriptions* depicts **Xie-**

bai San as: "The fire heat impairs Qi, for which three methods can be adopted for treatment of the lung: in case there is typhoid fever, the pathogenic heat will impair the lung, then **Baihu Tang** can be used for relieving restlessness, which is a temporary solution to cure the symptoms; in case there is internal deficiency, the Yin-fire will impair Yin, then **Shengmai San** can be used for replenishing Yin, which is for a complete cure of diseases; in case the healthy Qi is not impaired, but the stagnated fire is very serious, **Xiebai San** can be used for clearing the lung-heat and regulating the Middle Jiao, which is to address both symptoms and root causes, and can give a remedy for the deficiencies of the first two formulas. " In case the fire heat impairs Qi, the fire heat may lie in the system of Qi, take **Baihu Tang** [containing the ingredients of Shigao (gypsum), Zhimu (rhizoma anemarrhenae) and Gengmi (polished round-grained rice)]. This is a severe cold formula that can clear heat very quickly, but it can merely relieve the symptoms of the disease; in case the deficiency fire impairs Yin, use **Shengmai San** [containing the ingredients of Renshen (ginseng), Maidong (radix ophiopogonis), and Wuweizi (fructus schisandrae chinensis)] to nourish Yin for a complete cure of the disease; **Xiebai San** can address both symptoms and root causes, making up for the deficiencies of the above two formulas.

Digupi (Cortex Lycii Radicis)

As a matter of fact, Digupi contained in Xiebai San is the root of Gouqi plant (lycium), which grows in the north of China. The Gouqi plants in Shanxi and Ningxia provinces in China grow quite well, bearing large pieces of Gouqi (fructus lycii). The Gouqi hangs on the twigs of the plant with rosy and lovely appearance and does not fall down to the ground even in the frost and snow of the severe winter, which shows its anti-aging image. In the season of winter, many things in the nature will get withered, but Gouqi does not. Therefore, many people insist that Gouqi fruits are able to resist aging. In a strong cold wind, its fruit does not fall but still keeps brightly red. As a medicine, it must be inclined to be warm and only the warm medicines can resist the severe cold.

The warm nature of Gouqi does not mean the other parts of the Gouqi plant as medicine are all warm. Its seed is inclined to be warm, but its root is cold and slightly bitter in properties. It is dry in the northwest of China, but the Gouqi plant can grow big with its roots going deeply into the earth to absorb the underground water. From this perspective, Digupi can also go deeper into human body, even to the inside of the bones. Again, it can clear the heat deep inside the bone on account of its bitter-cold property.

Let us see the three Chinese characters "地骨皮" ("Di Gu Pi", cortex lycii radices in English). The first character "地" ("Di", means earth) signifies that it goes to the Middle Jiao. The earth is subsumed to soil, and the soil is subsumed to the neutral. Therefore, according to the **Wuxing Doctrine**, "地" ("Di") is corresponding to human being. "骨" ("Gu", means bone) signifies that it goes to the kidney, which is in the Lower Jiao. So, "骨" ("Gu") is corresponding to the place at the bottom, i. e. to the earth. "皮" ("Pi", means skin) signifies it is corresponding to the lung since the lung dominates the skin and hair, and the lung is corresponding to the nature. And therefore, Digupi is a medicine with a broad sense.

The Chinese name of this medicine "Digupi" implies that it can enter the Middle Jiao to help transportation and transformation (T&T) since it grows out of the earth and it draws the spleen and stomach as the saying goes "like draws to like". When it goes to the kidney, it can clear the pathogenic fire in the Lower Jiao and clear the deficiency-heat in the bone. As the cuticular layer of the root of the Gouqi plant, it can also go to the lung, the skin and hair to disperse the deficiency heat out.

第四章　桑寄生与桑白皮

桑寄生

真品桑寄生为何难得

在南方，大桑树的枝桠之间偶尔会长出一种小植物，两三尺高，叶子明显跟桑树不一样，这就是桑寄生。它的叶微圆，比桑叶厚，而且很柔，背面有薄薄的一层绒毛，当它枯死以后，就呈淡黄色。

桑寄生在四川、两广一带比较多。它必须在不怎么采桑叶的树上才有，如果经常被采桑叶，这棵桑树的精气不足了，就不容易长出桑寄生。桑寄生是一种寄生植物，感桑树的精气而生。一些桑农在桑树上看到桑寄生，往往会把它拔掉，怕它伤害桑树，所以真正的桑寄生就比较难找。

现在我们一般用的桑寄生，其实都是杂寄生，是其他树上长的一些寄生，它虽然形状跟桑寄生很像，甚至就是寄生在不同树上的同一种植物，但它的药力远远不及桑寄生。纯粹的桑寄生我们现在很难找到，杂寄生也还是有一些作用的。最可恶的是现在有很多人用榕树枝来冒充桑寄生，这就一点作用都没有了。

祛风上行

桑寄生枝叶都可以入药，甘平，入肝肾两经，驱风化湿，强筋壮骨。

桑寄生依然是祛风的，因为它是感桑树的精气而生，它跟桑树有很相通的地方，跟桑枝也有一些相似的功能，但是桑枝主要走四肢，桑寄生主要走脊背，驱脊背间的风。所以很多强直性脊柱炎经常用到桑寄生，如果得到真正的桑寄生，效果会非常好的。

我们知道，植物的根都要扎到泥里，但桑寄生的根扎在树里面。上面有风露在滋养它，下面有桑树的精气在滋养它，不沾泥土的污浊，它是一种比较干净、清虚的植物，所以古人说它能"滋养血脉于空虚之地"。

往上走，所以它祛风明目，而且还能够让牙齿、头发坚固，还能长须眉。有人眉毛掉得比较厉害，或者胡子掉得比较厉害，都可以考虑用这个。髪为血之余，必须血液充足，然后才能长头发，长胡子。有的做了化疗或者放疗的人，头发、眉毛和胡子都掉了，为什么？因为伤了血。

上次我们讲了如果眼睛里面有翳障的话，可以用蝉蜕来褪掉翳障。但桑寄生就不能用。切记：如果眼睛里有翳障，千万不要用桑寄生了。

桑寄生何以能安胎

桑寄生在《神农本草经》里列在上品。它是寄生的，有"子象"。"子"就是孩子，怀孕时孩子是寄生在母亲的身上的，就像桑寄生是寄生在桑树上一样，他们都是一种寄生，同气相求，所以桑寄生能安胎。一般配上阿胶、艾叶，治胎动不安，效果非常好。

当然，安胎的药还有很多，如黄芩、白术、砂仁都可以用。

为什么用黄芩呢？黄芩是一味清热的药，在这里用炒黄芩。产前宜凉，产后宜温。因为在产前是母子两个人挤在一起的，容易产生热，黄芩正好清热。

白术是一味健脾的药，孩子能够在胎里安住，要靠脾气的统摄，所以经常要用到炒白术。

砂仁是一味芳香的药。孕妇一般很忌讳用芳香。如果必须用芳香，首选就是砂仁。砂仁虽然芳香，但它的芳香并不伤胎元。伤胎元的香味只有麝香和冰片。尤其是麝香，走蹿力度太强了。砂仁虽然也芳香，也能走蹿，但力度不大，而且它还有升提的作用。胎最怕的是往下掉，现在用白术一固，用砂仁再略微把它往上升提一点，这样孕妇会感觉很舒服，往下坠的感觉就会轻一些。

用药中的形象思维

桑寄生的安胎作用，我们从它的形象上就可以看出来。很多药都是如此，从外形上能感知它的作用。

施今墨老先生曾经讲过另一味安胎药：蚕茧。蚕茧里面有一个蚕蛹，不也像孩子在母亲的子宫里吗？蚕蛾破壳而出，也就像胎儿以后要出生，而且蚕茧像网兜一样，它能够给你兜住。施老先生经常讲，不是这个胎怕掉吗？我用蚕茧把你给兜住。

后来，包括施老的有些弟子都不相信这个了，或者说都把这个当一个笑话来讲，这就很可惜了，其实这也是传统中医用药的一些独到之处。只不过是现在我们已经科学化了的中药学就不讲这个，要么是不屑于讲，要么是不敢讲，其实这些都是自然之理，它们同气相求，在形象上有相似之处，在作用上也有相通的地方。这点值得我们去思考和运用。

我们要用一种共鸣、理解的思维去看，而不能因为它不科学就一棒打死。就像儿子长得肯定像父亲，至于为什么像，这就是一个形象跟形象之间的一种联系，你可以说它是基因。蚕茧长得像胎盘，或者说蚕茧有胎盘的形象，桑寄生是寄生，跟这个孩子怀在母亲肚子里边这样的寄生，也有相似之处，所以它们的作用有相通的地方，我们可不可以说它们有某种共同的基因呢？

杜仲寄生

杜仲跟寄生经常一起用，祛风除湿，补益肝肾。

在北京植物园有一种大树，它底下都围着一个三米多高的筒形的铁丝网，这就是杜仲。它的树皮可以入药。为防止有人来偷刮树皮，下半截就用铁丝网罩起来。杜仲树杆的皮剥下来后，里面是紫色的，掰开后会发现它有丝，非常柔韧，得费点力气才能拉开。看到丝会让我们联想到人体的筋，色紫入血分，筋属肝，所以杜仲是一个入肝经血分的药，甘温，比较善于驱下焦的寒湿，同时它是树皮，皮就会走表，所以能驱寒湿达表。杜仲和寄生都偏于驱逐风湿之邪的，它补益的作用并不大，但为什么我们经常会用它来补益肝肾呢？

《黄帝内经》讲，"邪之所凑，其气必虚"，很多人感到腰酸、腰痛、腿软，大家就说肝肾阴虚，或者直接说肾虚。肾虚容易闪着腰，肝虚容易扭着脚。因为肝肾虚了，外邪就更容易侵袭腰部及下体。风湿之邪就寄居在下身，让人感觉很不舒服。又因为这个风湿的邪气一直在腰在膝盖，就会消耗掉人的很多能量，让你的肝肾更加亏虚，用杜仲和寄生主要还是把缠绵不去的风湿驱除出去。这样，肝气就能充分生发开来，肾气也不会做无谓的亏耗，所以用杜仲和寄生来补益肝肾，其实是通过驱邪来达到补益的目的，它本身的补益力量很小。

杜仲引气血下行

杜仲能引气血下行。那么，气血上行是什么？气血并走于上，人往往会呈现高血压。杜仲引气血下行，不正好可以降压吗？杜仲主要降下焦有风寒邪气的那种高血压。高血压患者出现腰膝酸痛，是因为肝肾阴虚，外邪入侵，肝肾进一步受困，同时导致肝阳上亢，肾阳不能潜藏，这样一来气血就会并走于上。杜仲引气血下行，还驱逐下体的风寒湿邪，用在这里最合适。

杜仲也有固胎的作用。从哪看出来呢？首先它是皮，有保护的意思，皮里面还有丝，像筋一样，也有保护的含义。

杜仲的使用禁忌

杜仲是味好药，但什么药都有不能用的时候。

一般来说，肾中有虚火就不要用杜仲，杜仲毕竟是温的，能助长肾中的虚火。

感冒的时候也不要用杜仲。杜仲是从里走表的一味药，它会先进入血分，进入肝肾，进入人体最深处。感冒的时候，邪气在表，你再用个杜仲，它会首先把邪气往里一拉，往下一拉。拉到肾里，就是肾炎；拉倒肝里，就是黄疸。

此外，要是舌苔比较厚腻，杜仲也要慎用。舌苔厚腻意味着中焦有湿热，中焦的湿热就得在中焦化掉，你用杜仲，把这湿热引到下焦去了，化起来会更难。

桑白皮

桑白皮的采集

桑白皮，在《神农本草经》里叫桑根白皮。

严格说来，取桑白皮，要选择十年以上的桑树，往东边长的嫩根上的皮。现在我们取桑白皮都是一棵桑树伐倒，所有根皮都入药。

刚挖起桑树根是青黄色，或金黄色的，但这个黄色只不过是一层很薄的表皮，把这层皮去掉，里面就是一层较厚的白皮，这才是入药的。

要用铜刀把外面的一层青黄的薄皮刮掉，为什么要用铜刀来刮呢？因为桑树忌铁器，用铁刀来刮它就会使其丧失药性。在取桑白皮的时候，会发现里面会有很多涎和汁，这也是桑树的精华，不能去掉。

桑白皮一般要用米泔水（即淘米水）来浸泡。因为它味微辛，略微有些燥性，用米泔水来泡，会让它变得更加的滋润。

何谓"杀人"

还有一点需要注意：露出土面的桑根是有毒的，在这种桑根上取的桑白皮，古书上讲它"可以杀人。""杀"人并不是让人马上就死，而是对人不好。

古人讲有很多东西都是"杀"人的。比如杏仁，一个杏核里本来只有一个仁，如果有两个，就叫双仁杏仁，古书里说，千万不要吃，这个是杀人的。这叫"物失其态"，对人就会有害。

有一次，一位朋友从新疆回来，给我带了很多杏仁，带壳的，我就在其中发现了几个双仁的杏仁。吃不吃呢？我故意把它吃了，看能不能毒死，当时想，实在中毒了我再治呗。吃过以后，一点事也没有，并没有被杀死呀。

古人在骗我们吗？再试一试，把露出地面的桑根白皮给吃了，可能也不会死。

人的生命力是很强大的，小小几颗杏仁，或几片桑白皮，哪能把人吃死呢？古人讲的"杀人"，并不是手起一刀，人头落地，而是"软刀割头不觉死"，在暗中消耗你的生命力，给你的身体造成损失。你根本感觉不到。

所以，古人的这些话我们不可小看或误解，不要轻易去试，更不要因为你吃一个双仁杏仁没被毒死就否定古人的说法。

桑白皮的作用

桑白皮，在四气上是寒的，在五味上是甘的，微微有些辛和苦。它色白走肺，甘寒就泻肺中之火，微辛则利肺中血气。辛入肺，甘入脾，加之它气寒，且是一味根部的药，所以又走膀胱。辛甘入脾肺，性寒入膀胱，能驱逐脾肺水气和邪热，使之从膀胱小便而出，这是它的作用。

肺为娇脏，不耐寒热，但肺里面有时会有一些虚热。肾里的虚热往上走，火克金，肾火入肺而克金。所以，肺里的虚火一时半会儿清不出去。桑白皮只用于清肺里缠绵不去、已经很深的热，如果是风寒感冒，肺里有一些临时的邪气，但不深，还未形成顽固的虚火，那就千万不要乱用桑白皮。

桑白皮是一味走里的药，能走到肺的深处。而感冒所受邪气产生的热是在肺比较浅表的地方，一旦用了桑白皮，就会把感冒的邪气往里带，到时候你再想把它带出来，就很难了。

桑白皮对于脱发、头发枯槁，也都有作用。一方面这是取其韧性，另一方面很多的脱发、头发枯槁、小孩流口水都跟脾肺有热有关，因为桑白皮能泻脾肺之热，所以能治本。

韧性

"桑皮纸"现在依然可以见到。在古代桑皮纸是一种非常好的纸，洁白而有韧性。

桑皮还是过去军用品中必备的一个对象，它可以搓成线，用来缝金疮。被刀砍斧剁枪刺致伤之后，如果创口太大，就要用桑皮线来缝。这对伤口是有好处的，同时还因为它有韧性，有生生之气。

有韧性的，还有蚕丝，而蚕丝也是跟桑叶有关的；春天桑树抽出的桑枝更有韧性，风再大也不会把桑枝刮断。这都是桑树生生之气的一种体现。

生生之气其实就是一种韧性，它百折不挠。人身上什么东西最有韧性？筋。当然骨骼也有韧性，因为得了肝气，得了生生之气。所以小孩子不怕摔，不会轻易骨折。老年人一摔，可能骨头就断了，因为他骨头太脆了。

我们看看这个"脆"字怎么写：一个骨肉旁，也就是"月"字，一个"危"字，就是指机体已经很危险啦，已经脆啦。

老年人，不但骨骼没有韧性了，血管也没有韧性了，血管一旦没有韧性，就容易破裂，尤其是毛细血管，一破裂，脑出血、中风啊就接踵而至。一般来讲，年轻人有生生之气，血管很柔，很少会中风。老年人没生生之气，所以骨头也脆了，血管也脆了，头发也脆了……

人的品格也是这样的，要有韧性，这个人才有生机。韧性，就是一种百折不挠的品格，一个百折不挠、能屈能伸的人，他前途会更好。

我们从桑皮、蚕丝的韧性，看到桑树的生生之气就体现在一个韧性上。人要健康，生理、心理也都要有韧性，如果缺乏，生理上就会生风，导致各种风病；心理上也会有风，导致不理智，甚至失控，我们写作"疯"。

泻白散

看到桑白皮我们会想起一个方子，叫泻白散。

泻白散

桑白皮一两，地骨皮一两，炙甘草半两，粳米一百粒，食后温服。

一两相当于三十克。泻白散是一种散剂，打成粉后不是一次性服完，每次只服一点点。桑白皮和地骨皮都要炒黄，然后和炙甘草、粳米一起打碎，做成散。

肺对应的颜色是白，泻白散其实就是泻肺散，用来泻肺中之火。

为什么要用地骨皮呢？地骨皮是一味入肾的药，能泻肾中的虚火，能清骨蒸痨热。有一种热，你会感觉它是从骨头里来的，这是阴虚生内热给人体带来的一种感觉。因阴虚导致长期低热，要用地骨皮来清。"肺为水之上源"，肾里面的水都是从肺里来的，肾里面的真精也是从肺里面来的。"肺金生肾水"，肺为肾之母，母亲总是把最好的东西给儿子，但儿子却往往给母亲带来烦恼，所以肾中的虚火容易传给肺，肺中的虚火往往源自肾。当肾阴虚的时候，肾阳就得不到封藏，肾火就会往上蹿，蹿到胃里、肺里，造成邪火。肾中真水源自肺是生理现象，肺中邪火源自肾是病理现象。有些年轻人有痨病，肺里有虚火，咳嗽，人特别瘦，原因之一在此。桑白皮和地骨皮能泻火。桑白皮主要泻肺里的火，地骨皮泻肾里的火。

桑白皮和地骨皮都是偏于甘寒的，它不是很苦。如果太苦，就会苦寒败胃。甘寒则既能泻火，又不会有苦寒败胃的副作用。实火可以通过暂用苦寒来清，虚火难清，用药的时间要长一些，所以只能用甘寒。

方中甘草也能泻火，还能缓中。甘草是甘甜的，入脾，如果用得少，它就是一味调和之剂，调和诸药。如果用得多，它就能泻也能清，清中焦之火。泻白散里的甘草算是用得比较多的，它也能泻火。同时甘味它就有缓的作用，甘能缓中，缓脾胃之急，一般当肺肾有火的时候，脾在中焦它就容易起急，上边是火，下面是火，脾在中间肯定急。

粳米清肺，养脾胃，扶土生金，还能养血。

肺里有虚火，但肺还不虚，可以用该方。如果肺虚，小便又特别多，就不能用泻白散了。

泻白散的方义

泻白散中虽然只有四味药，但它体现三才：天、地、人。桑白皮走肺，对应天；地骨皮是走地的药，走肾，往下走。炙甘草和粳米走中焦，对应的是人。这个方子的药味虽然少，但是思路非常广阔，是一个很大气的方子。古人的很多方子都是如此。

《古今名医方论》是这样解释泻白散的："夫火热伤气，救肺之治有三：伤寒邪热侮肺，用白虎汤除烦，此治其标；内虚阴火烁阴，用生脉散益阴，此治其本；若夫正气不伤，郁火不甚，则泻白散之清肺调中，标本兼治，又补二方之不及也。"如果是火热伤气，火热在气分，就用白虎汤：石膏、知母和粳米。这是一个大寒的方剂，清热特别快，但只是用来治标。如果是虚火伤阴，则用生脉散：人参、麦冬、五味子。这是养阴治其本的。而泻白散是标本兼治的，能补以上两个方子的不足。

地骨皮

泻白散中出现的地骨皮，我们再重点讲一讲。地骨皮是枸杞的根。枸杞，南方没有，北方有，陕西宁夏那里的枸杞长得特别好，树特别大。枸杞有一个特点，就是在严冬的霜雪之中，枸杞的果实依然红润可爱，在枝头不掉下来。这是一种抗衰老之象。冬天很多东西都衰老了，凋零了，枸杞不凋零。所以现在很多人说枸杞子能够抗衰老。在那么凛冽的寒风中不掉下来，而且还红通通的，这味药肯定是偏温。偏温它才能耐大寒。

枸杞子是偏温的，但不意味着整个枸杞树其他入药的部位都偏温。它的子是偏温的，但是它的根是寒而微苦的。西北是缺水的地方，但枸杞树依然能长得很大，因为它的根扎得特别深，能够吸很深的地底下的水。在我们的身体里，地骨皮也能够走得很深，到达骨头深处。又因为它是苦寒的，所以能清热，所以它能把骨头深处的热给揪出来清掉。

我们看"地骨皮"这三个字：地，说明它走中焦，地属土，土是属中的，所以它对应人。骨，走肾的，肾在下焦，它对应最底下的地方，也就是对应地。皮，是对应肺的，肺主皮毛，肺对应的是天。所以地骨皮也是很大气的药。

从这个药名我们可以看到：地骨皮能走中焦，帮助运化，因为它是土里面长的，跟人的脾胃同气相求；走肾，能清下焦的邪火，清骨头里面的虚热；因为它是枸杞树根的表皮，所以走肺与皮毛，能把搜出来的虚热之邪，通过肺与皮毛给透出去。

Chapter 5   Sangshen (Mulberry Fruits) and Sangpiaoxiao (Mantis Egg-Case)

Sangshen (Mulberry Fruits)

Shape of Sangshen and its Processing

The life quintessence of mulberry trees is condensed into Sangshen. The mulberry tree begins to bear fruits in the month of April, which is the best season in a year when Yang in the universe is the most vigorous, and the vitality of mulberry trees also reaches its utmost.

Generally, Sangshen is purple black in color and very juicy. When getting ripe, the fruits will drop to the ground very easily, so the ripe fruits must be collected just before they fall to the ground. Before it is ripe, Sangshen is sour in taste; and only when the fruits become purple black in color, will they become sweet.

The purple black fruits can dry up so easily in air since they contain too much juice. Therefore, they must be steamed first and then be dried up for preservation on shelf.

There is another way to store Sangshen, i. e. to extract the juice and then boil it in a stone pot until it is condensed into paste like Qiuligao (autumn pear syrup) for storage. Attention: the mulberry fruit juice cannot be boiled in the iron pot since iron can restrict Sangshen and reduce its overall medical effect.

Nourishing Yin and Dispelling the Wind

Sangshen, when used as a medicine, can nourish the liver-kidney Yin. Its black color signifies that it goes to the kidney and enters the system of blood. Its sugar content is so high that it can nourish Yin and dispel pathogenic wind. In addition, the mulberry tree itself collects the vital life essence from the Jī star. All the herbs related to the mulberry tree have the efficacy of dispelling pathogenic wind. Sangshen has a very good effect in nourishing the liver and dispelling pathogenic wind.

Many ancient health maintenance books wrote, "It is suitable to drink the mulberry liquor in April, which can help dispel hundreds of winds". How to make mulberry liquor? Is it brewed with Sangshen? Or, is it to use mulberry fruits to soak in liquor? In reality, there are many ways for brewing mulberry liquor according to the ancient records, but the easiest way is to boil the mulberry fruit juice into paste. Whenever needed, just put some paste into liquor and blend up them into mulberry liquor. The mulberry fruits are perishable, but the thick mulberry paste will have a longer shelf life. In fact, the ancients also used antiseptic substance, but not so highly technical as it is today. By the way, liquor was often used by the ancients as antiseptic substance. Some liquor mixed into the mulberry paste will be helpul for anticorrosion. Sangshen can nourish Yin and dispel wind, and a little liquor added can motivate the mulberry vigor to move faster in limbs, blood vessel, bones and the internal organs in order to dispel various winds. In brief, Sangshen can nourish Yin and dispel wind, functioning to nourish blood for ceasing the endogenous wind, which proves the saying, "for dispelling wind, the first thing to do is to nourish blood; and when blood circulates smoothly, the endogenous wind will blow itself out".

Improving Vision and Maintaining Health

A piece of mulberry fruit holds a lot of small seeds, each of which is just like a black blinking eye. Such an image naturally suggests that it can improve eyesight. The liver opens at eyes, and nourishing the liver, kidney and Yin can improve eyesight, too.

Sangshen can help blacken and multiply hair, activate the internal organs, benefit all joints, and help one see and hear well. In a word, Sangshen is a fantastic fruit.

The older the mulberry tree is, the better fruitsit will bear, since it is filled with deposits through time and tide. In Daxing district, Beijiing, there is an orchard, where all the ancient mulberry trees are hundreds of years old. In May every year, many people go there to pick mulberry fruits for health maintenance purpose. It cannot get effect instantly. Nourishing should be carried out bit by bit while life is going on.

Mainly Dispelling the Endogenous Wind

The majoreffect of Sangshen is to dipel the endogenous wind, which can be compared more or less with the natural world.

The wind in spring is gentle, and it can blow all things on earth to grow; The wind in fall is called metal wind (autumn wind), and it brings coolness, though, it blows off leaves and dries up all grasses. The autumn wind is chilly, and it blows the season into the severe winter step by step.

So is the human body. While one is growing up, he or she is always energetic with flexible tendon and blood vessel, and the endogenous wind is like a gentle breeze; when he/she is getting old, he/she will become exhausted and the life essence and vigor has been drying up, and his or her tendon and blood vessel will become with thin and brittle. By that time, the endogenous wind in his or her body would be like the autumn wind. Therefore, when he/she himself/herself is flexible and strong enough, all the wind in his or her body, whatever is, will be just like a gentle breeze. But on the contrary, if he/she himself/herself becomes weak physically, the wind, whatever it is, will bring trouble to him or her. The key point is not what the wind is like, but how he/she should nourish Yin and dispel wind in order to help the physical body become flexible and strong enough.

This is like a complicated legal case in the Chan sect: the streamers are fluttering in the wind, for which a monk said it was the wind that was blowing, while another monk said it was the streamer that was fluttering. At last, the master Huineng said that neither the wind nor the streamer were moving, but the hearts of the kind-hearted persons were moved. Whether one's heart is moved or not does not depend upon the wind or the streamer but on oneself. So it may be also said here it is neither the gentle wind nor the autumn wind that decides, but it is the human physical conditions, flexible or strong, that decide.

Sangpiaoxiao (Mantis Egg-Case)

Uses of Animal Medicines Should be Controlled

The animal medicines are generally discussed at the end of the Herbal Books since the ancient time like the herbal classic **Shennong Bencao Jing** that was arranged according to the three grades of medicines, i. e. the upper grade, the middle grade and the lower grade. For each grade of medicines, the metal and stone medicines always come first; and the next come the herbs; and the animal medicines always come last. The intention of such arrangement is to remind the users of trying to avoid using animal medicines since the heaven always takes pleasure in the welfare of living things and all the animals are living creatures. For sure, plants have life in them, too, but in any case, plants are different from animals.

Sangpiaoxiao was listed in the upper grade in the book of *Shennong Bencao Jing*, which, however, puts quite few animal medicines in the upper grade category, especially the worm medicines are generally listed in the middle or lower grades of medicines. *Shennong Bencao Jing* describes Sangpiaoxiao as: "salty and sweet in taste with mild nature, it is mainly used to treat the spleen and stomach Qi in the Middle Jiao, hernia-conglomeration, impotence, infertility, a-menorrhea, lumbago, relaxing the five types stranguria, and inducing urination".

Shape and Formation of Sangpiaoxiao

Sangpiaoxiao is the eggs laid by mantis on Sangzhi. Mantis lays eggs on many different plants, but only the eggs on Sangzhi are called Sangpiaoxiao. Surely the eggs on the other plants may also be used as Sangpiaoxiao, but it is not so effective as that on Sangzhi, which is similar to Sangjisheng discussed in the above section.

Mantis looks very strange. A french writer named Fabre wrote *Souvenirs Entomologiques*, in which he observes the mantis very carefully. He says that two days after mating the mantis will lie on the twig of a tree with its head adown and discharge something from its tail, which at the very beginning is not foam, but in air it will be foaming like the foaming agent used for house decoration. Then mantis lays eggs in the foam that will dry up in the air to form a case sticking to the twigs. That is called Sangpiaoxiao in which there are lots of mantis eggs.

Ferocity of the Wild

Fabre says mantis is an age-old and very fierce creature. As it is always said that even a vicious tiger will not eat its cubs. That is to say, no animal is so vicious that it will eat that of the same spacies alive, but mantis is. At the time of mating, a femal mantis will eat the male mantis alive from head to belly even the forelegs with only some debris of wings and hindlegs being left over. The femal mantis is bigger than the male one. Before discharging eggs, a femal mantis usually mates with many male mantises and eats up many of them simultaneously while mating.

There is a Chinese idiom saying "a mantis trying to stop a chariot" (which implies "to kick against the pricks"). A mantis has two powerful forelegs like two knives, though, it is impossible for it to stop a chariot anyway. This idiom implies that a mantis is very brave and fierce with only brute courage. By the way, there is another idiom saying that the mantis stalks the cicada, unaware of the oriole behind (which means "to covet gains ahead without being aware of danger behind"). A mantis in size is not much bigger than a cicada, but it is brave enough to catch a cicada. A mantis is of a carnivorous animal, and it is able to vanquish the creature bigger than itself. The "the oriole behind" in the above idiom tells that the mantis is careless and unaware of the oriole behind, or it may also tells that mantis is too brave to mind the oriole behind and focuses on stalking the cicada.

The brutality and ferocity of a mantis shows its multiplying property. The mantis itself enjoys the nature of vitality. The eggs are for producing new generation, which proves the strong vitality. Furthermore, the eggs laid on the mulberry twigs gain the vigor of the mulberry tree, and will have much stronger vitality.

The mantis is a creature with multiple larvae. A femal mantis is able to ovulate out lots of eggs, some of which will be eaten by some other insects, though, many larvae will be hatched.

Mantis is green in color. Green color signifies that it can enter the liver. Green color is also the symbol of ferocity and vigor for multiplying. For instance, Qingpi and Chenpi, the former is stronger and more fierce, and it can relieve stagnant Qi. When orange becomes yellow, it will become mild, too. It can then regulate Qi circulation for eliminating phlegm.

Astringency of Sangpiaoxiao

The mantises lay eggs in late autumn. The nature follows the law of birth in spring, growing in summer, harvesting in autumn and storing of gain in winter. The mantises exactly follow such a law. The mantis eggs are indeed an indication of harvesting in autumn and storing in winter. When the mulberry leaves fall completely in winter, some bulging things can be seen on the twigs, which are Sangpiaoxiao. All the eggs will experience the frost and snow in the long winter season, and will be hatched into the mantis larvae till the season of Mangzhong (grain in ear) next year when it is summer, i. e. April or May in Chinese lunar calendar when Yang is in the most sufficient state and the little larvae will then be hatched out. The mantis eggs are enclosed and stored for such a long time and have to experience the severe winter, indicating that there should be some temperature inside though *Shennong Bencao Jing* describes that Sangpiaoxiao is salty and sweet in taste and mild in nature. Overall, it is inclined to be warm and it is endowed with a strong astringency. Its major effect is to reinforce the kidneys.

Astringency of Sangpiaoxiao is corresponding to the harvesting in autumn and storing of gain in winter. One may have the doubt about the contradiction between its multiplying property mentioned above and its property of astringency referred here. The two properties appear to be contradictory to each other, but in essence, the multiplying property refers to its nature in itself. However, when used as medicine clinically, it shows the property of astringency. Its astringency is not a bad thing. In the corresponding seasons of harvesting and storing of gain, the vital essence should be astringed and recuperated. In autumn, in response to the astringency required by the season, doctors often fill a prescription of some seasonal medicines like Sangpiaoxiao, Shanyurou (common macrocarpium fruit), Wuweizi, Yizhiren (bitter cardamom) etc. based on the syndrome differentiation in order to astringe and control the vital life essence of human body.

Meanwhile, one may also use its property of astringency to cure the diseases like spermatorrhea, sperm released with urine, and femal leukorrhagia, all of which are related to the kidney Qi not being astringed. By the way, it will be more effective to use Sangpiaoxiao plus Longgu (ossa draconis) for astringing purpose.

Of course, this is mainly to cure the deficiency-cold syndromes. The spermatorrhea may take place due to deficiency or excess. If it is due to excess, the ministerial fire disturb the sperm chamber and the sperm would then be released, manifesting spermatorrhea in a dream, a fleeting illusion, and a thready and rapid pulse, signifying vigorous pathogenic influence. While the spermatorrhea taking place without dreams is often resulted from weariness, it may manifest a thready and slow pulse, which is related to the deficiency-cold. And in such a case, the seminal fluid is white and turbid, so Sangpiaoxiao may be used. If necessary, Fuzi, Rougui, Wuweizi, Longgu, Nuomi (sticky rice) may also be added to make into pills for use.

The children's bed-wetting (enuresis) at night is also a manifestation of unconsolidation of kidney-Qi. A child himself is sensible and he does not want the bed-wetting, but due to the unconsolidation of the kidney-Qi, he fails to hold in. For such a case, just a little Sangpiaoxiao will do.

Doubtlessly, one should try to avoid using the animal medicines if there is any other effective recipe available. In each mantis egg-case, there are thousands of lives. Therefore, the less one use animal for medicine purpose, the better it would be for life of animals. *Newly Compiled Chinese Materia Medica*, an excellent book written by Chen Shiduo, a medical expert in Qing dynasty, called for sympathizing with even the puny lives, which tells us the importance of showing respect to lives.

Chinese Medicinels not Inflexible

Sangpiaoxiao has the property of astringency, and then why does *Shennong Bencao Jing* says that Sangpiaoxiao "can induce urination"? Generally, once it is astringent, urinary obstruction will arise.

In reality, the effect of Sangpiaoxiao inducing urine is primarily to induce the stagnated urine due to deficiency in the Lower Jiao. The kidney takes charge of releasing both urine and faeces, When trapped by the deficiency-cold in the Lower Jiao, the urine may not be easily released. In that case, Sangpiaoxiao can be used to consolidate the vital life essence, and the function of Qi transformation of the kidney will become more powerful. As such, urine can then be induced naturally. The kidney likes to be consolidated and storing, which can then help the kidney to function well and release the waste fluid smoothly.

Sangpiaoxiao is salty and sweet in taste and mild in property. Its salty taste can help soften hard mass, and its strong ferocity can help harmonize blood, disperse blood stasis and eliminate blood stagnation. **Shennong Bencao Jing** says Sangpiaoxiao can be used for hernia-conglomeration. The hernia actually is colic, and conglomeration is actually a lump in the abdomen due to Qi-stagnation and blood stasis in the body. Sangpiaoxiao can also be used for curing amenorrhea. It can break up the pathogens and take in the healthy Qi as well, which shows its reconciliation and breaking power, i. e. , it has recuperating and curing effects simultaneously.

As a matter of fact, even if a medicine is astringent, it does not mean it only plays the function of astringency. It is often able to astringe the healthy Qi and discharge the unhealthy Qi. This is quite a natural process rather than a rigid or inflexible process. If it were a rigid or inflexible process, it might either astringe all things indiscriminately, or induce or release all things, good or bad. In fact, only TCM medicines can have a balanced effect to astringe the good and release the bad since they are the natural produces.

Channel Tropism and Contraindications

After knowing the effects of Sangpiaoxiao, one may know what meridians it can enter. The properties of its vital ferocity, reconciling blood and consolidating the kidney confirm that it can enter the liver and kidney meridians; Relaxing the five types of stranguria and inducing urination indicate that it can enter the bladder meridian. Its effects of tonifying the vital life essence and inducing urination signify that it can supplement the healthy factors and drive out the unhealthy factors simultaneously without any confliction.

Although **Shennong Bencao Jing** says Sangpiaoxiao is sweet in taste and mild in nature, yet it is warm with multifying effect. However, Sangpiaoxiao must not be used when endogenous heat occurs, especially, the heat in the kidney, bladder, and there is frequent and urgent urination and yellow urine, or even burning hot feeling in the urethral orifice at the time of urination. Sangpiaoxiao should not be used either in case of fire arising from Yin deficiency. Sangpiaoxiao can be used for treatment of spermatorrhea. However, if the spermatorrhea takes place in a dream, that often attributes to the deficiency fire that disturbs the sperm chamber. In that case, when Sangpiaoxiao is added for astringing purpose, the fire may be trapped in the sperm chamber, which will then worsen the spermatorrhea, or even result in some red and white turbidity and the like. Therefore, in spite of its mild nature, Sangpiaoxiao must be used with caution.

第五章 桑葚与桑螵蛸

桑葚

桑葚形状及制法

桑树的精华集中在桑葚上，桑葚挂满枝头，正值人间四月天，这是一年中最美好的季节，是天地之间阳气最旺盛的时候，桑树的生发之气也在此时达到极致，终于结出了它的果实，这就是桑葚。

桑葚一般都是紫黑色，汁特别多，成熟后特别容易掉到地上。我们应该在它掉地上之前采收，同时又必须保证它成熟了。桑葚还没有成熟的时候是红色的，比较酸，只有当它已经变成紫黑色，才会很甜。

把紫黑色的桑葚采下来，晾晒，是不会干的，因为它里面的汁太多了。必须先蒸熟，它才容易晒干。这是一种保存的方法。

还有一种保存方法，就是把它的汁榨出来，放在石锅里慢慢熬成膏，就像秋梨膏那样的，留待慢慢享用。为什么不能把它放在铁锅里熬呢？因为桑葚也是怕铁的，跟铁在一起，它的作用就大打折扣。

养阴祛风

桑葚是养肝肾之阴的一味药，它长在桑树上，跟肝有关；呈黑色，必定入肾，入血分，而且糖分那么多，必然养阴，养阴又可以驱风，加上桑树本身又是箕星之精，桑树上的东西都有驱风的作用，所以桑葚养肝驱风的作用非常好。

"四月宜饮桑葚酒，祛百种风。"古代很多养生书都这样讲。常有人问我，桑葚酒到底怎么做？是用桑葚来酿呢？还是用桑葚来泡酒呢？其实桑葚酒在古人记载中有很多种做法，最简单的还是先将桑葚汁熬成膏，到了用的时候，加酒一兑，就是桑葚酒了。桑葚膏要是浓稠的话，保质期就会长一些，否则容易腐烂，怎么防腐呢？古人也有防腐剂，只不过是没有今天这么高科技。在桑葚膏里面兑入适量白酒就可以防腐了，酒就是古人用的防腐剂。桑葚养阴祛风，再加一点酒，引动桑葚，在四肢、血脉、百骸、五脏里，让它跑得更快，这就能祛百种风，所以桑葚的作用是养阴祛风，或者说是养血息风。这又印证了我们以前讲的：治风先治血，血行风自灭。

明目养生
一个桑葚含有很多小籽，每一粒籽就像一颗乌黑的眼睛，闪闪发亮。我们很自然就能想到：它能明目。的确如此。而且，肝开窍于目，养肝肾滋阴也能明目。

桑葚还能乌发、生发，能利五脏、利关节，能让人耳聪目明。总之这是非常好的一种水果。

越古老的桑树上结的桑葚越好，因为其中饱含岁月的积淀。在北京大兴有一个古桑园，那里的桑树都是几百年的。每年 5 月份，都会有很多人到那里去摘桑葚，这是一种养生。当然，它的作用也不是打了鸡血一样立竿见影。前面我们讲，杀人是不知不觉慢慢的进行的。

主祛内风
桑葚主治内风。何谓内风，我们依然可以用自然界来做比喻。

春天的风是和风，它吹生了万物。秋天的风叫金风，金风虽然送爽但同时它也吹落了树叶，吹枯了百草，是肃杀之风，它把季节吹到严冬。

人体也是这样的，当人体在生长的时候，真精充足，筋脉柔韧，体内的风是和风，人体在衰老的时候，真精枯涸，筋脉脆薄，体内的风就是秋风。这似乎并不在于风而在于我们自身。当我们自身足够柔韧的时候，不管什么风，都是和风。当我们身体脆弱，经不起风的时候，那么不管是什么风都可能把我们吹坏，对于我们的身体来说，这风就是要命的风了。所以关键不在于它是什么风，而在于把我们自己养好，养阴祛风，使机体足够柔韧。

这就是禅宗里面的那则公案：风吹幡动，一个和尚说是风动，一个和尚说是幡动，最后慧能说：既不是风动也不是幡动，而是仁者心动。你的心动不动不是取决于风或者幡，而是取决于你自己。现在我们在这个问题上也可以讲，不是和风也不是肃杀之风，而取决于我们的身体是不是柔软，是不是坚韧。

— 221 —

桑螵蛸

动物药须用之有节

自古本草书讲动物药，一般都会放在最后。《本草纲目》就是这样的；《神农本草经》是按上中下三品来分的，每一品都是先讲金石类药，再讲草木类，最后才讲动物类的药。其用意，在于提醒我们不要轻易地用动物药。因为天有好生之德，动物是一条生命，当然植物也是一条生命，但是毕竟动物和植物还不一样。

桑螵蛸在《神农本草经》中被列为上品，而《神农本草经》中上品的动物药是很少的，尤其是虫类药，基本上都在中品和下品。《神农本草经》这样描述桑螵蛸："味咸甘平，主伤中，疝瘕，阴痿，益精生子，女子血闭，腰痛，通五淋，利小便水道"。

桑螵蛸的形状及形成

桑螵蛸是螳螂在桑枝上产的卵。螳螂会在很多植物上产卵，但是只有在桑树上产的卵才叫桑螵蛸。当然在其他树上产的卵，也有人采来当桑螵蛸用，但它的作用是没有桑螵蛸好的。这类似前面讲的桑寄生。

螳螂长得很奇怪。法国的法布尔，写了一套书叫《昆虫记》。他对螳螂的观察非常仔细。他说，螳螂在交尾后两天，会趴在树枝上，头朝下，从尾部排出一些东西，刚排出来的时候本来还不是泡沫，但见了空气就会发泡，像我们装修的时候用的发泡剂。然后把卵产在泡沫里面，泡沫在空气里慢慢风干了，就形成一个囊，紧贴着树枝，这就是桑螵蛸，其中有许许多多螳螂产的卵。

野性的刚猛

法布尔讲，螳螂是一种非常古老又非常野蛮的动物。我们讲虎毒不食子，再狠毒的动物一般都不会活活的吃掉自己的同类，但螳螂就是吃自己同类的一种虫子。在交配时，雌螳螂会把雄螳螂活生生吃掉，从头开始吃，一直吃到肚子，最后吃得只剩翅膀和小腿的残片，连大腿都啃掉了。雌螳螂比雄螳螂要大一些。而且一个雌螳螂在排卵之前要跟很多的雄螳螂交配，同时也就要吃掉很多的雄螳螂。

有个成语叫"螳臂挡车"，螳螂有两个大刀一样的臂，非常有力气，

— 222 —

但用来挡车，注定是要失败的，不过这也说明螳螂勇猛，有匹夫之勇。还有"螳螂捕蝉，黄雀在后"，螳螂的个头并不比蝉大，但它敢去捕蝉。它是肉食动物，能够降伏比自己体积大的动物。黄雀在后，怎么理解呢？螳螂是马大哈没注意到后面有黄雀吗？可能不是的，还是因为它胆子大，一心来捕蝉，黄雀在后它不在乎。

螳螂这种野蛮、刚猛的性质，就是一种生发之性。螳螂本身具有生发之性；卵是用来生下一代的，升发之性更足；加之又在桑树上排卵，得桑树的生发之气，它的升发之气可想而知。

螳螂多子，它每次要排很多卵。虽然有一部分会被其他小虫子吃掉，但是能够孵出的小螳螂还是很多。

螳螂是绿色的。绿色通肝，也是刚猛和生发之气的象征。比如青皮和陈皮相比，青皮更加刚猛，力性更大，用于破气。等到橘子黄了，就要温和一些了，因为黄色主土，它就会平和一些，故用于理气化痰。

收摄之性

螳螂是在深秋产卵。我们知道，大自然的规律是春生夏长，秋收冬藏，螳螂符合这一规律，它产的卵是秋冬季节收藏之象。在冬天，桑树的叶子落光以后，我们在枝头能看到有一些鼓鼓囊囊的东西，那就是桑螵蛸。漫长的寒冬，它在那里忍受霜雪。直到第二年芒种的时候，才孵化出小螳螂来。芒种都是夏天了，农历四五月份，是阳气最足的时候，螳螂才破壳而出。螳螂的卵，要封藏那么久，而且要经历严冬，说明它里面就有一定温性，虽然在《本经》上讲它是味咸、甘、平，但是它总体来讲依然是偏温的而且有很强的收摄性，能固肾，这是它的主要作用。

收摄性跟秋收冬藏相应。有人会说，你不是说它有生发之性吗？怎么现在又说它有收摄之性呢？二者看似相反，其实，生发之性是说它本身，而在药用上则是有收摄性。收摄其实也不是坏事，秋收冬藏的季节，精气应该收敛、静养。秋天，为了应季节的收敛之气，我们经常会给病人在辨证处方的基础上，配一些应季的药，如桑螵蛸、山萸肉、五味子、益智仁等，用来收摄人体的精气。

我们还可以利用它的收摄之性，来治疗那些不能收摄的病。比如遗精、精随小便而出、女子白带过多，都跟肾气不能固摄有关，用桑螵蛸配上龙骨来收摄，效果会非常的好。

当然这主要是用于治疗虚寒性的病症。遗精有虚实之分，如果是实，是相火扰动精室，精也会出来，往往表现为有梦而遗，一场春梦，遗精了，其脉细数，这是邪气盛；无梦而遗，往往出现在比较累的情况下，其脉细缓，这跟虚寒有关。虚寒的遗精、白浊，咱们就可以用桑螵蛸，在必要的情况下，还可以加上附子、肉桂、五味子、龙骨、糯米，做成丸药服用。

小孩子晚上尿床，也是肾气不固的表现。他已经懂事，本不想尿床，但是因为肾气不固，没能控制住，到早上起来的时候，追悔莫及。这种情况单用一点桑螵蛸就可以了。

当然，如果能用别的办法，咱们还是尽量不用动物药。一个桑螵蛸里有成千上万的生命，咱们还是少用为好。陈士铎的《本草新编》"怜其细小"，告诉我们还是不要用为妙。

中药的作用不是机械的

有人可能要问，既然它是有收摄性的，《神农本草经》为什么又讲它能"利小便水道"呢？按理说，一收摄应该会出现小便不通啊。

其实，桑螵蛸利小便，主要是利下焦虚滞的小便。肾司二便，被下焦虚寒所困，所以小便下不来，用桑螵蛸，精气一固，肾的气化能力足了，小便自然就利了。肾是喜欢固，喜欢封藏的。你让肾封藏好了，它自身的各种功能就会很好，水邪就自然能排出来。我们要这样来认识它。

桑螵蛸味咸甘平，咸就能软坚，它又有刚猛之气，能和血、化瘀、逐瘀。《神农本草经》讲，疝瘕可以用它，疝就是疝气，瘕就是体内因为气滞血瘀而产生的一些硬块。女子血闭也可以用它。它能把邪气打散，又能收摄正气，且和且攻，刚柔相济。

即使是一味收摄的药，也不会一味收敛。它把正气给你收敛住，邪气依然排掉。这是一个自然的过程，而不是一个机械的过程。如果是一个机械的过程，那么它就不加分辨全都收摄住了，要通利就好的坏的都给你通利出来。只有中药才有这种作用，因为它是自然的产物。

归经与禁忌

我们知道桑螵蛸的作用，也就知道它能归哪些经了。生机刚猛，和血固肾，肯定入肝经肾经；通五淋，利小便，入膀胱经。一边补益精气，一边利小便，补正和驱邪是并行不悖的。

虽然《神农本草经》上说它是一味甘平的药，但它仍然有温性，善生发，当我们遇到有内热，尤其是肾、膀胱里面有热，出现尿频、尿急、尿黄，甚至排尿的时候感觉尿道口发烫，就千万不要用桑螵蛸了。阴虚多火的也不要用。桑螵蛸虽治遗精，但如果是有梦而遗的，往往是虚火扰动精室，清火还来不及呢，加点桑螵蛸一收，那这个火收在精室里，可能会加剧遗精，甚至导致赤白浊之类的。这味药虽然平和的，但用的时候还是要非常注意。

Chapter6　Baijiangcan (Stiff Silkworm) and Wind Dispelling Medicines

Baijiangcan (Stiff Silkworm)

Shennong Bencao Jing describes Baijiangcan (stiff silkworm or silkworm lava) as "salty, pungent, mild and non-toxic, it has the effects of curing night cries of babies due to convulsion, eliminating the three common parasitic diseases in the intestines of babies, and removing the dark spots to beautify the complexion and cure the pruritus vulvae of men."

Source of Baijiangcan

Those who have the experiences in rearing silkworms must know that they have to exercise great care and keep the silkworm nursery clean, and dare not say any unlucky words. Some of the silkworm breeding families even hold some activities to offer sacrifices. In a word, they do all these things for fear that the silkworms fall sick and get stiff (dead), which means financial losses for them.

Silkworms are quite different from the other creatures when they die in that the remains of the other creatures will get rotten and go stink soon after they die, but the silkworms will become stiff and not get rotten or go stink. As such, the dead silkworms are called Baijiangcan (stiff silkworm).

As medicine, Baijiangcan must be stiff silkworm that dies from illness. In the hot summer, mosquitoes like to bite the silkworms, causing the silkworms to die and become black and useless.

Making the Best Use of Silkworms

TCM gives much stress on the properties of all herbs to the greatest extent and making use of them to the utmost.

The farmers breeding silkworms is for obtaining the silk cocoons. If silkworms die and become Baijiangcan, they will sell it to the drugstore.

TCM always takes a humble attitude of mercy and reverence towards using

Chinese traditional medicines. For example, the sandalwood and rhinoceros horn, only the leftover bits and pieces or offcut materials are used for medicines.

Baijiangcan Subsumed to Metal, Medicines Associated with Metal Restraining the Wind

Baijiangcan is white in color, subsumed to metal from the perspective of **Wuxing Doctrine**, and it can enter the lung. Meanwhile, stiffness is also subsumed to metal. Metal in **Wuxing Doctrine** is of *Jiehua*, which means to become stiff. All things that are associated with metal can become stiff. Stone is hard, and it is subsumed to metal, so is the turtle shell. Besides, Baijiangcan has gained the energy of mulberry while it was growing, so it can restrain the pathogenic wind.

In fact, the mulberry is also subsumed to metal. After all the leaves fall off, the mulberry tree will be in white color that actually is subsumed to metal. In the previous parts, the mulberry has been defined to be subsumed to wood because it grows vigorously in spring with life vitality, and also it is able to dispel the pathogenic wind, all of which are the natures of wood. With vitality of life and the effect of dispelling pathogenic wind, mulberry comes under the category of wood genera physiologically. However, mulberry can also restrain wind; wind is subsumed to wood; and metal restricts wood. Therefore, mulberry is subsumed to metal pharmacologically.

Baijiangcan Cures Baby Night Cries due to Convulsion

All the effects of Baijiangcan are about dispelling wind. The baby's night cries due to convulsion are often related to the liver wind. Generally, baby cries take place at midnight from 11 p. m, to 1 a. m. or from 1 a. m. to 3 p. m. since Qi and blood flow into the liver and gallbladder channels in these periods of the day when the liver wind is stirred up and the gallbladder heats up, babies will become so agitated and irritable that they will start to cry. In such cases, Baijiangcan can be used for dispelling the wind and calming the liver. But now, Chantui (cicada slough) and the like is used instead, or the physiotherapy methods like Tuina (massage) or back pinch (holding between the fingers) are adopted instead of medication, which is also effective. In case that it is very serious and influenced by wind, Baijiangcan may be considered in line with syndrome differentiation and treatment. If any heat is associated, some Chantui may be added, too.

The "convulsion night cry" mentioned in **Shennong Bencao Jing** refers to the night cry arising from convulsion, for instance, the accompanying twitch of wind manifestation in crying. In that case, Baijiangcan may be used; but in other cases, try to avoid using Baijiangcan.

Baijiangcan Kills the Three Parasites

The silkworm is also a kind of worm. Worms usually come into being and grow in the wind. They like to attract the wind and can function to dispel the wind.

Parasites in human body must be treated by way of dispelling pathogenic wind. **Shennong Bencao Jing** says, Baijiangcan can "kill three parasites" ("three" in Chinese here refers to many or various), that is, it can get rid of various parasites. The worms grow in wind, and parasites survive inside human body, indicating that there is wind in the body. When such wind is gentle and soft, the parasites will stay in their places without any disturbances, the human may feel nothing; But if there is the endogenous pathogenic wind, the parasites inside the body will become discontented and poke their noses everywhere and even give birth to some pathogenic things that will then make people feel ill or suffer from pain.

Let us see the Chinese character "风" (feng, means wind in English). In the middle is a "worm". the ancients started to be aware that worms come into being in wind, and wind contains worms. Some people may claim that wind can be classified into endogenous wind and exogenous wind. In fact, both of them contain worms. The wind-cold type common cold and the wind-heat type common cold (anemopyretic cold) appear to be unrelated to the worms. However, from the ancient complex font of "風" (feng, means wind), it can be understood clearly that virus hides in the wind and comes into being with the wind. The virus is also a kind of worm simply because they are invisible to our naked eyes. The endogenous wind sometimes manifests wind that is formed from blood deficiency, which stirs up some pathogenic worms.

I once heard a story from a military doctor about his experience of rescuing and curing a wounded soldier: in the war times, the wounds were pretty scary. Because of the large surface of wounds and delayed treatment, some wounds would breed grub worms, but some would not. One may think the wounds with grubs being bred would be more serious. But in fact, it is not true. The wounds with grubs looked terribly sick, if properly cleaned, disinfected and bound up, the wounded soldiers would survive. However, those whose wounds did not breed any grubs died finally since the wounds without breeding grubs indicated that the wounded soldiers had lost vitality of life. The wind on the one hand signifies the existence of worms, but on the other hand it also signifies the vitality of life.

It may also be asked how to comprehend the grub breeding on the corpses. As a matter of fact, there are two different systems for comprehending the living and the dead, which tell us the grub breeding on the wounds is an entirely different matter from that on the corpses.

Baijiangcan is Used as a Major Beautifying Medicine

How can Baijiangcan remove the dark spots to beautify the complexion?

Those who have reared silkworms would have the knowledge that silkworms will experience ecdysis, which shows it can help remove dark spots or stripes on the face like the ecdysis of silkworms to beautify one's complexion.

The silkworms will experience 4 ecdyses in their life. What does "four" mean? According to the principle of the Earth-Four generating metal(originated from ancient observation of celestial phenomena), the number "four" is subsumed to metal, which means the silkworm is related to metal, so it is able to dispel the wind. The formation of dark spots on the face is also related to wind. The skin of a person may be pretty delicate and tender, but the face quite easily goes dark. On the one hand, the face is exposed to the outside and has to suffer from the exogenous wind. In the modern time, it has to suffer from another hurt of radiation from computer screen. The endogenous wind of the body goes upwards, carrying the endogenous heat to scan the face. Hence, both the exogenous and endogenous winds act on the face, bringing punching ravages, which will definitely leave some traces, like dark spots behind on the face.

Baijiangcan is used for dispelling wind. Baijiangcan is subsumed to metal and it is white in color, which means it can go into the lung. However, the lung dominates skin and hair. Besides, Baijiangcan can enter the stomach meridian of foot-Yangming, and the face is subsumed to the meridian of Yangming. Therefore, Baijiangcan can bring about a very good effect on dispelling wind over the face, removing the dark spots and achieving a beautifying effect.

Baijiangcan is a quite effective medicine for beautifying purpose. It was recorded that **Yurong San** (Jade-like Face Beauty powder) that was used in the royal palace in Qing dynasty also contains the ingredient of Baijiangcan.

In line with the peculiarity of the silkworm ecdysis, can it be proved to have some other medical effects? The answer is "Yes". Gnerally speaking, the skin of babies is delicately tender and smooth, but some babies have a scale-like rough trace on the skin, which is called embryo scale in TCM theory. Such embryo scale is actually resulted from Qi and blood deficiency, and lung Qi obstruction, which can be cured by washing with Baijiangcan decocted water.

Processing ofBaijiangcan

The top-quality Baijiangcan is white in color, and each piece of them is perfectly intact. Generally, the silkworms should be soaked in rice-rinsed water for a whole day to soak off mulberry saliva, which is a kind of substance to be formed inside silkworms after eating mulberry leaves. While in soaking, saliva will percolate slowly out of the mouths of silkworms.

After soaking, dry it in the sun. It may be suggested to parch on fire to dry up, but not advisable. The silkworm is subsumed to metal, and fire can restrict the metal. If parched on fire, its property of metal will be destroyed. Even though decocting is done over fire, that is a different thing since both water and fire are used while in decocting, which is totally different from that of fire to be used solely.

Compatibility of Baijiangcan with Dilong(Earthworms)

Baijiangcan is often used together with Dilong (earthworm or lumbricus), i. e., rain worms.

The silkworms always raise their heads. When Baijiangcan is used as medicine, it will goes upwards. While the earthworm behaves on the contrary, it digs into the earth. So, when the earthworm is used as medicine, it will go downwards.

The silkworm likes neat and tidy environment. They only live on the mulberry leaf, which is also quite clean; while the earthworm lives underground, it is not quite clean.

Baijiangcan and the earthworm are of two different worms, and their medical properties are opposite to each other.

The earthworm is salty-cold with slight toxicity in property, so it is for descending and it can alleviate water retention and dredge meridians. Furthermore, because of its salty-cold property, it can also bring down a fever. Taking a piece of earthworm in hand and pulling it, one will find it is elastic, which looks like a blood vessel, indicating that the earthworm can intenerate blood vessels. As for many spasms, especially the head spasm, Baijiangcan is often used together with earthworms for treatment.

Baijiangcan goes upwards, so it can guide the medical effect of the earthworm upwards. When a patient suffers from pathogenic wind, he may also suffer from the accompanying heat and much disharmony, and therefore, the blood vessels would become indurated or hardened. In such a case, if the pathogenic wind again stirs up Qi and blood, it may easily burst out blood vessels, resulting in cerebral hemorrhage or fundus hemorrhage etc. The stiff silkworm used together with earthworm can intenerate blood vessels simultaneously while they are used for dispelling the pathogenic wind. As a matter of fact, Baijiangcan can also intenerate blood vessels, as one can see the silkworm is very soft and its silk is soft, too. When Baijiangcan is used together with earthworm, it will become more effective for treatment. And furthermore, earthworm can bring down the heat as well.

Baijiangcan used together with earthworm can cure the phlegm-damp and the stagnated blood in meridians and collaterals. One of the Chinese patent medicines named **Huoluo Dan** (veins and artery relieving pill) contains the major ingredient of stiff silkworm, earthworm, Chuanxiong (ligusticum wallichii), Caowu (radix aconiti agrestis), Wuxiang (dutchmanspipe root), Moyao (myrrh) etc.

Qianzheng San

Qianzheng San contains Baifuzi (rhizoma typhonii), Baijiangcan (stiff silkworm) and Sheng Quanxie (crude scorpion), all of which are in equal dosage.

Facial Paralysis

Qianzheng San, just as its Chinese name (Qianzheng) implies, is to set righ what is distorted. When suffering from illness of stroke (apoplexia), some patients may have facial paralysis, but some others, even without suffering from illness of stroke or facial paralysis, may have a tilted tongue. When one is warned of his tilted tongue, he may deny it and try to prove it by putting tongue out, which is true sometimes. But after a while, he puts out tongue without intention, the tongue becomes tilted again. Such a case is also called facial paralysis. Regardless of the endogenous wind or exogenous wind, whenever the facial paralysis arises, **Qianzhen San** may be used. But for use of this medicine, a general rule should be followed, that is, stop using it when the facial paralysis is cured, and never use it for a long time. In a prescription for a decoction, when the three medical ingredients contained in **Qianzheng San** are needed, each of them must not exceed 3 to 6 grams.

The reason that the mouth becomes twisted is that the pathogenic wind phlegm obstructs the meridians and collaterals, especially the Zuyangming meridians encircling the lips. When there occurs the pathogenic wind phlegm retardation, Qi of the Zuyangming meridians will be disturbed, to which the mouth will give response, resulting in twitching or twisting depending on its seriousness.

Baifuzi (Rhizoma Typhonii)

In additionto Baijiangcan, **Qianzheng San** contains Baifuzi and crude scorpion.

Baifuzi and Fuzi are different plants with different effects, but only their roots and seedlings look similar in appearance. Baifuzi goes to the stomach meridians, and it is more effective for removing the wind phlegm. The wind always goes upwards to head and faces intangibly to form "moving wind over head and faces", which is like guerrilla warfare without any specific settling spots. Such wind wonders around head and faces as roving doctors in the past or monks who always travelled here and there without a specific foothold. The moving wind cannot be caught with the common medicines, but only Baifuzi, which can search and drive it away gradually.

It may be argued that Chuanwu (aconite root) can also catch the moving wind. Baifuzi is used here instead of Chuanwu since the former goes upwards while the latter goes downwards. Chuanwu is generally used for treating rheumatism in lower limbs (legs). For instance, ischialgia can be treated with Chuanwu, and the wind on faces should be treated with Baifuzi instead.

Yurong San, which was always used for beauty purpose in the royal palace in the past, contains Baifuzi since this herb is effective for dispelling the moving wind on the faces in order to achieve the expected beautifying effects. Baifuzi is often used together with Baizhi (radix angelicae), which can penetrate into muscle, extend to skin, dispel pathogenic wind and remove dampness. Both Baifuzi and Baizhi are inclined to be warm-dry. If they were to be used too much or too long, they would consume Qi and blood. Therefore, some nourishing and mostening herbs must be added in order to keep nourishing and dispelling pathogenic wind at the same time.

Scorpion

The whole scorpion also has curing effects on dispelling wind. When writing a prescription, doctors sometimes write "Quanchong" (which means "the whole bug" of scorpion). It is unpleasant for the patients to hear of scorpion, so doctors often call it "Quanchong" in a euphemistic way. The power of scorpion is on the tail, i. e. , the joints. Some doctors will only take the part of the tail when using scorpion as medicine. The whole scorpion means to take the scorpion as a whole for medicine use. Those who are particular about the medicine of scorpion will cut off the feet. By the way, the scorpion produced in Qingzhou city in Shandong province of China is usually taken as the best of all.

Scorpion is a kind of blue green black bug. The blue green color goes into the liver, signifying a strong and fierce Qi. If stung by a scorpion, one will feel very painful, which means the strong and fierce Qi is functioning. As for curing and treating the scorpion's stinging, In case it is only on the surface, some saliva of snails applied to the wound will work well; but in case the stinging is deep, the crushed snail juice applied to the wound will help to recover more effectively. In a word, everything has its vanquisher.

All medicines of worms and the like are adept in moving and searching, and have the functions of guiding medical effects to go deeply into various joints of human body.

When the wind pathogen lies in meridians and collaterals, the scorpion may be used. However, one should try to avoid using it as possible since scorpion has strong toxicity and it could impair Qi and blood. Just for this reason, many medical books write that **Qianzheng San** should not be used for the patients who are suffering from stroke (apoplexia) due to Yin deficiency. In fact, it is another matter in clinical practics, and it depends on the extent to which the medicine is used and what herbs it may be used together with.

About Wind-Pathogens

Wind pathogen is a term covering a very extensive concept. If the pathogenic wind is on the surface, the proper way is to guide it off with the herbs represented by Sangye (mulberry leaf) for dispelling wind and relieving exterior symptoms. In case the wind is in meridians and collaterals, the proper way is to drive it out with the herbs represented by Sangzhi (mulberry twig) for dispelling the wind. In case the wind lies inside due to deficiency of Yin, the proper way is to put it out with the herbs represented by Sangshen (the mulberry fruits) and the like. All winds are called "wind" in spite of their great differences. They definitely have some similarities as to symptoms, so, there will be some similarities of medication for treatment, too.

All in all, Yang without gaining its Yin will become pathogenic wind, and

Yin without gaining its Yang will become phlegm. When there is pathogenic wind, phlegm will arise. So those who are struck by stroke (apoplexia) will show some symptoms of phlegm. Even the cold due to the exogenous wind will also bring some phlegm. Regardless of the endogenous or exogenous winds, they share some similarities in the way of treatment. The wind due to deficiency of Yin may result in an excessive symptom (a physically strong patient is running a high fever, etc.). In such a case, we may refer to the treatment of dispelling pathogenic wind. The wind in between skin, meridians and collaterals, blood vessels and bones may also consume Yin and blood, so in such a case, what could be done is to nourish Yin to quiet down the wind.

Snakes

In TCM, scorpion always naturally remind of snake since they share some similarities in medical effects of moving and searching for pathogens in human body.

Properties of Snakes

The snakes to be used as medicines include zaocys dhumnade and long-noded pit viper, but for dispelling wind-damp, the latter one comes the first in effects. Among the long-noded pit vipers, the agkistrodon is the best one. In China, the agkistrodon produced in Qichun county of Hubei province is considered to be the best when used as an herb. Qichun county enjoys a good reputation for some well-known herbs like Qi'ai (Chinese mugwort), Qishe (long-noded pit viper), Qi-bamboo and Qi-turtle.

In the market of herbs or in drugstores, the long-noded pit vipers are all dead and dried up, so how can one distinguish the long-noded pit viper from the other snakes? Some people may make the judgement from the abdominal patterns, which in fact cannot be relied upon too much. Generally speaking, after the snake dies and dries up, its eyes will close up and sink down. But for the long-noded pit vipers, when they are dried up, their eyes will not close up or sink down.

All the snakes live in the dark pits or holes with gloomy and poisonous environment. Such environment underground will deposit toxins in snakes. Similarly, the wind could be pervasive and changeable and move here and there in human body. The snake is also characterized with crawling and getting in holes and openings. In the shady, damp and perilous opening, there might be snakes. When the wind enters the dark and damp joints in human bodies, it is usually hard to be driven out with the common medicines. In such a case, the long-noded pit viper can work well and it can even run into the deepest spots to ferret out the pathogenic wind.

Snake Soaked with Liquor Has Better Effects

Many books of materia medica say "snake used with liquor gives better effects", which means that snake used together with liquor will turn out to be more effective since liquor can also be moving and spurting here and there in the human body to dredge meridians and collaterals. Snake and liquor together can bring out the best effect in each other. Many people often soak liquor with snakes, but attention is required that those who just drink the snake-soaked liquor should try to avoid the exogenous wind and sit at home with all windows closed since the snake-soaked liquor not only can open the hair pores of human bodies but also leave ossature and meridians and collaterals in certain permeable state. As such, when the internal pathogens is running out, the exogenous wind, if any, can drive deep into skin even the meridians and collaterals and the ossature at the same time, which will be terribly troublesome.

There was a story that a man put the living snake into a jar of liquor. After a certain period of time, the snake looked dead. However, when he opened the jar for drinking the liquor, the snake suddenly came out and gave him a bite. Snakes usually have very strong vitality of life. Such a case warns that even if a dead snake is soaked in liquor, one must try to keep away from it at the time of opening the jar. In particular, do not try to look inside or smell it at the mouth of the jar since it is unhealthy at the moment of opening the jar.

Shetui (Snake Slough)

The snake goes into Yin and blood systems and can worm its way into shady and dark joints in human body. The slough is on the surface of a snake, so this image suggests that it goes through the exterior, and then into the darkest points in human body to drive out the wind-pathogens and dispel the pathogenic wind in blood.

Especially, some skin diseases, in the process of healing up, may cause long-lasting rubefaction and itch, which means heat and wind still exist in blood. The snake slough can help to remove it. For sure, Chantui is also effective if the skin disease is not so serious. Suppose the pathogenic factor mainly lies in Qi system, Chantui can be workable; but when the pathogenic factor is lingering and moving in the blood system, the snake slough must be used, or the two may be used simultaneously.

While purchasing the snake slough in drugstores, try to select the slough in silver white color. In fact, the snake slough should be essentially white regardless of yellow snake or black one. Generally, a substance loses its right state or origi-nal condition, it will become poisonous. Therefore, the black or yellow slough should not be used as medicine since it may be the slough from the sick snakes.

A snake generally exuviate five times a year, so the output of snake slough is considerably large.

Leave Some Leeway When Writing a Prescription

When the wind pathogen lies in between meridians and collaterals, the last resort is to use the long-noded pit viper.

As discussed previously, when wind-cold-damp pathogen lies in between meridians and collaterals and skin, Qianghuo, Duhuo, Sangzhi and Sangjisheng etc. can be used to dispel the wind and eliminate the damp pathogen. All of these are herbal medicines. In case the pathogen goes deeper inside, these herbal medicines may not work effectively. And then, some animal medicines like scor-pion, scolopendra and the like should be used. If such animal medicines fail a-gain, the last resort might be the long-noded pit viper, which not only can dispel the wind in the joints of bones, but also cure the leprosy or the serious wind pathogens. An article named *Discourse of the Snake-Catcher* written by Liu Zongyuan in Tang dynasty, in which it says, "In the field of Yongzhou lives a peculiar kind of snake, which is able to cure the leprosy". The pathogenic wind in leprosy is very fierce, for which strong medicine, i. e. , the snake (the long-noded pit viper), must be used. Generally, the snake medicine should be avoided unless it is a must. On the one hand, it is out of mercy; on the other hand, try to avoid using medicine to the extreme at the beginning.

For writing a prescription, especially for newly diagnosed and confirmed patients, it is important to leave some leeway in prescriptions. Do not use the medicine of the long-noded pit viper when the pathogenic wind is first diagnosed though it is quite effective. But what if it is not so effective as expected? There would be no alternative available. Once, there was a patient suffering encephalanalosis. At the first visit, I told him that I only wrote the prescription for 70% effect. He then felt as if I didn't try my utmost. I tried to explain that it was his first visit and I, just like carrying some weight, was not so sure of the weight at very beginning and had to have a try with 70% of my capability to move it. When I was sure of its weight, I would then try my best as needed to carry the weight!

Too much water will drown the miller. This tells us a truth that nothing should go to the extreme, neither should the use of medicines.

Banxia Baizhu Tianma Tang

The pathogenic wind, if lying in beween the skin, meridians and collaterals, are normally the exogenous wind in most cases. Of cause, sometimes the endogenous wind is included. Suppose there is merely the endogenous wind, the calming wind medicines should be used for treatment.

To calm wind is a little different from dipelling wind that has been discussed in the above sections. Dispelling wind is to drive out the pathogenic wind, while to calm wind is to let the wind quiet down itself, which is also called stabilizing wind, that is, try to keep the wind calming down and do not stir it up any more.

Properties of Tianma (Gastrodia Elata)

Among the medicines for calming wind, Tianma (gastrodia elata) always comes the first. It can enter the liver meridian system. For medicine use, the root of Tianma should be is taken, and the wild Tianma will be far better.

When Tianma begins to sprout, a red and straight plant like an arrow will grow up. Therefore, it is also called Chijian (red arrow) or Dingfeng Cao (stabilizing wind grass). It is said that the wind cannot move it, but it always shakes itself when the wind calms down. Besides, Qianghuo and Duhuo have the similar properties to Chijian, which is written in some books, but I never saw such a thing before. However, what one should keep in mind is that Tianma is associated with wind.

Tianma as a medicine is partially dry, so, can it be used for treatment of endogenous wind due to deficiency of Yin? In fact, it can be used in such a case, but the critical point is to make sure what medicine it will go with. If used with the medicine for nourishing Yin, it will have the effects of both nourishing Yin and dispelling wind. If used with the medicines for reducing phlegm, it will function to remove the wind phlegm. For instance, Tianma used with Banxia (pinellia ternate), Nanxing (arisaema heterophyllum blume), and Baizhu (white atractylodes rhizome) can dispel wind phlegm. There is a very typical formula called **Tianma Banxia Baizhu Tang**.

Analyses of Banxia BaizhuTianma Tang Formula

Generally, pathogenic wind always arises simultaneously with phlegm. Human body actually contains half Yin and half Yang, which are closely intertwined with each other. If Yin and Yang become inharmonious, and intend to separate from each other, Yang and Yin will lose balance. If Yang fails to gain its corresponding Yin, it will turn into pathogenic wind or fire; if Yin fails to gain its corresponding Yang, it will then turn into phlegm. Some tangible substances, if they could not obtain the necessary energy, may function improperly and become phlegm, while the corresponding energy will give no play to its function and then become pathogenic wind or fire that may act wildly.

Tianma for calming wind, and Banxia, Baizhu, Chenpi and Fuling (these four herbs used together to make a formula called **Erchen Tang**) for removing phlegm, are used together as the main ingredients to make a formula called **Tianma Banxia Baizhu Tang**. There are many different versions about this formula, but it is here to introduce the version covered in the book of *Yixue Xinwu* (Medical Insights) written by Cheng Zhongling.

Banxia Baizhu Tianma Tang contains the herbal ingredients of Tianma (gastrodia elata), Banxia (pinellia ternate), Baizhu (white atractylodes rhizome), Chenpi (pericarpium citri reticulatae), Fuling (poria cocos), fresh ginger, Gancao (liquorice), Dazao (jujubae), and Manjingzi (fructus viticis).

Tianma can quiet down pathogenic wind and **Erchen Tang** can remove phlegm. Therefore, the cases of the wind or fire stemming from Yang failing to gain its corresponding Yin, or the phlegm stemming from Yin failing to gain its corresponding Yang will be eliminated. It is not enough to get rid of the wind and phlegm only, and it is also critical to have Yin and Yang intertwined with each other again. For this purpose, Baizhu must be used since it can tonify the spleen and mobilize the Middle Jiao to work properly, which will help Yin and Yang intertwine with each other. In a word, the intertwining of Yin with Yang, to a great extent, depends on T&T functions of the spleen.

Ginger, Gancao and Dazao are used as the reconciling substances in the Middle Jiao. The fresh ginger can also be used as corrigent medicine for Banxia since it can mitigate the toxicity of Banxia on the one hand and calm the adverse-rising energy, tonifies the spleen, and warms to reduce the phlegm on the other hand. Dazao may be removed in case of abdominal distension.

Manjingzi is used with Tianma for dispelling the pathogenic wind around head and faces. Especially, when the dizzy giddy symptom occurs, Manjingzi used with Tianma (gastrodia elata) will bring a very good effect. But in the case of no dizzy giddy symptoms, Manjingzi may be removed from the formula.

Banxia Baizhu Tianma Tang is a typical and fundamental formula for removing the wind phlegm. Generally, when one suffers from serious phlegm and high blood pressure at the same time, he or she usually would have serious pathogenic wind, too. In that case, **Banxia Baizhu Tianma Tang** can be used for treatment.

Tianma enters the Qi system of the liver meridian. **Banxia Baizhu Tianma Tang** enters the Qi system, too. If the endogenous wind goes deep into the blood system, Chuanxiong should be added to the formula to dispel the pathogenic wind there. By the way, Tianma and Chuanxiong are commonly used medicine pair.

Tianma Gouteng Yin

Tianma Gouteng Yin is another famous formula related to Tianma. It contains the herbal ingredients of Tianma (gastrodia elata), Gouteng (uncaria), Shijueming (concha haliotidis), Chuan Niuxi (radix cyathulae), Shanzhi (cape jasmine), Huangqin (scutellaria baicalensis), Yimucao (motherwort), Duzhong (eucommia ulmoides), Sangjisheng (parasitic loranthus), Yejiaoteng (tuber fleeceflower stem), Zhufushen (cinnabar poria cum ligno hospite).

Tianma Gouteng Yin (In Chinese "Yin" means "drink", but in fact here means "decoction") is not named as **Tianma Gouteng Tang** (in Chinese "Tang" means "soup", but in fact hear means "decoction", too) because of the difference in the way of drinking. "Tang" must be taken regularly, for instance, twice a day, a bowl of it once, while "Yin" refers to drinking it like tea. When in decocting it as "Yin", more water may be added to make the decoction light in taste, then drink it whenever one wants to. There are many formulas named as "Yin", for example, **Shengmai Yin** (i. e. pulse-activating decoction), **Zuogui Yin** (left restoring decoction), **Yougui Yin** (right restoring decoction), **Sansheng Yin** (three life decoction), all of which can be taken as tea.

Compatibility of Tianma (Gastrodia Elata) and Gouteng (Uncaria)

Tianma is always used together with Gouteng. Gouteng enters the liver meridians and the pericardium meridians to quiet down the wind and quench the fire. Actually, the wind and fire often act in collusion with each other, where the wind assists the fire and vise versa. Meanwhile, the wind can eliminate dampness, but in case the wind inside human body is powerful, it will consume and impair Yin fluid, resulting in deficiency of Yin and blood. Furthermore, the deficiency of blood will then cause wind and fire. All of these form a vicious circle with the wind and fire fanning each other and getting stronger and stronger mutually. Thus, both the fire burns up and the wind swirls upwards to lift Qi and blood upwards then, causing "Qi and blood to go upwards simultaneously" to give rise to some symptoms like dizziness, headache or high blood pressure etc.

Gouteng is used here since it can calm pathogenic wind and clear fire. Some senior TCM doctors in the past, especially imperial physicians of the royal palace in the Qing dynasty, for example Zhao Wenkui etc. prescribed medicines with great subtlety. Once encountering the heat symptoms, they would use Gouteng since once the fire occurs, the wind will occurs accordingly, that is, the fire can result in wind and vise versa, and they fan each other. The ordinary doctors generally give treatment of fire for fire, but the more experienced doctors will actually give more concerns on preventing fire from leading to wind, so they are able to add some Gouteng at the proper time when writing a prescription.

Properties of Gouteng and Its Selection

When Gouteng is used with Tianma, its capacity for quieting down wind and quenching fire will become stronger and give rise to an effect of "one plus one making greater than two. "

Gouteng is growing on the vine with two hooks to hook up to the branches and twigs of trees by which it then extends further while swinging in the wind. Of course, some Gouteng only have a single hook, whose efficacy may not be so effective. Now doctors, when writing a prescription, usually write double-hook Gouteng, i. e. two hooks are required. Well, in some areas, the Gouteng even have no hooks at all but only the peduncles. Such a Gouteng is the worst in medical effect.

For selection of Gouteng, the first and the most important point is to examine the two symmetrical hooks. The second point is to select the tender Gouteng, which is better and green in color, but it will become black when it is dried up, whereas the old Gouteng is yellow in color. In the previous sections, it has been mentioned that the herbs, when they are green in color, are always strong and fierce in effect, and they can enter the liver, so is Gouteng. The tender and green Gouteng can enter the liver, but when it grows old and becomes yellow in color, it will then go to the spleen. Thus, its function for dispelling wind will become less effective. What's more, the section of the rattan between the two hooks for the tender Gouteng is in square form. However, when it grows old, this section will become round. So, in the process of selecting Gouteng, try to take the square-rattaned Gouteng.

Shijueming (Concha Haliotidis) and Conch Medicines

Shijueming (Concha Haliotidis) is in fact the shell of abalone (sea-ear). As an herb, it is covered in the category of conch, with a character of heavy texture. It can be used to improve eyesight, suppress Yang and calm the liver wind.

Shijueming, as its name implies, "Shi" (means "stone") explains that it is very heavy, which is close to a substance like a stone; "Jueming" ("Jue" means "to decide"; "ming" means "to clear eyesight") explains it can go to eyes to improve eyesight. There is another similar herb called Caojueming (cassia occidentalis), i. e., Juemingzi (cassia seed), which also has the effect of clearing the liver and improving eyesight. The only difference between them is on its herbaceous property. Shijueming has holes in it, but the best is the bigger one with 9 holes in it and is more effective as an herb. Shijueming with 7 holes is still good, and the worst is the one with only 5 holes in it.

Zhenzhumu (concha margaritiferallsta or nacre mother of pearl) is another herb that is similar to Shijueming. Many of the shells for growing pearls are interconnected with pearls. After the pearls are removed, all the leftover parts are Zhenzhumu. The herbs like Shijueming and Zhenzhumu are actually calcium carbonate when they are examined and analyzed with the help of modern chemical analysis, but they have different uses. Both Shijueming and Zhenzhumu are quite hard with certain toughness, whose main function is to quiet down pathogenic wind. However, Muli (concha ostreae) is little more course, which feels dry without the fine and smooth sleekness manifested in both Shijueming and Zhenzhumu. Muli is inclined to inducing astringency and surpressing wind. Besides, Sheng Waleng (raw concha arcae) and Haigeqiao (concha meretricis seu cyclinae) and the like are inclined to resolve hard lump and reduce thick phlegm.

Searching for and Capturing the Pathogenic Wind

Shijueming is a repressing medicine, and it can guide the liver Qi downwards and repress to calm the liver and quiet down the wind.

Tianma and Gouteng go upwards. The wind swirls upwards so the medicine may also follow the wind to go upwards. But after the medicine swirls up, the wind must be caught and repressed dowards, for which Shijueming is used.

Chuan Niuxi is used to guide the Qi and blood to go downwards, and it can work together with Shijueming to repress pathogenic wind downwards.

Therefore, for the high blood pressure due to the liver wind agitation or hyperactivity of liver-Yang, it should be considered to use such four herbs as Tianma, Gouteng, Shijueming and Niuxi. But if the blood stasis is more serious, Chuan Niuxi (radix cyathulae) should be used instead; if not so serious, Huai Niuxi (achyranthes root) can be used since Chuan Niuxi is more effective for promoting blood circulation to remove blood stasis, whereas Huai Niuxi is inclined to nourish the liver and kidney. Tianma and Gouteng go upwards, which is equivalent to chase after. Shijueming and Chuan Niuxi go downwards to repress, which is equivalent to remand the captive. These four medicines come first in the formula since they are the major herbs.

Ancillary Medicines Used in Tianma Gouteng Yin

The pathogenic wind may cause fire that in the human body manifests as rapid pulse, yellow furred tongue, red eyes and yellow urine etc. So, Zhizi (fructus gardenia) and Huangqin (scutellaria baicalensis) should be used to clear the heat. Zhizi can clear the lingering fire in the Tri-jiao, and Huangqin mainly clears the lung fire. Such fire generally wonders in the Upper Jiao, so two bitter medicines are used to clear them. Yimucao (motherwort) is used here as an ancillary medicine for cooling and nourishing blood and eliminating blood stasis.

The endogenous wind often goes with deficiency of liver-Yin and kidney-Yin. "The defensive Qi comes from the Lower Jiao". If the Lower Jiao becomes deficient, the defensive Qi will become weak too, and then some exogenous wind will get in by taking advantage of the weak defensive Qi, to act in collusion with the endogenous wind to infringe upon the waist and lower limbs of human body. Many aged people always complain about soreness of waist and unease of the lower limbs because of senility on the one hand and the exogenous pathogenic infringement on the other hand. Under such circumstances, Duzhong and Sangjisheng should be used since they can nourish the liver, and the most important function of these two herbs is to eliminate the wind-damp pathogen out of the liver and kidney mildly and smoothly and to nourish the healthy Qi of the liver and kidneys. Furthermore, Duzhong can guide Qi and blood to go downwards.

Yejiaoteng in the formula can tranquilize and allay excitement and cure insomnia. When it is used with Shuanggouteng (uncaria laevigata), they can bring the best effect in each other.

Fushen (poria cum ligno hospite) is to help the consciousness to lurk down without moving outside in order to help fall asleep. Zhufushen actually is Fushen dyed with Zhusha (cinnabar) since Zhusha can also function to tranquilize mind. Therefore, Zhufushen will become more effective in tranquilizing mind.

Both Yejiaoteng and Zhufushen can help one fall asleep. As it can be seen many aged people sleep less every day because of pathogenic wind in the body. When the wind disturbs, they would not fall asleep. In fact, sleeping helps Yin and Yang interwine with each other, which not only helps nourish Yang, but also nourish Yin. Less sleeping will fail Yin and Yang to interwine naturally with each other, causing pathogenic wind and phlegm. In that case, Yejiaoteng and Fushen are used to help Yin and Yang intercommunicate with each other, and then have the heart and kidney intercommunicate, too. Therefore, a sound sleep can help one obtain nourishment to build up his health. By the way, even without suffering from insomnia and having normal sleep, one may also use some Yejiaoteng and Fushen to help Yin and Yang to get interwined.

Zhengan Xifeng Tang

The formula of **Zhengan Xifeng Tang** contains the ingredient herbs: Huai Niuxi (achyranthes root) 1 *liang*, Sheng Zheshi (raw ochre) 1 *liang* (rolled thin and fine), Sheng Longgu (raw ossa draconis) 5 *qian* (crushed), Sheng Muli (raw oyster shell) 5 *qian* (crushed), Sheng Guiban (raw turtle shell) 5 *qian* (crushed), Baishao (radix paeoniae alba) 5 *qian*, Xuanshen (radix scrophulariae) 5 *qian*, Tiandong (asparagus cochinchinensis) 5 *qian*, Chuanlianzi (szechwan Chinaberry fruit) (crushed) 2 *qian*, Sheng Maiya (raw malt) 5 *qian*, Yinchen (oriental wormwood) 2 *qian*, Gancao (liquorice) 1. 5 qian.

Unnecessary Change of Medicine Sequence in Zhengan Xifeng Tang

Zhengan Xifeng Tang is a very famous formula in the ***Records of Traditional Chinese and Western Medicine in Combination*** written by Zhang Xichun, a leading medical expert in late Qing Dynasty. The Medicine sequence in **Zhengan Xifeng Tang** above remains unchanged as its original sequence.

The ***Records of Traditional Chinese and Western Medicine in Combination*** is a nice book. First of all, Zhang Xichun was quite a broad-minded and selfless person who liked to share what he has with the others. His ***Records of Traditional Chinese and Western Medicine in Combination*** collects numerous medical monographs of his, and some of his speech scripts, letters and even poems in order to make his monographs integrated. He tried his utmost to present all his teaching scenes to the readers. So, he always tirelessly explained formulas, herbs/medicines and medical principles in combination, and especially, paid much attention to answering questions and solving puzzles to his disciples. He often wrote letters to his disciples to explore into some medical knots. By the way, he often kept the same medicine sequence in his prescription without changing the sequential order of medicines, which is different from many other doctors who often rearrnge the medicine sequence in different prescriptions, and cause some misunderstandings by the others.

Manifestations of Excessive Vigor of the Liver Qi

Sometime, one may be in good physical conditions to some extent, or even in a robust condition, or at least he is not in a state of being apparently strong and actually weak. However, the following phenomena may suddenly occur: the endogenous wind rises; his blood pressure becomes very high; his faces become specially red; and his pulse beats very rapidly and vigorously, which seems to challenge the fingertips of the doctor who is taking his pulse. This is called "vigorous pulse challenging the fingertips", which is a manifestation of excessive vigor of liver Qi. In such a case, he will need **Zhengan Xifeng Tang** for treatment.

The liver is an organ of the "General" with very fierce and tough properties. When the pathogenic wind stirs up in the liver, it may indicate that the General is in rage and may turn renegade. In that case, actions must be taken to repress it.

Heavy Repression

Huai Niuxi is heavy in property, and it goes downwards. In the formula of **Zhengan Xifeng Tang**, Huai Niuxi is used with 1 *liang*, which is quite a large dosage. Sheng Zheshi is a kind of rufous rock that can enter the system of the liver meridian and blood. When entering the liver meridian, it can repress the liver Qi. Sheng Longgu and Sheng Muli not only have the repressing effect, but also have the astringent function so they can restrain the up-going Yang. When the liver Qi is vigorous, Yang is sure to go outwards. In this formula, Sheng Longgu and Sheng Muli are used to repress the liver wind and restrain the up-going and floating Yang.

Sheng Guiban 5 *qian* is used here since it is of the raw shell of the river turtle, used as a medicine, which effectively functions to nourish the primordial Yin (i. e. the kidney Yin). Attention: mountain turtle shells are toxic, and the sea turtle shells can not be used as medicine. Strictly speaking, both of them are useless. In clinical practices, sometimes they are found to have a little effect but are quite far from the effects of the river turtle shells. Furthermore, Sheng Guiban must be the bottom part of the river turtle shell, and the best part is that with regular patterns like the Chinese character "王" ("Wang", means "King"). The turtleback, if having hexagon patterns on it, cannot be used as medicine, either.

Sheng Guiban has repressing effect. When used together with Huai Niuxi, Zhishi, Longgu, and Muli, it seems to bear down on one with the weight of Mount. Stones, grass herbs, bones, conches and shells are all used to press down in order to repress the liver wind. In case of hyperactivity of liver-Yang, the only way to do is to repress it. Wind is the primary pathogen of all diseases, and the liver is a traitor among the five internal organs (heart, liver, spleen, lungs and kidneys). Wind is the source that may cause various diseases. Physiologically, the liver is a good organ, as in TCM called "the organ of General", "liver storing blood", "liver housing soul", "liver controlling dispersion". However, when the liver falls sick, it will become a traitor and start to hurt the other internal organs. Therefore, impairment of all the five internal organs is always related with the liver, like a General who rebels will commit murder and arson, causing a great destruction. Under that condition, a large number of troops will have to be deployed to carry out repression.

Combination of Hardness with Softness for Appeasement

To repress with force is not the best way, and to "kill" the General (referring to the organ of liver) is not the final target, since the "organ of General" is still expected to return to work continuously. So, one should think over why the General (the organ of liver) starts to rebel? It may be that the owner does not take good care of it, or may impose too much assignment on it, or does not give it favourable treatment. Liver is subsumed to Yin in nature and Yang in function. Hence, the herbs like Danggui and Baishao should be used to nourish it, after which the liver will restrain itself properly.

While one is trying to repress the liver, he must appease it, too. In fact, Chuan Niuxi and Guiban used in the above formula shows the concept of alternate kindness in the process of repression. And then, 5 *qian* Baishao is used, which is actually a large dosage targeting at nourishing the liver and Yin since the sour taste of Baishao can enter the liver. With this medicine, the General (the organ of liver) would feel very comfortable. Xuanshen (radix scrophulariae) is added to nourish the kidney, which can then nourish the liver further, letting the liver feel more comfortable.

Where can the liver and kidney obtain their Yin? Yin cannot arise from nowhere. That is why Tiandong is added in the formula to nourish the lung Yin in order to promote the secretion of saliva or body fluid. When the lung is fully nourished, it can then promote the kidney to make up sufficient fluid to the liver and kidneys. This goes like it rains from the sky, and all plants on the earth will obtain enough water supply. All these processes are the necessities for appeasing the General. With both severity and kindness, the General organ (the liver) would be appeased finally.

While taming the General organ, one may still feel worried about the "lingering anger" of the liver. Hence, Chuanlianzi is used here to give a last blow, i. e. to relieve the liver Qi.

The next appeasement is to improve the General's living surroundings and environment. Sheng Maiya (raw malt) can soothe the liver, tonify the spleen and upbear the stomach Qi. The medical classic ***Jingui Yaolue (Synopsis of Golden Chamber)*** says, "In case of the liver diseases, try to consolidate the spleen at first since the liver can infect the spleen," Sheng Maiya can satisfy such a requirement. For soothing the liver, Chaihu (radix bupleuri) is not used since the patient may suffer from deficiency of the liver Yin at the moment when he needs **Zhengan Xifeng Tang**. Chaihu can impair the liver Yin, resulting in more serious deficiency of the liver Yin, and causing the patient to suffer dysthesia. Hence, it is only Sheng Maiya that can be used here to soothe the liver. Sheng Maiya refers to the wheat that is just to sprout and then is dried in the air. The wheat (malt) dried in this condition has a strong vitality of life. Therefore, it can be used for soothing the liver. Yinchen (oriental wormwood) may be used to soothe the liver and eliminate the dampness and heat, too. The liver is most afraid of dampness and heat. When there is deficiency of the liver Yin and hyperactivity of liver-Yang, the dampness and heat will be very easily accumulated. Meanwhile, under the conditions of dampness and heat, the hyperactivity of liver-Yang may also occur. As such, Yinchen must be used to eliminate the dampness and heat in order to improve the living environment of the liver.

So, on the one hand the liver is repressed, and on the other hand, the stasis is relieved. The dampness and heat are also eliminated and nutrients are provided. When all these conditions are satisfied, the liver would play its functions obediently, which is like appeasing the General in the army. The TCM principles are similar to that of the nature, and that of the human power management, too.

Zhengan Xifeng Tang is often used in clinical pratices, but attention must be called to that this formula can not be used long. When the General (the liver) gives in, the repression should not be enforced any further. Otherwise, the patient may become weak and listless, and some other diseases may come up. Stop using the formula right after the patient gets better.

第六章 白僵蚕与祛风息风类药

白僵蚕

《神农本草经》这样描述白僵蚕："咸、辛、平，无毒，主治小儿惊痫夜啼，去三虫，灭黑点，令人面色好，男子阴痒病。"

白僵蚕的来源

有过养蚕经验的人应该都知道，养蚕人家都是小心翼翼的，蚕室要保持卫生，甚至连不吉利的话都不敢说，还有人家要举行一些祭祀活动，总之生怕蚕生病，蚕生病就会死，死了就意味着没有收入。

蚕死后跟别的动物是不一样。别的动物一死，尸体很快就会烂，发臭；而蚕死后，尸体会变得很僵硬，不腐烂，不发臭，我们叫它白僵蚕。

用来入药的白僵蚕，必须是因病自然死亡的蚕。夏天蚊子喜欢叮蚕，一叮就死了，而且会发黑，这就不能用了。

物尽其用

咱们中医讲究物尽其性，任何一种事物都要物尽其性，物尽其用。

民间养蚕，是为了取蚕茧，做蚕丝。如果养蚕不顺，蚕中途死了，变成了白僵蚕，那就卖给药店。

中医用药的态度，充满了谦逊、慈悲和敬畏，是很怜惜万物的。比如檀香和犀牛角，用的往往都是边角料。

僵蚕属金，金药治风

白僵蚕，色白属金，入肺；坚硬，也是属金，金在五行中"从介化"，介化就是变硬。跟金相关的都会硬，石头那么硬，是属金的，还有乌龟背上的硬壳也属金。且僵蚕又得桑之气，因为它是吃桑叶长大的，所以又能治风。

其实桑也属金，桑树叶子掉光以后，我们会看到它呈白色，白属金。

— 250 —

可能有人会问，前面不是一直说桑属木吗？它旺于春季，有生生之气，而且，它还治风，这些不都是木的特征吗？现在怎么又突然说它属金呢？其实这不矛盾，它有生生之气，可以治邪风，所以可以说它在生理上是属木的；但它又能治风，风属木，金克木，所以它在药理上是属金的。

白僵蚕治小儿惊痫夜啼

白僵蚕的一切作用，都是围绕祛风。小儿惊痫夜啼，往往跟肝风有关。晚上哭，一般是在子时、丑时，气血流注于肝胆经。这时肝风动了，胆热起来了，小孩就会非常得烦躁、易怒，就会哭。所以用白僵蚕来驱风平肝。但现在一般不这么用，现在小儿夜啼的话，往往用蝉蜕之类，有时候连药都可以不用，转而用推拿、按摩、捏脊等手法，也可以。只有在比较严重的时候，在辨证论治的基础上，有风的话，才考虑加一些僵蚕。如果气分有热的话，可以加一些蝉蜕。

《神农本草经》所谓"惊痫夜啼"。就是因为"惊痫"而发生的夜啼，比如在哭的时候伴随抽搐等风象，这时候可以用僵蚕。其他时候不要轻易用这味药。

杀三虫

蚕是一种虫子，虫得风而生，与风同气相求，所以有驱风之用。

当我们身体有虫的时候，也要通过祛风来治。《神农本草经》讲白僵蚕能够"去三虫"，也就是祛除各种寄生虫。虫得风而生。我们体内都有寄生虫，因为身体里有风啊，当这个风是和风时，这些虫都安分守己，不乱动，你也就感觉不到；当身体内有邪风的时候，体内的这些虫就不安分了，到处乱窜，甚至还会生出邪虫，人就会很难受。

我们看"风"字，里面就是一个虫。虫得风而生，风里就有虫，古人早就意识到了，不用你现在去研究。有人说风有内风外风啊，其实内风外风里都有虫。现在讲风寒感冒，风热感冒，好像跟虫没有关系，但你写繁体"風"字就能悟到：病毒来了，它躲在风里面啊，病毒也是一种虫，只不过你看不见而已。内风有血虚生风，也引动一些虫。

听一位老军医讲他以前救治伤员的事情：在战争年代，伤员的伤口往往都很吓人，由于创面大，时间长，有的人伤口上会生蛆，有的人的伤口上则不生蛆。你以为伤口生蛆虫的更严重吗？不是的。伤口生蛆看起来很恶心，但你进行适当清理、消毒再包扎后，这个人就活过来了。反而是那些伤口不生蛆的伤员死了。为什么？因为伤口都不生蛆了，说明他的身体里面没有生生之气。风一方面意味着有虫子，另一方面也意味着一种生生之气。

有人问，尸体也会生蛆，如何理解？其实，理解死人有一套体系，理解活人又是另一套体系。伤口上生蛆和尸体上生蛆也是两回事。

美容要药白僵蚕

那白僵蚕为什么能够"灭黑点，令人面色好"呢？

养过蚕的人都知道，蚕是要蜕皮的。它也是能够让人像蚕蜕皮那样把脸上一些黑点、斑纹褪掉，令人面色好。这是第一层意思。

蚕一生要蜕四次皮。四是什么？地四生金，四是属金的，这又意味着蚕跟金有关，能够祛风。脸上的斑点的形成，也跟风有关。人全身可能皮肤都比较细嫩，就是脸不争气，很快就会变得又黑又焦。这是为什么呢？一方面是因为脸在外边，每天都要经受外风；现在又多了一重，要经受计算机屏幕辐射。体内的风也是往上走的，携带者体内的内热，游走于面部。外风内风同时作用于你的脸，这样蹂躏，当然老得快，而且会留下各种痕迹，也就是那些斑点。

我们用僵蚕来驱风。僵蚕属金，色白入肺，而肺主皮毛；僵蚕还入足阳明胃经，而面部恰属阳明。所以它驱脸上的浮游的风效果非常好，所以它能够灭黑点，能美容。

僵蚕是一味很好的美容药，在清朝宫廷的玉容散里，就用到白僵蚕。

根据蚕能够蜕皮的特性，还有没有别的作用呢？有。一般来说，婴儿的皮肤会特别细嫩光滑，但有的婴儿身上跟长了鳞似的，摸上去都碍手。中医称为这叫胎垢。这是因为气血不足，肺气不宣。可以经常用僵蚕煎汤来洗。

白僵蚕的炮制

优质的白僵蚕是白色的，一条一条，很直很完整的。一般先用淘米水把僵蚕浸泡一天，把桑涎给泡掉。桑涎就是蚕吃了桑叶后在体内形成的一种类似痰涎的东西，泡的时候会有一些涎沫从蚕的嘴里慢慢透出来。

然后把它晒干。有人说用火炒，这是不可取的。蚕属金，火克金。用火炒过，它的金性就会被破坏掉。当然在熬药的时候用火熬又另当别论，因为熬药时是既有水又有火的，这和纯粹的用火炒不一样。

僵蚕地龙配伍

经常跟僵蚕相配的是地龙，也就是蚯蚓。

蚕的头都是往上抬的，僵蚕入药往上走；地龙则相反，它是往土里边钻的，入药就往下走。

蚕喜欢干净的环境，它只吃桑叶，桑叶也很干净。地龙则生活在土里，吃的也是土，很不干净。

僵蚕和地龙是两种不同的虫子，它们有相反的性质。

蚯蚓性咸寒，有小毒，主降，能利水、通经。因为咸寒，所以它还能退热。你拿一条蚯蚓，用手拉一拉，会发现它很有一些弹性，这像什么呢？像血管。蚯蚓能软化血管。对于很多痉挛，尤其是头部痉挛，经常用僵蚕地龙相配。

僵蚕往上走，把地龙的药性往上引。当一个人有风的时候，就会伴随着热，也会伴随着很多的不柔和，血管由此硬化，风再鼓动气血，就容易冲破血管，导致脑出血、眼底出血等。僵蚕配地龙，在驱风的同时还能够软化血管。其实僵蚕也有软化的作用，蚕也是很软的嘛，而且蚕吐的丝也是软的。与地龙相配，作用更大，而且地龙还能退热。

僵蚕配地龙，还用于治经络中的痰湿死血。活络丹的组成，就是僵蚕、地龙、川芎、草乌、五香、没药这几味。

牵正散

牵正散

白附子、白僵蚕、生全蝎，等分。

口眼歪斜

牵正散，顾名思义，就是哪里歪了，它都能给你牵正。有的人中风，口眼歪斜，还有的人没有中风，没有口眼歪斜，但舌头伸出来是歪的，你一提醒他，说你舌头都歪了，他说不歪啊，再伸出来真不歪了，等下次无意一伸舌头，又歪了，这也算歪。不管内风外风，只要出现了歪，都可以用牵正散。用这个方有一个原则，就是中病即止，且不能久用。一般我们在汤药里面开到牵正散，三味药每味大概用 3 – 6 克就够了。

嘴巴为什么会歪？是因为风痰阻滞经络，尤其是阻滞足阳明经。足阳明经绕唇口一圈，当风痰阻滞，足阳明经气被扰动，嘴巴就会有反应，轻则抽搐，重则歪斜。

白附子

除了白僵蚕以外，牵正散还用了白附子和生全蝎。

白附子与附子，并不是同一种植物，作用也不一样，只是它们的根和苗有些相似而已。白附子入胃经，最能化风痰。风往上走，走到头面部，若有若无，形成"头面游风"，就像打游击战那样，没一个准儿地方。还像过去那些游医、游僧那样，今天在这里，明天在那里，你根本找他不到。头面游风，用一般的药抓它不住，只有白附子能把它慢慢搜到、赶走。

有人会说川乌不也是收游风的吗？这里为什么不用川乌，而用白附子？因为白附子往上行，川乌则是往下行。所以川乌一般治疗下肢的风湿，如坐骨神经痛，可以用川乌。风在脸上就要用白附子。

过去宫廷里常用来美容的玉容散，其中用到白附子，就是因为它善祛头面之游风，有美容的作用。它往往跟白芷同用，白芷能深入肌肉，外达皮肤，散风化湿。这两者都偏燥，用多了、用久了就会耗伤气血，所以又要加入滋润之品，且散且补。

蝎子

全蝎也是治风的，开方有的时候写作"全虫"。蝎子，说出来挺难听的，叫全虫要委婉一点。蝎子的力量主要在尾部，那一节一节的就是。有的大夫用蝎子，就只用蝎尾。全蝎，就是整个蝎子都入药，如果你讲究一点，还可以把脚去掉。青州的蝎子最好。

蝎子是一种青黑色的虫子。青色入肝，还意味着有刚猛之气，蝎子蜇人特别疼，就是这股刚猛之气在发挥作用。怎么治呢？伤口比较浅的，把蜗牛吐出来的涎沫涂在上面就会好；如果伤口比较深，就得把蜗牛砸碎，绞出汁来涂在上面，就会慢慢好转。效果非常神奇，一物降一物呀！

虫类药都善于走窜、搜剔，而且有引药深入的作用，子善于深入人体各种缝隙，把其他药引进去。

风邪在经络，也可以用蝎子，但是咱们尽量不用。因为蝎子是属于大毒之品，能伤人的气血的。也正是如此，很多书都讲，遇到阴虚类中风，就不要用牵正散了。其实，在实际运用中可以另当别论。可以用，只不过看你用到哪个份上，而且要注意配伍。

风邪概要

风邪是一个很广的概念。风在表，宜宣之，这就是我们讲的以桑叶为代表的疏风、解表类药；风在经络，宜祛之，这就是我们讲的以桑枝为代表的各种祛风的方法；如果风在里，是阴虚的风，则宜熄之，这就是以桑葚为代表的一系列药。各种风，差异很大，但既然都叫风，就有相通的地方，在症状上有类似，在用药上也相通。

总而言之，阳不得其阴则为风，阴不得其阳则为痰。有风的时候，痰就会出现。中风的人都会有痰象，就连感冒，伤了一点外风，接着也往往有痰。不管是治内风外风，在治疗上都有相通的地方。阴虚生风也可能产生实症，我们可以参照驱风法。风在肌肤经络筋骨之间也会消耗人体的阴血，也可以参照养阴息风法。

蛇

说到蝎子我们又会想到蛇。它们的作用也比较相似，能走蹿、搜邪。

蛇的性能

入药的蛇，有乌梢蛇、白花蛇，在祛风湿方面，以白花蛇最好，白花蛇中又以蕲蛇为最好。蕲蛇产于湖北省蕲春县。蕲春县有几个很有名的药材：蕲艾、蕲蛇、蕲竹、蕲龟。

怎么来区分蕲蛇和其他的蛇呢？我们在药材市场或是在药店里看到的蕲蛇都是死的。有人说从腹部的纹路上可以分辨是不是蕲蛇，其实这都不足为凭。一般的蛇死了以后眼睛就闭上了，晾干后眼睛就陷下去了。蕲蛇晾干后，眼睛不会闭，也不会陷下去。

蛇是生长在"土穴阴霾之处，秉幽暗毒疠之气"，它生长在地下非常阴暗、有毒的地方，蛇本身也是有毒的。风会在人体走蹿，"善行而数变"，无孔不入；动物之中也有同样善于走蹿、无孔不入的，这就是蛇。哪里阴、哪里潮、哪里湿、哪里险恶，蛇就往哪里钻。风在人体内走到阴湿的缝隙中，用一般的药就不容易把它赶走，这个时候就要用到蕲蛇。蛇能够走蹿到人体最幽暗的地方，把风给揪出来。

蛇得酒则良

本草书中说蛇"得酒良"，跟酒一块用比较好。因为酒也是走蹿的，能通经络，与蛇的作用相得益彰。人们经常用蛇泡酒。但要注意，喝了用蛇泡的酒以后不要见外风，得坐在家里，窗户都不能开。因为蛇泡的酒不但容易打开人的毛孔，而且能让你身上的骨骼、经络都处于某种通透状态，好让内在的的邪气往外透，这时候要是见了外风，外风会长驱直入，深入你的肌肤甚至经络、骨骼，那就麻烦了。

有人把一条活蛇放到坛子里，泡了一段时间，看样子蛇已经被泡死了。有一天，他想喝酒了，把酒坛打开，里边的蛇突然蹿出来，把这个人咬了。是有这种情况的，蛇的生命力很强。同时，这个故事也告诫我们：即使是泡了一条死蛇在坛子里边，在开坛的一霎那，都要离远一点，尤其不要一开坛就把脸凑过去看、闻。因为刚开坛的时候，喷出来的那一阵酒气对人体不好，人要离远一些。

蛇蜕

蛇走阴分、血分，能够钻到最阴暗的地方。蛇蜕在蛇的体表，则能走表的，它能够钻到人体最阴暗的地方，把风邪发散出来，能散血中之风。

尤其是一些皮肤病，在快好又没好还剩一些的时候，皮肤发红、发痒，久久不散，这就意味着还有血热，血中还有风，可以用一些蛇蜕。如果不是太严重，用一些蝉蜕也行。当邪气主要在气分的时候，用蝉蜕，当邪气依然缠绵在血分的时候，就必须用蛇蜕了。也可以二者同用。

从药店里面买蛇蜕要选银白色的，蛇蜕本来它就应该是白的，不管黄蛇也好，黑蛇也好，它的蛇蜕必须是银白色的。黑色的或者发黄的都不要用，可能这个蛇本身它就是病的。物失其态它就有毒。

一条蛇一年大概要蜕五次皮，所以蛇蜕的产量还是比较可观的。

处方用药，要留有余地

当风邪在经络间的时候，用蕲蛇，就基本上用到顶端了。

前面我们讲，当风寒湿邪在经络肌肤间的时候，可以用羌活、独活来散它；用桑枝、桑寄生等，可以祛风散湿透邪。这些都是植物药。当邪气已深，植物药不管用了，可以用一些动物药，全蝎、蜈蚣之类的，当这些还不管用的时候，那就得用到蕲蛇了，蕲蛇不但治骨骼之间的风，还治麻风、大风等。中学的时候学过柳宗元写的一篇文章叫《捕蛇者说》，说"永州之野产异蛇……可以已大风"。大麻风是风里面非常厉害的，在用药的力度上必须非常大，所以得用到蛇。但一般的时候，能不用蛇，我们尽量不要用蛇，既是出于慈悲心，更重要的是，用药不能一上来就用到极致。

开方子的时候也是这样的，尤其病人在初诊的时候，开方用药一定要留有余地。不要见风就用蕲蛇，虽然用蛇会有效果，但万一没有达到预期效果呢？你再想用别的，就没有别的用了。曾经有一个病人，患的是脑萎缩，初诊的时候我跟他说，我给你开的方子只用了七分力，他就觉得好像我没尽心似的。我说，这是咱们第一次看，就好比我要搬动一张桌子，我不知道它到底有多重，先要试着搬一下，用七分力，然后我就知道这桌子有多重了，下一次我就该用多大力用多大力，这个桌子不就搬起来了吗！

"满招损、谦受益"，这是一个真理。什么东西都不要满，用药同样如此。

半夏白术天麻汤

当风在肌肤经络之间的时候，往往以外风为主，有的也夹带一些内风。如果纯粹是内风，那怎么治呢？咱们后面就要讲息风药。

息风和前面的驱风略有不同，驱风是要把风赶走，息风是要让风自己停下来，也叫定风，就是把风定在那里，不要再刮起来。

天麻的性能

息风类药，首推天麻，它入肝经的气分，入药用根，野生天麻会更好。

天麻发芽后，会长出一支红色的、笔直的植物，就像一支箭插在那里，所以又叫赤箭。赤箭又叫定风草，据说风刮它不动，倒是在没有风的时候，它自己在那里摇一摇。还有很多植物，比如羌活、独活，也是这样的。我没有亲眼见过，但是书上都是这样记载的。我们记住天麻要和风联系起来。

天麻是一味偏燥性的药，那么遇到阴虚的内风是不是就不能用了呢？其实还是可以用的，关键是看天麻跟什么药跑。它跟着养阴的药，就会有养阴祛风的作用；跟着化痰的药，就有化风痰的作用。比如，天麻跟半夏、南星、白术配伍，就能祛风痰，有个代表的方子叫天麻半夏白术汤。

半夏白术天麻汤方义

有风就会同时有痰。本来，人体阴阳参半，而且紧紧交抱在一起，现在人体阴阳不和谐了，有分离之势，有多少阳得不到阴就有多少阴得不到阳。阳不得其阴，就成了风，成了火；阴不得其阳，就成了痰。有一部分物质的、有形的东西在那里，得不到能量，不能正常地运行，就成了痰，而与之相应的那一部份能量也无用武之地，就胡乱作祟，成了风和火。

咱们用天麻来息风，用半夏、白术、陈皮、茯苓，也就是二陈汤，来化痰，这就是天麻半夏白术汤。当然这个方子有很多版本，咱们这里以我们新安医家程钟龄先生《医学心悟》的版本，这也是现在比较被大家公认的天麻半夏白术汤。

半夏白术天麻汤

天麻、半夏、白术、陈皮、茯苓、生姜、甘草、大枣、蔓荆子。

天麻息风，二陈汤化痰。于是，阴不得其阳、阳不得其阴的产物去掉了。光把风和痰化掉还不行，还得让阴阳重新交抱起来，那就得用白术。白术健脾、运中，中焦一运转起来，阴和阳就更容易交抱。阴阳的交抱很大程度上取决于脾的运化功能。

姜、草、枣，也是入中焦的调和之品。生姜还可以反佐半夏的。在很多用到半夏的地方，会用生姜来减轻它的毒性，此其一；其二，生姜有降逆、化痰和健脾的作用，它还能温化痰饮。如果腹胀，可以去掉大枣。

蔓荆子也是一味祛风的药，是来配天麻的，它可以祛头面之风。尤其是当出现头晕之类症状的时候，蔓荆子配天麻效果非常好。如果不头晕，可以把蔓荆子去掉。

半夏白术天麻汤是化风痰的代表方、基础方。比如，如果一个人痰象比较重，同时血压比较高，风象也比较严重，那可以用半夏白术天麻汤。

天麻走肝经气分，半夏白术天麻汤也是走气分的，如果内风深入血分，怎么办呢？再加川芎，就能驱血中之风了。天麻、川芎，也是常用的对药。

天麻钩藤饮

跟天麻相关的还有一个很有名的方剂，叫天麻钩藤饮。这个方的药味稍微要多一些。下面是比较公认的一个版本：

天麻钩藤饮

天麻、钩藤、石决明、川牛膝、山栀、黄芩、益母草、杜仲、桑寄生、夜交藤、朱茯神。

"天麻钩藤饮"为什么不叫"天麻钩藤汤"呢？因为饮跟汤还是有一些区别的。汤得定期喝，比如说一天两次，每次一大碗。而饮则是当茶喝的，你可以多加水，煮得稍微淡一点，想喝的时候就喝。叫"饮"的方剂也很多，比如说生脉饮、左归饮、右归饮、三生饮，都是可以慢慢喝，当茶喝的。

天麻、钩藤配伍

天麻、钩藤这是经常用的一个搭配。钩藤是入肝经、心包经的，能够熄风、静火。风和火往往狼狈为奸，风助火势，火助风威。风能燥湿，当人体风盛时，就要耗伤阴液，造成阴虚、血虚，血虚又生风生火，如此恶性循环。风火相煽，越煽越大，火性炎上，风性上旋，就把气血往上提，造成"气血并走于上"，导致头晕、头痛、高血压等症状。

这里用到钩藤，是因为它能息风，也能清火。过去很多老中医，尤其是清代的太医，比如赵文魁等人，用药非常精到，一旦遇到热象，就会用钩藤。为什么呢？一旦有火，就会相应地起风，火能生风，风也能生火，于是风火相煽。一般的医生也就是见火治火，但水平比较高的大夫，见火就会注意防止生风，所以及时地在方中加入钩藤。

钩藤的性能及选择

当钩藤与天麻配伍的时候，息风静火的能力就能大为增加，起到一加一大于二的效果。

钩藤是长在藤上的，有两个钩，藤随风摇摆，在摇摆的过程中，会挂在一些树枝上，借力向上攀登生长。当然也有单钩的，作用就没有那么好。现在我们一般在开方的时候写"双钩藤"，要求有双钩。有些地方，药材质量非常不好，你抓的钩藤根本就没有钩，全部都是一些梗子，这就更不好了。

选择钩藤，首先看有没有对称的两个钩，其次，钩藤是嫩的好，嫩的时候它是青的，晒干了会发黑，老了就变黄了。我们之前曾提到，当一个东西颜色很青的时候，就入肝，而且有一股刚猛之气，钩藤也是这样的。嫩时色青入肝，老了发黄，就入脾了，所以驱风的力量就会大为减弱。再者，就是看两钩之间的那一截藤茎，嫩的钩藤，茎是方的，老的钩藤茎，茎就变圆了。我们要选方茎的。

石决明与贝壳类药

石决明，其实就是鲍鱼的壳，是贝壳类的，质地很重，作用是明目潜阳、镇肝风。

石决明，顾名思义："石"说明它很重，是一种跟石头比较接近的东西；"决明"明说明它通眼睛，能够明目。还有一个药叫草决明，也就是决明子，也有清肝明目的作用，只不过它是草本的。石决明上有孔，以九个孔的最好，叫九孔石决明，比较大，那种小的石决明，七个孔的也行，最差的也得有五个孔。

跟石决明类似的还有珍珠母。产珍珠的那类贝壳，很多珍珠都是跟贝壳连在一起的，把珍珠抠出来以后，剩下的部份，都是珍珠母。像石决明、珍珠母这类药，通过现代化学分析，都是碳酸钙，但是它们的作用却不一样：石决明、珍珠母比较坚硬，有韧性，主要作用是息风；牡蛎则比较粗糙，没有石决明和珍珠母那么细腻润泽，它给人一种很干燥的感觉，所以偏于收涩，也有一定镇风的作用；还有生瓦楞、海蛤壳这样的药，作用又偏于软坚散结化顽痰。

追捕与解回

石决明在这里是一个重镇的药，它能够把肝气往下引，往下压，平肝息风。

天麻和钩藤是往上走的。风往上旋，药跟着往上旋，这是顺风势而动。药往上旋了以后，还要把风抓回来往下压，所以用了石决明。

川牛膝也是一味引气血下行的药，跟着石决明一起把风往下压。

所以凡是肝风内动、肝阳上亢的高血压，这四味药不能丢：天麻、钩藤、石决明、牛膝。瘀血比较重的时候用川牛膝，瘀血不重的时候用怀牛膝，川牛膝能很好地活血化瘀，怀牛膝则偏于补养肝肾。天麻、钩藤往上走，相当于去追捕；石决明、川牛膝在往下压，相当于把俘虏押回来。这四味药是主药，所以我把它排在前面了。

天麻钩藤饮中辅助药物

风能生火，在人身上的表现就是：脉数、舌苔黄、眼睛红、小便黄，等等。所以用栀子、黄芩来清热。栀子能清三焦浮游之火，黄芩主要去肺火。这种火一般都在上焦，用两个苦药来清。益母草是一个凉血、养血、化瘀的药，它也能够祛风，在这里是个辅助性的药。

内风往往伴随着肝肾阴虚，"卫气出于下焦"，下焦亏虚则卫气弱，一些外风趁虚而入，跟内风狼狈为奸，侵犯人体的腰部、下肢。所以很多老年人总是说腰酸，下肢也不太舒服，这一方面是因为人本身衰老；另一方面就是因为外邪趁虚而入。所以我们这时要用杜仲和寄生。它们能养肝肾，但主要的作用还是驱逐肝肾的风湿邪气，它们驱邪的力量，平和而舒缓，不仅能够祛肝肾之邪，又能够养肝肾的正气，而且杜仲是能够引气血下行的。

后面是夜交藤，能镇静安神，治疗失眠。它与双钩藤配合，效果相得益彰。

还有茯神，就是要让人的神潜伏下去，神潜伏下去了，不再外越，人也更容易睡着。朱茯神就是用朱砂染过的茯神，朱砂也是镇心安神的，朱茯神镇心安神的作用就更大了。

夜交藤和朱茯神是让人睡觉的。我们看，很多老年人睡觉就少，因为体内有风，风一扰动他就睡不着。而睡觉是阴阳相交，既是养阳，又是养阴。当睡觉少的时候，自然阴阳就不交了，阴阳不交，就会生风生痰。所以咱们用夜交藤和茯神来交通阴阳，交通心肾。让人睡个好觉，在睡觉中得到补养。即使这个人不失眠，觉睡得还行，这两个药也可以用，这是取它交通阴阳的意思。

镇肝息风汤

镇肝息风汤

怀牛膝一两，生赭石一两（轧细），生龙骨五钱（捣碎），生牡蛎五钱（捣碎），生龟版五钱（捣碎），生杭芍五钱，玄参五钱，天冬五钱，川楝子二钱（捣碎），生麦芽二钱，茵陈二钱，甘草一钱半。

镇肝息风汤的药序无需调整

镇肝息风汤是非常有名的一个方子，它来自张锡纯的《医学衷中参西录》。镇肝息风汤用药顺序我没有调整，因为不用调整。

张锡纯的《医学衷中参西录》是一本很好的书。张锡纯是很坦荡、很豁达、很无私的一个人。他愿意把自己的东西全部拿出来跟大家分享，《医学衷中参西录》收了他的很多专著，为了弥补专著的不足，还收录了他与弟子的很多演讲、信件甚至诗词。他想尽量地把他师承传道的现场呈现给读者，所以不厌其烦，讲完方再讲药，讲完药再讲医理、再讲病案，而且他都能结合起来讲，他还特别注重给学生答问解疑，给学生写的信，也是在探讨医学的问题。他是一个不保守的人，他的方子也没有打乱。而过去有很多人的方子都是故意打乱，让人看不懂的。

肝气过旺的表现

当一个人需要用镇肝息风汤的时候，他体质往往还是不错的，甚至比较强壮，至少也得外强中干。忽然，内风起来了，高血压很高，脸特别红，脉很弦，很大，跳得很快而且有力，把脉的大夫甚至都能够感觉这个脉正在挑衅他的指尖，这就叫"弦大搏指"，是肝气过旺的表现。

肝为将军之官，其性刚猛、刚烈。肝风内动，就可能是将军正在大怒，要叛变了。怎么办呢？当然要镇压啊！

泰山压顶，重兵镇压

怀牛膝质地很重，是往下走的，这里用到一两，剂量很大。生赭石是一种红褐色的石头，入肝经血分，能走肝经的镇压肝气；生龙骨和生牡蛎也能重镇，同时还有收摄作用，能够收敛往上走的阳气。肝气旺，阳气肯定也在往外越，所以用龙骨、牡蛎来镇压肝风，也收摄往上奔越的浮阳。

还用生龟版五钱，生龟版是生的河龟龟版，是大补真阴的一味药。注意：山龟版很多是有毒的，海龟版是不入药的，严格地讲，都没有用。但现在在临床上也能看到有一点作用，但是作用比河龟的差多了。而且，生龟版只能用乌龟的底板，也就是腹部的，有规则的王字纹的最好。背上的叫龟甲，花纹是呈六边形的，也不能用。

生龟版可以重镇，连同前面的牛膝、赭石、龙骨、牡蛎，给我们一个感觉，就是泰山压顶。石头、草木、骨头、贝壳、甲壳，一起重重地往下压，镇压肝风，这就叫镇肝，肝阳上亢，只能镇压！风为百病之长，肝为五脏之贼！风是百病的源头，可以导致各种病。肝在生理状态下是好东西。"肝为将军之官，谋虑出焉"，"肝藏血"，"肝藏魂"，"肝主疏泄"。但当肝病了的时候，它就不好了，成了五脏之贼，能伤害五脏。五脏之伤跟肝都有关系，这就好比将军叛乱了，到处杀人放火，破坏力很强。这当然要重兵镇压了。

刚柔相济，好生安抚

但重兵镇压并不是办法，不能把将军镇压到死，咱还得指望它回到岗位好好工作呢！所以我们要想想：将军为什么会造反？那是因为你对它不好，给他的任务太重，待遇却不够优厚。肝是"体阴而用阳"的，要用当归、白芍这些养阴的药去养它。当肝得到了充分滋养的时候，肝阳就会收敛。

我们在镇压它的同时，还得好好地安抚它。其实前面用的牛膝、龟版就于镇压中有安抚之意了，接着，白芍五钱，用量比较大，酸以入肝，是在柔肝养阴。用了这味药，将军会很受用。再来一味玄参，滋水养肾，肾水生肝木，也会让肝很舒服。

肝肾之阴从哪里来？从天上来，所以加一味天冬。天冬是补肺阴的，补肺生津，把肺补足了，肺金生肾水，能给肝肾补足水分。就像先把水放在天上，天上一下雨，地上的树不都湿了嘛。这些都是对将军进行的必要的安抚。一打一摸，他就会慢慢地伏贴一点。

你在驯服的同时怕它余怒未消，还要适时打击一下它的气焰，所以加一味川楝子。川楝子是破肝气、泄肝气的。

接着，再继续安抚，改善将军的生活环境。生麦芽疏肝，而且还能健脾，升发胃气。《金匮要略》一开始就讲，"见肝之病，知肝传脾，当先实脾"，生麦芽恰合此意。疏肝，我们不用柴胡，因为当人体需要用镇肝息风汤的时候，他的肝阴已经比较虚了，柴胡劫肝阴，可能导致肝阴更虚，人会烦燥，所以只用生麦芽疏肝。生麦芽，就是在小麦刚发了一点芽的时候就把它晾干，这个时候的麦很有生发之气，可以用来疏肝。茵陈也可以疏肝，而且能清利湿热，肝最怕湿热，在肝阴不足、肝阳上亢的时候，湿

— 263 —

热最容易聚集，而在湿热的情况下也有可能导致肝阳上亢，所以茵陈一定要用。把湿热去掉，也是在改善肝的生活环境。

一方面狠狠地镇压你，另一方面，郁结给你解开了，湿热给你去掉了，滋养给你增加了，你怎么办？是继续作对还是乖乖投降，做你的太平将军呢？说白了就是威逼利诱，这就跟摆平一个人是一样的道理。所以说，医理通于自然之理，同时也通于人事。

镇肝息风汤现在在临床上会经常用到。但这个方子是不能久用的，将军都就范了，你就不要再打压他了，否则，整个人都会蔫掉，甚至再生出其他的病，用这个方，一定要见好就收，适可而止。

Chapter 7　Silkworm Excrement and Formulas for Improving Vision

Silkworms eat mulberry leaf, after which the faeces to be defecated is called Cansha (silkworm excrement). Cansha is also one of the medicines in the category of the mulberry of genera.

Late Silkworm Excrement

Upbearing the Clear and Descending the Turbid and Dispelling the wind

In a prescription, Cansha is often written as "Wancansha (late silkworm excrement) ", which refers to the excrement defecated by silkworms at the moment when the silkworms are ready to spin silk. Such kind of Cansha is of the top quality. Though Cansha is a kind of faeces, it does not stink, and it gives out a puff of fresh scent. Silkworms eat nothing but the simple food of mulberry leaf nor drink water, so they are quite clean creature, and in fact, their excrement is the neatest and tidiest faeces.

The functions of Cansha have been introduced a lot in many related medical books. For instance, it can dispel the wind, eliminate the dampness, cure arthralgia and hemiplegia, eliminate the gastrointestinal turbid dampness, cure cholera twitch, damp-warm syndromes, pantalgia and rubella etc.

Cansha is just the output of an intensive processing of mulberry leaf by silkworms. In essence, it is another form of mulberry leaf. Mulberry leaf can dispel wind, and so can the silkworms and Cansha. Furthermore, Cansha can upbear the clear and descend the turbid.

For instance, Cansha can elinminate the turbid dampness out of the intestines and stomach. As it is known that the spleen dominates the ascending of the clear, and the stomach dominates the descending of the turbid. The transportation and transformation of the life essence of water and grain by the intestines and stomach is a process of upbearing the clear and descending the turbid. To upbear the clear is to transport the life essence of water and grain and the nutrient substances to the whole body. The functions of the spleen are also incarnated in both the small intestine and the large intestine. The spleen is not just an organ, and it is also a kind of function. The small intestine digests the life essence of foodstuff and transports the waste liquid and the residues to the bladder and the large intestine respectively. "Digestion of the life essence of foodstuff" shows that the spleen is functioning, while "transportion of the waste liquid and the residues" is to push the turbid to the large intestine, which shows that the stomach Qi is functioning. When the spleen and stomach are not good enough to upbear the clear and descend the turbid, the clear Qi and the turbid Qi will be intertwined in the intestines and stomach to form the turbid dampness. In that case, the medicines like Cansha for upbearing the clear and descending the turbid will be needed to give a push. When the clear Qi is elevated in a smooth and proper distribution, the turbid will naturally go down and the waste will be excreted. Then, the intestines and stomach will become refreshing again. That is the process that Cansha eliminate the damp turbidity of the intestines and stomach.

Again, Cansha can cure cholera twitch. Cholera ("Huoluan" in Chinese Pinyin) is a common disease in summer and autumn, which, just as its Chinese name implies, means the spleen and stomach are suddenly in complete disorder. Under such a circumstance, the spleen does not upbear the clear Qi but the turbid Qi instead. When the turbid Qi goes up, it will cause vomiting; and when the stomach does not descend the turbid Qi, it may descend the clear Qi instead. When the clear Qi goes downwards, it will cause diarrhea. Cholera will cause vomiting and diarrhea, which will make the patient feel weak all over. The long-lasting vomiting and diarrhea will devitalize the healthy Qi, causing twitch or cramp in legs since the spleen is governing the limbs. Twitch or cramp in legs remind of great seriousness of cholera. For the treatment of cholera, Mugua (pawpaw) and Cansha should be used for guarding against cramp in legs.

In addition, for its functions of upbearing the clear and descending the turbid, Cansha can cure the pantalgia that stems from the pathogenic warm-dampness in the body. Besides, Cansha can cure rubella, too, since it can dispel pathogenic wind.

Clearingthe Liver and Improving Vision

Cansha can clear the liver and improve vision. As the ancients said, "The life essence of the five internal organs (heart, spleen, liver, lungs and kidneys) and the six hollow organs (gallbladder, stomach, large intestine, small intestine, bladder, and Tri-jiao) of the human body goes upwards to pour into the eyes. " It is not an easy matter to keep bright eyesight. Only when all the vital organs of the human body is supplied with sufficient life essence, will the eyes not become nearsighted or longsighted, but become quite clear and bright. The condition of eyes can predict the state of one's health conditions. If the life essence is not sufficient in the vital organs, or too much turbidity stays in the body, one may become dim-sighted. Especially when the turbid prevails in the body, it may cause some other eye diseases. Cansha can dispel wind, upbear the clear Qi and descend the turbid Qi, hence it can do the good to eyes and improve one's vision.

The liver is most sensitive to the turbid dampness and heat, and Cansha can descend the turbid dampness so to clear the liver. When the turbid dampness is descended, the eyes will naturally become bright. For example, when the oil is insufficient, the light of the oil lamp will become dim. Similarly, the deficiency of Yin will result in dim and blurry eyesight. When the lamp core is getting dirty, the lamp may also become dim. Under that circumstance, removal of the ash slag on the top of the lamp core will make the lamp become bright again, which is like clearing the liver for improving vision.

In addition, Cansha is often used to fill in the pillow to clear mind and eyes, dispel wind and soothe nerves. If Cansha is used together with some adjuvant herbs, it can become more effective.

Cansi Tang

Concerning the use of silkworm excrement for cholera twitch treatment, there is a very well-known formula called **Cansi Tang** recorded in the book of ***The theory of cholera***.

Cansi Tang contains the ingredient herbs of Cansha (silkworm excrement), Mugua (pawpaw), Wuyu (fructus evodiae), Dadou Huangjuan (semen sojae germinatum), Yiyi Ren (coix seed), Huanglian (coptis chinensis), Huangqin

(scutellaria baicalensis), Zhizi (fructus gardenia), Banxia (pinellia ternate) and Tongcao (tetrapanax papyriferus).

This formula is used for curing cholera, which primarily arises from the damp-heat stagnated in the Middle Jiao, causing disturbance of Qi circulation, disharmony between the ascending and descending, vomiting and diarrhea, and even twitch. In such cases, it needs to eliminate dampness and heat, upbear the clear Qi and descend the turbid to open up channels of Qi circulation so that the spleen and stomach can function in their normal physiological conditions.

Cansha functions as the monarch medicine in this formula since it can upbear the clear and descend the turbid, and especially it is effective for eliminating the gastrointestinal turbid dampness.

Huangqin, Huanglian and Zhizi are all bitter cold. The bitterness can eliminate dampness, and the coldness can clear heat, so they function as the ministerial medicines in this formula. Huangbai (phellodendron amurense) is not used in this formula since it goes though the Lower Jiao, but the pathogenic influence of cholera mainly takes place in the Middle Jiao. Huanglian is used here to clear the Middle Jiao, and Huangqin is used to clear the Upper Jiao. Zhizi is used to clear the floating heat in the Tri-jiao, but it tends to go to the Middle Jiao.

Both Wuyu and Banxia can descend the turbid, and control nausea and vomiting. Banxia is featured with acrid opening and bitter downbearing; it can descend the stomach Qi, tonify the spleen and reduce phlegm. From the perspective of the curative effect, they can assist Cansha for treatment of diseases. Cansha, Huangqin and Wuyu are all partially cold and cool in property. However, "The spleen, like the wet soil, can only carry on its T&T functions in warm state", and it does not like coldness and coolness. Therefore, Wuyu and Banxia can be used as corrigent medicines against the cold and cool properties of Cansha etc.

Cholera often causes twitch in legs, for which the twin herbs of Wuyu and Mugua can work effectively. These two herbs enter the Middle Jiao and go downwards, too.

Dadou Huangjuan, Yiyi Ren and Mugua all have dispersing effect. Therefore, they are used to soothe the Middle Jiao, eliminate dampness and relax muscles.

Tongcao is light in both smell and taste, and it can invigorate Yang and excrete dampness. After the dampness is excreted, heat will be easier to be dispersed.

Other Dung-Type Medicines

As for dung-type medicines, two of them are introduced here: Yeming Sha (bat dung) and Wangyue Sha (hare dung).

Yeming Sha (Bat Dung)

Yeming Sha (bat dung) is of the dung of bats, which can be seen in some grottoes, or on the windowsills of some old houses or under roofs of houses.

When examined carefully, many small heads and eyes of worms and even some crushed wings can be seen in the crushed Yeming Sha. The bats eat small worms, most of which will be digested. However, the eyes of the worms are hard to be digested, and then reserved in the dung. The objects of the same function as like draws to like, so Yeming Sha has some effects for treatment of eye diseases. Furthermore, the dung medicine can descend the turbid and purge fire, so Yeming Sha has the effect of improving eyesight.

Bat is a flying mammal, and it takes flying insects as food. The flying creatures are all related to wind. Hence, Yeming Sha can dispel wind, too.

Wangming Sha (Hare Dung)

Wangyuesha (hare dung) isthe dung of wild hares. The dung of the domestic rabbits has no such effects as that the wild hares since the domestic rabbits live on feed.

The wild hare is subsumed to wood, to be exact, to the wood of Yin. It gets out of its cave at night, which is also subsumed to Yin. Furthermore, the wild hare gets out of its cave to look up at moon and absorbs the vital life essence of moon. The moon is of the lunar vital essence, which is cool and moist. Therefore, Wangyue Sha is cold, and it can clear heat.

It is said the wild hare likes to eat pipewort, after which its dung will become effective for eyesight since pipewort as herbal medicine can improve eyesight.

The genuine Wangyue Sha includes a lot of foreign materials like broken grasses and the like. Its surface is not quite smooth, from which it can be distinguished from the dung of the domestic rabbits.

Moving without Holding to Purge Fire

The medicines of dung and the like, such as Cansha, or Yeming Sha, or Wangyue sha all push down without holding since dung itself comes out of the cacation channel. Therefore, when such medicine is taken, it will help push down the waste easily.

The medicines of dung often contain gallbladder bile with the taste of bitterness. The bitter substances help descend and clear fire. Furthermore, the gallbladder governs descending. It may be asked whether the silkworm has a gallbladder, or any bile is included in Cansha. It is hard to say, but it is quite sure that the dung of all large animals, including human excrement, contains the bile. That is why the excrement always tastes bitter. Whenever it is necessary to purge fire quickly, the medicines of dung might be one of the choices.

But one thing should be kept in mind that medicines of dung are not advisable for the pregnant women due to the following two reasons:

In the first place, all the medicines of dung have foul smell for they are dreggy excrement. When in pregnancy, the women would have to take in the clear Qi (fresh air) as the most precious thing and keep away from the dirty things in order to nourish the fetus.

In the next place, the medicines of dung and the like are for the purpose of descending. When in pregnancy, the women will expect Qi to rise, so they usually use some Baizhu and Sharen to tonify their spleen in order to keep the spleen astringed and the embryo Qi rising, and then, the fetus will become stable.

However, the medicine of dung may be used after delivery of baby since some dreggy things inside the body after delivery may not be completely discharged or eliminated. In that case, when necessary, Cansha and the like may be used in order to upbear the clear Qi and descend the turbid.

Other Medicines for Clearing Liver and Improving Vision

Gujingcao (Pipewort)

Gujingcao has been mentioned above as a medicine for improving vision. It is quite common in the rice field in the south of China. Generally, in September of Chinese lunar year, after the rice is harvested, a lot of grasses will overgrow in the field. Gujingcao, as its Chinese name implies, receives the life quintessence of the rice and studs around in the field. On the top of each piece of the pipewort sprouts out a little white ball.

Gujingcao is light in texture and insipid in taste. Lightness implies that it can fly upwards, which means its medical effects will run up to eyes. Insipidity implies that it can penetrate downwards and guide the deficiency-heat to run downwards. Gujingcao is growing up in the rice fields under the nourishment of the remaining life quintessence of grain. It can harmonize the stomach. Meanwhile, it is growing in the golden season of September, in correspondence with Metal in **Wuxing Doctrine**, gaining the features of metal, so it also has the effect of soothing the liver and dispelling wind.

Gujingcao is pungent, sweet and slightly warm in properties. It is a special medicine for treatment of eye diseases, removing nephelium of eyeball, especially removing the "flying stars" before eyes. When in deficiency of vital life essence, or with floating fire in eyes, it always seems to have some bits and pieces of stuff fluttering in eyes, which can be swept off with Gujingcao. Whenever "flying stars" occurs in the eyes, true or false, Gujingcao can be used for treatment.

Gujingcao, as a commonly used medicine in the ophthalmology department, is often used together with herbs like Juhua (chrysanthemum), Mimenghua (butterflybush flower), Shengdi, Juemingzi (cassia seed) and so on.

Mimenghua (Butterflybush Flower)

Mimenghua, as its Chinese name implies, is used to cure eye diseases. When one feels unclear like a veil of mist in his eyes, Mimenghua may be used for treatment.

It not only clears heat, but also smoothens and moistens the liver meridian and puts out the endogenous wind, so it is quite good for eyes. For the treatment of different eye diseases, especially eye diseases of the aged people due to deficiency of liver-Yin and kidney-Yin or fire excess, Mimenghua and Gujingcao are often used together, with some liver and kidney nourishing medicines like Shengdi and Shanyurou (common macrocarpium fruit) added or some Juhua added, too, if necessary. In fact, Juhua has the similar effect to Mimenghua.

Mimenghua plus Gouqizi (fructus lycii), Shengdi, Shajili (astragali complanati semen), and Gujingcao makes a super-duper formula for the treatment of nearsightedness due to dificiency of liver-Yin and kidney-Yin. For children, their eyesight might recover gradually if at the early stage of nearsightedness or in the case of pseudomyopia, since over eyestrain may result in disorder of blood on account of excessive use of eyes, which will then do harm to liver-Yin and kidney-Yin, causing failure of supports from the vital life essence and energy. Under such a circumstance, this formula is quite effective.

Mimenghua used together with Huanglian (coptis chinensis), Chishao (radix paeoniae rubra), Jingjie (schizonepeta), Fangfeng (radix sileris), Juhua (chrysanthemum) and Longdancao (radix gentianae) can cure dim eyesight, eye itching and eye sting resulted from wind-heat and dampness-heat etc.

Mimenghua has a lot of tomentum and fluff on it. The ancient classics mention that it should be wrapped up with silk cloth for decocting. Silk cloth is woven with natural silk, which also has the effect to dispel wind and relieve rheumatic pains.

Juemingzi (Cassia Seed)

Juemingzi is also a common medicine for curing eye diseases. It is quite common in the south of China and it looks like beans with each pod contiaining a number of seeds. The leaves of Juemingzi have a special feature, i. e. , they open in the daytime and close tightly at night like the eyes of human beings.

Juemingzi is collected in autumn. They can enter both the liver and spleen meridians with a little nourishing effect. They can purge the liver fire and tonify the kidney fluid. When fluid rises,. the fire will retreat, and then, eyes will become bright and clear. Juemingzi is tasteless, light in texture and floating, so it can dispel the wind-pathogens and stop tears and pains.

Juemingzi has another name called Caojueming (cassia occidentalis). By the way, there is another medicine called Shijueming (concha haliotidis). These two medicines have the similar efficacies, so both of them are called Jueming (cassia tora).

Now, many people take Juemingzi as tea, claiming that it can reduce the "Three Highs" (i. e. hign blood pressure, high blood sugur, high blood fat). Such a saying might be right, but don't drink too much. Once an old man came to visit me, and told me that his excrement had always been dry and hard. After some time of drinking Juemingzi tea, he got much improvement and his excrement was not dry and hard any more. Juemingzi can clear liver-fire and tonify the kidney fluid. After the liver-fire is cleared, the excrement will definitely not be dry and hard any more. When the kidney is tonified, it will become much stronger to cope with excrement and urine. Besides, Juemingzi is cold and cool in properties. Actually, all seeds will fall downwards when they are ripe and whaterever they are, so Juemingzi, as a seed-type medicine, definitely has the effect to help relieve the bowels. However, the above-mentioned old man started to bleed in his eye ground after long-lasting drinking Juemingzi. Juemingzi does have the effect of clearing the liver-fire and dispelling the wind, but if it is used too much, it may cause some other impairment.

So Juemingzi tea should not be drunk for too long time. Those who are in liver deficiency or blood-insufficiency will suffer from disturbacnce of endogenous deficiency wind if keeping on drinking Juemingzi tea for too long time. Besides, the above-mentioned old man is also suffering from diabetes mellitus, so too much and long drinking Juemingzi tea results in bleeding in his eye ground. Those who suffer from the spleen deficiency or diarrhea should not use Juemingzi, either, for it can cause thin sloppy stool, which, after long use of Juemingzi, may sap Qi of the Middle Jiao or cause Yin depletion due to diarrhea.

Juemingzi has another effect, i. e. detoxication of snake venom. Gnenerally speaking, when a snake bites, the snake venom will first get into the liver meridian. Juemingzi can clear the liver, so theoretically, it can help to clear the snake venom.

By the way, Juemingzi should be crushed before decocting. Juemingzi dislikes Huomaren (fructus cannabis). As a matter of fact, Huomaren can also relieves the bowels, but neither of these two medicines likes each other. However, among the Chinese patent medicines, there is one formula called **Juemingzi-Huomaren Oral Liquid**, which is for relieving the bowels. They dislike and defend against and restrain each other, but the mutual inhibition of medicines sometimes does not mean a bad thing.

Cijili (Tribulus Terrestris)

Here is another medicine Cijili, which is quite common in the northwest of China, especially in Xi'an city. On the ground extend its vines upon which grow leaves orderly and pieces of thorned seeds like that of spinach. Cijili is generally collected in the winter time.

Cijili, as a vine plant, always extends on the ground and stops at nothing. Its thorns can hook the hair or feather of animals or birds and are taken to distant places to grow. This shows it is good at "travelling".

Cijiliis good at breaking. It has thorns all over its vines, so it can pierce to break something. As a medicine, it can pierce stagnation of blood stasis. Cijili is always used to treat lobular hyperplasia and hyperplasia of mammary glands of breasts. It is also able to relieve the red eye swelling, that is, to break the swelling and dispel the stagnated dampness and heat. For those who are in poor health, Cijili should be used with caution because it grows thorns and has the effect of dispelling wind. And with such an effect, it may also dissipate or consume Qi of liver and lung and even some blood. Therefore, only when in the necessary or unavoidable circumstances can Cijili be used.

Cijili not only can eliminate and dispel liver wind, it can also discharge the lung Qi. Sometimes Beichaihu (honewort) is used to soothe the liver. For those who are relatively weak in physical health, especially the intellectuals who do their brain work with concentrated attention and blood consumption, when the liver stagnation occurs, Chaihu (radix bupleuri) is always used for soothing the liver. However, after Chaihu is used for too long time, it may plunder the liver-

— 274 —

Yin. In such cases, Cijili will be used to substitute for Chaihu. In spring time when the liver Qi is vigorous, the liver is strong enough for catharsis by itself, Beichaihu is not needed again in order to avoid any over dissipation, and then, Cijili may be used instead. Similarly, in the formula of **Xiaoyao San**, Chaihu sometimes may also be substituted with Cijili.

There is another type ofCijili called Shayuan Jili (astragali complanati demen), which is partial to nourish the liver and kidney. In fact, Shayuan Jili and Cijili are the different thing though they share the similar Chinese name. This will be discussed in the following part regarding restorative medicines.

Ophthalmological Diseases and Doctors

A series of medicines have been discussed above related to eyes. It is sure that eye diseases are involved with physical strength and weakness, coldness and heat. When the blurring of vision arises from deficiency of Yang, the medicines with properties of coldness like Juemingzi and those medicines of dung and the like should be used with much care, otherwise, they may worsen the symptoms, leading to blindness by the end.

Gujingcao and Mimenghua may substitute mutually, but it depends upon the compatibility of medicines. By the way, Tusizi (semen cuscutae) is also quite effective for treatment of eye diseases. It can improve eyesight through warming and invigorating the liver and kidney.

For treatment of eyes diseases, ophthalmology in Chinese medical tratment also takes references to the theories related to the five viscera (heart, spleen, liver, lungs and kidneys) and the six hollow organs (gallbladder, stomach, small intestine, large intestine, bladder and Tri-jiao) of the human body and follow the concepts about treatment based on syndrome differentiation.

Regarding ophthalmology, the TCM expert Fu Renyu in the Ming dynasty wrote a very nice book named as **Shenshi Yaohan**, which is a comprehensive work about ophthalmology of TCM. This book can by and large help the readers to understand and solve the problems on eyes diseases.

In modern times in China, there were two experts with very high ophthalmological skills. They were Wei Wengui in Beijing and Lu Nanshan in Shanghai, who were more active and well-known experts in TCM before 1960s. And now their medical works, with great reference value, are still available in many bookstores.

第七章　蚕砂与粪便及明目类方药

蚕食桑叶，排出的粪便，就是蚕砂，因此，蚕砂也属于桑之属。

晚蚕砂

升清降浊而祛风

开中药的时候，蚕砂写作"晚蚕砂"，就是蚕到了快要吐丝的时候的排出的蚕砂，这是最好的。蚕砂虽然是一种粪便，但它并不臭，反而有一股清香。因为蚕的饮食非常单一，只吃桑叶，不吃别的，也不喝水，因此蚕是比较清净的动物，所以蚕砂算是最干净的粪便了。

蚕砂的作用，书上讲得很多，比如它能祛风燥湿、治痹症、治半身不遂、化肠胃的湿浊、治霍乱转筋、治湿温身痛、治风疹，等等。咱们不用都记住，我们要从书中列的这些症状，看到它背后的东西。

其实，蚕砂只不过把桑叶经过了一道深加工，被蚕吃了，消化了，再排出来，其实本质上还是桑叶。桑叶能驱风，蚕也能驱风，所以蚕砂依然是驱风的。蚕砂还能升清降浊。

比如说，蚕砂去肠胃湿浊。我们知道，脾主升清，胃主降浊。肠胃运化水谷，就是一个升清降浊的过程，升清就是把这些水谷精微、营养物质输送到全身。脾的功能在小肠、大肠里依然有体现。脾并不仅是一个器官，而且是一种功能。小肠泌清别浊，这依然是脾胃的功能起作用，"泌清"就是脾在起作用，"别浊"就是让浊气往大肠走，是胃气在起作用。当脾胃升清降浊的能力欠佳的时候，清浊之气在肠胃中交织在一起，形成湿浊。这时候就需要有升清降浊能力的药来促进一下，蚕砂就可能用到，清气升起来了，输布出去了，浊气往下排掉了，肠胃就清爽了，所以说它能化肠胃的湿浊。

再比如，治疗霍乱转筋。霍乱是夏秋季节很常见的一个病，顾名思义，就是脾胃霍然一时乱了套。脾不升清，反而升浊气，浊气往上升就会呕吐；胃不降浊，反而把清气往下降了，清气下陷人就会拉肚子。所以霍乱的症状就是上吐下泻，人没有力气，吐泻久了，伤了正气，腿就会抽筋，因为脾主四肢。霍乱到了腿抽筋的时候就很严重了。在治霍乱的时候，即使腿没有抽筋我们也要用一些防止腿抽筋的药，比如木瓜、蚕砂。

还有，治湿温身痛。湿温身痛是湿温之邪困在身体里造成的，通过升清降浊也可以把它去掉。至于治疗风疹的原因，就很简单了，因为它有驱风的功能。

清肝明目

蚕砂还能清肝明目。古人讲："五脏六腑之精气皆上注于目。"拥有一双明亮的眼睛很不容易。你五脏六腑的精气必须很足，才能既不近视，也不远视，眼睛还特别清澈、明亮。一看人的眼睛，就知道这个人的健康状况。当五脏六腑的精气不够的时候，或者当人体的浊气太重的时候，眼睛会昏花。尤其是当体内浊气盛时，还可能生出其他眼病。蚕砂能祛风，又能升清降浊，所以它对眼睛有好处，有明目的作用。

肝最怕湿热浊气，蚕砂把这股湿浊之气迅速往下降，起到清肝的作用。浊气降了，眼睛自然就亮了。眼睛就好比一盏灯，当这盏灯里油少了的时候，灯火就暗淡，这就是阴虚导致眼睛不亮。还有可能是灯头太脏，灯火也会晦暗不明，咱们可以修剪一下灯头，把灯芯的灰剔掉，然后再把灯芯打亮一点，这就相当于一个清肝明目的过程。

此外，蚕砂还经常用来填充枕头，可以清利头目，散风安神，如果跟着别的药，配伍起来一块用，效果会更好。

蚕矢汤

蚕砂治霍乱转筋有一个很有名的方子，就是《霍乱论》中的蚕矢汤。

蚕砂、木瓜、吴萸、大豆黄卷、薏苡仁、黄连、黄芩、栀子、半夏、通草。

这个方子就是用于治疗霍乱的。霍乱主要是因为湿热阻滞在中焦，扰乱了气机，导致升降失调，上吐下泻，甚至出现转筋，这就要清利湿热，升清降浊，以打开气机，恢复脾胃正常的生理运转。

蚕砂是升清降浊的，尤其善于化肠胃的湿浊，所以做君药。

黄芩、黄连、栀子都是苦寒的，苦能燥湿，寒能清热，作为臣药。为什么不用黄柏呢？因为黄柏是走下焦的，而霍乱的主要邪气在中焦，不要惊动下焦了。黄连是清中焦的，黄芩是清上焦的，栀子清三焦浮游之热，它也是走中焦比较多。

吴萸和半夏，都能降浊止呕。半夏辛开苦降，能降胃气，健脾化痰。在疗效上，它们对蚕砂有帮助。而在性质上，蚕砂和黄芩、黄连、栀子，都是偏寒凉的，而"脾为湿土，得温则运"，不喜欢寒凉，吴萸和半夏这两味温药，可以反佐蚕砂等药的寒凉之性。

霍乱往往会导致腿抽筋，而防治腿抽筋有一对药非常好用，就是吴萸和木瓜。这两味药也都是入中焦的，而且都能往下走的。

大豆黄卷、薏苡仁和木瓜，都有宣化的作用，能够调畅中焦，还能够利湿、舒筋。

再加上一味通草。通草气味俱淡，能升阳、渗湿。湿渗掉了，热也就容易散掉。

其他粪便类药

粪便类的药咱们再讲两味，一是夜明砂，还有一个是望月砂。

夜明砂

夜明砂就是蝙蝠的粪便。在一些岩洞里，老房子的窗台上、屋檐下，经常可以看到。

蝙蝠的粪便很容易碎，仔细地看，你会发现其中有很多小虫子的小头和小眼睛，还有一些碎了的翅膀。蝙蝠吃小虫子，虫子吃进去后，很多都消化掉了，唯独小虫子的眼睛最难消化掉，所以蝙蝠的粪便里有很多小虫子的眼睛，同气相求，它就对人的眼睛有一定的作用，加之它是粪便，能降浊泻火，所以有明目之功。

蝙蝠是一种能飞的哺乳动物，它吃的是飞虫，能飞的动物都跟风有关，所以夜明砂也能祛风。

望月砂

望月砂，必须是野兔的粪便；家兔喂的是饲料，它的粪便就没有望月砂的作用了。

兔子是属木的，而且是属阴木，它夜间出来活动，也是属阴。而且，兔子夜里会出来望月亮，得月亮的精气，月亮是太阴之精，其精气是凉润的。所以，兔子的粪便是寒凉的，能清热。

有人说，野兔特别喜欢吃谷精草，吃了谷精草以后，它的粪便就会更加明目了。因为谷精草也是一味明目的药。

真正的望月砂，里面有很多碎草之类的杂质，表面不是很光滑，通过这些我们就可以区别于家兔的粪便。

走而不守，迅速泻火

粪便入药，不管是蚕砂、夜明砂，还是望月砂，都是走而不守往下降的，因为本身就是从这条路上出来的，所以吃下去，再次往下通，就能轻车熟路。

粪便类药中，往往含有胆汁，故其味苦，苦又能降，能清火，而且，胆也是主降的。当然，有人会问，蚕有没有胆？蚕砂里有没有蚕的胆汁？这就很难说了。但是，只要是大型动物的粪便里肯定有胆汁，人的粪便里也有胆汁，所以粪便会略带苦味。你若想迅速降火泻火，就可能用到粪便类的药。

有一点需要注意，粪便类的药，孕妇都是不宜用的。原因有二：

首先，粪便类的药都有浊气，哪怕它再干净它也是粪便，也是污浊的，怀孕养胎，以清气为贵，尽量不要接触这些污浊之物。

其次，粪便类的药都是往下降的，怀孕时正愁气不能升提呢，往往用一些白术、砂仁来健脾，健脾是为了使脾能固摄住，使胎气往上升，胎气一升，胎就比较稳固，不容易下坠。

当然，产后可以用这类药的，因为产后体内往往还有一些污浊的东西没有排干净，在必要时，可以用蚕砂之类的，升清降浊。

其他清肝明目药
谷精草

刚才我们提到谷精草，是一个明目的药。谷精草在南方的稻田里很常见。一般在农历九月，割完稻以后，稻田里剩下一些草，这些草在稻子收割之后会长得非常快。

谷精草，顾名思义，它得到了谷物的精华。稻田里的谷精草星星点点，每根草上都会长个小白球。

谷精草质地非常轻，味很淡。轻就会上浮，会引药上行，入眼睛；淡就会下渗，导虚热下行。而且它是得谷物余气生出的草，又能和胃气。它

— 280 —

生在金秋九月，得金气，又有疏肝驱风的作用。

谷精草辛、甘、微温，是目疾专药，可以除翳障，尤其是它可以"去星"。精气不足，或是眼中有浮游之火的时候，眼睛里会感觉有星星点点的东西在飘，这就叫"星"，谷精草能把这些去掉。只要是眼中有星，无论虚实，都可以用谷精草。

谷精草经常配合菊花、密蒙花、生地、决明子等中药一块使用，是眼科常用的一味药。

密蒙花

密蒙花，一看名字也会感觉到它应该是治眼睛的，眼睛迷蒙不清，可用密蒙花。

密蒙花生长在树上，味甘，色紫，能入肝，而且它有润性，性微寒。

它能清热，还能平润肝经，平熄内风，对眼睛非常好。我们在治很多眼病，尤其是在治老年人肝肾阴虚、火比较旺的眼病时，经常会把密蒙花和谷精草一起用，还可以再加一些滋养肝肾的药，如生地，山萸肉，还可以加一些菊花。菊花跟密蒙花有相似的作用。

密蒙花配上菊花、枸杞子、生地、沙蒺藜、谷精草，是治疗肝肾阴虚近视非常好的一个方子。小孩子刚刚近视，或假性近视，说是能够慢慢恢复过来。往往是因为用眼过度，久视伤血，继而伤了肝肾之阴，精气不能上承导致的。这个方子常常一用就灵。

密蒙花跟黄连、赤芍、荆芥、防风、菊花、龙胆草这些药一起，能够治疗风热、湿热导致的眼花、眼痒、眼睛刺痛等。

密蒙花有很多毛，所以古书上面都说要"用绢包煎"。绢是蚕丝织成，也有祛风的作用。

决明子

治眼睛的常用药还有决明子，它长得像豆子，在南方有很多，一个荚里能够结很多籽。它的叶子有个特点，就是昼开夜合，而且一合上就合得特别严实，跟人的眼睛一样，早上就开了，晚上就合了。

决明子是秋冬季节采，入肝、胆两经，略微有一些补，能泻肝火，益肾水。水生火退，眼睛自然就亮了。决明子气味很淡，力薄气浮，能升散风邪，收泪止痛。

决明子又叫草决明，前面我们还讲了一味药叫石决明，它们有相似的作用，所以都叫决明。

现在很多人在喝决明子，说决明子能降"三高"。有这个说法，也是对的，但是不能喝太多。我上周有位老人，我问他大便怎么样，他说大便一直都干结，后来他就喝决明子泡的茶，大便就不干结了，能解下来。这是什么道理呢？因为决明子能清肝火、滋肾水，肝火清了，大便就没那么干结了，肾水得到滋润，肾司二便的能力也强了。而且决明子是寒凉的，不管什么"子"，都是向下坠的，所以，决明子就能促进大便解出来。但是，再后来他眼底出血了，这就是喝决明子喝得太多了的缘故。决明子清肝清得太厉害了，疏风疏得太过分了，反遭风害。

所以喝决明子不能喝时间太长。如果是肝虚血弱的，喝多了就会导致虚风内扰。刚才我说的这位老人还有糖尿病，所以他喝多了眼底出血。脾虚腹泻的人，也不能用决明子，它能够让大便变稀，用久了，大伤中气，哪天大泻亡阴了，会拉得收不住。

决明子还有一个作用，那就是解蛇毒。一般来说，被蛇咬到了，蛇毒首先入肝经。决明子能够清肝，蛇毒随之而解。咱们纯粹从理论上是讲得通的。

决明子要捣碎了熬，而且决明子恶火麻仁，其实火麻仁也是通大便的。偏偏有一个中成药叫"决明子火麻仁口服液"，就是用来通大便的，它们俩互不喜欢，互相防着，互相制约，所以说，药物相恶并非坏事。

刺蒺藜

我们再讲一味药：刺蒺藜。

这味药，西北比较多，西安最多。它是蔓生的，藤贴在地上长，藤上有很整齐的叶子，上面生出一个个像菠菜籽那样的种子，带着很多的小刺儿，一般在冬天采。

蒺藜善行。它是藤生的，藤在地上蔓延，无所不至，是善行的表现。蒺藜的刺能够挂在动物的皮毛上，被带到很远的地方去播种。这也是它善行的一种表现。

蒺藜还善破。它有刺，有刺破之意。它可以刺破一些瘀血、积聚。所以常用来治乳房小叶增生、乳腺增生。它能退眼睛的红肿，把肿给刺破，让郁积的湿热散掉。如果人的身体比较虚的话，就连刺蒺藜这样的药也要少用，毕竟它还是长了刺的，能够祛风散风的，在发挥这些作用的时候，它消耗肝肺之气，还会消耗一定的血。所以要到有必要的时候才用。

刺蒺藜平散肝风，还能泄肺气。我们有时候用北柴胡来疏肝。如果这个人比较弱，尤其是知识分子，平时用心耗血，如有肝郁，用柴胡来疏肝，但柴胡用久了就会劫肝阴，这时候就要用刺蒺藜来代替柴胡。当春天肝气比较旺的时候，肝本身疏泄能力比较强，那么就不要用北柴胡了，以免发散太过，可改用白蒺藜。包括逍遥散里，有时候也可以把柴胡去掉，用刺蒺藜来代替。

还有一种蒺藜叫沙苑蒺藜，偏于补肝肾，我们在后面讲补药的时候要讲到。这是两种不一样的药。

眼科病与眼科医

上面我讲的一系列的药都跟眼睛有关。

当然，眼病有实有虚，有寒有热，如果是阳虚的视力模糊，那么，那些寒凉药，如草决明，还有那些粪便类的药就要慎用了，否则，会让精气越来越弱，最后瞎了。

谷精草和密蒙花是能够通用的，要看跟什么药配伍。还有一味非常好的眼科药就是菟丝子，它也能明目，而且通过温肝肾达到明目的作用。

眼科往往也是参照五脏六腑，用的依然是中医辨证论治的思想。

关于眼科，明朝医家傅仁宇的《审视瑶函》，文字写得非常美，它是中医眼科集大成的著作。看通了这本书，眼睛的问题基本上就能够掌握了。

近现代有两个人眼科水平非常高：一个在北京，一个在上海，北京的叫韦文贵，上海的叫陆南山，他们都是民国时期到五六十年代比较活跃、很有名的中医眼科大夫。现在我们能买到他们的书，也非常有参考价值。

Volume 3
Cassia of Genera — Fire-categorized Formulas and Medicines

Chapter 1   Introduction of Warm and Hot Medicines

Fire-categorized formulas cover the warm and hot medicines represented by Guizhi (Cassia twig) and Rougui (cassia bark). First of all, let us briefly introduce the warm and hot medicines.

Functions of Warm and Hot Medicines

Warm and hot medicines mainly have the following functions:

Driving out Coldness

One important function of warm and hot medicines is to eliminate coldness from the human body. As it is known that coldness is a kind of bleak and stern Qi. By the season of deep autumn and winter, coldness will become deeper and stronger, causing things on earth to wither. In the early spring, there is still chill in the spring air, grasses and trees could not sprout or bloom. Only when the chill in the spring air fades away completely will the land be covered with green. Coldness impairs Yang-Qi (the positive energy) and the vitality of human body. Because of this, there comes a saying: "All diseases arise out of coldness." From the perspective of human vitality, it is so indeed. But when one says "arising out of coldness", it does not really mean diseases directly arise from coldness, but means that diseases arise from the absence of healthy Qi or vitality in the human body, and from the bleak and stern Qi. Whatever the diseases are, cold diseases, warm diseases, or hot diseases, they all have bleak and stern Qi, which makes human body wither.

But where does the coldness come from? It definitely comes from the outside first. The cold pathogen can impair human body. In the first place, it attacks the surface to hurt the triple Yang meridians, i. e., Taiyang meridian, Yangming meridian, and Shaoyang meridian, which have been clearly stated in the classic of **Shanghan Lun (Treatise on Cold Pathogenic Diseases)**. The Taiyang meridian is in charge of the surface of the whole body, and the cold pathogen will hurt Taiyang meridian. So, in case of cold pathogen hurting the surface of body, **Mahuang Tang** (ephedra decoction) may be used. When the cold pathogen goes to Yangming meridian, **Gegen Tang** (radix puerariae decoction) should be used. In case the cold pathogen goes further to Shaoyang meridian, **Xiao Chaihu Tang** (radix bupleuri decoction) will have to be used for harmonizing purpose. Mahuang (ephedra), Guizhi, Gegen (radix puerariae), and Chaihu (radix bupleuri) are all pungent and warm medicines for dispersing purposes. The exogenous cold pathogen may also go into the triple Yang meridians, i. e., Taiyin meridian, Shaoyin meridian, and Jueyin meridian. The impairment of Taiyin meridian actually hurts the lung and spleen (primarily hurts the spleen); the impairment of the Shaoyin meridian actually hurts the heart and kidney, since the hand Shaoyin is subsumed to the heart meridian, and the feet Shaoyin is subsumed to the kidney; the impairment of the Jueyin meridian actually hurts the liver. Therefore, when saying the cold pathogen hurts the triple Yin meridians, to put it simply, we may take it as the cold pathogen hurts the liver, spleen and kidney directly, but it also has to be noted that these two statements, in fact, are not, strictly speaking, identical.

In summary, for treatment of the bleak and stern cold pathogen, the warm medicines have to be used.

Rescuing Patients from Collapse by Restoring Yang

The second function of the warm and hot medicines is called "rescuing patient from collapse by restoring Yang". When the bleak coldness wreaks havoc in human bodies, it threatens to engulf us just like an ominous storm, and inside a body it will become shady and dismal with apparent cold wind rage, so Yang Qi will soon be gone. Under such a circumstance, the hot medicines must be used to rescue the patient from collapse by restoring Yang, which is the final push at death's door.

If the patient still has a beating pulse, but the pulse is somewhat weak, **Dushen Tang** (Ginseng Decoction) will do; if the patient's pulse is quite feeble, only faintly discernible, **Shenfu Tang** (Ginseng and Radix Aconiti Carmichaeli Decoction) will have to be used to restore Yang; if the patient looks pale, add some E-jiao (donkey-hide gelatin) in **Shenfu Tang**. When the patient is dying, or he/she is even about to sweat, and Yin and Yang are about to separate from each other, add some Shanyurou (common macrocarpium fruit) in **Shenfu Tang** additionally. In case that the patient cannot afford ginseng, a large dosage of Shanyurou plus Dangshen (codonopsis pilosula) can also help to rescue him out of danger. Similarly, serious illness may also be treated in such a way. If the shady and dismal coldness is very vigorous prior to a serious illness, a large dosage of Fuzi (radix aconiti carmichaeli) or ginseng should be used to restore Yang in order to rescue the patient from collapse, which is similar to the fight with the back to the river. Such a "fight" is often commanded by a "great general" (a medical expert) since an ordinary doctor seldom has the courage and ability to control such a situation.

In the process of restoring Yang, it is also necessary to guard against interactive sudden swashes of cold and heat. It is like a glass just taken into a room from the cold outside, which is still very cold. But at this moment, if one pours boiling water into the cold glass, it may suddenly crack at the bottom, which is called "cold-heat swashing". The same is true to the human body. While the bleak cold is in an extremely serious state, lots of hot medicines are used at the same time, the patient may not stand them quite well, and will then react with them very badly, such as vomiting. Therefore, some cold and cool medicines, like Zhudanzhi (pig bile), are often added for restoring Yang in the formulas such as **Sini Tang** (decoction for treating Yang exhaustion) and the like. Zhudanzhi is a cold medicine, which, to be used together with the heavily hot medicines, will not affect restoration of Yang, but on the contrary, it can help the human body adapt to the hot recipe.

Warming for Tonification

"Warm and hot medicines" is actually a general term, but there are in fact some differences between the warm medicines and hot medicines. Dispelling the cold and restoring Yang are the major functions of the hot medicines, while the warm medicines are primarily warming to make tonification and to activate meridians.

"Warming" does not just mean to heat up, it also refers to the vitality, with which health may be maintained. Therefore, general tonic medicines are often partial to warmness in order to perfuse the human body with vitality, which is taken as warm tonification. It is not a mechanical mass-for-mass supplement, but a mobilization and cultivation of vitality of human bodies with their own warmth. This is the fundamental difference between TCM and the western medicine. As to the western medicine, the amount of glucose or amino acids to be made up is fixed, while TCM is not the same, for example, TCM uses Dihuang (rehmannia) to nourish Yin. Dihuang is a greasy herb, but if used well and properly, it will not be greasy but will help patients to have a good appetite. Generally, only a hundred grams of Dihuang to be used in the formulas for nourishing Yin may help the patient to increase weight far more than a hundred grams, showing the Yin-nourishing effect of Dihuang since it mobilizes the body vitality and helps the patient to gain energy from most basic diet every day. However, what Dihuang itself can directly give the patient is something quite fractional.

Moreover, to tonify is not the same as to nourish in that the former is much quicker while the latter is quite slow. Therefore, as for human bodies, only at the moment of terrible weakness can tonification be made. In the normal cases, it will be sufficient to carry out nourishment step by step. Thus, many health maintenance methods do not seek quick success and instant benefits, but aim for long-term effects, which is called health maintenance. Usually, the warming tonification also implies the meaning of warm nourishment, which means to nourish with warmth in order to restore vitality and help the body slowly return to its normal condition.

Warming for Activating Meridians

It is a common sense that "coldness can result in coagulation", and can easily cause solidification of things. The same is true with regard to our human bodies. While in chills, the blood circulation of the human body will slow down, easily causing obstruction of blood vessels. The obstructed Qi can easily form phlegm, and the obstructed blood can easily produce stasis, both of which stem from coldness. However, as it develops, it will no longer be just coldness since longer obstruction will be transformed into heat. Phlegm may take shape and arise from coagulation of Qi due to chills. The phlegm as a foreign matter in the body will then be transformed into fire if it stays inside the body for a long time. From the Chinese character "痰" ("tán", means phlegm), it can be seen two components of "火" ("huǒ", means fire) inside the Chinese character "痰" (phlegm). As for blood stasis, it is likely that the blood slows down in circulation in the vessel, and then coagulates inside. If it coagulates for too much long time, it will then become a foreign matter staying inside the blood vessel, and begins to catch fire. Phlegm and blood stasis possibly stem from coldness or heat. But with time passing by, there will be signs of transforming into fire, so the "six pathogens" (i. e. the six exogenous factors including wind, coldness, heat, dampness, dryness and fire, which cause diseases) are all transformed from fire. Therefore, one must consider the appropriate way to clear the fire.

Coldness can result in coagulation. When Qi and blood does not circulate smoothly, it may make a person's spirits droop and bring about a lack of vitality. Then, the method of warming to activate meridians may be adopted to vitalize Qi and blood so that Qi and blood can circulate smoothly and transformation function can be invigorated. The spleen is the source of Qi-blood generation and transformation. When the spleen is warmed up, it will speed up the T&T function, and then, some phlegm and blood stasis will be removed. This process is called **Wentong**, which can improve the capacities and functions of human body.

The way of **Wentong** is quite frequently used in TCM. For instance, Aijiu (moxa-moxibustion) is one of the basic methods adopted in TCM treatment. Fundamentally, it is one of the **Wentong** methods, but such a **Wentong** method is very particular about the location on the body. Aiye (folium artemisiae argyi) is also a herb for warming through meridians. But for Aijiu treatment, Airong (mox-a) should be substituted for Aiye because Airong is made of Aiye by the way of repeatedly pounding with a pestle until all the mesophyll turns into ash. And then, shaking off all the ash, the remaining fluffy material is actually the leaf vein and retinervus of Aiye, which is featured with warm property of Aiye. The leaf vein and retinervus can function in the meridians, so Airong can warm through meridians and collateral.

Warming for Transformation

Warm medicines have another function, i. e., warm dispersing. The formulas for dispersing blood stasis often contain warm medicines, like Danggui Wei (Angelica sinensis tail). And the formulas for reducing/resolving phlegm also contain many warm medicines, like **Erchen Tang** [Decoction of Banxia (pinellia ternate), Juhong (exocarpium citri rubrum), Baifuling (white poria) and Gancao (liquorice)], it is the most fundamental formula for reducing phlegm, in which both Banxia and Juhong are warm, and Gancao is also partially warm.

In fact, phlegm and blood stasis is like oil film remaining in the plates that have contained fried dishes, which are oily and hard to clean without using cleansing detergent. However, detergent alone does not work well; it is also necessary to use water, preferably hot water to help cleanse the plates quickly. The detergent to be used for cleansing plates is like the key medicine for reducing phlegm, and the hot water to be used for cleansing is like the medicines for promoting the secretion of saliva or body fluid while reducing phlegm. For instance, add some Lugen (rhizoma phragmitis), Tianhua Fen (radices trichosanthis) and the like, or even add some moistening medicines like Shashen (adenophora stricta), Maidong (radix ophiopogonis) to the formulas so that phlegm may be reduced much more quickly without impairment of Yin. In a word, to use hot water for cleansing plates is just like using warm medicines to reduce phlegm.

The same is true for dispersing blood stasis, for which there are many different medicines like Honghua (safflower carthamus), Taoren (peach kernel), Sanqi Fen (notoginseng powder), and Danshen (radix salviae miltiorrhizae) and so on. In the process of dispersing blood stasis, additionally put in **Siwu Tang** [Decoction of Danggui (angelica sinensis), Baishao (radix paeoniae alba), Chuanxiong (ligusticum wallichii), and Shengdi (dried radix rehmanniae)]. Dispersing blood stasis itself comes at the cost of blood consumption, so it is necessary to nourish blood at the same time when dispersing blood stasis is done. New blood is generated and the blood stasis is washed away, which is equivalent to adding water while using detergent. All these medicines are playing the warming function like hot water for cleansing plates.

In the phrase "温化" ("Wenhua", means "warm transformation" in English), the character "化" ("hua") does not mean to reduce phlegm and disperse blood stasis only. When talking about spring, summer, growing summer, autumn, and winter, one should keep in mind that they are corresponding to life, growth, transformation, harvest, and storage respectively. In the whole process from life to storage, there is one step of "transformation". Furthermore, "化" (Hua) also refers to "change", "transportation and transformation" (T&T), which is corresponding to internal organ of the spleen. The spleen dominates T&T. when T&T is being carried on efficiently, Qi and blood will be easily generated. From water and grains to Qi and blood, the process relies upon T&T of the spleen. When the T&T functions well, many diseases can be transported away, or otherwise, many diseases may not be transported away. Therefore, Li Dongyuan, one of the four medical experts in the Jin and Yuan dynasties, attached great importance to the spleen and stomach, not only because the spleen and stomach are the foundation of the acquired constitution, but also because the healthy T&T of the spleen and stomach can tackle the pathogenic factors and generate Qi and blood. The T&T processes are involved with the spleen, and are in need of energy and temperature. As the saying goes, "The spleen is wet soil, and it will start its T&T function only when it is warm."

So is the nature. Let us take a look at the earth in spring. After the season of Beginning of Spring comes the season of Rainwater according the Chinese lunar calendar. By this season, the earth has not been warmed up yet, but it starts to have more and more rain. In spite of more rain, the earth is still lifeless, even the winter jasmine does not blossom either since only water is not enough, and warm temperature is necessary, too. Wet soil fails to grow grass, and trees fail to sprout. They are eager to being warmed up. Then slowly, when the following seasons like the Waking of Insects, Spring Equinox, Qingming (Clear and Bright) come one by one, the earth begins to warm up, and then, it becomes lively and full of vigor immediately with sprouting trees and blossoming flowers. The universe and earth transform and generate all things, which is also the result of warming temperature, that is, the process of transformation can only be carried out at certain temperature.

For health maintenance, in fact, it is to foster the body's capability to carry on T&T, for which warm medicines are often needed.

Abuse of Warm Medicines

Where there is anything that works, soon its abuse will follow.

Abuses as Aphrodisiac Medicines

Abuses of warm medicines are common. Among the abuses, the first is the medicines for aphrodisiac use, which is neither a kingly way nor a bossy way, but a tricky way that is quite inadvisable.

In the volume of Mulberry of Genera, I have not mentioned the male silkworm moth since this medicine is not suggested to use. The male silkworm moth refers to a male moth that has just come out from the silkworm cocoon and has not experienced mating. Its wings and feet were cut off, stir-parched slightly in a pot, soaked with wine or directly ground into powder to fill in capsule for consumption. Those who take it can improve their sexual capacity rapidly because of its aphrodisiac effect.

But this is not advisable since it can seriously impair health, too. The male silkworm moth as a medicine is warm, but warm medicines are able to consume Yin. Those who take it will be motivated by sexual passion. Excessive lust will impair the life essence physically, and the momentary joy will have to be repaid without failure since it is terribly difficult to make it up once the life essence is consumed up.

Hot Medicines are inadvisable for Health Maintenance Purpose

In fact, the human body represents a process of life, but life keeps changing and transforming all the time. Each of us wishes that life would be transformed into a more and more healthy and beautiful state. For health maintenance, never try to seek quick success and instant benefits. It is impossible for a farmer to harvest the rice immediately after he transplants rice seedlings the day before. It takes time to change and transform. The same is true of the human body, for which one has to be patient enough in order to maintain health. Never try to solve all problems with just a snap.

Medicines like Fuzi (radix aconiti carmichaeli) can only be used to drive out coldness, or to rescue the patient by restoring Yang, but it must not be used for health maintenance purpose. Anyone that takes Fuzi as food for health maintenance will definitely be hurt. No doubt, in certain specific environment in a particular area, it may be used as necessary. In fact, the ancients adopted warming and nourishing methods more for health maintenance purpose, for example, they used Lurong (pilos antler) and Lujin (deer's sinew). In *Shennong Bencao Jing*, deer, as an animal medicine, is listed on the top, and it is a flesh and blood product that is much better for health maintenance. Please keep in mind that just a little will be helpful and workable. When the ancients used the top-grade medicines or the flesh and blood product, they would stop it where necessary. Try to avoid using Fuzi, which is listed in the category of low-grade medicines. If used without restriction, it would inevitably destroy physical health.

Of course, Fuzi can play its role in the body when it is used. For instance, after taking in the patent medicine of the **Fuzi Lizhong Pill**, one will feel energetic and ready for action. Why is it so? Because it can stir up Yang of the body and then cheer one up. But one should not rely on medicines to brace himself up since **Fuzi Lizhong Pill** is just like a hormone. It may temporarily mobilize a person's energy at the cost of consuming both the kidney Yin and kidney Yang. So whatever one does, he/she has to do it with the long-run effect in mind. The effects that a certain medicine takes temporarily will be insignificant in the long run, and he/she should take into consideration the effects after one year, five years or even thirty years. That is to say, when one is using a medicine, he/she should never keep his/her eyes on its quick effect since there is ample time for his/her life afterward.

Slight Fire Generates Qi and Sthenic Fire Consumes Qi

There are many similarities between warm and hot medicines, but also there are differences. In many books regarding herbs, out of the commonly used medicines, there are quite few hot medicines, and most of them are warm medicines. In practice, doctors rarely use extremely hot medicines, which are only to be used under certain circumstances. For common diseases, if the hot medicines are really necessary, the cool medicines or even the cold medicines must be used simultaneously for corrigent compatibility, or otherwise, only a very small dosage of hot medicines is to be used. *Huangdi Neijing* repeatedly states: "Slight fire generates Qi, and sthenic fire consumes Qi". "Slight fire" refers to a small fire, which is able to stir up the vitality of human body, full of vigor like the season of spring. The sthenic fire refers to an excessive fire, which on the contrary, is able to consume human body fluid and blood. So hot medicines can only be used for a short period of time, either to rescue life by restoring Yang, or to drive long-lasting coldness out of the body, but they should not be used for a long time. Even the warm medicines cannot be used for long, or in case they have to be used for long time in some cases, it may be necessary to add "water", that is, when the warm medicines are used, one should pay attention to nourishing blood and generating Qi, which is the most basic principle of using warm medicines.

The sunshine, rain and dew in the nature are the foundation for the growth of all plants. The temperature of sunshine cannot be too high; 20 degrees is the best, 30 degrees can be endured, but 40 degrees will be very hard to withstand. Meanwhile, the sun alone will not work well, and rain is also necessary, or otherwise, drought will take place. This is why the warm medicine and Yin nourishing medicine should be used together, which is not only the law of nature, but also the principle of disease treatment and health maintenance.

第三卷 桂之属－火部方药

第一章 温热药概论

火部方药是以桂枝、肉桂为代表的温热类药。首先我们要对温热药做一个大体的说明。

温热药的作用

温热药，主要有以下这些作用：

逐寒

逐寒，就是把寒气从人体驱逐出去。我们知道，寒是一种阴惨肃杀的气息，到深秋、冬天，寒气渐深，万物随之凋零；早春虽然节气已至，但若依然春寒料峭，草木也不会那么早发芽开花，必须等到春寒全部褪尽以后，才有大地春回。寒能够伤人的阳气，伤人的生机，所以有一种说法叫"百病皆起于寒"。从人体生机的角度看，确实如此，但"起于寒"并不是说直接起于寒气，而是说百病起源于人体没有正气，没有生机，起源于人体内的肃杀之气。不管什么病，寒病也好，温病也好，热病也好，它都包含一种肃杀之气，让人走向凋零。

寒是从哪儿来的呢？首先是从外界而来。寒邪伤人，首先是犯表，伤三阳经：太阳、阳明、少阳，这在《伤寒论》里都讲得非常的清楚。太阳主一身之表，寒伤太阳，寒邪在表，用麻黄汤；如果传到阳明，那么就用葛根汤；如果在少阳，就要用小柴胡汤来和解。麻黄也好，桂枝也好，葛根、柴胡这些都是辛温发表的药。外界的寒邪还有可能入三阴：太阴、少阴、厥阴，伤了太阴其实是伤了肺和脾，主要是伤了脾；伤了少阴其实就是伤了心和肾，因为手少阴之心经，足少阴之肾经；伤了厥阴经是伤了肝。寒邪伤三阴，说白了就是寒伤肝、寒伤脾、寒伤肾。咱们私底下可以这样简单地理解，但也要知道这两种说法之间不是严格等同的。

要治阴惨肃杀的寒，得用温煦的药。

回阳救逆

温热药的第二个作用叫回阳救逆。当人体内阴寒肆虐的时候，就像黑云压城城欲摧，体内是阴惨惨的，寒风怒号，阳气马上就要没有了，这时候就要用热药来回阳救逆了，这是垂死之际的最后一搏。

如果病人的脉还在跳，没有脉息欲绝的话，光用独参汤就可以了；当他脉息非常微弱，若有若无的时候，就要用参附汤来回阳了；如果这个人脸色惨白，在参附汤里面还要加阿胶；当这个人快要死了，甚至汗都快要出来了，阴阳快要离绝的时候，在参附汤里还可以加山萸肉。如果遇到很穷的人家，用不起人参，可以用大剂量的山萸肉加党参来给他救脱，它也能把人从垂危挽救回来。大病也是这样的，如果大病前面的阴寒非常盛，就用到大剂量的附子或者人参来回阳救逆，这就相当于背水一战了，指挥这样作战的往往是大将，一般人没有这个胆识和操控能力。

在回阳救逆的时候，还要防止寒热相激。就像一个玻璃杯刚从外面拿进来，很凉，你现在急着要喝水，就把刚烧开的开水倒下去，杯底就裂了，这就叫寒热相激。人体也是这样的，如果阴寒太重，你用很多的热药，病人可能马上受不了，会产生不好的反应，如呕吐等，所以往往在四逆汤之类的回阳救逆的方子里面还要略微加进去一些寒凉的药，比如说猪胆汁。猪胆汁是一味寒凉的药，它跟大热一块并不影响回阳救逆，反而让人体能够接受这个大热的方子。

温补

温热药其实是温药和热药的总称。温药和热药还是有差别的。驱寒和回阳救逆主要是热药的作用，温药的作用则主要体现在温补和温通。

温，就意味着暖，意味着有生气，有生气才可以有健康。所以，一般补养的药往往都偏温，以给人体灌注生生之气，这就是温补。它并不是机械地以物质来补物质，而是以自己的温性来调动人体的生气、培植人体的生机。这是中医跟西医补法最根本的区别。西医给你补进去多少葡萄糖就是多少葡萄糖，补进去多少氨基酸就是多少氨基酸。中医则不一样，比如说，给你用地黄养阴，地黄是滋腻的东西，但是地黄如果用得好，吃了以后你不但不觉得滋腻，反而觉得饭量变大了。可能，这几剂药里面地黄只有一百克，给你养阴，却让你增加了远远超过了一百克的体重，这就是地黄养阴的作用，它是调动你身体本身的生机，让你身体从日常最基本的饮食里去吸取能量，地黄本身能直接给你补充的东西，只是一小部分而已。

而且，补跟养还不一样，补是很快的，养是很慢的。我们的身体，只有在大虚的时候才可以补，平时就不要补了，但是要养，慢慢地养。所以很多养生的方法都不是急功近利的，都要在一个很长的时间段里才能看出效果，这就叫养。我们讲平时温补，也有温养的意思，通过温来养它，使其恢复生生之气，慢慢地恢复正常。

温通

我们都知道"寒则凝"，寒容易使东西凝固。人体也是这样的，遇到寒气，血流动的速度就会减缓，这样就容易堵，气堵住了就容易成为痰，血堵住了就容易产生瘀。这在根源上都是因为寒，但是后来在变化中就不再是寒了，郁久又会化热。痰可能是因为气寒，气不能通而形成的，痰作为身体的一个异类在这里久了就会化火，所以痰字里面两个火。瘀，可能是因为血跑得慢了，凝在那里了，凝久了就成为身体或者血管里面的一个异物，也开始着火了。痰和瘀在源头上可能是寒也可能是热，但是时间一长，都有化火的迹象，所以"六淫皆从火化"，那就得考虑到适当清火。

寒则凝，气血不行，使人精神萎靡，缺乏生机了，如果用温通的方法，可以鼓动气血，使气血运行和生化的速度加快。且脾为气血生化之源，得温则运，在气血的加速运行和生化中，一些痰和瘀滞会被化掉，这是温通，它能提高人体的各种能力、各项功能。

温通的方法在中医里用得非常多。比如艾灸，是中医治病的一种基本方法，从根本上讲，就是温通的，只不过温通的部位是很有讲究的。而艾叶也是一个温通之剂。为什么艾灸要用艾绒，而不是用艾叶呢？艾绒是把艾叶反复捣，叶肉就全部变成灰了，把那些灰全部抖掉，剩下的绒毛状的物质其实就是艾叶的叶脉叶络，它有艾叶的温性，又以络走络，所以它能温通经络。

温化

温药还有一个作用，叫温化。我们知道化瘀的药里面往往带有温药，比如当归尾。化痰的药里面也有很多的温药，比如二陈汤，它是化痰最基本的一个方剂。其中半夏是温性的，陈皮也是温性的，甘草也是偏温的。

其实痰和瘀就像装过菜的碗，里面油滋滋的不好洗掉，得用洗涤剂。但光用洗涤剂还不行，还得加水，最好加热水，才能洗得快。用洗涤剂就好比化痰用的主药，用水好比在化痰的时候要注意生津，比如加一点芦根、花粉之类的，甚至要加一点沙参、麦冬这些很滋润的药，化痰化的更快而不伤阴，而用热水好比用温药。

化瘀也是这样的，化瘀有很多药，红花、桃仁、三七粉、丹参等，在化瘀的同时我们还要加进去四物汤，当归、白芍、川芎、生地。化瘀的本身是以伤血为代价的，所以，我们要一边化瘀一边养血。新血出来了，瘀血被冲掉了，这也相当于一边用洗涤剂一边加水。这些药偏温就好比是用热水。

温化的"化"还不仅是化痰化瘀的意思。我们讲春、夏、长夏、秋、冬，它们对应的是生、长、化、收、藏。从生长到收藏，中间有一个"化"的过程。"化"就是变化、运化，对应于五脏是脾，脾主运化。如果运化非常得力，那么气血就非常容易生化出来。从水谷到气血，它是靠脾运化过来的。脾运化功能好很多病都能被运化掉。当人体脾运化不行的时候，很多病化不掉。所以李东垣他非常注重脾胃，这不仅仅是因为脾胃是后天之本，而且因为脾胃的健运能够化解病邪，化生气血。所有的运化，都跟脾土有关，都需要能量，需要温度，"脾为湿土，得温则运。"

自然也是这样的。我们看看春天的大地，立春完了是雨水，大地还没有回暖，雨水开始变多，虽然雨水多，但是大地依然很萧条，连迎春花都没有开。因为光有水还不行，还得有温度。湿土上面依然不能长草，树依然不发芽，它迫切地需要温度，慢慢地，惊蛰、春分、清明，大地才开始回暖，马上就生机勃勃了，发芽的发芽，开花的开花了。天地化生万物，也是温化的结果，要有温度才能化。

我们养生，其实养的是人体运化的能力，也经常用到温药。

温热药的滥用之处

任何东西，只要有用，就会有滥用。

壮阳、催情

温热药的滥用之处很多，首先是用来壮阳、催情，这不是王道也不是霸道，而是诡道，我们非常不提倡。

上次讲桑之属的时候，我就没有讲雄蚕蛾，因为这个药是不能用的。雄蚕蛾就是从蚕茧里面刚出来的雄的蚕蛾，还没有经过交配的，把它的翅膀和脚都剪掉，放在锅里稍微炒一下，泡酒或者直接碾粉装胶囊，人喝了就可以壮阳、性能力会迅速提高。

这是不提倡的，因为它非常伤身体，这味药本身是温热的药，温热的药耗阴，喝了以后情欲被催动，然后淫欲过度又会伤精，你一时痛快了，等到你得病以后再想把它补回来就非常难了。

大热之药不可用于养生

其实人体是一个生命的过程，而生命是处在变化当中的，生命一直是在化，我们希望生命越化越美好，所以在养生上千万不要有急功近利的心态。你今天插了秧，明天就可以收稻子吗？这是不可能的。它有一个慢慢变化的过程，身体也是这样的，你得有耐性。而不要企图通过一把火就解决问题。

像附子这样的药，只能用来驱逐寒气，或者用来回阳救逆，绝不能用来养生，你要是把附子当饭吃，肯定是要伤人的。当然特定的地区有特定的环境，大家可以用这个。用温补养生的方法古人用得很多。比如说古人经常用鹿茸、鹿筋，在《神农本草经》里面鹿是列在上品的，这是一个动物药，而且是血肉有情之品，你用这个来补多好啊，而且又不需要用太多，用一点点就行了。他们用上品的药、用血肉有情之品都是适可而止，何况用附子这种下品的药，你要是不加节制，伤人会伤得很快的。

当然附子吃下去以后是有效果的。像附子理中丸这个药，你吃一颗以后浑身来劲，觉得特别有精神。为什么？它把你阳气振奋起来了。但人不能靠药物来振奋，因为附子理中丸只相当于一个激素，它临时把你的精力调动起来了，这是以消耗你身体里的真阴真阳为基础的。所以我们做一件事情一定要有长远的眼光，吃了这味药，当时会怎么样，这个是小问题。一年以后会怎么样，五年、十年、三十年以后会怎么样，我们都要考虑到。用药不要取快于一时，因为人的生命是来日方长的。

少火生气，壮火食气

温药和热药有很多相通的地方，但是也有很大的区别，不能混淆。各类本草书中，常用的药，热药很少，大部分还是温药。在实际运用中，我们很少用到大热的药，即使用热药也要分场合。对一般的疾病，如果要用到热药的话，必定要用凉药、甚至是寒药来反佐它，要么就是用的剂量非常小。《黄帝内经》反复讲一句话，叫"少火生气、壮火食气"，"少火"就是小小的火，它能让人体有生机，像春天一样；壮火，就是很大的火，反而消耗人体的津液、血液。所以热药只能用于一时，要么用于回阳救逆，要么用于驱逐身上的陈寒，不能久用。哪怕是温药也不能久用，如果必须久用，也要一边温一边加水。用温药的时候要注意养血生气，这是用温药的一个最基本的原则。

我们经常讲，大自然的阳光雨露，这是万物生长的基础。阳光的温度不能太高，20多度最好，30多度也能忍，到40度就受不了。光有太阳还不行，还得下雨，否则就是干旱。这就是温药和养阴的药一块儿用的道理，是自然之理也是治病养生之理。

Chapter 2   Gui (Cassia)

In this volume, Gui (cassia) is taken as a typical example instead of Fuzi (radix aconiti carmichaeli). Gui (cassia) includes Guizhi (cassia twig) and Rougui (cassia bark), which are listed as the top-grade medicines in ***Shennong Bencao Jing***. In this book, the top-grade medicine is selected as the typical example for each category of medicines.

Gui is a plant that grows in the south of China, and it remains green throughout the year. The Chinese character "桂" (guì, means cassia) is formed with a "木" (mù, means wood) in the left and "圭" (guī, referring to a sort of jade ware to be held by the ancient emperors or dukes for certain ceremonies) in the right. The character "圭" (guī) looks like a leaf with one vertical stroke in the middle like the longitudinal leaf vein, and the four horizontal strokes like the horizontal leaf veins. The horizontal veins of Gui tree leaf are particularly obvious. Some people claim that the right side of "桂" (guì) signifies that "桂" ("guì") is "like a messenger holding a jade ware to take a lead for all medicines. "

There is a couplet, of which the first line reads "What is moving? It is the apricot flower in February and the osmanthus fragrans in August", and the next line reads "Who is pressing? It is the bright lighting at midnight and rooster crowing at dawn. " From the perspective of TCM, February is in the season of spring when the earth starts dispersing. In this season, the human body is also in a state of dispersion, therefore, the normal Qi circulation must be maintained. The apricot flower, white-color-oriented with a slight pink, having rising and dispersing functions, can enter the lung to help human body to carry on dispersion so that Qi can move and circulate smoothly in the body. Hence, it is said the apricot flower in February is most moving/touching. Autumn is a depressing, cooling and cold season when people will feel depressed, but the osmanthus fragrans is warm and sweet-scented, which can bring a ray of warmth in such a depressed and cold season, so it is also moving/touching. One may feel that time is passing by so quickly, and he does have a sense of urgency, so "the bright lighting at midnight and rooster crowing at dawn" can remind him of hard working/study. This couplet implies the meanings of both "restrain and relax", which tells that one not only plays to his heart's content by seeing and smelling apricot flower and osmanthus fragrans, but also should work hard as reading books by midnight and rise up upon hearing the crow of a rooster to practise the sword skill. This reflects the ancients had the ability to restrain and relax themselves, enjoy the psychological disposition and physical practicality, and fully understand aestheticism and possess realistic feelings.

The moon in autumn is always the most beautiful since the moon represents the life essence of Taiyin (alternative name given to the moon by the ancient Chinese). It is also a kind of negative thing, corresponding to the stern and depressing atmosphere of autumn. Hence, the moon in this season will be extraordinarily bright and clear. The moon in autumn is beautiful indeed, but it shows a heavy, stern and depressing atmosphere, so, with the help of the warmth of osmanthus fragrans, the season of autumn is becoming balanced. At the Mid-Autumn Night in the full-moon atmosphere, the ancient poet Bai Juyi in Tang Dynasty left us the beautiful poem line "Staying at Lingyin Temple to search for osmanthus seeds in the moon". While enjoying the glorious full moon, we are accompanied by the osmanthus fragrans. The full moon night is the time for reunion. The cassia tree has its sons (seeds), but it is much harder to search for the seeds hanging in the tree. Of course, the man who was searching for the seeds but failed to find them would have the sense of loss. The full moon is beautiful, but when it is accompanied with a slight sense of loss, it would appear poetic, showing that the ancients had given much thought to it.

However, "桂" (gui) exists in many different forms, but the Gui tree with its twigs and barks being as medicines is not the same plant as that with blossom of osmanthus fragrans in spite of the same name being used in Chinese for them. The former is called cassia tree and the latter is called osmanthus fragrans tree. There are similarities but also great differences between the two. What is going to discuss in the following part is about cassia tree.

Guizhi (Cassia Twig)

Guizhi refers to the twigs of the cassia tree, the best of which are the tender twigs on the top of the tree. As a medicine, Guizhi is usually picked and collected in February, August, and October.

Guizhi is pungent, sweet, and warm in its medicinal properties. It mainly goes into the lung and bladder meridians. In the lung meridian, it is able to regulate circulation of Qi; in the Taiyang bladder meridian, it is able to transform Qi and metabolize the fluid. In case the cold-strike symptom of Taiyang meridian arises, the herb of Guizhi will be the necessary choice.

Guizhi for Limbs

Guizhi, as a medicine, goes upwards to the upper limbs, and horizontally to the shoulder and arms. The pain in the shoulder due to cold strikes, and the pains in head and neck can be treated with Guizhi since it affects the foot Taiyang bladder meridian, and goes to shoulder and arms.

Twigs are all going upwards, so Guizhi gets into the upper limbs more. If legs require warming up, some other medicines may be added to guide the effects of Guizhi downwards. Guizhi is also able to enter collateral, similar to the function of Sangzhi (mulberry twig). However, Sangzhi is mild in property, whereas Guizhi is hot. They have different medical properties for different purposes. Guizhi has the functions of warming and activating meridians, so it can warm through the meridians and blood system to disperse the wind-cold, but also to eliminate the cold coagulation and blood stasis. Gizhi is widely used, not only for treatment of the cold due to wind-cold, but also for treatment of diseases like rheumatism.

Guizhi for Blood System

Guizhi is red in color. Theoretically, red things can enter the heart and the blood system, so Guizhi can disperse the cold in the blood system.

Guizhi is often usedtogether with Mahuang (ephedra) since Mahuang has a lighter smell, entering Qi system, while Guizhi smells more intense than

Mahuang, entering the blood system. When Mahuang and Guizhi are used together, they will cooperate with each other to invigorate Qi and blood, showing a strong capacity to induce sweat.

However, it is inadvisable to use Guizhi when a patient suffers from Yin deficiency, mass formed by blood stasis or endogenous heat because of its properties of warming and activating blood circulation. Therefore, when a patient suffers from rapid pulse or very dry feces, Guizhi should be used with special caution. It should not be used in a large dosage, or some other corrigent medicines are to be used with it. Otherwise, it may bring a consequence of "Guizhi killing due to excessive Yang". When the excessive Yang arises with vigorous endogenous heat, use of Guizhi is like pouring oil on fire, or holding the candle to the devil.

Guizhi Tang

Guizhi Tang (Cassia Twig Decoction) is taken as the No. 1 formula in *Shanghan Lun (Treatise on Cold Pathogenic Diseases)*. *Yizong Jinjian (the Golden mirror of medicine)* hailed **Guizhi Tang** as "the Originator of All formulas", i. e. the forefather of all formulas. How did it win such a good reputation?

Zhang Zhongjing's Illustration about Guizi Tang Modifications

Zhang Zhongjing used **Guizhi Tang** as an example for showing the way of modifications (addition and subtraction of herbs to/from formulas). There are many formulas in *Shanghan Lun*, such as **Longmu Guizhi Tang, Daqinglong Tang, Xiaoqinglong Tang, Guizhi Jiagui Tang**, and so on, which are all derived by way of addition to and subtraction from Guizhi Tang. Zhang Zhongjing just took **Guizhi Tang** as an example to show that the formulas are ever changing now and then. In the book of *Shanghan Lun*, many formulas have the ingredient herbs of Guizhi, and Baishao, and especially, Guizhi is more commonly used. What the readers should do is to learn the variable compatibility of Guizhi and how formulas are modified. Zhang Zhongjing set an example to demonstrate modifications of **Guizhi Tang**.

Later, whenever in some other new situations, we probably do not need to use **Guizhi Tang** or the herb of Guizhi, but we should follow the concept that

Zhang Zhongjing taught us. In fact, many modified formulas are made according to Zhang Zhongjing's method, or enlightened by him.

Therefore, instead of saying **Guizhi Tang** is the originator of all formulas, it might be taken as a good demonstration for writing medical prescriptions as well.

Harmonizing Ying and Wei and Regulating Qi Circulation

Guizhi Tang has the effects of inducing perspiration, eliminating the superficial pathogens and regulating Ying Qi and Wei Qi, which is able to make itself the forefather of all formulas. If we get down to analyze the problems regarding human bodies from the four levels of "Wei, Qi, Ying, and Blood", many of them will become clear and incisive. "Wei" is on the skin layer of the body and it is like a defence shield, which can be taken to protect the body. Under "Wei" is Qi, and then comes "Ying". As to "Ying", it can be compared to "military camp" located inside the body. "Blood" is the innermost part. So when just attacking the "Wei" system, the pathogenic factors might be very light and superficial; if the pathogenic factors attack the Qi system, it signifies that the pathogenic influence goes deeper, then again to the "Ying" system, which means the invaders have gone into the military camp. When the pathogenic factors get into the blood system, that would be much more serious. Maybe the camp is full of invaders who are going to make an attack at the command post.

Guizhi Tang can regulate "Ying" and "Wei", which is very important to harmonize the system of Qi in the whole body, so it is the "**Forefather of All Formulas**", and many other formulas are derived and evolved from it.

Guizhi Tang for Treatment of Taiyang Cold

Regarding **Guizhi Tang**, *Shanghan Lun* states: "As to Taiyang diseases, headache, fever, sweating, and fear of wind, **Guizhi Tang** can be used for treatment. " The foot Taiyang bladder meridian dominates the surface/exterior of the whole body since its main part is on the back that is of Yang.

When the wind-coldimpairs Yang, it stays on the surface of body. In that case, the patient generally has a "headache" at the back side of the head.

As to "fever", it is a manifestation of confrontation between the healthy factors and the evil/pathogenic factors.

As to "sweating", it is a manifestation of discord between Ying and Wei. When the wind pathogen has entered pores, it wants to go in further, but the body's healthy factors guard against it, and then both of them refuse to budge at the pores. The pores are in an open state and sweat cannot help going out.

A burnt child dreads the fire. Those who catch a cold will dislike the wind-cold, so **Guizhi Tang** can be used for treatment. **Guizhi Tang** is able to regulate Ying and Wei, and in fact, it is to support the healthy factors to resist against the pathogenic factors, i. e. to express support for the body's healthy factors, through which Qi and blood are invigorated to drive away the wind pathogens on the surface of body.

Harmonizing Ying And Wei for Treatment of Sweating Syndrome

Shanghan Lun again states: "If the patient does not have any other diseases in his internal organs, but only has a fever now and then or sweats a little now and a little then, and is not cured, that is attributable to discord within Wei (defensive Qi), which can be cured by inducing sweat with **Guizhi Tang** in advance. "

That may not be caused by the wind-pathogens on the body surface but caused by some other factors resulting in the discord between Ying and Wei. Therefore, it can be treated by inducing perspiration with **Guizhi Tang** to harmonize Ying and Wei before the body sweats irregularly itself. When Ying and Wei become harmonious, sweating will take place regularly again. Hence, **Guizhi Tang** is frequently used in many cases of sweating syndromes.

Original Formula of Guizhi Tang

According to the original version of **Guizhi Tang** in *Shanghan Lun*, **Guizhi Tang** contains the herbal ingredients:

Guizhi (peeled cassia twig) 2 *liang*, Shaoyao (paeonia lactiflora) 3 *liang*, Gancao (liquorice) 2 *liang*, Shengjiang (fresh ginger) 3 *liang*, and Dazao (jujube) 12 pieces (cut opened)

The units of weights and measures adopted in Chinese successive dynasties are different. In the time when Zhang Zhongjing was living, *Liang*, as the weight unit, was not the same as it is presently used in China, and is even different from that used in the Ming and Qing Dynasties. One *liang* at the time of Zhang Zhongjing was only equivalent to two *qian* in Ming and Qing Dynasties, or equivalent to present three grams, so three *liang* of that era is only equivalent to six *qian* in Ming and Qing Dynasties or eighteen grams now. Zhang Zhongjing in his prescription noted that "decoct the herbs with seven liters of water until three liters decoction is left. Drink it while it is warm, one liter at a time", which means to decoct the prescribed herbs with seven litres of water into three litres of decoction, and then, drink one litre only at a time. After drinking **Guizhi Tang**, the patient should have a bowl of hot porridge since the hot porridge can harmonize and stir up the stomach Qi in order to speed up inducing perspiration from the body, which helps to disperse the wind pathogens out of body. In addition, after having hot porridge, the patient should lie in bed for a rest under the cover of quilt till he is slightly sweating. At that time, the pores open easily, and if not covered with the quilt, the patient may have pathogenic wind enter the body again. If suffering from pathogenic wind again while in sweating, the patient will become worse. After drinking one-litre **Guizhi Tang**, if the patient still does not have sweat, he can drink one more liter. But if the patient starts to sweat after drinking, he should stop drinking the remaining two liters, i. e., stop taking the medicine as soon as it strikes the disease.

Medication and treatment have their rules and processes to follow. Use of **Guizhi Tang** needs to take such a process: Guizhi functions to promote blood circulation, disperse the superficial pathogenic factors, induce perspiration, and stir up Qi of the spleen and stomach; Shaoyao, as a medicine, is for astringing purpose, when used together with Guizhi, it can invigorate Qi of the spleen and stomach, and regulate Ying and Wei, not only going to the exterior but also defending the interior. The other three herbs of Shengjiang, Gancao and Dazao all go into the Middle Jiao, and especially, Shengjiang can play warming and dispersing functions as well. They work together by way of stirring up the healthy factors of the spleen and stomach to improve circulation of all the systems within human body, and then drive out the pathogenic factors. In this process, the spleen and stomach are especially relied upon. Hence, the three herbs as Shengjiang, Gancao and Dazao are added in the formula.

Key Herbs in Guizhi Tang

Whenever a TCM doctor sees a formula, he or she should have the ability to spot the key herbs in it. In the formula of **Guizhi Tang**, the key herbs are Guizhi and Shaoyao, which involve a lot of background knowledge.

Shaoyao as a medicine with a taste of sour has the efficacy of astringency. It can regulate Wei (the defensive system) and converge Yin. Meanwhile, Shaoyao is able to go into the liver. Guizhi as a medicine is pungent and dispersing. These two herbs show their opposite characteristics: one for dispersing and the other for converging. Therefore, in the process of dispersing by Guizhi and converging by Shaoyao, Ying and Wei become harmonized. With Shengjiang, Gancao and Dazao added, the spleen and stomach will have sufficient energy as a foundation, and then, Ying and Wei will be regulated and harmonized more easily.

In spite of the astringency property of Shaoyao, when it is properly used, it will not converge the pathogenic factors. Guizhi can regulate Ying and eliminate the superficial pathogens, but it will not impair Yin. Guizhi is used in this formula instead of Sangzhi since Sangzhi is mild in property and it has no such effects as inducing perspiration or dispersing.

Guizhi is warm and is subsumed to Yang, while Shaoyao is cold and cool, and is subsumed to Yin. Guizhi and Shaoyao enjoy the different properties of warmth vs cold, astringency vs dispersion, and Yin vs Yang. They mutually restrain themselves to play their functions of regulating and harmonizing Ying, Wei, Qi and blood. Furthermore, Guizhi appears reddish in color, so it is able to go into the heart to uplift the heart Yang; Shaoyao can guide the effects of Guizhi into the liver to uplift the liver Yang; Meanwhile, Guizhi can guide the effects of Shaoyao into the heart to converge Yin and blood of the heart.

The matching of Guizhi with Shaoyao gives expression to the theory of Yin and Yang. And addition of Shengjiang, Gancao and Dazao to the formula reflects the concept of the Three Superpowers of Sky, Earth and Human Being.

That Guizhi goes upwards, so it can be taken as the medicine of Sky; and that Shaoyao goes downwards, so it can be taken as the medicine of Earth; Shengjiang, Gancao and Dazao functioning as material bases in between the Sky and the Earth are to supply energy and power to the spleen and stomach, so they are taken as the medicine of Human Being. This formula embodies the thought of the Three Superpowers of Sky, Earth and Human Being. We should fix our eyes upon the Sky and Earth, and of course we have to take Human Being into account, too.

Examples of Clinical Uses of Guizhi (Cassia Twig) and Shaoyao (Radix Paeoniae Alba)

As it is a common sense that sweat is the fluid of the heart. When one suffers from being uneasy in mind or nervous, he may be sweating easily since at this moment he is unable to keep calm. To keep a calm state of mind is very important since the mind controls the normal operation of the human body. In case one is in a panic state of mind, he will then be in a "state of utter stupefaction", which will then result in many physiological abnormal conditions like sweating or shivering. Under such circumstances, use Guizhi to soothe and calm the nerves, which in turn can constrain sweat. Many formulas for treatment of sweating symptoms contain seeds of wild jujube, which is also to restrain the mind, and then constrain sweat.

Guizhi and Shaoyao are often used for treatment of obstruction of Qi circulation in the chest and symptom of chest pain. Many patients with heart troubles have a very slow pulse beat, and sometimes feel very much oppressed in the chest. Whenever they are entangled with even small troubles, they will get flustered with accelerating heartbeats and feel out of breath. In those cases, they can be treated based on syndrome differentiation plus relatively large dosage of Guizhi and Shaoyao. Guizhi has the effect of going into the heart to activate the blood circulation so to help the pulse beat a little faster, which means it can help the blood circulate faster. As such, much Qi will start to disperse and the blood stasis will also be broken through, and then the patients could feel relaxed in their mind. So Guizhi, Shaoyao, Gualou (trichosanthes kirilowii maxim), and Xiebai (allium macrostemon) are often used together for treatment of heart troubles of thoracic obstruction, which is found very effective. In fact, many heart troubles are caused by failure of the lung Qi falling and heart Yang deficiency, causing obstruction of Qi circulation in the chest, which then results in chest oppression. Under that circumstance, Guizhi and Shaoyao should be used for treatment. It is quite sure that rapid pulse can also cause chest oppression, but the treatment for such a case will be a different matter since Guizhi and Shaoyao target the heart troubles of slower pulse beats.

Guizhi and Shaoyao are also frequently used to treat abdominal pain due to the discord of Qi and blood, for which, to some extent, Ying and Wei are to be regulated and harmonized, and especially the abdominal pain of deficiency-cold may be treated with.

Guizhi can go into limbs to accomplish its function and Shaoyao can follow Guizhi to go into limbs, too. Meanwhile, Guizhi will follow Shaoyao to go into the five viscera, implying that the two medicines can cooperate mutually to pass through the whole body when they are used together. So whenever there arise the symptoms of pain and numbness in limbs, or failure of limbs to stretch out, Guizhi and Shaoyao can be used for treatment since Guizhi can warm up the anadesma and Yang as well. Shaoyao, sour in property, can nourish the liver and Yin in that "the liver dominates the anadesma". Under the guidance of Guizhi, the sour taste of Shaoyao will play its function on anadesma so to help stretch out limbs. Hence, many diseases related to limbs are frequently treated with Guizhi and Shaoyao.

Furthermore, Guizhi and Shaoyao are also used for treatment of the diseases related to meridians. Guizhi can warm to activate meridians, and it can especially dredge the collateral. In prescriptions, Guizhi is often written as "Nen Guizhi" (tender cassia twig) by doctors. A piece of "Nen Guizhi" hangs in a cassia tree, looking like the collateral in the human body. It can go into the meridians of the human body, and stimulates blood vessels to improve the blood circulation and break the stagnation of collateral.

A cold deficiency of the spleen and stomach due to chronic dysentery is normally attributed to the disorder of Qi and blood circulation, and disharmony between Ying and Wei as well, so Guizhi and Shaoyao can also be used for treatment. Shaoyao tastes sour, and it has effect of astringency for treatment of dysentery. As mentioned above, Guizhi has the effects to warm up and activate meridians. Guizhi and Shaoyao can work side by side to drive out and disperse the cold pathogenic factors through warming treatment on the one hand, and converge the healthy factors and prevent them from falling on the other hand so that the regular viscera functions will be restored. Guizhi can enter the liver meridian, and along with Shaoyao, it can also enter the spleen meridian to invigorate the spleen Yang. Guizhi and Shaoyao have been proved effective for treatment of chronic dysentery. In addition, Guizhi and Shaoyao may function differently when they are used with other medicines, for instance, they are sometimes used with **Xianglian Pill**, and sometimes with **Baitouweng Tang**.

In the cases of numbness and pain in limbs, or pain at joints, Guizhi Mu (peeled cassia twig) is used to substitute for Guizhi. But it has to be clarified that the so-called "peeled" twig is different from that described by Zhang Zhongjing. What Zhang Zhongjing called the peeled Guizhi refers to removing the outer coarse bark, but now we use the tender cassia twig, so it can be used directly and it is unnecessary to peel the twig again. Guizhi Mu means that the outer bark has to be peeled off completely with only the wood inside to be remained and used. The outer bark has strong scent while the wood inside only smells a little. Therefore, when Guizhi Mu is needed, a large dosage will have to be used, around 20 grams. But if the limbs are severely cold, and Guizhi Mu is not strong enough to warm up and activate the meridians, Fuzi (radix aconiti carmichaeli), or the processed Fuzi can be used with just a small dosage, but it should be decocted for longer time since the limbs is treated by means of the dispersion and outreaching attributes of Fuzi. With a small dosage, it goes to the limbs; too much of it will go to the five viscera instead, especially to the kidney.

Guizhi Tang and Modifications of the Formula

Let us take **Guizhi Tang** in *Shanghan Lun* as an example to illustrate the method of addition and subtraction of herbs to/from formulas. For instance,

Shanghan Lun states: "When suffering from Taiyang diseases, the patient will dislike wind, have difficulty in urination, or have a limb spasm with difficulties of curling and stretching out freely and smoothly, **Guizhi plus Fuzi Tang** will do. " Excessive diaphoresis may result in more perspiration. The patient dislikes wind since his or her pores can close up, which is also due to the disharmony between Ying and Wei. Therefore, the patient has to use Guizhi Tang. But why does the patient find it difficult to urinate? On the one hand, the waste fluid has run off from the sweat pores, and on the other hand, there might arise the kidney Yang deficiency. Excessive diaphoresis may lead to the extent of internal impairment of the kidney Yang and external Yang depletion. In such a case, **Guizhi Tang** is used with a piece of Fuzi added for stopping perspiration and restoring Yang.

Shanghan Lun again states: "Use the burning-warm acupuncture needle to induce perspiration, but the needle point may suffer from cold, swell up and form a red nucleus, where a blast of air seems to rush from the lower abdomen up to the chest, which should be treated with **Guizhi plus Tang** (it means to add more cassia twig in **Guizhi Tang**) ". Probably in the era when Zhang Zhongjing was living, some doctors might adopt more barbaric methods to give treatment of diseases. *Shanghan Lun* often says "by fire", indicating that fire was used to make people sweat. The people at that time might be physically stronger and more robust. When the wind cold stayed in the body surface, it might be dispersed by warming the patients with fire. But Zhang Zhongjing might not have thought that method was a better way. Another way was to use acupuncture therapy to induce perspiration, which is called a "burning needle", that is, burn the acupuncture needle and then puncture into human body, or heat the needle after it is punctured into human body, through which heat is transmitted into body. For the physically stronger and robuster patients, the shock of such a hot needle would induce perspiration, but for the physically weak patients, such a method would cause a syndrome of "needle point being cold", which means the patients might suffer from cold again from/at the acupuncture point", where there would arise a lump swelling, or "rushing piglet air" in the body. The so-called "rushing piglet air" refers to a blast of air in the lower abdomen like a piglet rushing upwards. When it rushes to the chest, the patient will feel especially uncomfortable. For such a case, use **Guizhi-plus Tang**, i. e. , add more Guizhi in the formula. The "burning needle" point catching a cold and swelling a lump gives a sign of disharmony of Ying and Wei, so **Guizhi Tang** has to be used continuously, but the dosage of cassia twig must be increased to two times of Shaoyao. By the way, for any of medicines, when the dosage is to be increased, its effects will be guided to go downwards. So, with Guizhi, if used for going on the body surface, one should decrease its dosage, which can be more effective. Now there arises a blast of air rushing upwards, indicating that the kidney Qi fails to be astringed. In the case that the kidney Qi is strong enough to pull downwards, the "piglet-like air" will not rush up any more. Now because the kidney Qi fails to hold itself, the dosage of Guizhi has to be increased to warm up the kidney. Of course, there is another saying that **Guizhi-plus Tang** is not formulated by adding Guizhi but Rougui (cassia bark) instead, which I believe is true since Rougui can directly warm the kidney, and that has been proved effective. However, It is certain that Guizhi can be used too since it also has the effect of calming the adverse-rising energy to suppress the uprush force.

　　Shanghan Lun says: "After Taiyang diseases are treated, and in case there occur rapid pulses and Qi rushing up to the chest, use **Guizhi Tang** (with Shaoyao removed) . " This is a remedy formula. Probably, the patient might have been treated with **Guizhai Tang** or **Mahuang Tang**, I suppose, however, he might have seen a quack doctor who would have given him a bad solution of treatment with Dahuang (rheum officinale) or Mangxiao (mirabilite) instead, which improved the constipation but also caused pathogenic factors to go in thereafter. Such a purgation of feces with an improper way would definitely impair the spleen Yang and cause bad T&T effects, which are attributed to the turbid accumulated in the chest, and Qi stagnation in the chest. When the superficial pathogenic factors are caught in the lung, there will occur a rapid pulse. Shaoyao, sour and bitter in taste, can help to gush diarrhea further under the previous diarrhea conditions, so it cannot be used again since its sour taste may bring about its function of converging the pathogenic factors. After Shaoyao is removed from **Guizhi Tang**, only the ingredients of Guizhi, Shengjiang, Gancao and Dazao are left. With the help of the pungent and sweet tastes of the remaining herbs, they may play a dispersing function and nourish Yang, invigorating the spleen Yang and activating the stomach Qi circulation to help drive out the pathogenic influences.

In case a patient often suffers from asthma, it is necessary to add the herbs of Houpo (Mangnolia officinalis) and Xingren (apricot kernel) in **Guizhi Tang**, for they can depress Qi and relieve asthma. For some Taiyang diseases, if mistreated, there will arise asthma, too, which can also be treated with **Guizhi Tang** with addition of Houpo and Xingren, but such an asthma should be that arising from the vigorous pathogenic factors. However, the asthma stemming from the kidney deficiency would be a different matter.

Guizhi Tang plus Yitang (maltose) will make **Xiao Jianzhong Tang**. Yitang is very good for nourishing the spleen and stomach, but people in modern time should not eat too much of it since it is indigestive. Now, **Xiao Jianzhong Tang** is seldom used since people in the modern time have a quite different physique from those in the past. All the people in the past had a plain life with only simple diets, and many people even were on short supply of food, and always cried piteously for food with empty stomach. Under that condition, taking some maltose, they would feel comfortable in the spleen and stomach and benefited from maltose. But now, many people eat their heads off, and therefore, they always suffer from the foul smell and fats in their stomachs. Under such conditions, if they take too much of sticky maltose, they may feel uncomfortable. Many other additions and subtractions to/from **Guizhi Tang** recorded in *Shanghan Lun* might not be suitable for the modern time. For instance, **Guizhi Tang plus Fuzi** for stopping perspiration and restoring Yang, that will not be the necessary case today. Most of the people in modern time suffer from Yin deficiency. If they take the above-mentioned hot medicines, they may get inflamed very easily.

Keep in mind that *Shanghan Lun* was written on the basis of cold impairment, i. e. its writing background was cold impairment, so Zhang Zhongjing took **Guizhi Tang** as the fundamental formula to make relevant modifications for making new formulas. People of that time in their physique and life style were quite different from the people of the present time, and even the climate and environment have also been changing now. Hence, for some medicines, people of that time could bear their effects, but people of present time may not necessarily withstand any more.

Guizhi Tang plus Longgu (ossa draconis) and Muli (concha ostreae) will make **Longmu Guizhi Tang**, which is usually used for restraining sweat. Longgu and Muli take the property of astringency, which has been proved effective for treatment of abnormal sweating syndrome arising from disharmony of Ying and Wei. Similarly, for the sweating syndrome arising from deficiency of both Qi and Yin in summer, **Shengmai Yin** plus Longgu and Muli can be used. For the sweating syndrome arising from endogenous heat, some other heat-clearing formulas plus Longgu and Muli may be used.

All in all, the addition and subtraction of herbs to/from **Guizhi Tang** is very flexible. Although we may not necessarily use all of them now, we should do research on them, from which we may understand and learn the methods of modifying formulas rather than blindly take the formulas to compare with the symptoms, which in fact is a very difficult thing. Some people always apply formulas in *Shanghan Lun* mechanically to a disease, and yell and praise the classic formula when a disease is cured, or keep quiet when failing to cure a disease. This is not correct approach. As to an empirical formula, if it is effective for curing a disease, one should take it as an example for analysis. Only in such a way can one improve his or her competence of curing diseases.

One should also respect the ancient medical classics while he or she is learning TCM. For example, *Shanghan Lun*, it is a clinical classic book in the history of TCM, which has laid the foundation of TCM syndrome differentiation and treatment. Hence, all the learners should show great respect to it, but must be neither bigoted or limited to it, nor admire the ancient things and belittle present achievements. Even the so-called stupid person may once in a while have a good idea. In case that one might collect all the good ideas given by such so-called stupid persons, that would be fantastic. Therefore, all the doctors should be open-minded and open to all people's great achievements in addition to Zhang Zhongjing's.

Never Limited to the Classic Formulas Only

There is a book called ***Book of the Living Man***, which was written in the

Song dynasty. It puts forward a lot of different views from Zhang Zhongjing's **Guizhi Tang**. The book says: "**Guizhi Tang** is good for the people in the northwest of China and proved effective in the four seasons all year round. However, it is not necessarily the case in the areas between the Yangtze river and Huaihe river, where it is only effective in the seasons of winter and spring. From the late spring to the time before summer solstice, if **Guizhai Tang** is used, Huangqin (scutellaria baicalensis) 1 *fen* to make into **Yangdan Tang**. But after the summer solstice, Zhimu half liang, Shigao (gypsum) 1 liang, or Shengma 1 *fen* should be added to **Guizhi Tang**. As for those patients who have a deficiency-cold physique, no modification (addition or subtraction) of **Guizhi Tang** is needed."

By the time of the Song Dynasty, some people found that **Guizhi Tang** was not that effective, so they started to put forward some new modifications, but also claimed that **Guizhi Tang** could only be effective for the patients in the northwest of China since the northwest is subsumed to Metal, and the north is subsumed to Water, geographically, referring to the areas of present Shaanxi and Gansu provinces and Ningxia Autonomous Region, where the weather is relatively cooler or cold, and the local people are endowed with a stronger physical fitness with a legacy left by the preceding generation of the Han Dynasty. At that time, **Guizhi Tang** was only suitable for the people in the northwest. But in the areas between the Yangtze river and Huaihe river, geographically referring to the areas of present Jiangsu, Anhui, and Zhejiang provinces, i. e. the middle and lower reaches of the Yangtze River, the local people are relatively delicate and physically weak, so some modifications were made, like Huangqin to be added for reducing the heat of **Guizhi Tang**. After the summer solstice, add Zhimu and Shigao, which are the key herbs of **Baihu Tang** for clearing heat; or Shengma, a cold and cool medicine. All the above modifications made are for the patients who essentially have endogenous heat. However, at that time, no pungent cool medicament like **Yinqiao San** was developed, so the only way was to add some cold and cool herbs in **Guizhi Tang** for clearing heat.

The ***Book of the Living Man*** was written in the Song Dynasty in 1108, about eight hundred years after Zhang Zhongjing. Obviously, the present situation has been changing over and over, so the **Book of the Living Man** reminds us of adapting ourselves to the changing circumstances. Regarding the formula like **Guizhi Tang**, it is still in use presently in the areas to the south of the Yangtze River, and even still popular there, but time has passed and circumstances have changed. As the saying goes: "Once on shore, we pray no more." Through exploration and inheritance from generation to generation, doctors and medical experts of the past generations have fished out a lot more ways for treatment of diseases, which we should not blindly reject.

Mahuang Tang

Guizhi can also be used together with Mahuang (ephedra), both of which form a medicine pair frequently used in Zhang Zhongjing's formulas. One of the typical formulas is **Mahuang Tang**.

Mahuang Tang contains the herbal ingredients: Mahuang, Guizhi, Xingren, Gancao.

Analyses of Mahuang Tang Fromula

Mahuang used with Guizhi can warm meridians and drive out coldness. Mahuang itself can induce perspiration, but if it is used together with Guizhi, it will become much stronger for inducing perspiration.

Normally, Mahuang goes to Qi system to induce perspiration, but it can only induce a little sweat since "sweat is the fluid of the heart", implying that sweat is induced from blood. Guizhi just goes into the heart and the blood vessels, so with the efficacy of Guizhi going into the blood system, more sweat will be then induced, indicating the pharmacological principles of compatibility of Mahuang and Guizhi.

Xingren purges the lung Qi and promotes circulation of the lung Qi. It helps Mahuang to purge the lung Qi so that pores will open. Hence, Mahuang and Xingren used together will play a more effective function for regulating and purging the lung Qi.

Mahuang Tang is mainly used to treat the syndromes of the superficial cold pathogens and closure of pores due to cold pathogens. "Coldness causes coagulation". Therefore, when the body surface suffers from the attack of cold pathogens, the pores will close up. As such, the heat inside the body cannot be dispersed out, and then the patient will feel rotten. Because of the cold pathogen in between the skin and meridians, there will arise a series of syndromes of pain in the body. So, **Mahuang Tang** is used to open the pores to let the body become permeable. At the same time, to induce some sweat can help drive the cold pathogens out of the human body. This is the implication behind the formula of **Mahuang Tang**.

Maxing Shigan Tang contains Mahuang and Xingren, which is mainly to take advantage of the function of promoting the lung Qi circulation. If Mahuang were not to be used with Guizhi, its effect for inducing perspiration would become weak. Of course, this refers to its strength relatively for the people of Zhang Zhongjing's time. Now, Mahuang is able to play its full function all the same with strong effect for inducing perspiration, especially, for the southern people, even without being coupled with Guizhi. Hence, the people in the south should take this formula with caution.

Following the *Wuxing Doctrine* to Soothe the Spleen

Gancao used in **Mahuang Tang** is for coordinating the actions of all the herbs in the formula. Meanwhile, sweet taste can enter the spleen (corresponding to Earth according to the *Wuxing Doctrine*), and the Earth can generate metal (corresponding to the lungs according to the *Wuxing Doctrine*), so Gancao also has the function of supporting the Earth to generate Metal. The three herbs of Mahuang, Guizhi and Xingren in **Mahuang Tang** are used for promoting and uplifting the lung Qi, inducing perspiration, regulating the lungs, and at the same time, soothing the spleen (earth), after which it would be much easier to regulate the lung Qi-circulation. This is the method frequently adopted according to the relationship between the elements of the *Wuxing Doctrine*, that is, the "mother" should be pacified before the "son" is to be cured.

While giving treatment of the liver diseases, one must give consideration to the spleen, too, since the liver (wood) restricts the spleen (earth). In the case of soothing the liver, the spleen (earth) must be pacified, too. Otherwise, in case it becomes tough, the liver may not be able to restrict it any more. Only when the spleen has been pacified before one starts to regulate the liver, will it become much easier to regulate the liver properly.

In short, one should give consideration to the spleen (earth) while giving treatment to different diseases related to the other internal organs since the spleen (earth) is located in the centre, where it has close link with the liver, heart, kidneys, and lungs.

Seeking for Mild Medication

The potency dimension of Mahuang to induce perspiration is obvious. Even in the era when Zhang Zhongjing was living, there arose a lot of accidental perspiration from the improper use of Mahuang, which then resulted in some terrible syndromes. Zhang Zhongjing's **Shanghan Lun**, to a large extent, is a book on the remedies for rescuing the improper treatments, serving to show that there existed a lot of mistakes in the medical field at that time, and also serving to show that **Mahuang Tang** was a very powerful formula even in Zhang Zhongjing's era. So, once it is wrongly used, it might lead to a consequence of life or death, i. e., quack doctors' murder.

Is there a better solution to avoid such an accident? Doctors of all dynasties have been trying their exploration and attempting to find a safer and milder treatment with the precondition of equal effects. Later, on the one hand, because of changes of the climate and people's physical conditions as well, and on the other hand, because of doctors of all dynasties having been exploring for safer, milder and more effective ways of treatment, Ye Gui (style name "Tianshi", a well-known medical expert in Qing dynasty) absorbed different opinions from other schools and established the febrile disease school. The formulas of the febrile disease school, such as those 60 methods listed in the book of **Shibing Lun** (**Treatise on Seasonal Diseases**), are all using very light and mild medication instead of heavy and fierce medication. Some people made a joke that the doctors of the febrile disease school are timid because of using some inessential medicines only like Lugen, Tianhua Fen, Doujuan (sprouted black soybean), Juhua, Sangye. These medicines do work to cure diseases. That is what patients dream of safe, mild and effective way of treatment, which is also the Chinese style of doing things, that is, skillfully deflected, and never confronting the tough with toughness.

Therefore, from *Treatise on Febrile Diseases* to *Treatise on Seasonal Diseases*, it shows the inheritance and development, but also reflects the pursuit of Chinese culture. One must not think that use of less and milder medicines by the febrile disease school is just due to timidness or lack of knowledge and experience. Such a view is definitely wrong.

Mahuang Jiazhu Tang

Mahuang Tang plus Baizhu (white atractylodes rhizome) makes the well-known **Mahuang Jiazhu Tang**. The book of *Jingui Yaolue (Synopsis of the Golden Chamber)* uses it to give treatment for those who suffer from smothery pain due to heavy endogenous dampness. Those who suffer from smothery pain due to the endogenous dampness plus exogenous pathogenic factors resulting in closure of pores may be treated with **Mahuang Tang** plus Baizhu since Baizhu can invigorate the spleen to eliminate dampness.

Baizhu and Mahuang is an excellently matched medicine pair, of which Baizhu goes to the Middle Jiao to remove the endogenous dampness while Mahuang goes to the body surface for inducing perspiration in order to eliminate the superficial dampness. Meanwhile, under the influence of the astringency of Baizhu, the potency dimension of inducing perspiration by Mahuang would become weak when it is matched with Baizhu. However, the potency dimension of eliminating the endogenous dampness by Baizhu would become stronger accordingly under the help of Mahuang. As such, the dampness can be resolved and eliminated easily from both the interior and the exterior simultaneously.

This method not only can be used for treatment of the smothery pain due to heavy endogenous dampness, but also it can be taken as a reference for treatment of many other diseases, such as arthritis, rheumatism, and skin diseases. Of course, some flexible modifications should be made necessarily.

If the dampness manifests an obvious symptom due to some excessive exogenous pathogenic factors, Cangzhu (rhizoma atractylodis) should be added in

Mahuang Jiazhu Tang since Cangzhu has a stronger potency dimension of removing dampness and its additional effect of inducing perspiration; Or Cangzhu and Baizhu may be added together in **Mahuang Jiazhu Tang** since Cangzhu can tonify the spleen to remove dampness while Baizhu can invigorate the spleen to eliminate dampness. When these two herbs are used together, they are able to bring out the best in each other for tonifying the spleen and eliminating dampness. In fact, there are many other modifications of **Mahuang Tang**, which will not be described in details here.

第二章　桂

讲火部方药，我们并没有以附子为代表，而以桂为代表。桂包括桂枝和肉桂，在《神农本草经》里列在上品。我们要选上品药作为一类方药的代表。

桂是生在南方的，四季常青。"桂"是"木"字旁加一个"圭"字，"圭"字就像一片树叶，中间的一竖是树叶的纵叶脉，四横就是横叶脉，桂树树叶的横叶脉特别明显。还有人讲右边的"圭"，意味着桂"如执圭之使，倡导百药"。

有一副对联，上联是"何物动人？二月杏花八月桂"，下联是"有谁催我？三更灯火五更鸡"。我们从医理的角度来考虑，二月的杏花为什么动人呢？因为二月是春天，大地在宣发，人体也在宣发，要生发就需要气机通畅，而杏花是以白色为主，微微泛一点粉红，是入肺的，有升散的作用，能够帮助人体宣发，让人气机畅达，所以二月杏花最动人。而秋季是肃杀的、寒凉的，在寒凉之中人心情就比较低落。桂花是温的，芳香的，在肃杀之季给人带来一丝温暖，所以它也是动人的。既看杏花又看桂花，是一种玩的心态，后边马上就收敛了："有谁催我"，感觉到青春年华韶光易逝，有紧迫感了，"三更灯火五更鸡"，要好好学习了。这幅对联也是有收有放，既能尽情玩耍，看杏花、桂花，又能勤奋努力，三更灯火攻书，五更闻鸡起舞，反应出古人能收能放，既有性情，也有实干，既懂唯美，又很现实的情怀。

为什么月亮到秋天最美？月亮是太阴之精，它也是一种阴性的东西，跟秋天的肃杀之气正好相应，所以秋天的月亮会分外的皎洁。秋月固然美，但肃杀之气太重了，配上桂花的温暖就平衡了。中秋月圆之夜，古人的诗里有描述"山寺月中寻桂子"。赏月的时候陪伴着桂花。月圆之夜是团圆之夜，桂是有子的，但是在月下寻找桂树的子是比较难的，找不到之后心情稍稍失落。月圆已经很美好了，再微微点缀一些失落，就会更有诗意。这也是古人用心良苦的地方。

不过，我们要说明的是，虽然都叫"桂"，但树枝、树皮入药的桂与开桂花的桂并不是同一种植物。开桂花的叫桂花树，而入药的叫肉桂树。二者有相通之处，也有很大差异。我们后面讲的桂树，是肉桂树，不是桂花树。

桂枝

桂枝是桂树的枝，以桂树顶上的嫩枝为最好。一般是二月、八月、十月的时候采摘。桂枝，药性辛、甘、温。它主要入肺经、膀胱经。入肺经它能利气，入足太阳膀胱经它能化气、行水。太阳伤寒就要用到桂枝。

桂枝，药性辛、甘、温。它主要入肺经、膀胱经。入肺经它能利气，入足太阳膀胱经它能化气、行水。太阳伤寒就要用到桂枝。

以枝入肢

桂枝是往上走的药，能行走上肢，横行肩膀、手臂。伤寒肩膀痛、头项强痛都会用到桂枝。这是跟足太阳膀胱经有关，也跟桂枝能行于肩臂的作用有关。

桂枝作为一种"枝"，它能入四肢。因为它是往上升的，因此桂枝入上肢多一些。如果要温下肢，可以加别的药把它往下引。桂枝是桂树上细小的枝条，它也能入络脉，这跟桑枝有相通的地方。不过桑枝是平性的，桂枝是热性的，药性不一样，用途用法也不一样。桂枝是有温通作用的，所以能温通经络、温通血分来散风寒，还能消除枝节间的寒凝血滞。桂枝不仅仅用在风寒感冒里，在治疗风湿类的疾病也会用到，它是一味运用很广泛的药。

桂枝入血分

桂枝是红色的，红色能入心、入血分，所以桂枝能散血分的寒。

我们经常把桂枝跟麻黄配在一起使用。麻黄气味比较淡，是走气分的；桂枝走的是血分，它的气味比麻黄要浓烈一些。麻黄跟桂枝一起使用，同时鼓动了气血，发汗的能力就强了。

但是桂枝性温，又能动血，所以阴虚、血症，还有内热的时候不宜用，比如说脉数或者是大便特别干用桂枝就要非常慎重。第一不能多用，第二你可以用其他的药来反佐它。如果在这些方面不注意的话，可能导致"桂枝下咽，阳盛则毙"。当你阳气比较亢，内热比较旺的时候再用桂枝，等于是火上浇油，助纣为虐。

桂枝汤

讲到桂枝我们就会想到桂枝汤，这是《伤寒论》的第一个方剂。《医宗金鉴》将桂枝汤誉为"群方之祖"，它是所有方剂的祖宗。为何有此美誉？

仲景以桂枝汤为例，指明加减大法

《伤寒论》里有很多方子，比如龙牡桂枝汤、大青龙汤、小青龙汤、桂枝加桂汤，等等，都是在桂枝汤的基础上进行加减变化而来的。仲景只不过是以桂枝汤的加减告诉后人：方子是千变万化的。《伤寒论》里很多方子都有桂枝、白芍，桂枝用得尤其多。所以我们要看它是怎么变化的，要掌握它的变化以及变化的方法。张仲景用桂枝汤的加减给我们做了一个示范。

以后我们再面对其他的情形，方可以不用桂枝汤，药可以不用桂枝，但是法我们都要依照这个精神。张仲景用桂枝汤的变化教给我们的是法，后人在方剂的加减变化中都是依据张仲景的这种变化之法而来的，或者说都是受到张仲景的启发。

所以，与其说桂枝汤是群方之祖，还不如说它是群方之范，是组方的范例。

调和营卫，整理气机

桂枝汤发汗解肌、调和营卫的作用，也足以让它成为群方之祖。

我们知道，人体的很多问题如果从"卫、气、营、血"这四个层面上来分析，会非常透彻。"卫"是在人体的最表层，就像保卫一样，我们可以把它比喻成卫兵。"卫"下面才是"气"，"气"后面是"营"。"营"我们可以把它比喻成军营，就是在里边了。"血"是在最里面的。所以当邪气犯了卫分的时候，这是邪气很轻很浅的，犯了气分就深一些，犯了营分就更深一步了，敌人都打到军营里面来了。入了血分，那就更严重了，可能营寨里面满是敌人，敌人都要攻击你的主将的大帐了。

桂枝汤能调和营卫，这对于调和整个人体的气机是非常重要的，所以它是"群方之祖"，很多方剂都是由它演变过来的。

太阳伤风，用桂枝汤

桂枝汤在《伤寒论》中是这样讲的："太阳病，头痛，发热，汗出，恶风，桂枝汤主之。"当风邪侵犯到足太阳膀胱经的时候，足太阳膀胱经是主一身之表，它的主要部分是在人的背上，而背为阳，所以说足太阳膀胱经是主太阳的。

当风寒伤阳的时候，风寒客于表，这时候的"头痛"一般是后脑勺痛。

"发热"，这是正气和邪气在相争。

"汗出"，这是营卫不和，风邪已经进入毛孔，还想继续进去，身体的正气挡住不让它进去，就在毛孔这里僵持着。毛孔就处在一种开的状态，汗就忍不住往外出。

人伤什么就怕什么，因为伤风了，所以会"恶风"。用桂枝汤主之。桂枝汤是调和营卫的，其实是在支持正气来抵抗邪气，给人体的正气一个声援，这样通过鼓动气血把在表的风邪驱逐出去。

调和营卫以治汗证

《伤寒论》又说："病人脏无他病，时发热自汗出而不愈者，此卫气不和也，先其时发汗则愈，宜桂枝汤。"

这可能就不是体表被风邪所伤了，往往是由于其他的原因导致营卫不和。所以"先其时发汗则愈"，就是在自汗之前你给他发一下汗，用桂枝汤调和一下营卫。营卫不和则汗出，营卫一和汗就会出得有规律，就不会自己出来了。所以桂枝汤在很多汗证中经常用到。

桂枝汤的原方

桂枝汤的组成在《伤寒论》的原书里是这样的：

桂枝汤

桂枝三两（去皮），芍药三两，甘草二两，生姜三两，大枣十二枚（擘）。

中国历代的度量衡是不一样的。张仲景时期的一两，与我们现在说的一两，与明清时期的一两，都不一样。张仲景的一两相当于明清时候的两钱，一钱相当于今天的三克，三两相当于六钱，十八克。仲景在方后讲，要"以水七升煮取三升，温时服，每次一升"。这就是说用七升水煮成三升，每次只服一升。喝完了桂枝汤以后要喝一碗热粥，因为热粥能调和和鼓动胃气，加速人体出汗，把风邪透出去，喝完热粥以后再盖上被子休息，等到微微汗出就可以了。因为这时候毛孔容易开，如果不盖上被子，可能又进了风，汗出当风，病还可能加剧。如果不出汗就再喝一升，如果出汗了，后来那两升就不要再喝了，中病即止。

用药治病，都有它的机理和过程。桂枝汤需要这样一个过程：桂枝是促进血液循环的，是发表、发汗、鼓动脾胃之气的；芍药是一味收敛的药，它和桂枝在一块，能够鼓动脾胃之气，能够调和营卫，既走表又守里；再加上姜草枣，这三个药完全是入中焦的，生姜能温能散。它们通过鼓动脾胃的正气，加速人体各方面的循环，从而把邪气驱逐出去。因为要依赖脾胃，所以加姜草枣这三个药。

桂枝汤的主药

我们在面对一个方剂的时候要有一个能力，就是抓住它的主药。桂枝汤的主药就是桂枝和芍药，这两个药有很多学问。

白芍是一味酸收的药，它能够和营敛阴，而且白芍是入肝的；桂枝则是一味辛散的药。这两味药一个酸收一个辛散，正好是相反的，在这一散一收之间，营卫就得到了调和。再加上姜草枣，给脾胃提供了足够的动力能量，有这个基础，营卫就更容易得到调和。

白芍虽然收，但用得好的话它并不敛邪，桂枝和营解肌但它并不伤阴，所以这里用桂枝而不用别的温热药。为什么不用桑枝呢？因为桑枝是平性的，它没有发汗发表的功能。

桂枝性温属阳，白芍寒凉属阴。桂枝和白芍一寒一温、一收一散，一阴一阳，互相制约，就收到了调和营卫气血的作用。而且桂枝呈红色，入心，能振奋心阳；白芍会把桂枝往肝里边引，又能振奋肝阳；桂枝也会把白芍往心里边引，又能收敛心阴、收敛心血。

桂枝配白芍，体现了阴阳的思想，再加姜草枣，又体现了天地人三才的思想。

桂枝往上走，是本乎天的，可以把它当天药；白芍是往下走，是本乎地的，我们可以把它当地药；姜草枣是给脾胃提供动力，提供物质基础的，相当于中间的，是人药。这个方子它体现天地人三才的思想，咱们主要抓天和地，至于人肯定也要兼顾到。

桂枝白芍临床应用举隅

我们知道"汗为心之液"，当心神不定、紧张的时候，人就容易出汗，因为这个时候是你的神镇不住。人的神非常重要，神指挥我们身体的正常运行、正常运转，如果神慌了，于是"六神无主"，人就会出现很多生理上的状况，或者出汗，或者哆嗦。这时就可用桂枝入心安神，安神就能敛汗。很多治疗汗症的方子里面有酸枣仁，也是通过收敛心神，继而把汗给镇住。

桂枝和白芍还经常用来治疗胸痹、胸痛。很多心脏病病人脉跳得特别缓慢，有时候心里就憋闷，遇到一点事心里就慌，心跳加速，感觉到气接不上，可以在辨证论治的基础上加上桂枝和白芍，量可以稍微用大一些。桂枝能够通心，振奋人的血脉，让脉搏跳得快一些，这意味着血液的运行加快了，很多气就会散开，很多瘀也会被冲开，这样人心里就松快。所以我们经常把桂枝白芍还有瓜蒌、薤白一块用，用来治胸痹型的心脏病，效果非常好。很多的心脏病因为肺气不降、心阳不振，全部堵在上面了，于是产生憋闷的感觉，这时都要用到桂枝和白芍。当然脉数也会让人感到憋闷，这时候的治疗就另当别论了。桂枝和白芍治疗心脏病主要是针对脉比较缓的情况。

桂枝和白芍还经常用来治疗腹痛。腹痛常常由于气血不调，而调和营卫在某种意义上讲就是调和气血，尤其是虚寒性的肚子疼，可以用到它们。

桂枝走四肢，白芍跟着桂枝一起，就走四肢；桂枝跟着白芍一起，又可以走五脏，所以这两味药在一起就能通行全身。四肢如果有酸楚、痛麻、伸不直，都可以用到桂枝和白芍。桂枝能够温筋、温阳，得到了阳气的温煦，原本伸不直的四肢，就能伸直了。白芍是酸的，能柔肝养阴，能柔肝就能柔筋，因为"肝主筋"，桂枝把白芍往四肢那一引，白芍的酸味对筋有很好的舒展作用，肢体就能舒展开了，所以治疗很多四肢的病也会经常用到桂枝和白芍。

络脉之病也要用到桂枝和白芍。桂枝能够温通经络，尤其能够通络，我们开方子的时候写的是"嫩桂枝"，一个嫩嫩的桂枝在一颗桂树上也就相当于络脉，所以它走人体的络脉，而且它又能振奋血管，提高血液循环的速度，打通络脉瘀积。

慢性的泄痢，导致脾胃虚寒，这往往也是因为气血失调，营卫不和，治疗中也可考虑用白芍和桂枝。白芍是酸收的，对泻痢有收敛的作用，桂枝有温通的作用，一边收一边温通，收是把正气收住，不让它往下坠，温通就是把邪气通出去，把寒气温煦过来，脏腑功能就能得到调整。桂枝入肝经，跟白芍一起既能入肝，还能入脾，温脾经、振奋脾阳，所以对很多慢性的泻痢有作用。它们跟不同的药配伍，作用也会有差别，有时候可以跟着香连丸一块跑，有时候可以合白头翁汤。

遇到四肢的麻木、酸楚、关节疼痛，我们会把桂枝换成桂枝木，桂枝木就是去皮的桂枝。这里讲的"去皮"跟张仲景讲的去皮是两回事。张仲景讲的去皮是去掉外面的粗皮，现在我们用嫩树枝，就不存在去外面的粗皮了，直接用就行。如果用桂枝木的话，就要把外面的那整个的一层皮全部去掉，用里面的木质。皮的味道很重，里面木质的味道很淡。所以，用桂枝木的话，用量就要大一些，用 20 克左右都可以。当四肢发凉很厉害，用桂枝木不足以温通时，我们还可以加附子，可用制附片，量要小，煎的时间要长一些。因为治四肢就要取轻清外达的属性，量少走四肢，用的量太大了反而走五脏，尤其是走肾。

桂枝汤与方剂的加减之道

咱们以《伤寒论》里桂枝汤来说明方剂的加减之道。比如《伤寒论》里说："太阳病，发汗，逐漏不止，其人恶风，小便难，四肢微急，难以屈伸者，桂枝加附子汤主之"。发汗发过了，一直往外漏汗，止不住。患者依然会恶风，因为这个时候毛孔关不住，依然是营卫不和，所以桂枝汤依然要用。为什么病人小便解不出来呢？一方面是水液从汗毛孔走掉了，另一方面可能还有肾阳虚。因为发汗太过，以至于内伤肾阳，外则大汗亡阳。这时候就要在桂枝汤里加一枚附子来回阳止汗。

《伤寒论》又说："发汗后，烧针令其汗，针处被寒，核起而赤者，必发奔豚，气从少腹上至心，灸其核上各一壮，与桂枝加桂汤主之"。可能在张仲景那个年代，某些医生治病的方法比较野蛮，《伤寒论》里面经常讲"被火"，就是用火来让人发汗。那时人的身体比较壮实，当风寒邪气在体表的时候，烤烤火就发掉了。张仲景并不认为那种方法好。还有用针灸让人发汗，叫"烧针"。把针放在火上烧，再扎进人体，或是把针扎入人体后再对其加热，这也是把热量传入人体，身体好的人通过这样一激，汗就出来了，身体不好的人就会出现"针处被寒"的情况，被针扎的地方又受到寒了，那地方就肿起一个包，体内出现奔豚气。"奔豚气"就是觉得小腹上面有一股气，像小猪似的突突的往上冲。冲到胸部，人特别难受，这时候，要用桂枝加桂汤，就是桂枝汤里面加重桂枝的用量。烧针的地方又受了风寒，还起了包，说明营卫依然不和，桂枝汤依然要用，只不过加重了桂枝的量，桂枝是白芍的两倍。任何一个药只要加重它的量，力量就会往下走。桂枝也是这样的，如果用于走表，少用点，药力反而强。现在有一股气在往上冲，这说明肾气不能固摄，如果肾气能在下面拉得住，那么这个"小猪"似的那团气也不会往上跑。现在因为肾拉不住了，就要加大桂枝的量，桂枝的量一加大，它就跑去温肾啦。当然还有一种说法，说桂枝加桂汤并不是加桂枝，而是加肉桂的。这个说法我是相信的，加点肉桂也会有效，因为肉桂直接就能温肾。当然，桂枝也有降逆镇冲的作用，用桂枝也没错。

《伤寒论》说："太阳病，下之后，脉促胸满者，桂枝去芍药汤主之。"这又是一个救误的方子，可能原来就是用桂枝汤或麻黄汤能解决的问题，遇到庸医了，用了下法，给你一顿大黄芒硝，大便虽然通了，但在表的邪气随之下陷，而且不当下而下之，脾阳必伤，运化势必不利，所以浊气积于胸中，造成胸满。表邪陷入肺中，所以有脉促。芍药是酸苦涌泄的，前面已经泻坏了，现在当然不能再用，何况酸收敛邪，当然不能再用，所以，去掉，就剩下桂枝和姜草枣，辛甘发散为阳，振奋脾阳，鼓舞胃气，逐邪而出。

如果这个人经常喘，那就要在桂枝汤里加上厚朴和杏仁，二者可以降气平喘；有的太阳病，如果误治，也会有点儿喘，也会加厚朴、杏仁。当然，这必须是实喘，如果是肾虚导致的虚喘，又要另当别论了。

在桂枝汤的基础上加饴糖，就成了小建中汤。饴糖很养脾胃，但是现在的人不宜多吃，吃多了不好消化。小建中汤我们现在用得不多，因为毕竟现在人的体质跟当时是有区别的。那时候大家吃的简单，素净，很多人甚至吃不饱饭，肠胃空虚，嗷嗷待哺，用点饴糖，脾胃那叫一个受用啊！现在的人饱食终日，肠胃中浊气、油脂多，再用饴糖，黏黏糊糊，人吃了会不舒服。《伤寒论》里桂枝汤的很多其他的加减法，我们现在都不是太适合，比如说用桂枝汤加附子来止汗回阳，这种情况现在遇到得少。现代人阴虚居多，再用这些大热的药就特别容易上火。我们要知道《伤寒论》是以伤寒为基础的，它的大背景是伤寒，所以仲景以桂枝汤为基础方进行加减。那时候的人，体魄、生活方式跟现在的人不一样，那时候的气候、环境跟现在也不一样，所以有些药，当时的人受得了，现在的人不一定受得了。

我们要知道《伤寒论》是以伤寒为基础的，它的大背景是伤寒，所以仲景以桂枝汤为基础方进行加减。那时候的人，体魄、生活方式跟现在的人不一样，那时候的气候、环境跟现在也不一样，所以有些药，当时的人受得了，现在的人不一定受得了。

在桂枝汤里加上龙骨、牡蛎，就叫龙牡桂枝汤，通常是用来收汗的。龙骨、牡蛎有收敛之性。对于营卫不和的汗证，效果很好。同样的道理，如果是夏天气阴两虚的汗证，我们可以用生脉饮加龙骨、牡蛎；如果是内热的汗证，我们可以把龙骨、牡蛎跟着其他清理热的方子一起用。

桂枝汤的加减非常灵活，虽然我们现在不一定都用得上，但是我们要通过研究它，从中领悟方剂加减的方法，而不能一味地拿方子去跟症状做对应，这是很难对应的。有些人，遇到病就拿《伤寒论》的条文和方子去套，治好一个病就哇哇大叫，说经方太神了，没治好的他就不吭声了。这很不好。验案要讲，没治好的病，更要拿出来分析，这样更有助于提高水平。

我们学中医要尊古。像《伤寒论》这样的古书，它是中医史上的临床经典，奠定中医辨证论治的基础，我们要尊重，但千万不要拘泥于它，更不要是古非今，觉得只有《伤寒论》好，只有张仲景好，我们现代都不行。愚者千虑，必有一得，我们把所有的愚者的这一得全部集中起来，那也是非常了得的。医家要有雅量，胸襟要宽广。你仅仅能容纳张仲景还远远不够。

不可拘泥伤寒古方

宋朝有一本《活人书》，对张仲景的桂枝汤提出过看法，书中说："桂枝汤治西北人，四时行之，无不应验。江淮间惟冬春可行，春末至夏至以前，桂枝汤可加黄芩一分，谓之阳旦汤，夏至后，可加知母半两，石膏一两，或升麻一分。若病人素虚寒者，不必加减。"

到了宋朝，有人就发现桂枝汤就没有那么好用了，所以他在这里提出来一些新的加减法，又说只能治西北人，西北属金，北部属水，都是比较寒凉的地方，像现在的陕甘宁这一带，人们身体素质较强悍，还有大汉遗风。当时桂枝汤只适合西北人，在江淮之间，只有在冬春才可以用桂枝汤。江淮地区也就相当于江苏、安徽、浙江一带，长江中下游，这一带的人要娇弱一些，所以他提出一些加减法，加黄芩减轻桂枝汤的热性。到了夏至以后还要加知母、石膏，这是白虎汤的主药，也是为了清热；或者加升麻，也是一味寒凉药，这都是治本来就有热的病人。当时还没有摸索出银翘散之类的辛凉之剂，就只能在桂枝汤的基础上加一些寒凉药，聊以清热。

《活人书》是宋朝的，成书于1108年，在张仲景后大概八百年。当时的情形就有变化，跟我们现在相差了又快有一千年了，现在又变了，所以《活人书》讲的这些也是在提醒我们要随机应变。桂枝汤之类的方剂，我们在江南依然在用，而且用得很广，但时过境迁，经过历代医家的探索传承，又摸索出了很多治病的方法，我们也不要盲目排斥。

麻黄汤

桂枝还可以配麻黄，这也是张仲景方子里面经常用到的一个药对，典型的方剂就是麻黄汤。

麻黄汤
麻黄、桂枝、杏仁、甘草。

麻黄汤方义

麻黄配桂枝可以温经散寒。麻黄本身就能发汗，和桂枝一起，发汗的力度会更大。平时麻黄走气分发汗，但只能发出一点来。因为"汗为心之液"，发汗是血里发出来的。桂枝正好入心，入血脉。用了桂枝，入了血分，发汗才会多起来。这是麻黄和桂枝配伍的药理。

杏仁是开肺气、利肺气的，它帮助麻黄来宣通肺气，肺气一宣毛孔就开了，所以麻黄配杏仁开利肺气的作用就会更大。

麻黄汤主要是治疗寒邪在表、寒邪闭表。因为"寒主凝"，体表受到寒邪的侵袭，毛孔就闭住了，体内的热就发不出来，人就会非常难受。寒邪在肌肤经络之间，又会出现身痛等一系列症状，所以用麻黄汤来打开毛孔让人体通透起来，同时发一些汗，让寒邪随着汗出来，这就是麻黄汤的作用。

麻杏石甘汤里面有麻黄和杏仁，这主要是取它开肺气的作用。麻黄没有配桂枝，发汗的力度就小了。当然，这是指在仲景的年代发汗的力度就小了。现在，麻黄不配桂枝，发汗的力度照样大，对于南方人尤甚。所以我们得慎用此方。

结合五行，安抚脾土

麻黄汤中用甘草，是为了调和诸药，而且甘能入脾，土生金，所以甘草又有扶土生金的作用。麻黄汤的前三味药开提肺气、发汗，是在对肺进行整治。同时安抚一下脾土，再来调理肺气，也会更容易。这就是根据五行关系经常用的一些手段，治其子则当安抚其母。

我们在治肝的时候也得兼顾到脾，因为肝木是克脾土的，所以在疏肝的时候要安慰一下脾土。因为脾是刚刚受过欺负的，你安抚好了它，它也强硬起来了，肝克不动它，我们再去调教肝，这样也容易把肝调教好。

总之我们在治很多病的时候都要兼顾到脾土。因为脾土在中间，在正中央就跟肝、心、肾、肺都有很密切的关系。我们在整治周围这四个脏的时候，都要兼顾到脾。

思考麻黄，追求平和用药

麻黄发汗的力度是有目共睹的。即使在张仲景那个年代，都有很多误汗的，就是不当用麻黄发汗而用麻黄发汗，就产生了坏证。张仲景的《伤寒论》很大程度上它是一部治坏症之书，是救误之书。足见当时的医学界有很多这样的错误，也足见麻黄汤即使在仲景的年代也都是很厉害的方剂，一旦用错了就会生死反掌，出现庸医杀人。

那怎么去解决这个问题呢？历代医家一直在探索，企图在保证同等疗效的前提下，寻求一种更安全、平和的治疗方式。

到了后来，一方面是因为气候、人的体质变化了，另一方面也是因为历代医家一直在探索更安全、平和、有效的治疗方式，叶天士集诸家之大成，温病派出现了。温病派的方子，比如《时病论》列的那六十法，用药都非常轻灵、平和，不怎么用猛药了。有人嘲笑温病派胆子太小，用的药都是无关紧要的，比如芦根、花粉、豆卷、菊花、桑叶，但它们确实能治病。这就是人们梦寐以求的安全、平和、有效的治疗方式啊！这也正是中国人的做事风格，喜欢四两拨千斤，不跟你硬碰硬。

所以，从伤寒到温病，体现的是继承和发展，也体现了中国文化的追求。我们决不能因为温病派用药用得少，用得平和，就认为没有胆量，没有见识，这是不对的。

麻黄加术汤

麻黄汤再加一味白术，就是有名的麻黄加术汤。《金匮要略》用它治疗湿家烦痛。病人平时身体有湿，再受了外邪，寒邪闭表，身体烦痛，咱们可以在麻黄汤的基础上加一味白术。白术健脾化湿。

白术和麻黄是一组非常好的对药。白术走中焦，主要化里湿，麻黄走表发汗，能化表湿。白术有一定的收敛性，麻黄配白术，发汗的力度就小了；白术配麻黄，化湿的力度也相应加强。这样，湿一面从表走，另一面从里走，就很容易化掉。

我们不仅用这个方来治疗湿家身烦痛，用它还可以治疗很多其他病症，像关节炎、风湿病、皮肤病都可以参照着使用，当然必须灵活变化。

如果是湿象比较明显的实证，麻黄加术汤中的术，就用苍术。苍术化湿的力度大一些，而且还有一定的发汗作用。还可以苍白术同用，苍术化湿健脾，白术健脾化湿，它们一块用，健脾和化湿的作用会相得益彰。

麻黄汤还有很多加减的方法，这里不一一赘述。

Chapter 3   Aiye (Folium Artemisiae Argyi)

Properties of Aiye

Authentic Aiye and Its Harvest Season

Ai (mugwort) is a pure Yang grass, a very important herb, which can drive out coldness. In most areas around China, the grass of Ai can grow, of which the best is produced in Qichun, Hubei province of China.

The shape of Aiye varies from place to place and even from season to season all year round. At the Dragon Boat Festival, the collected Aiye, when spread out, looks like a cluster of flickering flames, which demonstrates its pure Yang Qi. Aiye picked before midday (the period of the day from 11 a.m. to 1 p.m.) on the fifth day of May according to Chinese lunar calendar will be the best for medical herb uses.

The twelve earthly branches are actually matched with the twelve months of a year. According to Chinese lunar calendar, the first month of the lunar year is Yin month, the second is Mao month, the third is Chen month, the fourth is Si month, and the fifth is Wu month. In the Si and Wu months, Yang Qi will be in a most vigorous state; and especially, on the fifth day of May of Chinese lunar year, which is close to the summer solstice, Yang will reach the peak point. So the Dragon Boat Festival is the best time to harvest Aiye. From its growing time, Aiye gains the pure Yang between the sky and earth. If the leaves are harvested by autumn or winter seasons, they would not be good enough in quality since their Yang would have been dissipated by then, that is, the pure Yang grass must be picked at the time when its Yang reaches the peak point.

Raw and Processed Aiye

Aiye smells aromatic, and tastes pungent and bitter.

Aiye is classified into the raw and the processed types. The former refers to the collected Aiye to be dried naturally in the shade, while the latter includes many different types, among which the first is made into Airong (moxa) through repeated kneading and pounding with a pestle; or another type is made by parching it black with vinegar, and even parching into charcoal of Aiye, known as processed Aiye.

The raw Aiye is warm in property while the processed Aiye will become stronger with a hot property. Meanwhile, the raw Aiye is partial to dispersion in nature, and it not only can enter the blood system, but also disperse the wind-cold and pathogenic dampness on the body surface. Once I did an investigation in Qichun, Hubei Province of China, the local people introduced me the advantages of Qi Ai (Chinese mugwort) , one of which is that whenever the local people catch a cold, or get wet in the rain, they just take a bath with the mugwort-boiled water and then would feel relaxed from head to feet. Aiye that the locals are using is of the raw Qi Ai.

Generally, the places along or around waters are heavily damp, so the people living near the waters will easily catch various rheumatic diseases, causing joint deformity or pain. Some patients may get more irritated when suffering from pains. The liver dominates anadesma. When the pathogenic dampness impacts anadesma inwardly from the outside and then goes further inwards, it will disturb the liver, which in turn affects the patient's emotion. Those patients who are suffering from the psychological and physiological pains are advised to grow mugwort, the pure-Yang grass, around their house, which would be beneficial to the health and also improve their living environment while they are given medical treatment. In such a way, the treatment might become more effective.

The processed Aiye is hot in property, and it has the securing and holding functions. Aiye itself is pungent, aromatic, dispersing and spurting in nature, but after it is pounded with a pestle into Airong that in fact is the leaf vein, it will be quite similar to the collaterals of human being. So, one can make the leaf vein go into the collaterals, even to the particularly fine meridians where the hot efficacy of Airong will be able to secure and remain there longer. Actually, it is still going in further even into the fine meridians but only slowing down inside because of the fine channels of the meridians. The positive side is that the more slowly it goes in, the longer it will definitely stay there.

The effect of the processed Aiye can be secured in the Lower Jiao. Fire always flames upward. When heat energy stays in the Lower Jiao, it can warm up the kidney Yang, and then the whole body. The processed Aiye is good at securing and holding, but also good at dispersing. It can enter the collaterals, different viscera, and go through anadesma into bones at the deepest points of human bodies, where the pathogenic factors are easy to hide inside, and the medical effect is not easy to get there. When medicines fail to target the diseases, the cure would be ineffective. The processed Aiye can permeate into the deepest points of human body to disperse the pathogens, especially, the cold dampness out of the deepest points. Permeating inside first and then dispersing the pathogens out are of the functions that the processed Aiye particularly has, but Fuzi and Rougui don't, so moxibustion can help cure a lot of diseases when it is used for warming and activating meridians and collaterals.

Moxibustion

Warm Property and Permeability of Qi Ai

Qi Ai is particularly strong in its effects for warming, permeating and dispersing pathogens. The effect of Qi Ai can also go downwards, while the effect of the other mugwort easily goes upwards. The so-called "fire flaming up" is referring to the natural fire. But the fire of Taiyang in TCM goes downwards, which is like the sunlight shining down from the sky. In human bodies, there exists fire that goes up, and also fire that goes down. The kidney fire always goes up while the heart fire goes down. So, if one wants to warm the kidney Yang, he has to guide the fire to go downwards. After the kidney-Yang is warmed up, make the kidney-fire go upwards. As such, the kidney Yang can be then really mobilized. However, if one uses the upgoing fire, the floating energy might be easily formed, and then it goes up to become a pathogenic fire. Such a fire is not the so-called slight fire that one normally needs to warm up the whole body to generate Qi.

Qi Ai enjoys a stronger permeability, and it even has the "power to permeate ceramic jar". One may fill a ceramic jar with liquor, and then grill the ceramic jar with Qi Ai, after which the liquor inside will taste the smell of Qi Ai. However, if the ceramic jar is grilled with some other types of mugwort, the liquor inside will not taste the smell of the mugwort at all, indicating that only Qi Ai is able to permeate the ceramic jar to transmit the fragrance and medical effect of mugwort to the liquor in it and the other types of mugwort won't have such a strong permeability. Furthermore, regarding "dispersion and permeability", only Qi Ai is able to permeate into meridians and collaterals and the five internal organs. For the other types of mugwort, it would be quite hard or even impossible.

Besides, as to the quality of mugwort, the more timeworn the mugwort is stored on shelf, the better it will be. Generally speaking, just over one year on shelf will be quite enough, and its heat power would be warm and gentle for generating Qi.

Requirements for Moxibustion

Some requirements regarding moxibustion should be followed. The first thing to do is to choose Qi Ai; and the second is to use the timeworn mugwort which has been on the shelf for over at least one year; and the last is to use the pestled Airong. Most of Airong sticks presently used, in fact, are not quite up to the standard since some of them do not contain Qi Ai but the other type of mugwort, and also the so-called "Airong" used is not the fiber of mugwort but the pestled whole stem of mugwort. Therefore, it has quite limited effect of permeating meridians and collaterals. In addition, some Airong sticks possibly contain no timeworn mugwort but newly produced mugwort. Failure to meet the above-mentioned three requirements may not bring about the effect as expected.

Moxibustion stresses on particular requirements besides what have been mentioned above. Proper moxibustion can bring the dying back to life. Even the representative of Yin nourishing school, the medical expert Zhu Danxi, one of the four medical scientists in the Jin and Yuan dynasties, had once used moxibustion at Shenque acupoint to cure the stroke prostration, which was a very serious case. Those patients who suffer from the stroke prostration will have enuresis unconsciously with eyes upturned. They will be dying, and will be very difficult to bring back to life. However, Zhu Danxi had rescued such a patient by means of moxibustion at Guanyuan acupoint according to the historical record.

Moxibustion, if abused, or improperly used, is bound to cause impairment to the life essence and blood. After all, moxibustion is in the use of fire, and fire can cause impairment of Yin. In **Shanghan Lun**, there are many bad cases resulted from the use of fire treatment. It was relatively colder in the era when Zhang Zhongjing was living than today, so the primary syndromes in that era were of cold pathogens. Under that circumstance, many patients who suffered from cold pathogens would be treated with the methods of fire, such as warming by a fire, burning needles, and moxibustion. These methods sometimes are effective, but sometimes they may cause bad consequences to the patients. In Zhang Zhongjing's era, such a thing could take place, how much more so now! People in modern times are somewhat weaker than those in the past, so moxibustion should be used with much caution. Of course, the hurt of improper moxibustion may last a quite long time with the bad consequences exposed bit by bit rather than just one or two days. In fact, many people are not conscious of the consequences of improper moxibustion when they have some sufferings.

Never Abusing Moxibustion at Guanyuan Acupoint

There are many stories regarding the capacity of moxibustion at Guanyuan acupoint to maintain health and longevity. Doucai, a doctor in the Song Dynasty wrote a book named "Bianque Xinshu" (Bianque Heart Book), having stressed the effects of moxibustion at Guanyuan acupoint on physical health of human body through a very legendary story. The story went like this: a soldier called Wang Chao in the Song Dynasty became a robber after retiring from military service, and later he met a miraculous person who passed to him a way of "Huangbai Zhushi" ("Yellow and White Way of Longevity", which is a way of keeping longevity by moxibustion at Guanyuan acupoint with a thousand moxa sticks in sequence at the turn of the summer and fall). By the age of ninety, he was still in fine fettle looking like a young man, physically well-developed and with perfect skin. He did evil things as a robber in the area of Yueyang city, Hunan province of China, and even committed a dozen rapes a day without feeling exhausted. Later, he was caught. Just before execution, the official at the execution asked him whether he had any invulnerability or exceptional function. He then disclosed his way, that is, moxibustion at Guanyuan acupoint with a thousand moxa sticks in sequence at the turn of the summer and fall. As time passed by, he could tolerate the cold and heat, and did not feel hungry for a couple days even without eating anything. He always felt fire-warm at the spot just below his navel, which attributes to the power of fire. Fire can bake the earth into bricks and wood into charcoal. The human body also needs such firepower. After Wang Chao was executed, the official at the execution ordered the soldiers to cut open his abdomen at the so-called warm spot. A stuff like a stone as silver white as jade was exposed, which was formed under the influence of moxibustion.

It seems effective according to this story, but it also hints lots of mishaps. If one does not make careful distinguishment and just follows it blindly like a sheep, it may delay cure of some diseases. First of all, one cannot take the ability of more sex as a sign of health. In fact, it is a pathological condition. According to TCM, this is called "Xianghuo Disturbance" ("Xianghuo" means "Ministerial Fire" that refers to the life-gate fire. It is corresponding to "Monarch fire", which refers to the heart fire) due to the kidney's failure to astringe the vital life essence. A ninety-year-old man, who did not stay at home in peace to enjoy his old age, had done evil things outside. That was undoubtedly disturbed by some diseases. Nothing could guarantee the effectiveness of his sperm if he really did a dozen rapes every day. I dare say all his sperms were dead and inferior ones. Even if Wang Chao's health and longevity was benefited from moxibustion at Guanyuan acupoint, yet his sexual capacity and fertility did not necessarily prove the real conditions of his health. In clinical practice, it can also be seen that many patients who suffer infertility, but in fact, they are very robust physically. Sometimes I feel that their health is maintained at the cost of their fertility. In the above story, it only tells us about Wang Chao's health and longevity but said nothing about his ability to give birth to and raising children. If he had children, he might not go to such an extreme to rape women over and again. Guanyuan acupoint is at the point three *Cun* below navel, and another point just besides is called Shimen acupoint.

If a woman were often to have moxibustion at this point, she might lose fertility to have children. The book of **A-B Classic of Acupuncture and Moxibustion** says women should not have the treatment of moxibustion at Shimen acupoint, which is also mentioned in the classics like **Medical Secrets from the**

Royal Library, **Qianjin** *Fang* (*Thousand Golden Prescriptions*), and **Compendium of Acupuncture and Moxibustion**. Therefore, those who want to preserve health or to cure infertility through moxibustion at Guanyuan acupoint must take it with caution. Once Shimen acupoint is affected, it may result in a complete failure of treatment of infertility.

Also, what Wang Chao said that the fire could turn the earth and wood into imperishable bricks and charcoal respectively. He hardly realized that the earth is better than bricks, and wood is better than charcoal, since the earth is alive with vitality to grow crops that are not able to grow out of bricks in that bricks are lifeless earth. Charcoal can be imperishable for thousands of years, but it is perishable wood, while the living wood has vitality. So, when a patient recovers his/her vitality, what will happen then? The so-called "Huangbai Zhushi" ("Yellow and White Way of Longevity") is nothing of the right way but a witchcraft. There are so many tricks and witchcraft in this world, which sometimes may achieve some effects, but it is deceptive and harmful. Moxibustion at Guanyuan or even all the other acupoints, if needed, must be done by the professional acupuncturists with great care.

Other External Applications of Aiye

Aiye has the effects of permeating inside and extending to the body surface, so, Aiye can search out pathogens at the deepest points in human body and then disperse them out through skin surface. The effects of Aiye can go through the whole body, especially into the liver, spleen and kidney meridians. The foot-Jueyin liver meridian, foot-Taiyin spleen meridian and the foot-Shaoyin kidney meridian all pass through the feet, so one can frequently have a footbath with Aiye-soaked water since feet are of the lowest parts, which are much easily contaminated. When the lower parts of the body are warmed up, the warmth will be transmitted to the upper parts. Warming up feet is equivalent to warming up the whole body. As it is always said that feet want keeping warm and head wants keeping cool. It does not mean to wash hair with Aiye-soaked water, but to wash feet with Aiye soaked water. It is advisable to use the clear and floating material like mulberry leaf or chrysanthemum water to wash hair, after which one will feel refreshed. For footbath, it is advisable to use the warm stuff, after which one will feel warm all over. Of course, if Honghua (safflower carthamus) is used together with Aiye, it can also promote circulation of blood; or Changpu (acorus calamus) can be added too, which can help induce refreshment. As such, the whole body will be regulated and nursed.

Aiyecan be put into a cloth sack to make a bellyband and wear it. Generally, the elderly people who suffer from stomach cold or ladies who suffer from cold coagulation and painful menstruation may wear such a bellyband around the navel or at the gate of vitality (the life gate) on the waist to alleviate syndromes of stomach cold and dysmenorrhea.

Airong can be put in socks for warming up feet and treating beriberi.

Of course, these methods are helpful to some extent. However, if the beriberi or dysmenorrhea is resulted from some more complex factors, the above method probably can only relieve the symptoms but not give a cure once and for all. The radical cure usually has to be done with medication based on syndrome differentiation.

Oral Administration Formulas containing Aiye

Aiye can be taken orally. For oral administration, it is often stir-fried with vinegar called fried Aiye or vinegared Aiye. In addition, Aiye may also be processed into charcoal, which is called Aiye Tan (folium artemisiae argyi charcoal).

There are two classic formulas for oral administration of Aiye. One is **Aifu Nuangong Pill**, and the other is **Jiaoai Siwu Tang**.

Aifu Nuangong Pill

This formula contains the ingredient herbs: Aiye Tan (Aiye charcoal), Zhi Xiangfu (processed rhizoma cyperi), Pao Wuyu (soaked fructus evodiae), Rougui (cassia bark), Danggui (angelica sinensis), Chuanxiong (Ligusticum wallichii), Jiu Baishao (liquored paeonia lactiflora), Dihuang (rehmannia), Zhi Huangqi (roasted radix astragali), Xuduan (radix dipsaci)

Aiye Tan is slightly mild, warm and clear in properties, and it has the efficacy of hemostasis. Xiangfu (rhizoma cyperi) is an herb for regulating Qi. Xiangfu and Aiye are frequently used as a medicine pair, which can permeate into collaterals and regulate Qi. In this formula, they play the function of warming the uterus. Wuyu and Rougui are hot medicines, used for warming up the liver and kidneys (it is inadvisable to use them in a large dosage). If Aiye and Xiangfu are supposed for merely temporary solution, Wuyu and Rougui can play the function of permanent cure. The symptom here shows the cold pathogen while the root of the problem is in the liver and kidneys. Xiangfu is for regulating Qi. In case the liver Qi is not smoothened, it will cause the imbalance of coldness and the heat. Only when the liver Qi is well regulated, will the coldness and heat become balanced naturally.

Danggui (angelica sinensis), Chuanxiong (ligusticum wallichii), Baishao (paeonia lactiflora), Dihuang (rehmannia) are the ingredient herbs of **Siwu Tang**, used for nourishing blood. Women take blood as the principal thing, so nourishing blood is very important for women while warm nourishing is adopted. If only warming up is done to activate meridians without nourishing the blood, the warm and dry medicines will cause disorder of blood.

Consideration must be given to regulating Qi while nourishing blood is being carried out. In addition, Qi will have to be slightly tonified while it is being regulated. For this reason, Zhi Huangqi must be used. To tonify Qi, the medical effects must be guided into the Middle Jiao, since the spleen is the "source of Qi and blood generation and transformation". Therefore, tonification of Qi will help promote Qi and blood generation and transformation. Huangqi and Danggui in this formula are the ingredient herbs of **Danggui Buxue Tang**, which is useful for enriching blood through tonifying Qi. And meanwhile, enriching blood in turn will also help to tonify Qi.

Xuduan is a very mild medicine. It is used in this formula for warming the liver and kidneys. It can also be used for miscarriage prevention. In case there are symptoms of fetus abortion or threatened abortion, Xuduan can be used as a remedy to prevent miscarriage. Xuduan has a good effect on bones and muscles, too. If there are fractures on the bones, Xuduan can be helpful for setting bones.

Aifu Nuangong Pill regulates Qi and blood circulation, warms the womb and regulates the menstrual function. Generally, it is used for treatment of menstruation delay or dysmenorrhea or even infertility due to deficiency coldness of uterus. When in dysmenorrhea, the patient may feel cold, and will desire to apply the warm band, which is also a reminder of the deficiency-coldness of uterus.

Jiaoai Siwu Tang

Jiaoai Siwu Tang is also a formula frequently used in gynecology department. In fact, there are many versions of it, and here the typical version is chosen for analyses.

Jiaoai Siwu Tang contains the following ingredient herbs:

E-jiao (donkey-hide gelatin), Cuchao Aiye (vinegar parched folium artemisiae argyi), Danggui (angelica sinensis), Chuanxiong (ligusticum wallichii), Baishao (paeonia lactiflora), Shudi (prepared rehmannia root), Puhuang (cattail pollen), Huanglian (coptis chinensis), Huangqin (scutellaria baicalensis), Shengdi (radix rehmanniae recen), Zhizi (fructus gardeniae), Diyu (sanguisorba officinalis), Baizhu (rhizoma stractylodis macrocephalae), Gancao (liquorice).

E-jiao and Aiye are a commonly used medicine pair. The former one is a Yin medicine for nourishing blood, while the latter one is a Yang medicine for Wentong (warming through meridians). The Yin and Yang medicines used together can warm blood, in the process of which it is necessary to nourish blood at the same time, so **Siwu Tang** is used in this formula.

There are a variety of modifications of **Siwu Tang** like additions of Danpi (cortex moutan radicis), Zhizi, and Shengdi for cooling blood; additions of E-jiao, Aiye for warming blood; additions of Taoren (peach kernel), Honghua for dispersing blood stasis; additions of Jingjie (schizonepeta) and Fangfeng (radix sileris) for dispelling pathogenic wind in blood.

With a special intention, a more complex version of **Jiaoai Siwu Tang** is chosen since this formula incorporates a lot of ideas. Cuchao Aiye matched with E-jiao can go into the liver to warm blood. In case blood has been cold for a long time, it may have blood heat included. Blood actually is very complex. One should not think that cold blood is just a cold, for the patient may suffer from heat syndromes in the other parts of the body. Or even if there are no heat symptoms for the time being, it may flash out right after one starts to warm up. This is no cause for concern. Huanglian, Huangqin, Shengdi, and Zhiziare used for clearing heat and cooling blood while the blood is warmed. In such a way, the medicine will be balanced, i. e. , while the warm and hot medicines are being used for warming, the cold and cool medicines are also added as corrigent, hence, the pathogenic heat will not arise.

This formula can also prevent miscarriage, in which Huangqin and Baizhu are the key medicines for miscarriage prevention. Whenever the fetal heat arises, Huangqin will be necessary. Baizhu is for tonifying the spleen, which is in charge of uplifting. So, to tonify the spleen will support the fetus. Diyu is used for clearing the large intestine heat, which is helpful for guiding the heat to go downwards. While a woman is pregnant, the prenatal mother and child hold together, which is particularly prone to generating heat. However, in such a case, the heat cannot be cleared with the severely cold medicine but in a way of purging the hollow viscera to eliminate the heat. For this purpose, a medicine like Diyu is often used. Those medicines for clearing the heat of the large intestine can also clear the lung heat since the lung and the large intestine are located up and down respectively inside the body, but they are linked and interacted mutually, playing the exterior and interior functions mutually. While they are in a clear and unobstructed state, a lot of pathogenic heat can be guided out of the body. Analogously, like chimney or sewer, where the chimneys and sewers are unobstructed, there won't be too much waste accumulated inside.

Of course, this formula may need further modifying (addition or subtraction) in clinical practice. For the treatment of hemorrhage of potential miscarriage, Puhuang Tan should be used instead, and the proportion of the warm medicines and the cool medicines in this formula must be adjusted accordingly in line with the specific symptoms of coldness and heat in the body. In the case of unobvious symptoms of heat, it is not necessary to use too many cold and cool medicines; Huanglian and Zhizi may even be taken out of the formula. In case the patient is relatively weak of Qi and blood, and is not able to withstand medical efficacy diffusion, remove Chuanxiong formula or just use a small dosage of it. Especially, for miscarriage prevention, Chuanxiong must be used with special caution.

Balance of Clinical Prescriptions

Jiaoai Siwu Tang also embodies the concurrent use of cold and heat medicines. Aiye is hot in property, while Huangqin, Huanglian, Shengdi, and Zhizi are cool in property. So, in writing a prescription in clinical practice, it is required to keep a balance of herbal uses, i. e. , to use the cold and hot medicines concurrently. As to the formulas for teaching purpose in classroom, different academic schools may take the hot medicines or cold and cool medicines respectively according to their different academic concepts, but the clinical prescriptions are often particular about medical balance, and will have to give consideration to many factors, that is to say, some differences do exist between the teaching and the clinical practice.

Diseases in fact also have their unique balance. Theoretically, a person in illness means he/she is suffering from a loss of balance. After all, the patient is not dead, but ill, which means there does exist certain temporary balance out of imbalance. Similarly, prescriptions not only have to remedy defects and rectify errors, but also keep a relative equilibrium, for which the cold and hot medicines are often used concurrently in prescriptions.

Besides, somepatients have heat in the upper part and coldness in the lower part while some others have endogenous heat and exogenous cold instead of mere coldness or heat. So, cold medicines should be used for diseases of heat, and hot medicines for diseases of coldness in the process of medication. Only in such a way can the balance be maintained inside of human body in order to promote the physiological functions to defeat the disease, which again involves the channel tropism of medical efficacies.

A medicine like Aiye can pass through and warm up the whole body. It is an excellent medicine for regulating coldness and heat in the human body, but it is hot in nature. It is often used together with the cold medicines for balance, but also help to direct the cold medicines into the parts where they should go.

第三章　艾叶

艾叶性能

地道的艾叶及其采收的季节

艾是纯阳之草，能驱逐寒气，是非常重要的一味药。全国大部分地区均产艾，以湖北蕲春的最好。

艾叶的形状，各地不同，一年四季也会发生变化。端午节时，将采来的蕲艾叶摊平，形状就像一簇蹿动的火苗，这意味着它的纯阳之气。五月初五端午节当天的午时之前采摘的艾叶是最好的。

十二地支跟十二个月是相配的，正月是寅月，二月是卯月，三月是辰月，四月是巳月，五月是午月，巳和午是阳气最旺的时候，尤其到了五月初五，接近夏至，阳气达到最高峰。所以端午节这天是艾叶采收的最佳时候。从艾叶生长的时间看，它得到的是天地之间的纯阳之气，你到了秋冬季节再去采，就不好了，它的阳气已经发泄掉了。纯阳之草必须在阳气达到顶点的时候去采摘。

生艾与熟艾

艾叶之气味，辛辣芳香而苦。

它有生熟之分：生艾叶就是把艾叶采来让它自然阴干；熟艾则有很多种，第一种是经过反复揉、捣，做成艾绒，还有就是用醋把它炒黑了，甚至炒成炭，也叫熟艾。

生艾叶是温性的，熟艾叶热性就更强了。生艾叶的性质偏散，能入血分，又能散体表的风寒湿邪。我在蕲春考察的时候，听蕲春人讲蕲艾的好处，其中之一就是，他们当地的人感冒了，或者说外出淋雨了，回来就用蕲艾煮水洗澡，洗完浑身轻松。他们用的就是生蕲艾。

水边湿气重，临水而居的人，容易得各种风湿病，湿流关节则关节变形、疼痛，有人甚至越疼心里越烦燥易怒，因为肝主筋，湿邪由外而内影响筋，又进一步深入，影响肝，影响情绪。心理和生理都很痛苦。对这样的患者，我往往建议他们在自己家周围多种艾草，虽然不是蕲春的艾，但依然是纯阳之草，对身体还是有很多好处的。在药物治疗的同时，改善一下生活环境，用药的效果就会更好。

熟艾叶性热，能守。为什么能守呢？艾叶是辛香发散、走蹿的。被捣成艾绒后，艾绒其实是艾叶的叶脉，它跟人体的络脉非常相似，以络入络，它能入特别细的络脉，艾的热性进入最细的络后，留得必然长久，所以说它能守，其实它本身还是在走的，只不过因为络脉比较狭窄，它在里面走得慢，所以留得长久。

熟艾还能守在下焦。火性炎上，当热量在下焦时，能够温肾阳，温煦整个人体。熟艾善守，也善透。它能入络、入脏、通筋、入骨，这些都是人体最深的地方，它有几个特点：一是邪气很容易躲在那里；第二是药力不容易进入。药和病不对称，疗效就差。熟艾能够透到人体最深处，把这些躲得很深的邪，尤其是寒湿之邪，透出来。先透进去再透出来，这是艾叶独有的一个作用，附子、肉桂都没有这个作用。所以，用艾灸来温通经络，常令百病回春。

艾灸

蕲艾的温煦和通透

蕲艾温煦和透邪的作用尤其强。

蕲艾的火力更能往下走，其他艾的火力则容易往上走。火性炎上，这是自然之火。但太阳之火则是往下走的，就像太阳光从天上往下照耀。人体有往上走的火，也有往下走的火。肾火往上走，心火往下走。我们想温煦肾阳，先要让火往下走。温了肾阳，再让肾火往上走。这样肾阳才能被真正调动起来。你如果用往上走的火，就容易构成一种升浮之气，火直接走上去成邪火了。这就不是能成为温煦全身的那种和缓的"少火生气"的火。

蕲艾通透的作用也要强一些。它有"透瓷之功"。用陶瓷罐子装的一罐酒，再用艾来灸罐子外表，如果用其他的艾来灸，罐里的酒依然是酒，不会有艾的味道。如果用蕲艾来灸，再打开罐子尝尝，会发现酒有艾味了。只有蕲艾能够透过陶瓷，把艾的芳香和温度传递给其中的酒，其他的艾没有这种强大的通透力。我们前面讲到的"散透"，能够透进筋骨，络脉，五脏，只有蕲艾有这个作用，其他的艾就很难说了。

还有一点，艾是陈久的比较好，一般来说，放一年以上就可以了，火力就会更加温和，火力温和才能"少火生气"。

艾灸的要求

所以艾灸是有一定要求的。首先必须是蕲艾，其次必须是储存了一年以上的陈艾，第三必须是捣碎的艾绒。现在我们用的艾条，其实都是不合格：它用的艾不一定是蕲艾，其中所谓的"艾绒"，其实并非艾绒，而是将整棵的艾全部打碎来用，透络的作用很小；还有，它可能不是陈艾。同时不符合这三个要求，我们就不要指望这个艾灸能有多大作用。

艾灸的讲究非常多，不仅是上述的这些。艾灸用得好，可以起死回生。就连滋阴派的代表人物、金元四大家之一的朱丹溪，都曾经通过艾灸神阙，救治中风脱证。中风脱证是很危险的，撒手遗尿，两眼上翻，即将死亡，很难挽回，朱丹溪通过灸关元，把人给救过来了。

艾灸如果滥用，或者用得不对的话，就必然要伤精伤血，毕竟艾灸是在用火，火能伤阴，《伤寒论》中就有很多用火治疗造成的坏证。张仲景那个年代比现在冷，是以寒邪为主，很多人受了寒邪之后就要用火法去治，比如烤火、烧针、艾灸。这些方法有时有效，有时反而把病人治坏了。在张仲景的年代都能把人治坏，何况现在呢？现在我们的身体比过去的人要柔弱一些，所以即使用艾灸都要非常谨慎，害人不是一天两天的，它可能慢慢地出问题，很多人出了问题，还不知道是怎么引起的。

灸关元不可滥行

关于艾灸关元能养生、长寿，有很多这样的说法。宋朝窦材有一本《扁鹊心书》，通过一个很传奇的故事，强调灸关元对人的身体作用之大：宋朝有个叫王超的军人，退伍后做了强盗，后来遇到奇人，传给他一个黄白住世之法。他到了九十岁的时候，依然像年轻人一样神采奕奕，身体丰腴润泽。他在岳阳一带为非作歹，做了江洋大盗，一天强奸十几个女人还不觉得累。后来他被抓住了，在临刑之前，监斩官就问他是不是有什么特异功能。他就把他的那个方法说出来了，说每到夏秋之交，就在关元上艾灸一千炷，久而久之就不畏寒暑，好几天不吃饭也不饿。到现在，他肚脐下边还有一块地方像火一样暖和，就是因为火的力量。火能使土变成砖，能让木变成炭。人体也需要这样的火力。王超死后，监斩官命人剖开他腹部温暖的地方，看到一个像石头一样银白如玉的东西，这就是用艾灸出来的。

这个故事非常好听，但其中有非常多的问题，我们如果不仔细辨别就盲从，就要误人的健康了。首先，咱们不能把性生活次数多看做是健康的一种表现。其实它是一种病态，用中医的话讲是"相火大动"，是因为肾不能固摄精气。一个九十岁的老人，不在家里安享晚年，还出来为非作歹，这明明是被病催的。他每天强奸十多个女子，谁能保证他精液的有效性呢。我敢说全是死精、败精。即使王超的健康长寿是得益于灸关元，但是健康跟生育也要区别来看，性能力和生育能力也不能等同于健康。在临床上，我们也可以看到，很多不能生育的人，其实身体都非常强壮。有时候我会感觉他们的健康就是以牺牲生育能力为代价带来的。这个故事里边只讲了王超健康长寿，也并没有讲他生儿育女，如果他有儿有女，他干嘛还出来做这种事？关元在脐下三寸这个地方，边上还有一个穴叫石门。如果女子经常无故灸这个地方就可能绝育。《针灸甲乙经》就讲：女子不能灸石门穴。《外台秘要》《千金方》《针灸大成》都这样讲。所以，有人他想通过灸关元来养生，或者来治不孕不育，一定要慎重。你一不小心灸到石门上去了，不但不能治，反而让你这个病永远治不了了。

还有，王超讲的，把土变成砖，把木头变成炭，就可以不朽，殊不知，土比砖要好，木比炭要好。因为土是活的，有生生之气，能长庄稼，砖上面是长不了庄稼的，砖是死了的土。炭虽然千年不朽，但它是死了的木头，活木头有生机多好啊。人得到火力会成什么样子，这很难说。所以说，这黄白住世之法，并不是一个正法，只不过是邪术而已。这个世界上邪术非常多，当然它也能达到某些效果，但它终究是诡道，是伤人的。所以说我们灸关元一定要小心，包括其他所有穴位的艾灸，在用的时候要非常的注意。你得懂才能用。

艾叶的其他外用方式

艾能够透里又能达表，能把人体最深处的邪气搜出来，然后再从体表散出去。艾叶能通行全身，尤其入肝、脾、肾这三经。足厥阴肝经，足太阴脾经，足少阴肾经都是经过脚的，所以，我们经常用艾叶来泡水洗脚，因为脚是人体地位最低的地方，而且也是最容易藏污纳垢的地方。把地位最低的地方温一下，就能够一直温到上面，温了脚也就等于温了全身。足宜常温，头宜常凉，我们没有说用艾叶来洗头，只能用艾叶来洗脚。洗头得用桑叶、菊花之类清轻上浮的东西，会洗得神清气爽。洗脚就要用温暖的东西，洗完了就浑身温暖。如果配上红花还能和血，配上菖蒲还能开窍，这样从下而上地调理人体。

艾叶还可以做肚兜，把它兜在一个布袋子里面，然后贴在身上。一般，老人胃寒或者女子瘀寒痛经，都可以做一个这样的肚兜，放在肚脐那儿，也可以放在腰上命门位置，对女子的痛经有缓解的作用。

艾绒还可以放到袜子里，用来温足、治疗脚气。

当然这些方法都是在某种程度上有用，如果脚气或者痛经的原因比较复杂，这个方法就只能有缓解的作用，而不能有彻底的治愈了，要彻底的治愈，还得辨证用药。

含有艾叶的内服方

艾叶还可以内服。内服的艾叶经常用醋来炒，叫炒艾叶或醋艾叶，还有把艾叶制成炭，叫艾叶炭。

艾叶内服，有两个很经典的方子。一个叫艾附暖宫丸，一个叫胶艾四物汤。

艾附暖宫丸

艾叶炭、制香附，泡吴萸、肉桂，当归、川芎、酒白芍、地黄、炙黄芪、续断。

艾叶炒炭后，性质就会稍微平和一些，温中有清，且有止血之用。香附是一味理气的药，跟着艾叶一起就能透络而理气，这是很常用的一个药对，在此温通胞宫。吴萸和肉桂都是大热之药，用于温肝肾，用量不宜大。如果说艾叶和香附是用来治标的，那么吴萸和肉桂就是用来治本的，标是胞宫有寒，本则在肝肾。何况香附是理肝气的药。肝气不顺，就会造成寒热不均，把气调通了，寒热自然就均匀了。

当归、川芎、白芍、地黄，这是四物汤，用来养血的。女子以血为主，在温养女子的时候要注意养血。若是光温通而不养血，那么这些温燥的药就会伤血。

治血必兼治气，理气必略补气，所以要用炙黄芪。补气，且入中焦，脾为"气血生化之源"，能促进气血生化。黄芪和当归叫当归补血汤，它通过益气来补血，在补血的同时益气。

后面，续断是一味很平和的药，用来温肝肾。它可以安胎，胎要掉了，或漏胎了，可以用它补救挽回。续断对筋骨也有很好的作用，筋骨折了、断了可以给你续上。月经断了，它也能给你续上。

艾附暖宫丸理气调血，暖宫调经。一般用于因胞宫虚寒引起的月经推后，痛经乃至不孕不育。在痛经的时候，身上感觉到冷，喜欢用热的东西敷，这也提示是胞宫虚寒。

胶艾四物汤

胶艾四物汤，也是妇科经常用到的方剂。它有很多版本，我们用的是比较有代表性的。

胶艾四物汤

阿胶　醋炒艾叶，当归　川芎　白芍　熟地，蒲黄　黄连　黄芩　生地　栀子　地榆　白术　甘草

阿胶和艾叶是常用的一对药。阿胶补血，是阴药；艾叶温通，是阳药。一阴一阳，能够温煦血液。温煦的同时需要养血，所以带上四物汤。

四物汤的加减非常丰富：凉血，加丹皮、栀子、生地；温血，加阿胶、艾叶；化瘀，加桃仁、红花；祛血中之风，加荆芥、防风。

我特意选了一个复杂一点的版本的胶艾四物汤，因为其中是有很多思想的。醋炒的艾叶配阿胶，入肝温血。血寒久了，又会夹杂着血热。血是非常复杂的，不要以为血寒就是寒，可能这个人身体的其他部位又有热象。或者没有热象，但你一温，热象马上就出来了。这时候该怎么办？咱们后面紧跟着黄连、黄芩、生地、栀子，在温血的同时再跟进去很多清热凉血的药，它们就扯平了。血得到了温煦，温热药又得到了寒凉的药作为反佐，不会产生邪热。

这个方子还有安胎的作用，其中黄芩、白术，是安胎的主药。胎热时黄芩是必用的。白术健脾，因为脾是主升提的，健脾就能固胎。地榆是清大肠热的，有利于导热下行。人在怀孕期间，母子交抱，两个人在一起，特别容易产生热。不能用大寒的药去清它，往往通过通腑泄热，像地榆这样的药会经常用到。清大肠的热就能清肺热，大肠和肺一个在上一个在下，它们互为表里，是相通的。当它们是通畅状态的时候，很多邪热都能导出。相当于烟囱和下水道，一个地方烟囱和下水道都是通的，里面就基

本上不会有太多垃圾堆积了。

　　当然，这个方子在用的时候还是得进行加减。如果治疗怀孕期间漏胎出血症，那么蒲黄就用蒲黄炭。还要根据具体寒热来调节方子温药和凉药的比例。若热象并不太明显，寒凉药就不必用那么多，黄连、栀子可以去掉。如果这个人气血比较弱，不耐走窜，川芎可以去掉，或者尽量少用。尤其是安胎，更要慎用川芎。

临床方平衡问题

　　胶艾四物汤还体现了寒热并用。艾叶是热的，黄芩、黄连、生地、栀子、地榆都是凉的。临床上开一个方子，要达成一种平衡，我们经常要寒热并用。用来作为教学的方子，可以一派热药，或一派寒凉药，但是临床的方子往往要讲究平衡，多方兼顾。所以说，从教学的方子到临床的方子，还是有一定距离的。

　　病，也有其独特的平衡。一个人病了，理论上说，是不平衡了，但实际上，这个人毕竟还没有病死，所以在不平衡之中又有某种暂时的平衡。方子也是这样的，它要补偏救弊，又要相对平衡，所以往往要寒热并用来达成这种状态。

　　何况，有人是上热下寒，有人是里热外寒，不是纯粹的一个寒或热。所以我们用药要把寒药用在有热的地方，把热药用在有寒的地方。这样去平衡人体，调动生理的功能，来战胜疾病。这就又涉及药物的归经等问题。

　　像艾叶这样的药，能通行全身，温煦全身。是一个调节人体寒热特别好的药。它本身是一个热药，但经常跟寒药一块用，它也能把寒凉的药带到它该去的地方。

Chapter 4　Rougui (Cassia Bark)

Rougui and Its Function of Warming the Kidneys

The Top Quality Rougui

Rougui is a very commonly used medicine. It is the bark of the cinnamon tree. The bark on the trunk close to the ground earth is considered to be the first-grade Rougui. Of course, the peel on the larger branches is also useful, but it is not so medically effective.

The cinnamon tree growing in Vietnam is called Thanh Hoa Gui, and the one that grows in Guangxi, China, is called Anbian Gui. This tree has a definitive puce color. The barks of both of them serve as a good source for pure Rougui. In addition, there is another Gui (cinnamon tree) called Guangui (royal cinnamon tree), which is said to be the superior Rougui, used especially by the emperors in the past. Another theory is that Guangui may be the bark of a kind of smaller cinnamon tree. Opinions differ on the subject. Whichever is correct does not warrant serious discussion here. When prescriptions are written, this medicine is always written as Ziyou Rougui, Ziyou Gui or Shang Rougui.

After the coarse tertia of the cassia bark and the membrane layer close to the trunk are scraped off, the remaining middle part of the bark is called Guixin (core of cassia bark).

Guizhi (cassia twig) extending at the top of the cinnamon trees is the best. It smells less strong, and has a tendency of rising (of medicinal meaning) within the body and dispersing throughout it. The bark on the trunk close to the earth is considered first-grade Rougui, and it has strong smell and taste with a tendency to move downwards in the body. It tastes sweet and pungent, indicating its property of Yang and dispersing function. Its pungent and sweet tastes are more intensive than Guizhi, and its heat is also intensive. Thus, it can go directly to and remain in the Lower Jiao to warm the kidneys and invigorate the primordial Yang. Rougui has many properties useful for warming the kidneys. In case there is deficiency-cold in the kidney, Rougui can be used to warm up the kidney Yang. **Ba-**

wei Dihuanng Pill is a very typical formula that can be used to accomplish this task.

Bawei Dihuang Pill

The formula of **Bawei Dihuang Pill** contains eight herbal ingredients:

Fuzi (radix aconiti carmichaeli), Rougui (cassia bark), Dihuang (rehmannia), Shanyurou (common macrocarpium fruit), Shanyao (Chinese yam), Danpi (cortex moutan radicis), Zexie (rhizoma alismatis), Fuling (poria cocos).

In fact, this formula contains the two herbs of Fuzi and Rougui, plus the herbal ingredients of the formula of **Liuwei Dihuang Pill**. The formula of **Liuwei Dihuang Pill** is formed by removing the two medicines of Fuzi and Rougui from the formula of the **Bawei Dihuang Pill** that was originally called "**Cui's Bawei Pill**", recorded in Zhang Zhongjing's *Jingui Yaolue* (*Synopsis of the Golden Chamber*). However, this formula was created before Zhang Zhongjing, and it might be passed down from Cui's family.

There are many other names used for **Bawei Dihuang Pill** like **Guifu Dihuang Pill**, **Jingui Shenqi Pill**, **Shengliao Bawei Pill**, **Jisheng Shenqi Pill** and so on, some of which use Guizhi instead of Rougui, or add Cheqianzi (semen plantaginis) and Niuxi (radix achyranthis bidentatae) in the formula of the **Bawei Dihuang Pill**. But the concept is consistent, and only a little modification had been made according to the specific symptoms or the quality of medicinal herbs at that time. For instance, if there appear serious cold symptoms, Fuzi and Rougui may be used more; If Fuling and Zexie are not so good in quality, Cheqianzi needs to be added to alleviate fluid retention. Therefore, a qualified TCM doctor must be quite familiar with medicinal herbs. Sometimes, even if the prescription is properly written, the inferior quality of herbs may erode its effectiveness. As a TCM doctor, one should not blame everyone or everything else but oneself, since the responsibility falls on the doctor for modifying the given formulas.

Bawei Dihuang Pill can warm and tonify the kidney Yang. In most cases, the kidney-Yin needs tonifying while the kidney Yang is tonified. That is why Fuzi and Rougui are used in addition to **Liuwei Dihuang Pill**, which is for tonifying the kidney Yin only. The kidneys store life essence. Impairment of life essence means impairment of the kidney Yin, which will then immediately result in impairment of the kidney Yang, too. Therefore, the insufficiency of the kidney Yang is always accompanied by deficiency of kidney-Yin.

Impairment ofthe Kidney Yang

Kidney Deficiency due to Exogenous pathogens

It is natural to question whether the kidney Yang will be impaired in case it is attacked by exogenous cold, resulting in deficiency of the kidney Yin. That is true! The kidney will catch cold directly in the case of kidney Yin deficiency, or otherwise it is unlikely to catch cold directly. Let us evaluate an extreme example. Mr. Zhao Enlong, a follower of Keemun Arm Boxing (ape-style forelimb boxing), is very good at Kungfu and also a master of Kungfu bone setting. He once told me that he has never caught a cold in all his life and is not afraid of cold weather, either. The first time when I saw him in the chill of early spring, he was wearing only the unlined clothes. He said that Beijing used to be colder than it is now, even that it would be enough for him to walk outdoors wearing one or two unlined clothes in winter. He is not afraid of the cold at all since he keeps on practicing Kungfu, which is an excellent way to nourish the muscles, tendons and the kidneys. The kidneys dominate the skeleton, which can be maintained perfectly if the kidneys are well nourished with sufficient life essence. Therefore, those who can maintain a strong skeleton can still walk fast and vigorously even by the age of 80. The Wei Qi comes from the Lower Jiao, and it can become powerful when the kidney life essence is sufficiently bolstered. Mr. Zhao Enlong is not afraid of cold weather, and never even catches a cold since he can defend against the attack from the exogenous pathogens. The reason why the kidney catches cold and the pathogenic cold can attack the foot Shaoyin meridians of the kidney is that the kidneys are suffering from the loss of life essence, as is described in *Huangdi Neijing*: "The pathogens always move closer to where Qi is in deficiency. " Therefore, when the kidney Yin is not in deficiency, the exogenous pathogens will not find any entry point into the body.

Some people claim that the coldness of melon and fruits can impair the spleen Yang first and then the kidney Yang gradually. This also happens due to the loss of kidney Yin. If the kidney Yin were sufficient, the kidney Yang would not be susceptible to any impairment.

Coldness After Sexual Intercourse Impairs the Kidney Yang Most

Improper sexual life can impair the kidney Yang, too. Some people may drink cold water or eat cold food immediately after sexual intercourse in summer, which is very risky since the kidneys are insufficient just after the sexual intercourse. At this time, the pathogenic cold particularly tends to enter the kidneys, causing impairment of the kidney Yang, and consequently causing infertility or even cold impairment due to Yin deficiency.

Now, a lot of peoplesuffer from infertility, which may have something to do with such conduct. Those who become infertile in this manner would have rapid pulse due to the endogenous heat in the body. In the case of common rapid pulse symptom, it is quite easy to cure, but for the rapid pulse stemming from infertility, it is very difficult to nurse these symptoms back to health. For such cases, what must be done is to soothe the liver first, and then nourish Yin. After that, some methods like softening hardness to dissipate stagnation should be used to cure the rapid pulse gradually. As soon as the pulse is no longer beating rapidly, warm tonification could be performed.

Cold impairment with Yin deficiency, if confirmed, is often serious and terrible. When taking cold food, the patient will have abdominal distension and feel extreme pain in the lower abdomen. In such a case, it is necessary to have a bowel discharge. The kidneys take charge of the two functions of urine and stool. The human body itself also has the function of rejection. When the cold pathogen accidentally enters the kidneys, it will drive the bad material into the large intestine as possible. At this moment, the patient must utilize the opportunity to purge it, but he should not use Dahuang (rheum officinale) since it is a cold medicine and should not be used while he is suffering from cold pathogens. Badou (croton), as a warm herb, can be the best choice for warming to purge.

Case of Cold Impairment with Yin Deficiency

Compilation of National Famous Clinical Cases records a clinical case of cold impairment with Yin deficiency treated by a doctor named Han Meicun, which says: a 40-year-old widow in Tai'an city fell in love and had sexual intercourse with a man, after which she had some watermelon, then the cold purslane pancakes and cold tea. By 10 o'clock in the evening, she fell ill. At the very beginning, she felt just a slight pain in the abdomen, but gradually she started to feel more and more pain and eventually she could not bear it. The cold pathogens went directly into the Shaoyin channel to impair the kidney Yang. The man gave her a massage. However, the more he did, the more painful she felt. Finally, she refused it completely since it hurt too much. A doctor was called in to write a prescription containing the herbal ingredients: Badou Shuang (defatted croton seed powder) 2 *fen*, Shexiang (musk) 1 *fen*, Xionghuang (realgar) 1. 5 *qian*, Guangyujin (radix curcumae) 2 *qian*.

Badou Shuang is useful for warming purge, and it is able to purge out rather than hold in, serving a purging and discharging function. Shexiang is aromatic with the ability to move and spurt, and it has a very strong permeability. Pain in the abdomen arises from the obstruction of Qi vitality by the cold pathogens, so Shexiang can purge the pathogens with its aromatic and permeating effects. Xionghuang is warm and severely dry, and it can drive out the coldness, while Guangyujin is used for eliminating blood stasis. Smash all these herbs into paste and seal it in beeswax, and swallow it down. The herbs are sealed in beeswax in order to prevent the medicine from starting to function in the stomach so that the medicine can go down as far as possible. As it goes far enough down, the beeswax melts and the medical effects take hold there. The woman mentioned before took 30 pieces with brown sugar and ginger-boiled water at a time. By the time before dawn, when the rooster started to crow, she had passed three stools like cow dung. At this point, the pain stopped. Therefore, whenever the Qi of Middle Jiao suddenly becomes deficient, **Shiquan Dabu Tang** can be used for nourishing. Fortunately, she had met with the experienced doctor Han Meicun, or else this side-effect would have proven fatal.

Heixidan Pill

If the pain is notso severe but the patient merely feels uncomfortable, or suffers from inexplicable fidgeting. That would indicate that the cold pathogens have entered the Lower Jiao and forced the kidney Yang to go upwards. For such cases, it is necessary to use the **Heixidan Pill** to warm the kidneys to dissipate the cold pathogens and tranquilize the floating kidney Yang.

Heixidan Pill contains the herbal ingredients:

Heixi (leadsulfide), Liuhuang (sulfur), Chenxiang (agilawood), Fuzi (radix aconiti carmichaeli), Huluba (fenugreek), Yangqishi (actinolite), Rougui, Poguzhi (fructus psoraleae), Huixiang (foeniculum vulgare), Jinlingzi (Szechwan Chinaberry fruit), Roudoukou (nutmeg), Muxiang (costustoot).

Heixi is a kind of heavy metal with a very firm texture, and it is more effective in tranquilizing and subduing hyperactivity than Longgu (ossa draconis) and Muli (concha ostreae). Liuhuang is a kind of stone with great heat in property and it can warm the Lower Jiao. It also has the effect of tranquilizing and subduing hyperactivity. Generally, fragrance floats upwards, but the fragrance of Chenxiang goes downwards into the Lower Jiao for warming and activating meridians. All the three medicines mentioned are used to subdue and activate Yang.

The herbs of Fuzi, Huluba, Yangqishi, Rougui, and Poguzhi are all used to warm the kidneys. Fuzi is sure to warm the whole body, but under the guidance of Huluba and Rougui, it will go downwards to warm the kidneys as well. Huluba is the seeds of the plant of fenugreek, which can warm the kidneys without impairment of Yin. Yangqishi is a kind of mineral, and it is able to warm the kidneys and support Yang. Normally, it should not be used, but it must be used in this formula. Rougui and Poguzhi are both used for warming the kidneys since Fuzi and Rougui are not enough to warm the kidneys here. The herbal seeds like Huluba and Poguzhi, warm but not dry, and the mineral medicine like Yangqishi are added together with the other herbs into this formula to warm Yang comprehensively and intensively, but also to keep Yang subdued as well.

Huixiang can warm the liver. Jinlingzi (Note: Jinlingzi is the same thing as Chuanlianzi), as the only bitter and cold medicine in this formula, is used for relieving the liver Qi. When used together with Huixiang, it is able to regulate the liver Qi. In this formula, all the other herbs are warm medicines except Jinlingzi, which is cold and used as a corrigent medicine.

Roudoukou and Muxiang are used in this formula for warming the spleen. At the time when the hyperactivity is subdued, the kidney, liver and spleen are all warmed. Moreover, the medicines used are mostly aromatic, and they can open all the orifices, activate Yang, and regulate Qi, which then activates Qi and causes it to circulate smoothly and distribute heat evenly to warm the body well. Otherwise, the cold and heat will become unbalanced, resulting in excessively endogenous heat. In a word, tranquilizing and subduing hyperactivity with the herbs of specific metal and stone for treatment of certain diseases is a unique knack that TCM doctors usually have for using the warm medicines.

If Renshen and Lurong are added to the formula additionally, they will make a new formula called **Shenrong Heixidan Pill**, in which Renshen can function to restore the primordial Qi from where nothing really exists and Lurong can restore Yang of Dumai (governor meridian) more effectively.

The function of **Heixidan Pill** is for warming and strengthening the lower primordial Qi, quieting down and subduing the floating Yang. Generally, it is used for treatment of deficiency of kidney Yang and kidney dysfunction in holding Qi. When the kidney Yang is insufficient, kidney Yin will flood upwards, causing the patient to suffer from an oily face and hair and excessive phlegm, sometimes including phlegm obstruction in lungs, making the patient unable to breathe. For such a case, **Guifu Dihuang Pill** may be workable. When the kidney Yin is insufficient, the kidney Yang will also run upwards. Many patients with kidney deficiency are susceptible to the excessively endogenous heat since there is no enough life essence to hold Yang. In case of failure to hold Yang, it will go up and become pathogenic fire. In this case, **Liuwei Dihuang Pill** can be used to nourish Yin and clear fire. In addition, when there are pathogens in the kidneys, especially the cold pathogens, that would be like a turtledove takes over the nest of a magpie, which would result in that the kidney Yang loses its position, and then runs outwards. In that case, **Heixidan Pill** should be used instead of **Liuwei Dihuang Pill**.

Heixidan Pill is different from **Zhengan Xifeng Tang**. By contrast, **Zhengan Xifeng Tang** is for tranquilizing and subduing the liver Yang, while **Shenrong Heixidan Pill** is for tranquilizing and subduing the kidney Yang. These are actually two different methods. Hence, when there arises Yang deficiency of the Lower Jiao, one must find out whether trouble is in the liver or in the kidneys.

Two Magic Effects of Rougui

Returning the Fire to Its Origin

In the formula of **Heixindan Pill**, Rougui not only warms the kidneys, but also guides the fire (here refers to "Yang") to return to its origin (i. e. , the kidneys), which cannot be done with the other medicines. Therefore, it is absolutely necessary to use the top-grade Ziyou Rougui (purple cassia bark) in the **Hexidan Pill**. The Rougui sold as cinnamon for spicing food use will not do any good.

Rougui can guide fire to return to its origin. Analogically, it is like putting-firewood into the stove. My teacher often said that the life sustaining fire of the kidney Yang is like the fire under a cooking pot. Only when the firewood under a cooking pot is slowly and continuously burning, can the food in the pot be cooked well. If the fire under the pot runs out, one can use a pair of tongs to put the burning firewood back into the stove. This concept is called "guiding the fire to return to its origin". The idea is to let the fire return to its place where it should be. The other warming medicines have little effect of returning the fire to its origin, and only Rougui has such unique effect since Rougui can restrain itself from being purged downwards and it can hold the warm Qi in the Lower Jiao constantly and dredge the collaterals. Hence, Rougui not only can warm the kidney, but also "guide the fire to return to its origin".

In the formula of **Bawei Dihuang Pill**, Fuzi and Rougui are usually used in a very small dosage. Only 5 to 10 grams of Fuzi and about 3 grams of Rougui will be sufficient since the modern people's fire is often stronger to the extent that they may have the accompanying fire though they sometimes suffer from the kidney Yang deficiency. It is important to give serious attention to the use of hot medicines. If the kidney is compared as a lamp, **Liuwei Dihuang Pill** would be like oil to be added to the lamp, and Fuzi and Rougui are like fire to ignite the lamp. Only when the oil is sufficient, can the lamp keep on lighting. Likewise, Dihuang, Shanyurou (common macrocarpium fruit) and Shanyao (Chinese yam) can be used as much as needed. For "ignition" purpose, the hot medicines should not be used too much, or otherwise, some unexpected consequences may arise, unless other corrigent medicines are used to bring the medical effect down quickly to completely eradicate the possible hazard.

Promoting Transformation of Qi in the Lower Jiao

Rougui also has a great use in promoting transformation of Qi in the Lower Jiao.

As it is analogized, the kidney Yang is like a fire that burns under the "cooking pot" of the spleen and stomach so that the spleen and stomach can function properly to decompose and digest food, and then the bladder can carry on pneumatolysis (i. e. , metabolism).

Huangdi Neijing says: "The bladder is like the governor organ at the state capital. When the body fluid is stored, the transformation of Qi can take place. " The bladder must have the function of pneumatolysis. Only when there is a fire under the pot, can the water in the pot be vaporized (this is what pneumatolysis means). One does not feel thirsty if he has saliva in his mouth since the kidney Yang is burning underneath and the bladder is carrying on pneumatolysis to transpire and transform the fluid. The excretion of urine also depends on the pneumatolysis of the bladder. In case the bladder fails in pneumatolysis, some troubles may occur to the saliva in the mouth and the urine. And then, one will feel either thirsty, or he may have much urine, or else he will urinate frequently, suffering from urgent urination or urinating incompletely each time. In particular, some elderly people often get up at night for urination, after which they want to drink some water because of dry mouth. That is a typical symptom of the kidney Yang deficiency and dysfunction of pneumatolysis. The fluid in the bladder cannot transpire into body fluid, but only be discharged, so they feel thirsty and urinate more and frequently. When there is an absence of phlegm or damp-heat in the Lower Jiao, **Bawei Dihuang Pill** can be used for treatment.

Wuling San

If dysfunction of the bladder occurs for Qi transformation, resulting in inability of releasing urine, **Wuling San** can be used.

Wuling San contains the ingredient herbs: Baizhu (white atractylodes rhizome), Fuling (poria cocos), Zhuling (grifola), Zexie (rhizoma alismatis), Guizhi (cassia twig).

This is the formula of **Wuling San** cited from Zhang Zhongjing's **Shanghan Lun**. The formula is simple: Baizhu enters the Middle Jiao and spleen (corresponding to the earth according to the **Wuxing Doctrine**). The earth (referring to the spleen) is able to restrict water (referring to the kidneys according to the **Wuxing Doctrine**); therefore, for treatment of water (the kidneys), it is necessary to tonify the spleen, which can then remove the fluid retention. The spleen dominates transportation and transformation. The pneumatolysis of fluid can be completed only when the Middle Jiao is properly functioning. There are three diuretic medicines: Fuling for removing water retention and tonifying the spleen; Zhuling, much stronger than Fuling for promoting diuresis; and Zexie, also for alleviating fluid retention, and specially the dampness in kidneys. After that, Rougui can be added to promote pneumatolysis of fluid. The diuretic medicines can activate Yang of the Lower Jiao, and Rougui directly warm and activate the kidney Yang. Hence, both of them can then bring out the best in each other.

Here, Guizhi is substituted for Rougui according to **Shanghan Lun**, in which Guizhi is used. However, in **Shanghan Lun**, the medication mainly targets the dysfunction of pneumatolysis caused by cold impairment in the Taiyang meridian, so Guizhi is used to warm the Taiyang meridian. Now, in case dysfunction of pneumatolysis is caused by the kidney Yang deficiency, Rougui should be used. The current *"Chinese Pharmacopoeia"*, concerning **Wuling San**, uses Rougui instead of Guizhi.

Zishen Tongguan Pill

Damp-heat disturbs the Lower Jiao, resulting in dysfunction of pneumatolysis, difficult urination, or very short, yellow, and even red urination with burning heat and pain at the urethra orifice at the same time. In such a case, the patient should take **Zishen Tongguan Pill**.

The formula of **Zishen Tongguan Pill** contains the ingredient herbs:

Huangbai (phellodendron amurense) 1 *liang*, Zhimu (rhizoma anemarrhenae) 1 *liang*, Rougui 5 *fen* (according to ***Secret Book in Orchid Chamber*** by Li Dongyuan, medical expert, one of the four medical scientists in the Jin and Yuan dynasties).

The dosage of the thre emedicines varies greatly. Huangbai and Zhimu are the main herbs for clearing the heat in the Lower Jiao. They are used in a large dosage that can sink down directly to the Lower Jiao. Rougui is simply used to promote pneumatolysis, and it cannot be used in a large dosage. Otherwise, it may promote pathogenic heat. The dosage of Rougui is very small. Under the influence of the large dosage of Huangbai and Zhimu, the heat of Rougui will not cause any impairment, but its effect for promoting pneumatolysis can still work well.

In case the Lower Jiao is very damp and hot, one should add Cangzhu and Niuxi, together with Huangbai, to create a formula called **Sanmiao Pill**. It is so called for the three herbal ingredients in that they will have a very good effect when used properly. Huangbai can clear heat and Cangzhu eliminates dampness. These two medicines used together will drive out all dampness and heat. Then Niuxi is added to guide the effects of the above two medicines downwards so that the dampness and heat in the Lower Jiao will be cleared away with much stronger potency.

Kidney Yin and Yang vs Dampness and Heat in Lower Jiao

Dysfunction of pneumatolysis of the kidneyscan lead to many diseases. As it is known, there are both Yin and Yang in the kidneys. The kidneys are just like a "坎卦" [Kǎn Guà; "坎"(Kǎn) means the sinking and uneven place or a pit, and "卦" (Guà) refers to a divinatory symbol. "坎卦" (Kǎn Guà) shows the possible changes under the condition of "坎"(Kǎn), i. e. under the conditions of sinking and uneven place or pit. The symbol of Kǎn Guà is 2: 2; the devinatory image is water, and the divinatory symbol is 2. Two drops of water mixed together still make water; i. e., the danger and difficulty of both sides put together are still dangerous and difficult.] Each person has two kidneys, one on each side for storing the life essence and dominating fluid. The two kidneys are equivalent to two "阴爻" (Yīn Yáo, which, in the ***Book of Changes***, refers to two symbols

"- -" for trigrams). In between is the life-gate fire, which is equivalent to a "阳 爻"(Yáng Yáo, which, in the **Book of Changes**, refers to the symbol "-" for trigrams, too, corresponding to Yīn Yáo symbol "- -". Guo Moruo, an outstanding historian, archaeologist, writer and poet in contemporary Chinese history takes the Yáng Yáo symbol "-" as the symbol of the male genital organ and the Yīn Yáo symbol "- -" as the symbol of the female genital organ). And in the above is a Yīn Yáo symbol "- -" and in the middle is a Yáng Yáo symbol "-". The primordial life essence in the kidneys is equivalent to two Yīn Yáo symbol "- -", while the primordial Yang hidden in the primordial Yin is the Yáng Yáo symbol "-". Yin and Yang hold and engage with each other perfectly and seamlessly. However, in case they fail to match up properly, Yang will become endogenous heat, and Yin will become the dampness. The dampness and heat will then be interacted, resulting in damp-heat in the Lower Jiao. Damp-heat lingering in the Lower Jiao will lead to dysfunction of pneumatolysis. In such cases, the **Sanmiao Pill** and **Zishen Tongguan Pill** are often used. The formulas of these two different pills contain only three medicines each, but they are greatly effective and also have very special significance.

A Medical Case of the Lower Jiao Transformation

About the year before the last, I had a relative who was confirmed to have kidney stones in a physical examination, but he didn't have any obvious symptoms, so he did not care too much about it. All of a sudden one day, he felt a little pain in his right waist. After a while, he felt more and more painful. Finally, the pain was too much to bear. Only then did he realize that he had not defecated or urinated for a whole day. He felt bloated and colic at the waist, and neither stool nor urine could be released. After examination in the hospital, there were three " + " signs for occult blood in urine and four " + " signs for glucose which is called the renal colic in the western medicine. An anorectal medicine pack was inserted into his anorectum, and he felt relieved a little bit. But after a while, he felt painful again. He called to ask me about the case. I was sure that it was damp-heat stagnation in the Lower Jiao, resulting in the dysfunction of pneumatolysis, which is very common in clinic practice.

"The kidney governs defecation and urination", which means that the defecation and urination are both related to the kidneys. In the clinical diagnosis, TCM doctors often ask the patients about their defecation and urination since these two things are involved with many factors. The state of pneumatolysis of the kidneys will reflect the conditions of stool and urine. "The liver governing dispersion" means defecation and urination depend on the regulating function of the liver. In case the liver fails to regulate its dispersion, stool and urine will not be released. The spleen governs T&T, in which the spleen controls the ascending of the clear, and the stomach controls the descending of the turbid. In case the spleen is trapped, and the ascending of the clear and the descending of the turbid cannot function properly, the stool and urine, especially the stool, will not be released smoothly. The lungs govern Qi circulation of the whole body, and also work together with the large intestine to serve the exterior and interior functions mutually. So, if the lung Qi fails to circulate smoothly, there will also be some troubles with defecation and urination.

The aforementioned disease is mainly due to the dysfunction of pneumatolysis of the kidneys, which results in the kidney failure to govern defecation and urination, and then obstruction of both defecation and urination; and the fundamental cause was damp-heat stagnation. Therefore, I gave him the following prescription:

Shang Rougui (top-grade cassia bark) 3g, Sheng Huangbai (raw phellodendron amurense) 10g, Sheng Zhimu (raw rhizoma anemarrhenae) 10g, Huashi Fen (talcum powder) 20g, Gan Lugen (dried rhizoma phragmitis) 30g, Daji (euphorbia pekinensis) 10g, Xiaoji (herba cepbalanoplosis segeti) 10g, Jinqiancao (lysimachia christinae) 12g, Haijinsha (lygodium japonicum) 10g, Sheng Zhizi (raw fructus gardeniae) 12g, Fendanpi (cortex moutan radicis powder) 12g, Bai Fuling (white poria cocos) 10, Jian Zexie (Fujian rhizoma alismatis) 10g, Jie Zhuling (grifola) 10g, Chao Baizhu (fried white atractylodes rhizome) 10g, Sheng Gancao (raw liquorice) 6g.

Zishen Tongguan Pill was taken as the main medicine to clear the dampness and heat in the kidneys to promote pneumatolysis. In addition, Huashi Fen and Lugen are used to target the kidney stones. Huashi Fen has heavy texture, and it can make the dampness and heat go downwards, which is useful for eliminating dampness and heat. Strictly speaking, it is the dampness that it makes go downwards. When the dampness is almost eliminated, the heat will be easily dissipated.

Lugen can promote the secretion of saliva or body fluid. Analogically speaking, to create fluid is like washing the encrusted grime in a thermos bottle. One should have to add some water while adding detergent for cleaning a bottle. Lugen here is equivalent to water. Lugen grows in water, indicating that it has a very strong ability to resist water and can replenish water, but it does not cause pathogens or induce phlegm. The water replenished by Lugen is fresh water. In addition, Lugen, to some extent, is also able to alleviate fluid retention.

Daji, Xiaoji, Jinqiancao, and Haijinsha are a combination of medicines frequently used for treating stranguria caused by stones. Sheng Zhizi can clear the floating heat in the Tri-jiao to induce urination. Stone and dysfunction of bladder pneumatolysis are both caused by heat in the Tri-jiao, so Zhizi is used to clear it. In the treatment of urinary diseases, attention and consideration should always be given to clearing the Tri-jiao, which is the main channel for fluid transfer.

Danpi and Zhizi are commonly used together. The formula of **Jiawei Xiaoyao Pill** is made by adding Danpi and Zhizi based on the **Xiaoyao Pill**. Zhizi is used directly after Danpi since there are three " + " signs in the occult blood in the report by western medicine examination. The occult blood means blood heat in TCM, which can be cleared with Danpi. Therefore, this treatment follows the TCM theory to deal with the medical reports given by the western medicine examination.

Fuling, Zexie, Zhuling, Baizhu, and Gancao all together make the formula of **Wuling San**, which can activate Yang and alleviate fluid retention in order to tackle the urination obstruction of the patient.

One hour after taking the medicine prescribed above, the above-mentioned patient started to urinate, and claimed no pain at his waist. Then after a short period of time, he also released stool. A check showed that the irregular stone had been discharged into urethra. And then, I told him to continue to take Chinese medicine and discharge the stone slowly, or use a laser to break the stone, which, however, might impair the Lower Jiao. Later, he took **Liuwei Dihuang Tang** plus some heat-clearing and dampness-eliminating medicines for one month, and then, his trouble of prostatitis was cured as well incidentally.

第四章　肉桂

肉桂及其温肾之功

最好的肉桂

肉桂是中医很常用的一味药，是肉桂树的皮，而且以靠近土的一节主干上的皮为最好。大树枝上的皮也有用，但是没有那么好。

产在越南的叫企边桂，我们国内还有安边桂，产于广西，颜色呈紫褐色，都是地道的好肉桂。还有官桂，有人说官桂就是最好的肉桂，是供奉给官家使用的，还有一种说法是，官桂是比较小的桂树的皮，说法不一，我们就没有必要深究谁对谁错。我们开方子时，常写作紫油肉桂、紫油桂或上肉桂。

把肉桂外面的那层粗皮和里面靠近树干的那一层薄皮刮掉，光留树皮最中间的部分，就叫桂心。

长在桂树顶上的桂枝最好，气味较薄，便于上行，升散。肉桂则以靠近根部主干上的为最好，这的肉桂气味俱厚，往下走。你尝尝，又甜又辣，辛甘发散为阳啊。其辛甘之味比桂枝更强，热性也比桂枝大。它能直达下焦，守而不走，温肾壮元阳。围绕温肾，肉桂有很多的作用。如果肾中有虚寒，可以用肉桂来温肾阳，典型方剂叫八味地黄丸。

八味地黄丸

八味地黄丸

附子　肉桂　地黄　山萸肉　山药　丹皮　泽泻　茯苓

前面附子、肉桂，后面是六味地黄丸。六味地黄丸就是在八味地黄丸的基础上减去附子、肉桂。八味地黄丸本来叫"崔氏八味丸"，始见于张仲景《金匮要略》，其实它在张仲景之前这个方子就有了，可能是某个姓崔的人家流传下来的。

前面附子、肉桂，后面是六味地黄丸。六味地黄丸就是在八味地黄丸的基础上减去附子、肉桂。八味地黄丸本来叫"崔氏八味丸"，始见于张仲景《金匮要略》，其实它在张仲景之前这个方子就有了，可能是某个姓崔的人家流传下来的。

八味地黄丸还有很多别名：桂附地黄丸、金匮肾气丸、生料八味丸、济生肾气丸等，其中有的把肉桂用成了桂枝，有的又加了车前子、牛膝。其思想都是一致的，只不过是根据具体病情，或是根据当时药材的质量，进行了一些灵机应变。比如说，寒象比较重的，附子、肉桂就可以多用；如果当时的茯苓、泽泻质量不是那么好，就要加车前子，加大利水的力度。所以，要做一个合格的中医，你得非常熟悉药材。有时候即使方子开对了，药材不好也会影响疗效，但你不能怨天尤人，可以在方子的加减上多下功夫。

八味地黄丸温补肾阳。补肾阳多同时要补肾阴，所以附子、肉桂后面紧跟着补肾阴的六味地黄丸。肾藏精，伤精就是伤肾阴，伤了肾阴接着就会伤肾阳。肾阳不足的同时，必有肾阴虚。

肾阳之伤

外邪伤肾，肾必先亏

当然有人说外寒侵犯肾，伤了肾阳了，也会有肾阴虚么？是的！肾直接受寒，往往是在肾阴虚的情况下。否则，肾不可能直接受寒。我们可以举一个非常极端的例子。北京的赵恩龙先生，是祁门通臂拳传人，武门正骨大师，功夫非常好。他跟我说，他这辈子从来没有感冒过，而且不怕冷。我第一次见到他的时候，正值春寒料峭，他只穿着单衣。他讲，北京过去的气温比现在要低，他冬天出门穿一两件就够了。他根本不怕风寒，为什么呢？因为他练功夫，中国的功夫是养筋、养肾的极好方法。肾主骨骼，肾精充足，骨骼就非常的好，到了八十岁的时候，还是健步如飞。卫气出于下焦，肾精足则卫气强大，所以他不怕冷，也不感冒，外邪根本进不来。肾之所以受寒，寒邪之所以能够直中足少阴肾经，前提就是肾精亏耗了。这就应了《黄帝内经》那句话："邪之所凑，其气必虚。"肾阴不虚，外邪拿你还真的没办法。

有人说吃瓜果，寒凉先伤了脾阳，然后慢慢再伤肾阳。这个也是以肾阴亏耗为前提的，你如果肾阴很充足的话，肾阳也没那么容易伤。

房事后误犯寒凉，最伤肾阳

不当的性生活，也很伤肾阳。有的人，夏天性生活以后马上喝凉水，或吃凉东西，这非常危险。因为性生活后，肾中空虚，寒凉之气特别容易入肾，肾阳受伤，轻则造成不孕不育，重则造成夹阴伤寒。

现在很多人不孕不育，都跟这个有关。这种不孕不育的人，脉象往往弦数。脉数是因为体内有热。一般的数脉，我们用一点药，很快就能调过来，但这种原因引起的数则很难调。必须先疏肝，然后养阴，还要用一些软坚散结的方法，才能慢慢把它拿下来。脉不数之后，才可大用温补。

如果是夹阴伤寒，那就会来势汹汹，非常危险。凉的吃下去，肚子就会特别胀、小腹绞痛难忍，这时候就得把它攻泻下来了。肾主二便，有时候寒邪入肾，人体自己也有排异功能，会把一些不好的东西，尽量往大肠里边排，这时候你必须顺势通一下。但不能用大黄，大黄是一味寒凉的药，人体正在被寒邪折腾得七死八活，哪还敢用大黄这样寒凉的药？这时可以用巴豆，巴豆是一味温药，温通泻下，正好派上用场了。

夹阴伤寒一案

《全国名医验案类编》中有韩梅村的一个夹阴伤寒的医案：泰安城中有个40岁的寡妇，"自由恋爱，妍识一男，一见即媾"（可惜这么精彩传神的句子，在后来的版本中被删了），有了性生活，完了她就吃西瓜，后来又吃马齿馅饼，也是凉的，吃完了又喝了一些冷茶，到了晚上十点钟，生病了，刚开始也就是肚子微微有点痛，后来越来越痛，以致不能忍受。这就是寒邪直中少阴，伤了肾阳。那个男的给她按摩什么的，越按越痛，最后就不让按了，因为一碰就疼。请来了医生。他开的方子是：巴豆霜二分、麝香一分、雄黄一钱五分、广郁金二钱。

巴豆霜温通泻下，走而不守，有摧枯拉朽的作用。麝香芳香走窜，极有穿透力。肚子疼是因为被寒邪闭住了气机，所以用麝香的芳香走蹿来通一下。雄黄温而燥烈，也能驱逐阴寒，广郁金是解郁化瘀的。把这些药捣成泥，用蜂蜡裹住吞下去。用蜂蜡裹住吞，是为了防止这味药在胃中就开始动。要让这味药充分往下走，走到下边，蜡化了，药力开始发挥作用。让她一次吃三十粒，用红糖姜水送下，到了鸡鸣的时候，拉了三次如牛粪一样的东西，这痛就好了。痛好了，中气骤虚，用十全大补汤收工。幸亏她遇到的是韩梅村这样的好医生，如果不遇到这样的好医生可能就死了。

黑锡丹

如果没有痛得那么厉害，只是莫名其妙难受、烦躁，那是寒入下焦，迫使肾阳上越，得用黑锡丹，一边温肾，散寒之寒邪，一边潜镇，收浮越之肾阳。

黑锡丹

黑锡、硫黄、沉香、附子、葫芦巴、阳起石、肉桂、破故纸、茴香、金铃子、肉豆蔻、木香。

黑锡是重金属，质地很重，比龙骨牡蛎更有潜镇的作用；硫磺大热，能温下焦，而且它属于石头，也能潜镇；一般的香气都是往上浮的，唯独沉香往下沉，能沉入下焦而温通。这三个药都是往下潜阳、通阳的。

附子、葫芦巴、阳起石、肉桂、破故纸，这几味药都是温肾的，附子当然全身都温，现在跟着葫芦巴、肉桂，它往下一带就温肾了；葫芦巴是植物的种子，温肾而不伤阴；阳起石温肾助阳，属于矿物，一般情况下不用，但这里必须用；肉桂、破故纸都是温肾的。在这种情况下，温肾仅仅靠附子肉桂是不行的，还要加上葫芦巴、破故纸这类温而不燥的种子类药物，加上阳起石这样的矿物药，全方位、大力度地温阳，并且时时不忘潜阳。

后面，茴香是温肝的。金铃子就是川楝子，是一味苦寒的药，它能破肝气，跟茴香一起则能理肝气。这个方子里所有其他药都是温药，用一味寒凉的药，有一个反佐地作用。

肉豆蔻和木香是温脾的。在潜镇的同时，温了肾，温了肝，温了脾，而且用药多芳香，芳香则能开窍、通阳、调气，让气流动起来，使热力分布均匀，更好地发挥温的作用。不然的话，就会寒热不均衡，导致上火。佐以金石潜镇、芳香流动，是用温热药的一个诀窍。

如果再加人参、鹿茸，就叫参茸黑锡丹，人参能回元气于无何有之乡，鹿茸能迅速回督脉之阳气。效果更佳。

黑锡丹的作用是温壮下元、潜镇浮阳。一般都是用于真阳不足，肾不纳气。肾阳不足的时候，肾阴就会往上泛，人就头面出油、多痰，甚至痰壅在肺里，气都喘不过来，这种情况尚可用桂附地黄丸；肾阴不足的时候，肾阳也会往上跑，很多肾虚的人容易上火，就是因为底下没有那么多真精把阳气固住，阳气固不住就会往上越，成为邪火，这种情况下，可以用六味地黄丸，养阴清火。此外，当肾中有邪，尤其是寒邪的时候，鸠占鹊巢，肾阳失其位，也会外越，这种情况下就用黑锡丹。

黑锡丹跟镇肝息风汤不一样。镇肝息风汤潜镇的是肝阳，参茸黑锡丹潜镇的是肾阳，二者方法是不一样的。所以，虽然同样是下焦阳虚，我们一定要弄清楚它到底是肝的问题还是肾的问题。

肉桂的两大妙用

引火归元

在黑锡丹中，肉桂的作用不仅仅是温肾，同时还引火归元，这是其他药不具备的。所以黑锡丹里面必须用上好的紫油肉桂，市场上我们常买回家做大料的那种肉桂是不行的。

肉桂引火归元，通俗的说，就是把柴火塞进灶里。我师父常说，人的肾阳命门之火就像烧饭用的锅底下的火。火只有在锅底下慢慢地烧，锅里面的东西才能熟。如果锅底下的火烧出来了，就用火钳夹住，连柴带火，一起塞回灶里，这就是引火归元，让火回到它应该去的地方。其他温药很少有引火归元的作用，这是肉桂独特的地方。为什么肉桂能引火归元呢？因为它守而不走，能够把温热之气一直留在下焦，还能通络脉。所以说肉桂不仅能温肾，而且还能引火归元。

在八味地黄丸里，附子和肉桂一般用得特别少。附子用上 5 到 10 克，肉桂用 3 克左右就足够了。为什么用这么少呢？因为我们现代人的火往往比较重，既使是肾阳虚，都可能伴随着火，所以，用热药就要注意一些。另外，如果说肾是一盏灯，那么，六味地黄丸好比给灯加油，而附子肉桂好比给灯点火。加油不怕多，地黄、山萸肉、山药你可以使劲用。点火则无需大，点到为止。当热药用于点火的时候，就要尽量少用；如果用得多了，就可能会出问题。除非你有其他的药为佐，把它迅速往下引，杜绝其危害。

促进下焦气化

肉桂还有一大妙用，促进下焦气化。

我们知道，肾阳好比锅底下的火，它在底下蒸动，脾胃才能运转，腐熟水谷、消化食物，膀胱才能气化。

《黄帝内经》讲："膀胱为州都之官，津液藏焉，气化则能出矣。"膀胱要有气化。锅底下有火，烧水的锅里才能冒出气来，这就叫气化。我们嘴里有津液，就不觉得渴，这是因为肾阳在底下蒸动，膀胱能够气化，把水液蒸腾上来，嘴里就有津液。小便能够排出来，这也取决于膀胱的气化。如果膀胱的气化功能不行了，那么嘴里的津液、下边的小便都可能出问题：要么就是口渴，同时尿多，要么就是尿频，尿急，尿不尽。尤其是有些老年人，晚上经常起夜，而且起完夜还得喝口水，因为口干了，这是典型的肾阳不足，气化不利。膀胱里的津液不能够蒸腾为津液，只能排出去，所以人会渴，小便也会多。在没有痰或下焦湿热的情况下，可以用八味地黄丸。

五苓散

如果膀胱气化不利，小便解不出来，则用五苓散。

五苓散

白术、茯苓、猪苓、泽泻、桂枝。

这是张仲景《伤寒论》中五苓散的方子。这个方子的方义很简单：白术是入中焦、入脾的，土能克水，治水须健脾，健脾可以利水。脾主运化，是水液运化的前提，必须让中焦运转起来，水的气化才能形成。紧跟着是三味利水的药：茯苓利水，健脾；猪苓利水的力度比茯苓还大；泽泻也是利水的，而且主要是利肾中的水湿。后边再加一味促进气化的药，就是肉桂。利水药可以同下焦之阳，肉桂直接温通肾阳，二者相得益彰。

这里，我是根据《伤寒论》才把肉桂写成桂枝的。《伤寒论》里写的是桂枝，但是《伤寒论》主要是针对太阳经伤寒导致气化不利，所以它用桂枝来温太阳经。如果现在是肾阳虚气化不利，那么就要用肉桂了。现在的《中国药典》上讲到五苓散，写的不是桂枝，而是肉桂。

滋肾通关丸

湿热困扰下焦，导致气化不利，小便不容易排出，或者小便可排但是非常短、黄，甚至发红，同时尿道口还会感觉热辣辣的痛，这时就要经常用到滋肾通关丸。

滋肾通关丸

黄柏、知母各一两，肉桂五分（李东垣《兰室秘藏》）。

三味药的用量悬殊非常大。黄柏、知母是清下焦之热，是主药，所以用量极大，量大则沉，直入下焦。肉桂完全是用来促进气化的，不能多用，多用则助长邪热。所以肉桂用量很小，在大剂量的黄柏和知母中，其热性已经不可能有任何危害了，但气化的作用还是可以施展的。

如果下焦湿热很重，再加苍术、牛膝，与黄柏一起构成三妙丸。叫三妙丸，就是因为这三个药如果用得好的话，效果会非常妙。黄柏清热、苍术燥湿，这两味药在一起湿热就没有了。再加牛膝，把它往下一引，清下焦湿热力度就更大。

肾阴肾阳与下焦湿热

肾的气化不利会导致很多病。我们知道肾里边有肾阴有肾阳，肾就是一个坎卦：一边一个，藏精主水的腰子，相当于两个阴爻，中间是命门之火，相当于一个阳爻。上边是一个阴爻，中间是一个阳爻。肾中真精，相当于两个阴爻，真阳藏于真阴之中，是为阳爻。阴阳交抱，配合得妙合无痕，如果配合得不好，阳就会成为热，阴就会成为湿，湿热就会交织在一起，导致下焦湿热。湿热缠绵在下焦，就会导致气化不利，三妙丸和滋肾通关丸会经常用到，这两个方子都只有三味药，但它们的作用非常大，意义也非常大。

下焦气化医案一则

大概是在前年的时候，我有一个亲戚，在体检的时候检查到有肾结石，但是他感觉没有什么明显的症状，也就没在意。忽然有一天他感觉到右侧腰有点痛，后来越来越痛，最后痛得实在不能忍了，才想到他已经有整整一天没有大小便了。他感觉腰很胀，绞痛，大便小便根本解不出来。到医院一检查，小便潜血有三个加号，葡萄糖有四个加号，西医说这个叫肾绞痛，用一个肛肠塞剂塞进去会有所缓解，但是过了一会就又会疼。他给我打电话，问这是怎么回事。这就是湿热壅滞在下焦，气化不利，临床上是很常见的。

"肾司二便"，大便小便都跟肾有关。咱们临证中一定要问大便小便，因为二者牵涉的东西太多了。"肾司二便"，肾的气化是不是顺利，二便会有所表现；"肝主疏泄"，大便小便能够出来，取决于肝的疏泄功能，如果肝疏泄不利，那么大小便也不会出来；脾主运化，脾主升清，胃主降浊，如果脾气被困住了，升清降浊来得慢的话，那么二便——尤其是大便，也不会那么顺畅；肺主一身之气，且与大肠相表里，肺气不利，大小便也会出问题。

这次这个病，主要是因为肾的气化不利，肾不能很好的司二便，所以大小便就都闭住了，根源都在于湿热壅滞。我出的方子是这样的：

上肉桂3、生黄柏10、生知母10、滑石粉20、干芦根30、大小蓟各10、金钱草12、海金沙10、生栀子12、粉丹皮12、白茯苓10、建泽泻10、结猪苓10、炒白术10、生甘草6。

以滋肾通关丸为君，清肾中湿热，促其气化。再加上滑石和芦根，这是经常用的一对药，能针对很多结石。滑石清利湿热，质重，能把湿热往下坠，严格地说，是把湿往下坠，当湿去得差不多的时候，热也就容易散掉。芦根生津，也就是补水，这好比洗热水瓶里面的水碱污垢，一边加洗涤剂，一边还得加水，用芦根相当于加水。而且芦根是生长在水里的，这意味着他抗水的能力非常强，能补水，但是不会敛邪，也不会生痰。芦根补出来的水都是活水。而且芦根在某种程度上来讲还有利水的作用，所以在这里也可以用。

大小蓟、金钱草、海金沙是治结石淋证经常用的一组药。生栀子能够清三焦浮游之热，利小便。结石、膀胱气化不利都是三焦有热，以栀子来清。治小便方面的病，经常要兼顾清三焦，三焦主通调水道。

丹皮是为了配栀子而用的，丹皮栀子是常用的对药。加味逍遥丸里就是在逍遥丸的基础上加丹皮栀子。这里为什么栀子后面直接带出一味丹皮？别忘了，前面西医检查的结果里边潜血还有三个加号呢。潜血，意味着有血热，恰好用丹皮来清。咱们要用中医的理论去统摄西医的检查结果。后面茯苓、泽泻、猪苓、白术、甘草跟前面的肉桂加起来就是五苓散，通阳利水。要知道，病人小便还不通呢。

后面茯苓、泽泻、猪苓、白术、甘草跟前面的肉桂加起来就是五苓散，通阳利水。要知道，病人小便还不通呢。

这个方子吃下去，一个小时后小便就解了，腰就不痛了。过了一段时间才解大便。一检查，说结石已经进入尿道了，形状很不规则，问我该怎么办。我说：你要是不急的话我们可以用中药让结石慢慢排出来。如果着急的话可以用激光把结石打碎了。但是激光碎石会伤及下焦，后面用六味地黄汤，略微加一些清热利湿的药，连吃一个月来善后。善后之后，此人连以前得的前列腺炎都好了。

Chapter 5　Other Medicines for Warming the Kidney Yang

Now let us get down to some other kidney-warming medicines.

To warm the kidneys is actually to warm the kidney Yang. As it is known, the liver, spleen and kidneys, especially the spleen and kidneys are in the Lower Jiao and under the control of Yin. Essentially, the five internal organs are all governed by Yin, and the liver, spleen and kidneys in the middle and Lower Jiao are even more under influence of Yin. The spleen is under the control of the foot Taiyin, which is the Yin of Yin. The liver is of foot Jueyin, and it belongs to Yin in physique and Yang in function. The kidneys are of Shaoyin, governing body fluid and belonging to Yin. The organs of Yin are susceptible to cold accumulation, so Yang must be maintained in Yin, i. e. , it is necessary to keep warming the Yang of Yin.

Both Yang and Yin of the kidneys should be taken into consideration. Yin and Yang are like an oil lamp. When the oil is burnt out and is about to dry, the lamp will become dim. Yin deficiency is like running low on oil, and Yang deficiency is like the lamp becoming dim. Therefore, in the process of warming Yang, that is, when trimming the lamp-wick, one also has to refuel the lamp. When the oil is sufficient, the lamp-wick is properly trimmed; ignite it with just a piece of match, and the oil lamp will then become vigorous. This is the principle of Yin and Yang. Zhang Jingyue, medical expert in the Ming dynasty, said: "Those who are good at nourishing Yin must seek Yin from Yang, and those who are good at nourishing Yang must seek Yang from Yin as well. " These words mean a lot indeed. For warming Yang, one must not be eager for quick success by using the hot and dry herbs such as Fuzi and Rougui and so on since "excessive fire consuming Qi" will lead to bad consequences. Hence, a lot of milder medicines are required in order to warm the kidneys.

Roucongrong(Cistanche)

Characteristics of Roucongrong

From the name "肉苁蓉" (Roucongrong, means cistanche), it can be determined that "肉" (Rou) in Chinese means "meat", which shows that it has nourishing attribute. Then regarding "苁蓉" (cōng róng), if the upper part "艹" of the characters "苁蓉" (cōng róng) is removed, the remaining parts will be "从容" (cóng róng), which refers to a kind of character of human behavior, i. e., "take things easy". Roucongrong, as a medicine, can nourish Yin and the kidney Yang as well.

Roucongrong is normally produced in the northwest of China like Xinjiang Autonomous Region, and Inner Mongolia. According to the ancient legend that Roucongrong was transformed from the horse sperms that fell to the ground. No matter this is true or false, we should connect in our minds that "horse" is subsumed to Yang, and it corresponds to "午" (Wu) in the twelve Earthly Branches, being the seventh in the rank. The horse is strong and it runs so fast, showing that horse is governed by Yang, but horse sperm is subsumed to Yin. Now that Roucongrong is so called to be transformed from the horse sperms, it means Yin and Yang are in one.

Roucongrong is sweet, salty, warm and moist in properties, black in color and scaly in appearance. The largest and top class Roucongrong can be sized as big as human arm. It can tonify the life essence of the kidney and the kidney Yang as well, but it always takes time to nourish.

Nourishing the Kidneys and Relaxing the Bowels

Roucongrong also has the function of smoothening intestines by nourishing Yin and warming the kidney Yang. When the kidney Yin and Yang are sufficient, the kidneys will become stronger to govern the defecation and urination so as to help people relax their bowels more smoothly. In short, it has the effect of pushing downwards, which means that those who suffer from the spleen deficiency and loose stool should use it with much caution. Meanwhile, Roucongrong is a little bit greasy, so those who have spleen deficiency and weak T&T function should stop using it.

On the other hand, many elderly people suffer from constipation with extremely dry stool because of Yin deficiency and blood depletion. They do not have sufficient body fluid to moisten the stool. Therefore, many elderly people need to use a glycerine enema pack for moistening the stool inside in order to release it. Those elderly people who are suffering from constipation can use Roucongrong.

The elderly people often suffer from kidney deficiency. Roucongrong not only can nourish kidneys and blood, but also relieve stool, thus, it serves multiple purposes. Generally, many elderly people have the trouble of constipation, but they have different methods of their own: some old people drink Dahuang (rheum officinale) (5 grams) soaked water every day, which can solve their troubles for the time being---but after drinking for a period of time, they will have problems of poor appetite. Some take Juemingzi (semen cassia) as tea. After drinking Juemingzi soaked water for some time, troubles with the spleen and stomach can occur, or endogenous deficient wind can cause the eye ground to bleed, since Juemingzi is cool and oily; Some other elderly people take Fanxieye (folium sennae) as tea, which can also help them for a while. However, all these medicines should not be used too long. Roucongrong is the only herb that can be used for an extended time to help relax constipation of dry stool that arises from blood depletion and Yin deficiency. In **Shennong Bencao Jing (Shen Nong's Herbal Classic)**, Roucongrong is listed as the top-grade medicine that can make a person feel energetic and help prolong his life if it is administrated continuously for long. However, Dahuang, Juemingzi and Fanxieye have no nourishing effect and cannot be used for an extended time.

Bajitian(Morinda Officinalis)

Characteristics of Bajitian

Bajitian is able to tonify Yang of Yin and is often used together with Roucongrong to bring out the best in each other. Actually, Bajitian is the root of a grass on the mountain. The herbal roots should generally be collected in the second or eighth months of the Chinese lunar year. In the second month of the lunar yeear, the grass has not sprouted out yet, and the root under the ground is poised for growing out. In the eighth month of the lunar calendar, the grass is withering and the life essence has been stored in the root, so the medical efficacy is at optimal strength. Bajitian is shaped like Danpi, with a thicker cortex outside and a core inside. As an herb, the core inside should be removed. Danpi is white (some are slightly reddish or yellow), while Bajitian looks a little reddish, and the inner core looks a little black.

Bajitian is pungent, sweet, bitter and warm in properties, and it enters the liver and kidney blood system for warming the kidneys, and tonifying Yang. ED (erectile dysfunction) often arises from a deficiency of kidney Yang failing to stimulate Qi and blood. Bajitiann is able to warm the kidney Yang.

Warming and Activating Effects of Bajitian

Bajitian can be used to treat various lumps and beriberi because of its warming effects. Its warm characteristic indicates that it can dispel the wind-cold-damp arthralgia of the whole body.

When kidney Yang deficiency occurs, Wei (defensive) Qi becomes weak accordingly, and exogenous pathogens are more likely to invade into the human body. Generally, the pathogens first attack the lower part of the body, causing soreness of waist and leg pain. Naturally, the pungent and dry medicines like Duhuo (radix angelicae pubescentis) will be used for treatment. However, some people can defend themselves against the attack from the pathogens since they are vigorous enough in the liver and kidney Yang, while some others succumb easily since they are too weak in the liver and kidney Yang to defend the pathogens. As it is often said, "Where the pathogenic factors flock together, Qi will definitely wither. "

Therefore, Bajitian can disperse pathogenic factors while it is tonifying the liver and kidney Yang. In reality, many medicines for warming the kidney Yang have such an effect.

Compatibility of Bajitian and Roucongrong

Bajitian is a medicine that can be nourishing, but it does not cause stagnation; it can warm up, but it does not cause dryness. The kidney dislikes dryness, but it becomes dry when it is warmed up, like things on a heater always become dry.

Comparatively speaking, Bajitian is warm, but it does not cause too much dryness. In spite of that, the real effect of warming will inevitably be somewhat dry. Roucongrong can further reduce the dryness of Bajitian since Roucongrong not only can warm up without causing dryness, it can also warm up and even moisten and nourish Yin at the same time. Therefore, Bajitian (tending to Yang) and Roucongrong (tending to Yin) are often used together to bring out the best in each other.

Yinyanghuo (Epimedium)

Yinyanghuo, also called Xianlingpi in Chinese, is mainly produced in the northwest of Sichuan province of China. This medicine, pungent and warm in properties, is able to enter Mingmen (life-gate), liver and stomach meridians in the Lower Jiao. It has medicinal ascending and descending effects.

Strongly Tonifying the Life-gate

Yinyanghuo is often used together with Chinese yam. Chinese yam used as an envoy medicine of Yinyanghuo can enter the spleen and lungs, and take Yinyanghuo to the place where it should go. When used with yam, Yinyanghuo can warm the Middle Jiao more intensively and better activate the function of the Middle Jiao. The Middle Jiao is the biochemical source of Qi and blood, and also the biochemical source of body fluid. To warm up the Lower Jiao needs to replenish Qi and blood, so the Middle Jiao must be invigorated first.

To enter the life-gate is to replenish the life-gate fire greatly. The life gate is in between the two kidneys. The life-gate fire is the driving force for the T&T of the spleen and stomach and the pneumatolysis of the bladder. Only when there is fire in the life gate can a person be full of vitality. If the life-gate fire is falling into a decline, one will then become withered. Yinyanghuo can be used to replenish the life-gate fire with great effect.

When the life-gate fire is falling into a decline, wind-cold damp pathogens can easily invade into the body. But after the life-gate fire is replenished, and is becoming stronger again, the wind-cold damp pathogens will be easily eliminated. Some people drink Yinyanghuo-soaked liquor branded "Xianlingpi", which is acceptable. It can warm the kidneys and the life gate to activate the healthy Qi of the human body for driving out the wind-cold damp pathogens with a better effect in treating rheumatism.

Estrus Promotion and Yang Tonification

Yinyanghuo can enter the liver meridian to activate the liver Qi. As it is known, the liver is the organ that governs emotions. The Chinese character "情" (qíng, means "emotion" in English) is composed of "忄"(means "heart") in the left, and "青"("qīng", means "green") in the right. The part of "忄" in the left implies that emotion is originated from the heart, while "青"(qīng) corresponds to the liver, implying that emotion also comes from the liver. So, it can be seen that "情" (qíng) is the result of interaction between the heart and liver. The heart controls mental activities, which is intangible; the liver stores blood, which is tangible. Emotion is a combination of the intangible and the tangible. On the tangible level, emotion depends on the liver. The sensitive parts of the human body, the positions where one feels emotional, are all on the liver meridian. Yinyanghuo enters the liver meridian to activate the liver Qi, by which it induces emotion.

At the same time, Yinyanghuo also enters the stomach meridian, which means it cancure ED (erectile dysfunction). The penis is called "宗筋" (zōng jīn, means "urogenital region" in English) in TCM. The liver governs the anadesma, and Zongjin (urogenital region) also belongs to the liver. The penis, in essence, is an anadesma that can carry on the family line, so it is called "宗筋" ["zōng jīn", "宗" ("zōng) in Chinese means patriarchal clan]. Zongjin also belongs to the stomach meridian. The stomach is a hollow organ with much Qi and blood. Only when the stomach gives much impetus and stronger foundation can the Zongjin become erect. Yinyanghuo also enters the stomach meridian to stir up stomach Qi, activate Yang of the liver and stomach, and stimulate Qi and blood, hence, the trouble of ED will naturally be overcome.

Yinyanghuo can enter the large intestine channel, which means it can descend since Qi in the large intestine is going downwards. This then helps stool to be released. Yinyanghuo is pungent and warm in nature, so, it can go upwards. Entering the liver meridian, it is also going upwards. In one word, Yinyanghuo can help to achieve medicinal ascending and descending effects. As an herb, it is relatively vivacious in nature, and easy to use.

Uses of Yinyanghuo in Formulas

Yinyanghuo warms the liver and kidney Yang, and it is often matched with Shajili (astragali complanati semen), Gouqizi (fructus lycii), Roucongrong, Wuweizi (fructus schisandrae chinensis), Niuxi (radix achyranthis bidentatae), Shanyurou (common macrocarpium fruit) etc., among which Shajili is for nourishing the liver and kidneys; Gouqizi is for warming the liver and kidneys; Roucongrong is for nourishing both the kidney Yin and Yang; Shanyurou, sour in taste, is for astringing the life essence, warming and nourishing the liver and kidneys; and Wuweizi is able to converge the life essence of the five internal organs.

When tonifying Yang, one must pay attention to convergence/astringency and storing. Tonifying Yin can subdue Yang. In case one only tonifies Yang but not Yin, fire may rise. Or in case one only tonifies Yang but does not restrain it, Yang will run out. This is the reason why Shanyurou and Wuweizi must be used to keep tonification and convergence going in parallel.

Shanyurou can mildly tonify Yin and Yang since it is sweet and sour in taste and partial to warmth in nature. In terms of specific functions, it not only can tonify Yin but also Yang in a very mild way. Therefore, Shanyurou is used in **Liuwei Dihuang Pill** and the case referred here as well. When these medicines are used together with Yinyanghuo, they not only will make Yinyanghuo tonify Yang but also take the tonification of Yin into account.

It should also be noted that in the process of tonifying the kidneys, one should try to guide the tonifying effects downwards since the kidneys are in the Lower Jiao. Only when the medical effect is guided quickly into the Lower Jiao, can it play its function on the right path.

Shajili, Shanyurou, Gouqizi, Roucongrong are all warm medicines for Yin tonification, while Yinyanghuo is also pungent and warm, and it helps tonify both Yin and Yang. Wuweizi is used here for astringency purpose and Niuxi for guiding medical effects downwards. Attention should be paid to the medical orientation in medication as Niuxi here is to guide medical effects downwards. Jiegeng (platycodon grandiflorum) must not be used here since it may cause the medical effects of the other herbs to go upwards. Otherwise, in case of the medical effects going upwards to the heart and lungs, the patients will get inflamed immediately and will feel rotten.

Contraindications of Yinyanghuo

Some men are especially excitable and prone to erection, but cannot maintain a course, which probably stems from a fire deficiency. Such a symptom cannot be treated with Yinyanghuo.

Yinyanghuo should also be used with caution in case a man suffers from nocturnal emission or spermatorrhea at night. Spermatorrhea can be divided into nocturnal emission in dreams and that without dreams. Spermatorrhea without dreams may arise from the kidney deficiency and failure to astringe the vital life essence, so Yinyanghuo can be used under appropriate circumstances. In case spermatorrhea is always accompanied by only a transient joy, or the so-called wet dream, that is probably due to fire in the kidneys. In such a case, tonics like Yinyanghuo should not be used again, or else, it will not only fail to tonify its primordial Yang, but will fuel its pathogenic fire instead.

In case urine is yellow or reddish in color, it is undoubted that endogenous fire is haunting in the Lower Jiao. In such a case, Yinyanghuo should be used with much caution, too.

In addition, attention must be given to the use of Yinyanghuo in the cases of the symptoms like dry mouth, Yin deficiency, and damp-heat in the Lower Jiao. Dry mouth means there is fire, and Yin deficiency is also prone to endogenous fire and even to damp-heat. Therefore, it is necessary to give priority to dispersing pathogens first, and then moisten and nourish the fire with mild medicines rather than tonifying fire in a hurry.

Xianmao (Rhizoma Curculiginis)

Xianmao can also enter the liver, kidneys, and the life gate to tonify fire and Yang.

Warming the Liver and Kidneys and Nourishing Anadesma

Xianmao is a kind of grass. According to the legend, it is said that sheep will have extra tendons if they eat such grass. The liver governing anadesma means that Xianmao can enter the liver to nourish anadesma. Sheep have flesh and tendons in their bodies. After they eat Xianmao, the sheep will have much more tendon volume, and the muscle and tendons in their bodies will become extremely thick and large. Thus, the sheep would become extremely strong. The meat of such kind of sheep is very helpful for warming life essence and blood. This reminds us that Xianmao can warm the liver and nourish the muscle and tendon.

Xianmao is milder in its medical property than Yinyanghuo, with its aphrodisiac effect being far less than Yinyanghuo, but it can warm the liver more effectively than Yinyanghuo.

Bawei Pill plus Xianmao Being More Effective

Xianmao can tonify the kidney Yang. Fuzi and Rougui are two standard and easily controlled medicines that are commonly used to tonify the kidney Yang, but Xianmao is somewhat weird in this aspect. Generally, when standard medicine fails to work quickly for treatment of a disease, some specific and weird medicines may be used for certain effects.

Days ago, an old man who was suffering from kidney Qi deficiency with frequent urination even could not restrain himself from urinating into his pants while coughing. Initially, a doctor gave him a prescription containing herbal ingredients of **Guifu Dihuang Pill** plus some astringent herbs, which took both the astringency and clarity of dampness into consideration. That was a very good prescription, but the patient did not recover after drinking over 30 doses. Then, on the basis of this prescription, I merely added Xianmao for him, he recovered by taking only a few doses.

How was it so? That in fact is just one of my tricks. **Guifu Dihuang Pill** plus Xianmao can intensify the potence of warming and tonifying the Lower Jiao with a quicker effect. That is also an empirical formula passed down from mouth to mouth regarding the combination of the weird and the standard medicines, which has never been systematically illustrated in medical books.

Buguzhi(Fructus Psoraleae)

Characteristics of Buguzhi

Buguzhi, also called Poguzhi, or Huguzi and other names with similar pronunciations. This medicine can warm the kidneys, while the kidneys govern the bone, so it means Buguzhi is good for bones, for which Buguzhi is generally accepted as its Chinese name.

Buguzhi is a kind of dark brown oblate seed, produced in Sichuan, Guangdong and Guangxi provinces of China. It is pungent, hot and dry in properties, aromatic in smell, bitter and sweet in taste. It is more descending than it is ascending in nature. It can tonify the spleen and warm the kidneys. Meanwhile, it is able to promote dampness and heat, therefore, those who suffer from serious dampness and heat, or Yin deficiency with heat should avoid using Buguzhi.

On Dampness and Heat

In case of damp-heat, it is advisable to clear the damp-heat first, and not to use the warm medicines rashly. Otherwise, when the heat gets worse, more dampness will converge, making dampness and heat intertwined. The human body is an organism integrating Yin and Yang, which is a physiological state. Only when Yin and Yang are held together can the human body have normal physiological activities. In case that Yin and Yang are incompatible, Yin will change into dampness and Yang will change into heat. In other words, dampness becomes the morbid Yin and heat becomes morbid Yang. Yin and Yang are intertwined, and dampness and heat can also be intertwined. Yin intertwining with Yang will be like husband embracing wife, showing warm humanity. However, entanglement of dampness and heat will be like adulterer and a prostitute conspiring together, which is bound to be immoral. Meanwhile, the dampness and heat, once intertwined, are not easily separated, which will certainly bring many adverse effects on the human body.

The liver has Yin and Yang. When the liver Yin and Yang are in harmony, the liver will be subsumed to Yin in nature and Yang in function. Yin in nature means that the liver stores blood. Yang in function means the liver governs dispersion and ascending, which is also related to sexual passion. When the two are not in harmony, damp-heat will arise. The liver is most afraid of damp-heat, and many liver diseases just arise from the damp-heat.

The kidney Yin and Yang should also hold together. All the five internal organs can store life essence that ultimately resides in the kidneys. The kidneys store the primordial life essence of the human body, requiring the kidney Yang to warm and nourish it in order to keep it active. The kidney Yang is the fire of the life gate between the two kidneys. It not only warms Yin of both kidneys, but also warms the bladder to promote the bladder to carry on pneumatolysis. Meanwhile, it is also necessary to warm up the spleen and stomach in order to promote the decomposition function of the spleen and stomach so that the spleen and stomach can maintain normal digesting function. This is the normal physiological state of kidney Yin and Yang. In case the state is broken or becomes disharmonious, part of the kidney Yin will change into dampness, and part of the kidney Yang will change into heat. The dampness intertwined with heat in the kidneys will result in various diseases like prostatitis and various stones, which are all related to damp-heat in the kidneys. Therefore, at the time of treatment of such diseases, one must never forget to clear the damp-heat in the kidneys.

Regulating the Fire of the Heart and Kidney

Buguzhi not only can warm and invigorate the kidney Yang, but also restrain the mind and make the fire of pericardium communicate with the fire of life gate in order to harmonize the endogenous fire in body.

The pericardium fire is actually the heart fire, and life gate fire is actually the kidney fire. The human body is a small universe or a small world of nature. Analogically, one may take the fire of nature as the fire of human body. The heart fire is just like the fire of the sun in the sky. The fire of the sun descends, and everything depends on the sun to grow. The kidney fire is like the underground fire, which is dispersing outwards. The two kinds of fire interact mutually to form a warm earth, unlike the other cold or hot planets. The heart fire and kidney fire intersect, just like the fire of the sun echoing the fire from the earth core. All changes on the earth, the passing of time, thunder, wind and rain are related to the mutual waning and waxing and interaction of the two fires. For instance, the information about the weather forecast regarding the weather changes is not only determined by the sky but also by the earth. It is the result of the interaction and compromise between Qi of the sky and Qi of the earth.

Buguzhi is aromatic in smell, entering the heart; it is bitter in taste, going downwards; acerb in taste, astringing the heart fire and guiding it downwards to warm the kidneys. It can also warm to nourish the kidney Yang to make the kidney fire flow upwards to the heart. And thus, the heart fire and kidney fire are regulated harmoniously.

Astringing Function of Buguzhi and the Qing'e Pill

Buguzhi can nourish the primordial Yang and enrich bone marrow. When both kidney Yin and Yang are sufficient and the kidneys are well nourished, the bone marrow will be enriched accordingly. Buguzhi is not only acrid, aromatic and dry, but also a little acerb, so it has the function of inducing astringency. Many kidney-warming medicines have the dispersing effect, like Yinyanghuo, a kind of leaf, which has a stronger dispersing effect but is not astringent. Therefore, those who take it will feel erotogenic. However, Buguzhi is different in that it can nourish the kidney Yang and induce astringency at the same time. Because of its astringing effect, it can restrain urination, astringe semen, and have many other effects. Thus, a well-known formula called **Qing'e Pill** comes into being.

The formula of Qing'e Pill contains the following herbs:

Yan Duzhong (salty eucommia ulmoides), Buguzhi (fructus psoraleae), Hutaorou (walnut meat).

In reality, there are many versions of **Qing'e Pill**. Here is the most typical version chosen for analysis. Hutaorou is actually the commonly-used Chinese name "Hetaorou". "Hetao" (walnut) has a very hard shell outside, just like the skull. Inside is the walnut meat like the human brain in shape with many folds. The brain is a sea of marrow, as it is always called, so walnut meat can tonify the kidneys and brain since they are similar in shape as similar things always attract each other. Walnut meat is mainly for nourishing Yin and replenishing fluid/water. Buguzhi is for nourishing Yang and invigorating fire. When the two medicines are used together, the fluid/water and fire will coordinate with each other, and Yin and Yang will promote mutually. Duzhong (eucommia ulmoides) enters the Lower Jiao, dispelling pathogenic wind, eliminating cold and dampness, and playing the function of warm tonification. The three medicines used together with the astringing, dispelling and tonifying functions will have good effects on the treatment of lumbago and soreness and weakness of waist and knees arising from kidney deficiency.

Sishen Pill

The formula of **Sishen Pill** contains the following herbs:

Buguzhi (fructus psoraleae), Wuzhuyu (fructus evodiae), Roudoukou (nutmeg) and Wuweizi (fructus schisandrae chinensis).

Sishen Pill is a famous formula for treating diarrhea before dawn, which usually arises from the factor that the kidney fire is insufficient to warm the spleen and the spleen is too insufficient to induce astringency. Buguzhi has the effect of inducing astringency and controlling depletion. Wuzhuyu warms the liver and also enters the spleen and stomach. Roudoukou warms the spleen. Wuweizi has the function of convergence.

The time before dawn (the period of the day from 3:00 a. m. to 5:00 a. m.) is the darkest moment when Yin is very vigorous and Yang is still weak. At this moment, the kidney fire cannot warm the spleen and Yang cannot ascend rapidly, because of which diarrhea will occur at this moment. Therefore, it is necessary to warm the liver, kidneys and spleen to support the Yang of the five internal organs from the three meridians, i. e., foot Taiyin spleen meridian, foot Shaoyin kidney meridian and foot Jueyin liver meridian, followed by inducing astringency, and then the diarrhea before dawn will be cured.

Of course, in the process of treatment, some other medicines may be added in this formula to give consideration to the treatment of other symptoms, since those who suffer from diarrhea before dawn usually have poor appetite with some symptoms like soreness of waist and abdominal pain, cold limbs, lack of vigor, as well as deep, slow and weak pulse, for which the **Sishen Pill** is quite effective. However, those who suffer diarrhea before dawn have extremely good appetite and the symptom of a surging pulse, which will indicate that those patients may have stomach heat. In such a case, Wuzhuyu should be used with caution, but corrigent such as **Qingwei San** may be needed to counteract it. In short, diarrhea before dawn should be treated dased on syndrome differentiation rather than according to the name of "Wugengxie" (diarrhea before dawn) by simply using **Sishen Pill**.

Sishen Pill is actually evolved from the formula of **Ershen Pill** that contains only two herbs: Buguzhi and Roudoukou. When the kidney fire is not sufficient to warm the spleen, Buguzhi can be used for warming the kidneys and Roudoukou for tonifying the spleen. This formula is a specific prescription for the case of kidney fire failing to warm the spleen. The two herbs are often integrated into the other formulas, like the **Liushen Pill,** which is will be discussed in the following.

Summary of Warm and Hot Medicines

Many kidney-warming medicines have been discussed so far. In fact, as to warming, it mainly refers to the process of warming from the lower parts, so there are many sayings in Chinese like "The foot wants keeping warm and the head wants keeping cool", or "The head won't be frozen to death, and the rear won't be warmed to death". After all, the foot is at the bottom of the human body, and the three channels of the liver meridian, spleen meridian and kidney meridian all pass through the feet. This is why "the foot wants keeping warm". To warm the feet means to warm the liver, spleen and kidneys. The warm medicines normally used are also for warming the liver, spleen and kidneys. There are also medicines for warming the lungs, but they are not so important as those for warming the liver, spleen and kidneys. After warming the kidneys, the fire will then slowly go up and warm the lungs and heart. Therefore, the warming process always starts with warming the liver, spleen and kidneys.

Many friends are concerned about Fuzi, which is "a valiant soldier" (a strong medicine). It plays a lot of roles, but it has to be used appropriately. So, it will be kept to the last: "the last but not the least". All the kidney-warming medicines introduced in the above sections are soft and mild and friendly to human bodies if appropriately used. As for Fuzi, of course, it has to be used properly, and it is better to use it for the cases where it is suitable, but it should never be used except when is necessary. The so-called "making good use of Fuzi" does not mean that it must be used, but only that it should be used where it is indeed necessary. Some doctors might have never used Fuzi in their whole life, but that does not mean they are not good at using it since they use it only when they feel it is necessary.

第五章　其他温肾阳的药

我们继续讲几味其他温肾的药。

温肾其实就是温肾阳，我们知道肝、脾、肾，尤其是肝肾是在下焦，是属阴。本来五脏都是属阴，肝脾肾在中下焦的就更属阴。脾为足太阴，为阴中之至阴；肝为足厥阴，体阴而用阳；肾是少阴，主水而属阴。阴脏容易有沉寒积冷，所以要阴中有阳，需要经常温一温。

我们讲过，要兼顾肾阳肾阴。阴阳就像一盏油灯，当油烧尽了，快要干的时候，灯火也会随之变得微弱，油快干了就好比阴虚，灯火随之变得微弱好比阳虚，所以在温阳的时候，在修剪灯芯的时候，也要注意加油，油足了，再修剪一下灯芯，再用火柴那么小的火把它点着了，油灯就很旺了，这是阴阳之道。张景岳讲："善养阴者必于阳中求阴，善养阳者必于阴中求阳"，这话很有深意。温阳，切不可急功近利，一下子用附子、肉桂等燥烈的大热药去温它，因为"壮火食气"，会导致不好的结果。这就需要有很多较为平和的温肾之品。

肉苁蓉

肉苁蓉性状

肉苁蓉，我们看它的名字：肉，说明它有补养的性质，苁蓉，如果去掉草字头，就是人的一种行为品格了，从容不迫。肉苁蓉能补阴，也能养肾阳。

肉苁蓉产在西北，现在蒙古、新疆这一带都有。古人讲，肉苁蓉是马精落地后所化，其真假，我们暂且不论，但由此，我们应该联想到：马是属阳的，在十二地支中对应的是午，马跑得那么快那么烈，这说明马是属阳的；而精又是属阴的。既然是马精所化，那么它是阳中有阴、阴中有阳的。

肉苁蓉的特点是甘咸温润，它的颜色是黑的，外表有鳞片。一个大的、非常好的肉苁蓉能有人的胳膊那么大，它能益肾精，壮肾阳，它补养的速度比较缓慢，比较从容。

养肾通便

肉苁蓉还有滑肠的作用，一是因为它养阴，养阴就能滑肠。二是因为它能温肾阳，肾阴、肾阳都充足了，肾司二便的能力变强了，会让人的大便更加通畅。总之，它有往下滑的作用，这意味着，脾虚便溏者要慎用。肉苁蓉是有一些滋腻的，脾虚，运化不动就不要吃它了。

反过来讲，很多老人都会便秘，大便特别干，往往是因为阴虚血枯，没有足够的津液去滋润大便，所以很多老人要用开塞露、水之类的来灌肠，把里边的大便滋润一下，才能解下来。这样的老年人便秘，就可以用肉苁蓉。

老年人往往肾虚，肉苁蓉既能够养肾，又能养血，还能通他的大便，一举多得。现在很多老年人便秘，他们私下里方法有很多：有的老人每天用5克大黄泡水喝，大便能解下来，但是喝久了就出现问题了，吃不下饭了；有的老人用决明子泡水喝，决明子也是凉的，油润的，但喝久了脾胃也喝坏了，或者虚风喝动了，眼底喝出血了；还有的老人用番泻叶泡水喝，也能够缓解一时。但这些药都是不能久用的。唯独肉苁蓉，如果真的是血枯阴虚导致的大便干结便秘的话，肉苁蓉是可以久用的。肉苁蓉在《神农本草经》中被列为上品，是久服轻身延年的一种药。而大黄、决明子、番泻叶都是不能久用的，没有补养的作用。

巴戟天

巴戟天性状

巴戟天能补阴中之阳，经常与肉苁蓉一起用，相得益彰。巴戟天是山上一种草的根。采根类药，一般在农历的二月或八月。二月，草还没有长出来，底下的根正蓄势待发，八月，草木凋零，精华已收藏在了根里，所以药力都比较足。巴戟天的形状很像丹皮，都是边有一层很厚的皮，里边有芯，用的时候要把里边的芯去掉。只是丹皮是白色的，有些稍微有点发赤或者发黄，巴戟天的外表有点发红，里边芯有点发黑。

巴戟天辛甘苦温，入肝肾血分，能够温肾，起萎强阳。阳痿往往是因为肾阳不足，无法鼓动气血，巴戟天来温肾阳。

巴戟天的温通作用

因为温通，巴戟天又能治各种疝块、脚气之类。温，就能散全身的风寒湿痹。

当肾阳虚的时候，卫气随之而弱，外邪就更容易入侵人体，首先入侵下体，导致腰酸腿痛，大家很容易想到用独活之类辛燥的药去治疗，殊不知风寒湿邪之所以只侵袭你而不侵袭别人，是因为别人肝肾之阳很旺，能够抵御更多的风寒湿邪，而你的肝肾之阳不旺，所以邪气也更容易侵犯你，"邪之所凑，其气必虚"嘛。

因此，在补肝肾阳虚的同时又能散邪，这是巴戟天一个独到的作用。其实，很多温肾阳的药都有这个作用。

巴戟天、肉苁蓉配伍

巴戟天是补而不滞、温而不燥的一味药。肾是怕燥的，一温就容易燥，好比放在暖气片上的东西，就会很干燥。

但温而不燥，也只是相对而言的。温肯定还是会燥，用肉苁蓉可以继续减小巴戟天的燥性，肉苁蓉不仅仅温而不燥，而且温而滋润、养阴，所以巴戟天和肉苁蓉会经常一起用，它们一个偏阳一点，一个偏阴一点，放在一起相得益彰。

淫羊藿

淫羊藿也叫仙灵脾，主要产在四川省的西北部。此药辛温，入下焦的命门、肝经、胃经，它可升可降。

峻补命门

一般，淫羊藿常配山药。山药是淫羊藿的使药，入脾、肺，它能把淫羊藿带到该去的地方。与山药一起用，淫羊藿温中焦的力度就会更大，更能调动中焦机能。中焦为气血生化之源，也是人体津液的生化之源，温下焦是需要气血去补充的，所以必须先调动中焦。

入命门就能峻补命门之火，命门在两肾之间，命门之火，是脾胃运化的动力，也是膀胱气化的动力。命门必须有火，人才能生气勃勃。命门火衰，人也就萎靡不振了。用淫羊藿可以峻补命门之火。

当命门火衰的时候，风寒湿邪就很容易入侵身体。命门的火补起来以后，火力壮了，风寒湿邪就容易被驱逐出去。有人用淫羊藿来泡酒喝，这是可以的，叫一味仙灵脾酒，它通过温肾、温命门来调动人体的正气，把风寒湿邪排出去，治风湿的效果比较好。

催情壮阳

淫羊藿入肝经，能动肝气。我们知道，肝是主感情的器官，"情"字就是一个竖心旁，一个青字，竖心旁意指情来源于心，青则对应肝，意指情也来源于肝。情，是心和肝相互作用的结果。心主神明，它是无形的；肝藏血，是有形的；情是无形与有形的一种结合。在有形的层面，情取决于肝。我们看看，人体的敏感部位，一摸就会动情的地方，都在肝经上。淫羊藿入肝经，动肝气，并藉此以催情。

同时，淫羊藿还入胃经，这意味着它能治疗阳痿。阴茎，在中医里叫宗筋。肝主筋，宗筋也属肝，阴茎在本质上就是筋，而且是一根能传宗接代的筋，所以叫"宗筋"。宗筋又属胃，胃为多气多血之府，必须胃给它动力、给它物质基础，它才能勃起。淫羊藿入胃经，能鼓动胃气。鼓动肝胃之阳，振奋气血，阳痿自然能勃起。

淫羊藿还能入大肠经，这意味着它能降，因为大肠之气是往下降的，大便因此才能出来。淫羊藿辛温，所以能往上升。入肝经，也是升的。所以，淫羊藿这味药可升可降，它的性质是比较活泼的，在运用的时候也比较好掌握。

淫羊藿的配伍方

淫羊藿温肝肾之阳，常配沙蒺藜、枸杞子、肉苁蓉、五味子、牛膝、山萸肉等。沙蒺藜是补肝肾的；枸杞子是温肝肾的；肉苁蓉既养肾阴又养肾阳；山萸肉酸收敛精，且温养肝肾；五味子能收敛五脏精气。

在补阳的时候，一定要注意收敛、潜藏。补阴则能潜阳，如果你只补阳而不补阴，就会补出火来。如果只补阳而不收敛，那么阳气就会外越。这就是要配上五味子和山萸肉的道理，边补边收。

山萸肉平补阴阳，本质上是甘酸偏温，但在具体的作用上，既补阴又补阳，补得非常平和。所以在六味地黄丸里面用到了山萸肉，在这里面也用到了山萸肉。这些药再配上淫羊藿，会让淫羊藿不只补阳，同时兼顾补阴。

还要注意，补肾把药力往下引，因为肾就在下焦，药力迅速归于下焦，才能补得其所。沙蒺藜、山萸肉、枸杞子、肉苁蓉都是补阴的温药，淫羊藿也是辛温，阴阳兼顾。然后用五味子一收，用牛膝往下一引。用药要注意它的方向性，这里，用了牛膝就把药力往下引了。千万不能用桔梗，否则会把药力往上提，提到心肺，人马上就上火，而且会很难受。

沙蒺藜、山萸肉、枸杞子肉苁蓉都是补阴的温药，淫羊藿也是辛温，阴阳兼顾。然后用五味子一收，用牛膝往下一引。用药要注意它的方向性，这里，用了牛膝就把药力往下引了。千万不能用桔梗，否则会把药力往上提，提到心肺，人马上就上火，而且会很难受。

淫羊藿使用禁忌

有的人，特别容易兴奋，容易勃起，勃起后又坚持不了多久，这很可能是有虚火，就不能用淫羊藿了。

晚上有梦遗、遗精的也要慎用。遗精分有梦而遗和无梦而遗。如果不做梦就遗精，这可能是因为肾虚不能固摄精气，在合适的情况下，淫羊藿倒还可以用。如果遗精总伴随着一场春梦，那是因为肾里有火，就不要用这些补阳的药了。否则，不仅不能补它的真阳，反而助长了它的邪火。

如果小便黄或者发红，明摆着是下焦有火无疑，也要慎用淫羊藿。

还有遇到口干、阴虚、下焦湿热的情况，用淫羊藿也要非常谨慎。口干意味者有火，阴虚也容易生火，而且容易导致湿热，要先以散邪为主，然后以平和之药润养，不宜急于补火。

仙茅

仙茅也是入肝肾、命门，补火壮阳的一味药。

温肝肾而养筋

它是一种草，相传羊如果吃了这种草，它身上的筋就会特别多。肝主筋，则意味着仙茅能入肝养筋。本来羊身上有肉也有筋，吃了仙茅，身上的筋就会变得特别粗、特别多，羊的力气就特别大。吃这种羊的肉，是非常温补精血的。此说是否属实，我没有考证，但至少，它提示我们，仙茅是能够温肝养筋的。

仙茅的药性，比淫羊藿柔和一些，催情的作用远远不如淫羊藿，但温肝的作用却比淫羊藿大一些。

八味丸加仙茅力量更足

仙茅能补益肾阳。附子、肉桂也补益肾阳，但附子、肉桂是最常用的、很正的、很老实的两味药，而仙茅则有点偏，往往，当正药不能迅速奏效的时候，用点偏药，能速建奇功。

前一段时间，有位老人，肾气虚了，小便特别多，老上厕所，到后来就小便不禁了，有时候一不小心，咳嗽一声小便都会出来，或者一不小心裤子就尿湿了。以前找的大夫给他开的就是桂附地黄丸的汤剂，再加一些收涩的药，有涩有利，寒温兼顾，方子开得非常好，一点都不错，但是他一直喝了三十多剂，病都没好。我在这个方子基础上加了一味仙茅，只吃了几剂，小便就收住了。

为什么？这其实是一个秘传的小窍门，只可意会不可言传。桂附地黄丸加一个仙茅，能够令温补下焦的力度变得更大，起效更快。这也是偏正结合的一个经验之谈，书里不可能系统给你讲，但这是师门口口相传的一些用药经验。

补骨脂

补骨脂性状

补骨脂，也写作破故纸、胡故子，等等，发音都相似，说明这是以字表音的。它能够温肾，肾主骨，所以对骨头又有好处，所以后来大家就公认"补骨脂"这个名字。

补骨脂是一种黑褐色的扁圆形的种子，产在四川、两广。它的性质是辛热香燥、苦甘并存、降多于升，能补脾、温肾。它能够助湿热，如果湿热严重，就不要用它了，阴虚有热的也不要用。

湿热论

遇到有湿热，宜先清利湿热，不要冒然的用这些温药，否则，热一加重，又会收敛更多的湿，让湿热进一步交缠。人体是阴阳，阴阳是一种生理状态。阴阳交抱，人体才有正常的生理活动。当阴阳不协调的时候，阴就成了湿，阳就成了热。或者说，湿就是病态的阴，热就是病态的阳。阴阳是交抱的，湿热也可以纠缠在一起。阴阳交抱，就像夫妇交抱，人道以成，这是很温馨的，而湿热纠缠，好比奸夫淫妇，狼狈为奸，必伤风化，它们在一起也不容易分开，给人体带来很多不利的影响。

肝有肝阴、肝阳，当肝阴肝阳协调的时候，肝就是体阴而用阳。肝体阴，就是肝藏血；肝用阳，就是肝主疏泄、主升发，而且关乎人的情欲。当这两者不协调的时候，湿热就产生了，肝最怕湿热，很多肝病都是湿热导致的。

肾阴肾阳也应该是交抱的。五脏皆能藏精，五脏之精又终归于肾，肾藏的是人体的真精，这真精需要肾阳温养着它，才有活性。肾阳是两肾之间的命门之火，它不但要温煦双肾之阴，还要温煦膀胱，促进膀胱的气化；还要往上温煦脾胃，促进脾胃的腐熟水谷，让脾胃能够正常的消化，这是肾阴肾阳的正常的生理状态。如果这个状态被打破了，不和谐了，那么一部份肾阴就变成湿，肾阳有一部份就变成热，湿热交织在肾里边，导致各种病，什么前列腺炎、各种结石，都跟肾里边的湿热都有关，在治这些病的时候，不要忘掉清利肾里的湿热。

调心肾之火

不仅仅温补肾阳，补骨脂还能收敛神明，让心包之火与命门之火相通，协调体内的火。

心包火其实就是心火，命门之火其实就是肾火。人体是一个小宇宙、小自然，我们可以用大自然的火来比喻人体的火，心火相当于天上太阳的火，它是往下降的，万物生长靠太阳；肾火相当于地底之火，它是要往外透散的。这两种火相互作用，才形成一个温暖的地球，而不是其他冷冰冰的或忽冷忽热的星球。心火和肾火是相交的，就好像太阳之火与地心之火的呼应。大地上的一切变化，寒来暑往，打雷、刮风、下雨都与这两个火的相互消长、相互作用有关。我们经常讲天气预报，其实天气不只是天决定的，也是地决定的，是天之气与地之气相互作用、相互妥协的结果。

补骨脂芳香入心，苦而能降，涩而能收，能收敛心火，使之向下而温肾；又能温补肾阳，使肾火向上而交于心。在一上一下之间，心肾之火得到调节。

固涩作用与青娥丸

补骨脂能养元阳，充实骨髓。当肾阴肾阳都足，肾得到了很好的滋养，骨髓自然充实。补骨脂不仅辛辣香燥，还有一点涩味，有固涩的作用。很多温肾的药都有发散的作用，比如淫羊藿是一种叶子，发散的作用较强，并不固涩，人吃了以后就会有控制不住情欲的感觉。补骨脂不一样，它补肾阳，同时还能固涩。有固涩的作用，那它的用处就大了：能固涩小便，固涩精液，固涩很多的东西，由此有一个很有名的方叫青娥丸：

盐杜仲、补骨脂、胡桃肉。

青娥丸有很多版本，这是很有代表性的一个。胡桃肉就是核桃肉，核桃外面有一层很坚硬的壳，就像脑壳一样，里面核桃肉就像人的大脑，有很多褶皱，既然像大脑，而脑为髓海，那么核桃就能益肾、补脑，它们同气相求。胡桃肉主要是补阴的，补水的；补骨脂是补阳的，补火的。这两味药放在一起，有水火既济、阴阳相生的意思。杜仲是入下焦的，能散风寒湿邪，又有温补之功。三味药一起，且涩且散且补，治肾虚引起的腰痛、腰膝酸软效果很好。

四神丸

补骨脂、吴茱萸、肉豆蔻、五味子。

四神丸是治五更泻的名方。五更泻，往往是因为肾火不足以暖脾土，且脾虚不能固涩而引起的。补骨脂有收涩固脱的作用；吴茱萸是温肝的，同时还入脾胃；肉豆蔻是温脾的；五味子收敛。

寅时是黎明前最黑暗的时候，阴气很重，阳气尚弱。此时肾火不能暖脾土，阳气不足以迅速升发，大便就要泻出来，需要温肝、肾、脾，从足三阴扶助五脏之阳，再顺势收涩一下，大便就出不来了，五更泻也就治好了。

当然，在治疗的时候，我们还可以加其他的药来兼顾一下。五更泻的病人通常会不太想吃饭，腰酸腹痛、四肢发凉、没有力气的感觉，脉沉迟无力，这时候很适合用四神丸。如果某个五更泻病人却特别能吃，饭量特大，脉也洪大，这意味着他可能有胃热，此时就要慎用吴茱萸了，还应加其他的药来反佐它，比如清胃散。总之，要辨证论治，不能看到五更泻就用四神丸。

四神丸是从二神丸演变过来的，二神丸是由补骨脂和肉豆蔻组成的。当肾火不能暖脾土的时候，可以用补骨脂温肾，用肉豆蔻健脾。这个方子专治当肾火不能暖脾土的情况。这两味药也是经常会合到其他方子里去。以后我们还会讲到六神丸，六神丸是另外一个药了，和四神丸、二神丸关系不大。

温热药小结

前面讲了很多温肾的药。其实，温，主要是从下边温，所以，"足宜常温，头宜常凉"，"冻不死的脑袋，热不死的屁股"。因为足在人体的最下面，而肝脾肾三经都经过脚，它们都需要温暖，所以足宜常温。温足也就是温肝脾肾，我们用温药主要也是温肝脾肾。温肺的药虽然也有，但是它没有温肝脾肾的药那么重要。温了肾以后，火慢慢往上走，也能够温到肺和心。所以，用温药要从温肝脾肾开始。

很多朋友开始着急，问我怎么还不讲附子，附子我们留到最后再讲。附子是一员猛将，它有很多作用，但是这员猛将要用得恰如其分、恰到好处。前面我们介绍了温肾的药，它们都很温柔、很平和，用得好的话对人也非常好，我们要善用这些药。至于附子，当然也要善用，而且更要善于在最合适、最必要的时候用，不必要的时候就不用。所谓"善用附子"，不是说非得用，而是该用的时候用，不该用的时候不用。有的人一辈子没用过附子，但他依然是善用附子的，为什么呢？因为他在不该用的时候不用，不用是更大的用。

Chapter 6   Medicines for Warming the Liver and Spleen

This chapter will focus on the medicines for warming the liver and spleen.

The spleen, in the Middle Jiao, is subject to the foot Taiyin meridian. The liver and kidneys, in the Lower Jiao, are subject to the foot Jueyin and foot Shaoyin meridians respectively. Yin needs Yang, so the three meridians of the liver, spleen and kidneys need warming for Yang.

Wuzhuyu is often used for warming liver; Ganjiang (rhizoma zingiberis), Doukou (cardamun) and the like are normally for warming the spleen.

Wuzhuyu(Fructus Evodiae)

Wuzhuyu is a severely hot medicine, which should be distinguished from Shanzhuyu (cornus officinalis). In prescriptions, Wuzhuyu is usually written as Pao Wuyu (soaked fructus evodiae) and Shanzhuyu is written as Shanyurou (common macrocarpium fruit). In the ancient poem line "Bian Cha Zhuyu Shao Yi Ren" (Wearing Zhuyu in hair, but they found one pal in nowhere). There has been a constant dispute about whether Zhuyu in this line refers to Wuzhuyu or Shanzhuyu. Some people claim that it should be Wuzhuyu in that it is good to wear for its fragrance. However, Shanzhuyu is a smaller wild fruit that becomes red in autumn, sour and sweet, so it may also be possible to remind people of nourishing Yin in fall and winter by wearing it.

Wuzhuyu is similar to Huajiao (pricklyash peel), and its plant is also similar to that of Huajiao tree. But Huajiao is prone to going into the spleen and lung meridians, while Wuzhuyu is prone to going into the meridians of all the liver and kidneys, spleen and stomach to "dispel the wind-cold of Jueyin, dry the dampness of the spleen, and lower Qi to remove stagnation, and descend the turbid".

Danggui Sini Tang

The main effect of Wuzhuyu is to warm the liver and disperse the coldness of foot Jueyin. Regarding Wuzhuyu, there is a typical formula called **Danggui Sini Tang**.

The formula of **Danggui Sini Tang** contains the herbal ingredients:

Wuzhuyu (fructus evodiae), Danggui (angelica sinensis), Baishao (radix paeoniae alba), Guizhi (cassia bark), Xixin (asarum), Shengjiang (ginger), Gancao (liquorice), Tongcao (tetrapanax papyriferus).

Danggui Sini Tang is mainly used to treat Jueyin cold limbs and weak or imperceptible pulse. In case the liver suffers from coldness, the blood system will become cold. And then, the liver will be short of power, resulting in the reverse coldness over the body. Wuzhuyu is used in the formula to warm the liver, but which is not enough. Danggui and Baishao (often used as a pair) are used to soothe the liver and nourish Yin additionally, through which the new blood is generated. The function of Wuzhuyu is equivalent to refueling fire and Yang to the liver; The function of Danggui and Baishao is equivalent to refilling fluid and Yin to the liver. The liver is subsumed to Yin in physique and Yang in function. Wuzhuyu warming the liver is to strengthen its function and Danggui and Baishao nourishing the liver Yin is to consolidate its physique. Only when the physique and function are both properly treated, can the liver work normally. In this formula, Wuzhuyu, Danggui, Baishao are the three main ingredient medicines.

Xixin used with Guizhi functions to warm the kidneys. Guizhi activates the bladder Yang and disperses the coldness in the bladder meridian. When the bladder meridian properly plays its function of pneumatolysis, it will in return have a warming effect on the kidneys since the kidneys and bladder are playing the exterior and interior functions mutually. Xixin works to disperse the wind-cold in the kidney meridian.

Shengjiang and Gancao enter the Middle Jiao to warm the spleen. In fact, **Danggui Sini Tang** not only warms the liver, but also gives the consideration to the spleen and kidneys at the same time.

The cold limbs not only need warming up, but also need the warmth to go through the whole body. Tongcao is used here since it can alleviate fluid retention, which means it can clear the bladder damp-heat. With the clearing effect of Tongcao and warming effect of Guizhi, the bladder will be able to fully play its pneumatolysis function.

Siwu Tang can be analyzed from the perspective of the monarch-minister-assistant-envoy theory. Wuzhuyu as the monarch medicine can warm the liver; Guizhi, Xixin and Shengjiang as ministerial medicines warm the spleen and kidneys; Danggui and Baishao as assistant medicines function to nourish the liver and Yin; Tongcao as envoy medicines work to alleviate fluid retention and activate Yang.

Treatment of Hernia with Salty Wuyu and Xiaohuixiang (Fennel)

After being parched with saline water, Wuzhuyu can go downwards and warm the liver and kidneys since salty materials enter the kidneys. Wuzhuyu baked in saline water is often used to treat hernia. Hernia usually arises from coldness in the liver meridian, which obstructs Qi circulation; therefore, Qi must be regulated in the process of warming the liver. In case a little boy suffers from hernia, his scrotum on one side will droop down and become extremely large, which means some Qi falls down. In the serious case, the boy will feel terrible pain if touched. The foot Jueyin liver meridian going around the genital, genital diseases are always related to the liver, which can be differentiated by the meridians. Now that the liver is cold, Wuzhuyu can be used to warm it up. Meanwhile, the trouble itself is related to the genital, indicating that it does have something to do with the kidneys. The genital organ is sometimes called the outer kidneys. There are two inner kidneys inside the body, and in between them is the life gate; the external kidney has two testes with the penis in the middle. Thus, the inner kidneys and the outer kidneys are corresponding to each other with some similarities and isomorphism.

The stir-baked Wuzhuyu with saline water used with Xiaohuixiang is a commonly used medicine pair for the treatment of hernia. Xiaohuixiang is pungent and warm in properties. It can slightly warm the liver, but it can regulate Qi with a strong effect. The combination of the two medicines can warm and activate meridians, regulating Qi, and eliminatng the liver coldness. Thus, the stagnation arising from the liver coldness will be removed. Sometimes, the patient does not need to use this medicine, and he can simply apply such medicines to the scrotum, lower abdomen or groin directly, which also have a good effect.

Wuzhuyu Used with Mugua (Pawpaw)

Many people may have had the experience of a cramp in their legs. When it hurts, they will feel involuntary muscular contraction, as if one tendon is about to break. That is because there is coldness in the shank. Coldness causes contraction, resulting in the involuntary muscular contraction of meridians.

Moreover, cramps in the legs are also related to blood coldness. Blood vessels are flexible. Flexibility is related to tendons, but the liver governs anadesma, so flexibility is also related to the liver. When the liver is cold, Wuzhuyu is used to warm it up, which subsequently warms the blood and the blood vessels, too.

Mugua goes to the lower limbs. It tastes sour, and it can relieve stress and soften anadesma. Wuzhuyu plus Mugua (i. e., warm plus sour) can warm and activate circulation of blood and soften blood vessels to cure the cramps in legs.

Wuzhuyu is usually parched with vinegar. It is used here to invigorate blood circulation since the liver stores blood, and the sour taste of vinegar can help enter the liver more. Once the liver has sufficient power, blood will circulate more smoothly.

Wuzhuyu Tang

Wuzhuyu has another effect, namely, to dry dampness of the spleen. It is aromatic and dry, while the spleen likes fragrance and dryness. Wuzhuyu parched with Huanglian-soaked water will have the effect of stopping vomiting, especially effective for the treatment of acid saliva regurgitation. There is a classic formula related to Wuzhuyu called **Wuzhuyu Tang** for stopping vomiting. The formula comes from Zhang Zhongjing's *Shanghan Lun*.

Wuzhuyu Tang contains the following herbal ingredients:

Renshen (ginseng), Wuzhuyu (fructus evodiae), Shengjiang (ginger) and Dazao (jujube).

Shanghan Lun says: "Diseases of Shaoyin, with some manifestations of vomiting, cold limbs and dysphoria, can be treated with **Wuzhuyu Tang**." It can also be used for treatment of "deseases of Jueyin, vomiturition, spitting ptysis and headache". In a word, **Wuzhuyu Tang** can be used for treatment of the syndromes of the liver and stomach deficiency-cold, especially vomiting.

There are two kinds of vomiting: cold vomiting and hot vomiting. **Wuzhuyu Tang** cannot be used to cure the hot vomiting, but to cure the cold vomiting. Vomiting is a rising sign, indicating the existence of fire. Although it is cold fundamentally, vomiting, whenever occurs, is always related to heat. For instance, when the liver is cold, it will fall into shortage of power. Essentially, the liverwood should restrict the spleen-earth. However, if the spleen and stomach are not restricted by the liver-wood, they would produce dampness and floating heat. Under the action of such floating heat, the patient will start vomiting. Thus, Wuzhuyu should be stir-fried with Huanglian soaked water, since Huanglian can dry dampness of the spleen and clear the floating heat of the spleen meridian, which addresses both symptoms and root causes.

Zuojin Pill

Wuzhuyu is aromatic and hot in properties, and it can dry the spleen dampness. Huanglian is bitter and cold in properties, and it can dry dampness. They are used in the formula to interact and restrict each other to tackle the symptoms and root causes at the same time. Wuzhuyu and Huanglian together make a formula called **Zuojin Pill**, which is often used for treatment of the acid regurgitation.

Sometimes, the patients may feel uncomfortable and noisy in the stomach and want to throw up, but fail to vomit anything. Occasionally, they may throw up a mouthful of gastric fluid, which is called acid regurgitation. Some people fail to spit out but swallow the gastric fluid unconsciously, which is called acid swallowing. Both acid regurgitation and swallowing in fact have the same name "acid regurgitation", i. e., a puff of gastric fluid flashing upward due to coldness or especially heat. Fire always inflames up, so the endogenous heat will cause the patients to throw up the staff in the stomach.

For the treatment of acid regurgitation, Wuzhuyu and Huanglian can be used based cold and heat syndrome differentiation. Generally speaking, Wuzhuyu is used in a smaller dosage of 2g while Huanglian is used in a relatively larger dosage around 5g. Previously, we mentioned the case of Wuzhuyu stir-fried with

Huanglian-soaked water, in which Wuzhuyu is the main herb, but here for curing acid regurgitation due to heat, Huanglian should be taken as the main herb and Wuzhuyu as the auxiliary herb.

Zuojin Pill is used to cure acid regurgitation. In case that it cannot stop acid regurgitation, add some Walengzi (concha arcae) and Haipiaoxiao (cuttlebone). Walengzi is a kind of shellfish that can relieve hyperacidity. Haipiaoxiao is the bone of cuttlefish, which has a very good effect of astringing ulcer. In most cases, severe acid regurgitation will be accompanied by gastric ulcer, so Haipiaoxiao used here can kill two birds with one stone.

While using Wuzhuyu, Li Shizhen normally did not add Huanglian but Fuling instead. For those who suffer from excessive phlegm or acid regurgitation due to phlegm and retained fluid, Wuzhuyu, Huanglian and Fuling can all be added in the formula. Those who suffer from acid regurgitation stemming from phlegm and retained fluid may not have too many heat symptoms, so Huanglian is not necessary. The phlegm and retained fluid often arise from the failure of T&T of the spleen. The spleen can carry on transportation only when it is warm. The spleen likes warm, dry, tasteless and permeable staff, but Huanglian is bitter and cold. In that case, Huanglian, if added, will run in the opposite direction. Therefore, in clinical practice, pathogenesis must be carefully examined and diagnosed so that the flexible actions regarding medication are to be taken accordingly.

Zuojin Pill and Wuji Pill

According to the *Wuxing Doctrine*, the metal restricts the wood, so, assistance to the Metal can make it more powerful to restrict the wood. The wood out of the Five Elements (metal, wood, water, fire and earth) correspond to the sour of the five tastes (sour, sweet, bitter, pungent and salt). So, to restrict the wood means to restrain the taste of sour. Hence, to put it simply and clearly, **Zuojin Pill** is a medicine for restraining the taste of sour.

The predecessor of **Zuojin Pill** is **Wuji Pill**, containing three herbs: Wuzhuyu, Huanglian and Baishao. These three herbs used together are mainly for curing vomiting and diarrhea with the help of the sour and bitter tastes, regulating the function of the liver and spleen, clearing heat and harmonizing the stomach. But this formula was seldom used. According to Zhu Danxi (medical expert in the Yuan dynasty), such cases as distention and fullness in the gastral cavity, acid regurgitation and noise in stomach are basically due to dampness and heat. Therefore, it is necessary to use Huanglian as the monarch medicine to e-liminate damp-heat in the Middle Jiao and purge the heart fire, plus a little Wuzhuyu as a corrigent medicine. He removed Baishao to make **Wuji Pill** into **Zuojin Pill**, which is pungent, bitter and descending for purging the liver of pathogenic fire, harmonizing the stomach, and clearing away the damp heat. Wuzhuyu is used to dry dampness of the spleen with its aromatic smell, and Huanglian is used to dry dampness of the spleen with its bitter taste and descend-ing property. These two medicines used together can function more effectively to clear dampness and heat in the spleen and stomach.

Descending Qi and the Turbid

Wuzhuyu can lower Qi and descend the turbid. The foul smell of turbidity floating in the upper part will cause vomiting. Wuzhuyu has the effect to stop vomiting since, to a large extent, it can induce the turbid to descend.

Wuzhuyu should be crushed into powder, and mixed with vinegar into paste. Application of the paste to the arch of the feet can help to conduct heat down-wards. In the case of sore throat, or mouth ulcers, especially those mouth ulcers arising from deficiency fire, such a method can be tried in case all the other rem-edies fail. There are many hot medicines, but not all can conduct heat down-wards by applying them to the arch of the feet. Some hot medicines with floating characteristics may cause the heat to go upwards instead of guiding the heat to go downwards if applied to the arch of the feet. In such a case, Wuzhuyu will be the best choice.

This method is called "guiding the dragon back to sea". The so-called "dragon" here refers to the floating fire, which stays in the upper part, causing various fire syndromes there. The application of the above-said paste to the arch of the feet will induce the floating heat downwards with the help of the warmth of Wuzhuyu itself. At the same time, the warmth absorbed at the arch of the feet will be transported to the whole body, after which it will then go down to descend the turbid and reduce the endogenous fire. In such a way, the deficiency fire will be guided downwards.

Wuzhuyu is often used for foot bath (foot massage). Feet should be kept warm since they are at the lowest point of the human body and are prone to getting cold. A lot of foul smell in the human body must be discharged through the feet, which makes feet smelly all the time. Both stool and feet are smelly. They are like human sewage channels. Wuzhuyu is warm and able to descend the turbid, so it is very good for foot bath.

Contraindications of Wuzhuyu

There are many contraindications in oral administration of Wuzhuyu, for instance, those who suffer from Qi deficiency should not use Wuzhuyu since it consumes Qi and also stirs up fire.

In addition, Wuzhuyu is pungent and dry, and too much of it will result in blurred vision and various sores or ulcers. Those who suffer from excess fire due to Yin deficiency or from endogenous fire in the internal organs should not use it. In case there arise heat symptoms, such as blurred vision, thirst, sore throat, or alopecia, etc. , great caution must be taken in the use of Wuzhuyu. Of course, all of these are just reminders regarding the use of Wuzhuyu, which are not absolute requirements in fact.

Ganjiang(Rhizoma Zingiberis)

Characteristics of Ganjiang

Ganjiang warms the spleen. It is not made by just drying the fresh ginger in the sun, but comes from the old ginger body. When ginger is planted in the ground, a lot of new ginger will grow out of it nearby. The original ginger will be the old ginger body that is very tough. Soak the old ginger body in flowing water for three days to eliminate the dryness-heat, and then scrape off the cortex and dry it in the sun, after which the dried ginger is called Ganjiang.

The cortex of the ginger must be scraped off since the cortex mainly governs dispersion, but what is needed for medicine is to borrow its warm property to warm the Middle Jiao rather than its dispersing effect. In order to ensure the warming property of Ganjiang and remove its dispersing property, it is necessary to remove the cortex as possible before it is dried in the sun. In fact, the holding property of Ganjiang is relatively weak since herbs with strong smell generally can disperse, while those with thick taste can hold on. Ganjiang enjoys both strong smell and thick taste, so it can hold and disperse simultaneously. However, compared with Fuzi, it has stronger holding property. Therefore, removing the cortex can intensify its property to take hold without dispersing.

The black parched Ganjiang, called Paojiang (processed ginger), is slightly bitter and mild in nature, and is not as hot as Ganjiang, but it has stronger potence to stay/hold. Paojiang enters the Ying blood system, and it is commonly used in medicines for warming and tonifying purposes.

Generally speaking, Ganjiang enters the spleen and stomach, driving out coldness and drying dampness. Coldness and dampness often go hand in hand. The spleen is of damp earth, and it starts its function of transportation whenever it is warmed. In case the spleen is not warmed, it will not transform the dampness. And then, the coldness may trap the spleen, causing the spleen Yang failure to ascend within the body, which will result in various symptoms of spleen Yang deficiency like listlessness, poor appetite, moderate pulse, loose stool or even diarrhea. When the Middle Jiao is warmed and the coldness is eliminated, the dampness will be transformed much faster.

Ganjiang not only enters the Middle Jiao, but it also passes through the six meridians (i. e., Taiyang, Yangming, Shaoyang, Taiyin, Jueyin, and Shaoyin), entering the heart, lungs, spleen, stomach, large intestine and kidneys. It mainly go to the Middle Jiao. the spleen and stomach can be closely linked up with the large intestine since it goes to the Middle Jiao and the spleen and stomach, and that is why it enters the large intestine meridian as well. Ganjiang can keep balance up and down. It can warm the lungs if used with Wuweizi; and it warms the stomach if used with Renshen.

Lizhong Tang

There is a typical formula regarding Ganjiang, namely **Lizhong Tang**.

Lizhong Tang contains the herbal ingredients:

Renshen (ginseng), Baizhu (white atractylodes rhizome), Ganjiang (rhizoma zingiberis), Gancao (liquorice).

Lizhong Tang can be used for curing vomiting, diarrhea, and even cholera due to deficiency and coldness in the Middle Jiao and the spleen failure to properly carry out transformation. If Fuzi is added, it will be made into another formula called **Fuzi Lizhong Tang**, which is more powerful for warming up the deficiency-cold of the five internal organs. Sometimes, even if the five internal organs are not cold, **Lizhong Tang** may help one become energetic due to the injection of warmth. However, **Lizhong Tang** cannot be abused, or used for long or misused. If the hot medicines like Ganjiang are misused or taken for a long time, they may impair Yin, or otherwise activate fire, which will impair vision, resulting in quick damage to the eyes. Therefore, although **Lizhong Tang** is a commonly used formula, it should be used with great caution based on syndrome differentiation.

Common Compatibility of Ganjiang

Ganjiang and Baizhu are often used together to dry dampness and tonify the spleen. Danggui and Baishao enter the liver to nourish the liver and Yin. Ganjiang, when added into the formula, can give warmth to Danggui and Baishao and make them enter Qi system for hematogenesis with greater potence.

Ganjiang and Gaoliangjiang (galangal) used together make a formula called **Liangjiang San**, which can warm the spleen. Whenever the spleen meridian has coldness, Ganjiang and Gaoliangjiang can be used for warming up, especially for the symptoms of coldness in the Middle Jiao, stagnation of Qi and disorder of spleen transportation. For such a case, it is unnecessary to use **Fuzi Lizhong Tang** since **Fuzi Lizhong Tang** contains many herbs of severe properties. Besides, Rensheng and Baizhu cannot regulate Qi but can easily obstruct Qi. However, **Liangjiang San** is an entirely different medicine, in which Gaoliangjiang is slightly reddish, aromatic and quite mild in nature, entering the blood system of the spleen. It not only warms the Middle Jiao, but also regulates Qi, warming and activating meridians, causing less adverse effects on patients. This formula is frequently used for treatment of deficiency-cold of the Middle Jiao, and it is often integrated into the other formulas.

Doukou (Cardamun)

Doukou in reality is not just a medicine, but refers to a series of medicines of the same category, such as Bai Doukou (amomum cardamomum), Cao Doukou (alpinia katsumadai), Rou Doukou (nutmeg), Hong Doukou (fructus galangae), and Caoguo (amomum tsao-ko). All the medicines in Doukou category can warm the Middle Jiao, but the functions of them are somewhat different, just like the five brothers who are quite similar, but each of them has his own advantages and disadvantages.

Bai Doukou(Amomum Cardamomum) and Sanren Tang

As to Bai Doukou, the character "白" (Bai) in its Chinese name "Bai Doukou" indicates that this medicine can enter the lungs. Indeed, Bai Doukou tends to go upwards to warm the lungs while it is warming the Middle Jiao. The lung governs Qi of the whole body, implying that Bai Doukou is inclined to promote the circulation of Qi, relaxing the Middle Jiao and promoting the T&T functions of spleen and stomach. One of the formulas related to Bai Doukou as the main ingredient is **Sanren Tang**. It is a classic formula used for the treatment of damp-warm syndrome.

Sanren Tang contains the herbal ingredients:

Bai Doukou Ren (amomum cardamomum kernel), Xingren (apricot kernel), Yiyiren (coix seed), Houpo (mangnolia officinalis), Banxia (pinellia ternata), Huashi (talcum), Tongcao (tetrapanax papyriferus), Zhuye (bamboo leaf).

Sanren Tang takes three kernels/seeds as the main herbs, i. e., Bai Doukou Ren, Xingren, and Yiyiren, all of which go to the lung. In addition, Baidoukou Ren can enter the spleen meridian and eliminate dampness aromatically as well while it regulates Qi. Xingren goes to the large intestine channel with the function of lubrication while moistening the lungs and depressing Qi. Yiyiren can go to the bladder meridian and alleviate fluid retention while clearing the lung pathogens. All these three kernels can eliminate dampness. This formula is quite effective for tackling the damp-warm syndrome of human body.

What is the implication of the damp-warm syndrome? Dampness always makes one feel sticky and clammy; Warmth always makes one feel lukewarm and stifling. Dampness is a Yin pathogen and warmth is a Yang pathogen. When they are intertwined, it will not be easy to make them separate again, from which the symptoms like slight fever and sweating will arise, but sweating does not lower the temperature. The patient may feel heavy all over the body and stuffy in the chest, have a poor appetite, and feel sweet or sticky in the mouth and unsmooth in urination. Meanwhile, there are also some other symptoms like thick and greasy coating on the tongue, and slow and slippery pulse.

When the warm pathogen is trapped by the damp and sticky pathogen, it will become much harder to be eliminated, and sweating cannot completely discharge the pathogen, and fever cannot be easily brought down. Just because of the dampness, the patient will feel very heavy all over his body. Dampness is trapped between the spleen and lungs, so the patient will feel stuffy and tight in the chest, losing appetite. The dampness also boxes up the bladder and lungs, resulting in urinary dysuria. The warm pathogen is partially hot, and essentially, it belongs to Yang pathogen that should have made the pulse beat faster. However, in this case, it is on the opposite side, and the pulse becomes slow, showing that it does not arise from coldness, but from dampness trapping the pulse. Thus, Bai Doukou Ren is used to promote the circulation of Qi and warm the Middle Jiao to activate the spleen and lungs to alleviate fluid retention and dissipate dampness. In addition, some pungent, bitter and tasteless medicines may be added for dispersing, descending and permeating in order to relieve the damp-warm syndrome.

Other Doukou(Cardamun)

Cao Doukou enters the spleen meridian, which tends to relieve Qi stagnation, warm the Middle Jiao to dry the dampness. It has much stronger aromatic scent than that of Bai Doukou.

Hong Doukou is actually the seed of Gaoliangjiang. It is similar to that of Gaoliangjiang in nature, but it is stronger in its hot property than that of Bai Doukou and Cao Doukou, so it has more intensive potence to warm the Middle

Jiao. Hong Doukou is rarely used in general, and sometimes Gaoliangjiang is used directly instead, if needed. Hong Doukou has little effect on promoting Qi circulation, and it is partial to warming the lungs and dispersing coldness, therefore, it tends to promote Qi circulation of the spleen to dry dampness.

Besides, Rou Doukou is partial togoing downwards to warm the kidneys, inducing astringency to the large intestine and stopping diarrhea. As such, it is used in the **Sishen Pill**.

Caoguo(Amomum Tsao-ko) and Dayuan Yin

Caoguo has a stronger effect of aromatic dryness than that of Cao Doukou, and it also is useful for reducing phlegm. The formula of **Dayuan Yin** takes advantage of Caodoukou to cure the hidden pathogen and malaria.

Dayuan Yin contains the herbal ingredients:

Binglang (areca-nut), Houpo (mangnolia officinalis), Caoguo (amomum tsao-ko), Zhimu (rhizoma anemarrhenae), Shaoyao (radix paeoniae alba), Huangqin (scutellaria baicalensis), Gancao (liquorice).

Binglang, Houpo, and Caoguo are the monarch herbs of **Dayuan Yin**. Binglang is very strong in its effects and it can drive the endogenous pathogens and stagnation out of the body. Houpo is aromatic in scent with the property of going downwards. It can eliminate the epidemic pathogenic factors if used together with Binglang. Caoguo is used to eliminate the hidden pathogens. All the hidden pathogens in human body can be driven out with Caoguo by way of warming the Middle Jiao and drying the dampness with its aroma. These three herbs can directly target the turbid to get rid of the pathogens. In some places, malaria is called "the spleen-cold syndrome", for which Caoguo can directly address to warm the spleen. However, such a case cannot be treated with the other warm medicines like Ganjiang since it holds to but does not move on, thus, the permeating and dispersing functions of Ganjiang are not so effective as that of Caoguo. Caoguo is aromatic and it can go downwards to warm the Middle Jiao with the advantages of permeating and dispersing effects.

The remaining ingredient herbs in this formula are for harmonizing purposes. Zhimu clears the heat of Yangming meridian. As the saying goes, "the spleen is damp earth, and it will start its T&T functions when it is warm." The spleen will be cold if not being warmed, but this does not mean the stomach is cold; in fact, the stomach may still be hot at this time. There is another saying, "the stomach as dry earth will be balanced only when its heat is relieved". Caoguo and Zhimu should be used together, for Caoguo warms the spleen Yang and Zhimu clears the stomach heat. This helps the spleen and stomach to gain what they need so that the Middle Jiao can function properly. In case the spleen is not warmed, the dampness will accumulate; in case the stomach fails to be cooled, the heat will accumulate. And then, the damp-heat will be trapped more and more in the Middle Jiao, resulting in fullness and stuffiness in the chest and abdomen. **Dayuan Yin** functions to harmonize the spleen and stomach, and eliminate the pathogens that stem from the disharmony between the spleen and stomach, for which Binglang and Houpo will play their role in the formula.

A formula can be analyzed and comprehended from many angles. The formula of **Dayuan Yin** can be analyzed from two different angles: in one way, the three herbs of Binglang, Houpo, and Caoguo are the monarch herbs, while the remaining herbs are only for harmonizing purpose; in another way, Caoguo and Zhimu are the monarch herbs with one for warming the spleen and another for clearing the stomach to regulate its coldness and heat. Binglang and Houpo are for driving out the pathogens, while Shaoyao, Huangqin and Gancao are used for harmonizing purpose.

第六章　温肝脾之药

我们今天主要讲温肝和温脾的药。

脾在中焦，为足太阴；肝肾都在下焦，分别为足厥阴和和足少阴，阴宜得其阳，所以肝脾肾这三经都需要温煦。

温肝，常用吴茱萸，温脾，常用干姜、豆蔻一类的药。

吴茱萸

吴茱萸是一味大热的药，我们要把它区别于山茱萸。开方子的时候，吴茱萸通常写成"泡吴萸"，山茱萸就写成"山萸肉"。古诗里讲"遍插茱萸少一人"中的"茱萸"，到底是吴茱萸还是山茱萸，历来都有争议：有人说应该是吴茱萸，它有芳香的气息，插在身上比较好；山茱萸是山上的小野果，秋天就红了，酸酸甜甜的，采来插在身上，提示秋冬养阴，也未尝不可。

吴茱萸和花椒有相似的地方，它的树也和花椒树有一点相似，但是花椒偏走脾肺，吴茱萸则偏走肝肾、脾胃之经，"散厥阴之风寒，燥脾家之湿。芳香，下气开郁，降浊"。

当归四逆汤

吴茱萸的作用，首先是温肝，散足厥阴的寒气。有一个典型的方剂，就是当归四逆汤。

当归四逆汤

吴萸、当归、白芍，桂枝、细辛，生姜、甘草、通草

当归四逆汤主治厥阴手足厥冷、脉细欲绝。因为肝寒，血分有寒，肝的动力不足，所以身上出现逆冷。所以用吴萸来温肝，但光温肝还不行，你还得给它滋养。当归白芍柔肝养阴，是常用的药对，肝藏血，当归白芍通过柔肝养阴而生血。吴萸相当于给肝补火、补阳，当归白芍相当于给肝补水、补阴，肝体阴而用阳，吴萸温肝以达其用，当归白芍养肝阴以滋其体，体用都兼顾了，肝才能正常，这三味是主药。

细辛配桂枝，是温肾的。桂枝通膀胱之阳，散膀胱经的寒。当膀胱经能气化了，对肾也有一定的温煦作用，因为肾与膀胱相表里。细辛则是散肾经的风寒。

生姜、甘草则入中焦，温脾。所以我们也不要以为当归四逆汤仅仅是在温肝，在温肝的同时它还是要兼顾脾和肾。

为什么要用通草呢？因为手足厥冷，不但要温，另一方面要让温度通向全身。通草能够利水，利水也就能利膀胱，通草和桂枝一起，桂枝温膀胱，通草能够通利膀胱，让膀胱的气化能够得到施展。

如果从君臣佐使的角度讲，我们又可以对当归四逆汤做另一番分析：吴茱萸温肝，为君；桂枝、细辛、生姜温脾肾，为臣，当归、白芍柔肝养阴为佐，通草利水通阳为使。

盐吴萸配小茴香治疝气

用盐水炒了以后，吴茱萸就能往下走，温肝肾。因为盐是咸的，入肾。盐水炒的吴萸经常用来治疝气。疝气常常是因为肝经有寒，把气机闭住了，我们在温肝同时还要理气。如果小男孩有疝气，一侧阴囊就会垂下来，变得特别大，有一些气坠下来了。坠得厉害的话，一碰就会疼得钻心。足厥阴肝经是要绕生殖器一圈的，生殖器这里有病，通过经络辨证，就知道它必然跟肝有关系。既然是肝寒，那么我们用吴萸。又因为它是生殖器的问题，跟肾有关系。生殖器有时就叫外肾。内肾在里面，有两个，中间是命门；外肾则有两个睾丸，中间是阴茎，这都是相对应的，有相似性、同构性。

用盐水炒的吴茱萸加上小茴香，是治疝气常用的一对药。小茴香也是辛温的，它温肝的力度略微小一些，但是有很强的理气作用。二者配合，温通理气，肝寒去掉了，因为肝气寒而造成的凝滞也化解了。有时候，这个药你甚至都不必喝，直接把它敷在阴囊、小腹或腹股沟部位，都有很好的作用。

吴萸配木瓜

很多朋友都有过腿抽筋的体会，一疼起来就感觉有一根筋像要断似的在收引。这是因为小腿部有寒，寒主收引，经脉就会收缩。

而且，腿抽筋还跟血寒有关。血管都是有柔韧性，柔韧性就跟筋有关，肝主筋，那么也跟肝有关。肝气寒，所以用吴茱萸温肝，温肝就能温血，温血也就能温血管。

木瓜是往下肢走的，味酸，酸就能缓急，能柔筋。吴茱萸和木瓜，一个温一个酸，温通血脉，柔化血管，这样就能治腿抽筋。

这里一般用醋炒吴茱萸，它还可以活血。因为肝藏血，醋是酸的，它就更能够入肝。肝的动力一足，血就更容易活了。

吴茱萸汤

吴茱萸还有一个作用，就是燥脾湿。它是一味香燥的药，而脾是喜欢香燥的。用黄连水炒吴萸可以起到止呕的作用。尤其是对于治疗吐酸水，效果非常好。吴萸止呕有一个经典的方剂，叫吴茱萸汤，它出自张仲景的《伤寒论》。

吴茱萸汤

人参、吴萸、生姜、大枣。

《伤寒论》讲："少阴病，吐利，手足逆冷，烦躁欲死者，吴茱萸汤主之，"它还治"厥阴病，干呕，吐涎沫，头痛"。总而言之，它就是治肝胃虚寒证，尤其是呕吐。

呕吐，有寒呕，也有热呕。如果是热呕的话，就不能用吴茱萸汤来治了；寒呕可以用。呕吐是上升之象，上升说明有火，即使是根本上是寒的，但只要是呕吐，也说明它还是跟热有关。比如，肝一寒，动力就不足了。本来肝木要克脾土的，肝木如果控制不了脾胃，脾胃就会生出湿，还能生出一些浮热。在这种浮热的作用下，人就产生了呕吐。既要温肝，又不能助长这些浮热，所以吴萸要用黄连水来炒，因为黄连能燥脾湿，还能清脾经的浮热，这就标本兼治了。

左金丸

吴萸香燥脾湿，黄连苦以燥湿，它们在一起，一热一寒，相互作用、相互制约，标本兼顾。在吐酸的时候，我们经常用到吴萸和黄连，这叫左金丸。

人有时候胃里面嘈杂，有一种要呕的感觉，但又呕不出什么东西来，偶尔呕出一口酸水，非常难受。有人能把这酸水给吐了，这叫吐酸；有人的酸水想吐还吐不出来，刚到喉咙又不知不觉被咽下去了，这个叫吞酸。

吞酸吐酸，都是胃里面有股酸水在往上泛，这可能因为寒也可能是因为热，但到底还是有热。有热，才会沤出酸来；而且火性炎上，有热，胃里面的东西才能够往上泛。

治吐酸，根据寒热，用吴萸和黄连。一般来讲，吴萸用量少，黄连用量大。吴萸用 2 克，黄连用 5 克左右，这就够了。前面黄连水炒吴萸，是以吴萸为主。这里如果治热性的吐酸，则是以黄连为主，吴萸为辅。

左金丸治疗吐酸，如果喝了还吐，里面可以加瓦楞子、海螵蛸。瓦楞子是一种贝壳类药，能制酸；海螵蛸就是乌贼骨，有很好的收敛溃疡的作用。往往，严重的吐酸会伴随着胃溃疡，这又一举两得了。

李时珍用吴萸，他往往不加黄连，而加茯苓，治痰多的人，或者痰饮造成的吐酸，吴萸、黄连、茯苓都可以加进去。痰饮造成的吐酸，热象没那么重，所以就不用黄连了。为什么会有痰饮呢？因为脾不能运化。脾得温则运，他喜欢温燥淡渗之品，你再加黄连这样一味苦寒药，就背道而驰了。所以，临床用药，一定要审察病机，灵活应变。

左金丸与戊己丸

吴萸、黄连这两味药配伍，为甚么叫左金丸呢？佐金平木，因为金克木，现在帮金一把，金的力度就会更大，它平木的作用就会更大。五行的木，对应五味的酸，平木就是制酸，左金丸说白了就是制酸丸。但明言制酸丸，窗户纸就捅破了，所以他要拐个弯。

佐金丸的前身是戊己丸，有三味药组成：吴萸、黄连、白芍。它们在一起，以酸苦涌泻为主，能调和肝脾，清热和胃。但这个方后来用的不是太多。朱丹溪认为，诸如胃脘痞满，吞酸、嘈杂之类，基本上都是湿热。因此需要用黄连为君祛中焦湿热，泻心火，再稍微用一点吴萸反佐一下就可以了。所以，他去掉芍药，使之成为辛开苦降、泻肝和胃、清化湿热的左金丸。吴茱萸和黄连，一个通过芳香一个通过苦降来燥脾湿。它们一块清脾胃的湿热效果非常好。

下气降浊，导龙归海

吴茱萸能下气降浊。浊气在上则呕，吴茱萸的止呕作用，很大程度上就是在把浊气往下引。

把吴萸打成细末，用醋一调，贴在脚心，能够导热下行。当咽喉痛，口舌生疮，尤其是那种虚火的口舌生疮，用很多方法都治不好的时候，你可以试试。热药有很多，并不是所有的热药贴在脚心都能导热下行。有的热药，轻阳上浮，贴在脚心它也可能往上走，不能导热下行了。吴萸这方面作用最佳。

这个方法叫导龙归海。"龙"就是浮越之火。火浮在上面，导致上部的各种火症，用醋调的吴茱萸贴在脚心，也就是人体的最下部，热和热同气相求，吴茱萸的热能够把上面的热往下拉；同时，吴茱萸通过脚心的吸收，运行至全身以后还是会往下降，降浊降火，把虚火往下引。

所以，吴茱萸还经常用来泡脚。脚宜常温，脚是人体地位最低的一个地方，容易发凉，而且人体很多浊气都要通过脚排掉，所以脚会臭。大便是臭的，脚也是臭的，它们就像人体排污道。吴茱萸温，又能够降浊，所以用来泡脚是非常好的。

吴茱萸使用禁忌

吴茱萸内服，有许多禁忌。比如，气虚的人不能用，因为吴茱萸耗气，还会动火。它辛燥，吃多了会目昏，还会生各种疮，心阴虚火旺的不要用，脏腑有热的人也不要用；如果出现了热症的，比如眼花、口渴、咽痛、脱发等，一定要慎用吴茱萸。这些是用吴茱萸的一些提示，但是也并不是绝对的。

它辛燥，吃多了会目昏，还会生各种疮，心阴虚火旺的不要用，脏腑有热的人也不要用；如果出现了热症的，比如眼花、口渴、咽痛、脱发等，一定要慎用吴茱萸。这些是用吴茱萸的一些提示，但是也并不是绝对的。

干姜

干姜性状

干姜是温脾的。干姜不是把鲜生姜晒干，而是用母姜做成的。把生姜种到地里，它旁边又会生出很多新的生姜来，原来的那一块就成了母姜，非常老。把母姜放流水里浸泡三天，把它的燥热之性泡掉，然后刮掉皮，再晒干，就是干姜。

为什么要把皮去掉呢？因为皮主散，而我们要取干姜的温性去温中焦，要温而不散。干姜守而不走，想确保干姜的这个性质，就要尽量把它往外散的性质去掉，所以要在晾干之前把它的皮去掉。实际上，干姜守而不走的性质比较弱，因为气味大的东西一般都能走，味厚的一般往往能守，干姜是气味俱厚，所以它能守能走。只不过跟附子比起来，它守的性能强一些，去掉皮，可以增强它守而不走的性质。

如果把干姜炒黑，那就是炮姜，有点发苦，没有干姜的大热，性质平和一些，守的力量也更强一些。炮姜入营血，一般用来温补的药里会用到炮姜。

总体来讲，干姜入脾胃，逐寒燥湿。寒与湿往往是相随的，脾为湿土，得温则运。如果脾得不到温，湿就不能化，寒仍是寒，脾被寒湿给困住，脾阳就不能升起来，人就会产生脾阳虚的各种症状：打不起精神，食欲不振，脉缓，大便溏泻甚至拉肚子。当温了中焦，逐了寒以后，湿也会化得更快一些。

干姜不仅仅是入中焦的。它可通行六经，入心、肺、脾、胃、大肠、肾，主要是以归中焦为主，既然归中焦、归脾胃，那么脾胃跟大肠他们联系比较紧密，它也能入大肠经。它会兼顾上下，所以它跟五味子一块就能温肺，跟人参一起就能温胃。

理中汤
用干姜有一个典型的方子，就是理中汤。
理中汤
人参、白术、干姜、甘草。

凡是中焦虚寒，脾不能健运，导致呕吐啊，拉肚子啊，甚至上吐下泻的霍乱，都可以用理中汤。如果再加上附子那么就是附子理中汤，力度更大，五脏的虚寒它都能温煦，即使五脏没有寒，吃了理中汤，在热力的作用下，人也会特精神。只是理中汤不能乱用、久用、误用。如果干姜之类的热药误用，或者久服误服，就会伤阴、动火，还会损目，让人的眼睛坏得特别快。所以，理中汤虽然是常用的一个方剂，但需要准确辨证，谨慎使用。

干姜的常用配伍
干姜跟白术经常一起用，能够燥湿补脾。
干姜同当归白芍一起，因为当归白芍是入肝的，能柔肝养阴，加干姜，能够给当归白芍这两味阴药以温度，让它们入气而生血，使生血的力度更大。

干姜跟高良姜一起，叫两姜散，是温脾的。凡是脾经有寒的可以用干姜和高良姜来温。当一个人既有中寒又有气滞，脾气凝滞不运，我们用干姜、高良姜更好，而没有必要用附子理中汤。附子理中汤药味多、性子烈，而且人参、白术补气易壅，没有理气之用。两姜散就不一样。高良姜是略微有点发红，入脾胃经的血分。它非常香，给人一种燥烈的感觉，但它的性质其实非常平和，不但能温中，还有一定理气和温通的作用，给人造成的不利影响比较少。这一般是中焦虚寒经常用的一个方，只有两味药，会混到其他方子里来用。

豆蔻

下面我们讲豆蔻。豆蔻其实不是一味药，而是一类药，比如白豆蔻、草豆蔻、肉豆蔻、红豆蔻，还有草果。豆蔻类的药都能温中焦，但它们的作用有所偏重，有所不同，就像兄弟五个，都挺相似的，但是又各有所长，各有所短。

白豆蔻与三仁汤

白豆蔻，一看白字，我们就知道它会入肺。确实，白豆蔻在温中焦的同时比较喜欢往上走，能温肺。肺主一身之气，白豆蔻偏于行气，一行气它就会宽中焦，促进脾胃运化。以白豆蔻为主的方子，有一个是三仁汤，是用来治湿温的一个经典方剂。

三仁汤

白蔻仁、杏仁、薏苡仁、厚朴、半夏、滑石、通草、竹叶。

三仁汤以三个仁为主药：白豆蔻仁、杏仁、薏苡仁。这三味药都会走肺，只不过白蔻仁在肺理气的同时还走脾，还香燥。杏仁在润肺降气的同时走大肠，能润滑。薏仁，它在清利肺邪的同时还走膀胱，能利水。三者都能除湿。它是能够解开人体湿温的一个比较好的方剂。

什么是湿温呢？湿给我们的感觉就是粘粘糊糊的，温也让人感觉到温温吞吞的，有种不利索的感觉。湿和温，一个阴邪，一个阳邪，它们缠绵交织在一起，不容易分开，其症状，往往身上发热，但热不是太大，会出汗，但是出了汗热也退不掉。身体非常重，胸中特别堵，什么东西也吃不下，嘴里可能会发甜，或发粘，小便还不利索。舌头一伸出来，舌苔很厚、很滑腻。脉比较缓、比较滑，这都是湿温的常见症。

温邪被湿粘腻住了，更不容易透散出来。即使出汗，邪也不能完全排出，热也不容易退掉。因为有湿，就会感觉身体特别重；因为湿困在脾肺之间，所以感觉到胸闷，堵得慌，食欲不振；因为湿困住膀胱和肺，所以出现小便不利。本来温邪是偏热的，它是一个阳邪，能够让脉变得快，但是这里不一样，脉反而缓，脉缓不是因为有寒，而是湿把脉给困住了。用白蔻仁来行气、温中焦，加速脾和肺的工作，让它们利水化湿的工作运转起来。再加上"辛开"、"苦降"、"淡渗"，达到解除湿温的效果。

其他豆蔻

草豆蔻是入脾的，它偏于破气开郁、温中燥湿。其香气比白豆蔻要浓烈一些。

红豆蔻其实就是高良姜的种子，性质跟高良姜有相似的地方，它的热性比白豆蔻、草豆蔻都要大，温中的力度也要大一些。红豆蔻一般很少用，有时直接用高良姜就行了。但红豆蔻行气的作用小，它偏于温肺散寒，偏于行脾燥湿。

还有肉豆蔻，偏于下行，能温肾，还能固涩大肠、止泻。所以四神丸用的就是肉豆蔻。

草果与达原饮

草果香燥的作用，比草豆蔻还要大，而且有化痰的作用，达原饮用它治疗伏邪、疟疾。

达原饮

槟榔、厚朴、草果、知母、芍药、黄芩、甘草。

槟榔、厚朴、草果是达原饮的君药。槟榔力度很猛，能把体内一些不好的气息、积滞摧枯拉朽一般往外赶。厚朴芳香，往下走的，配槟榔能破除戾气。草果是除伏邪的，邪气潜伏在人体，用草果的温中香燥去除它。这三味药直捣巢穴，化浊驱邪。有的地方把疟疾叫作打脾寒，草果正好能温脾，你不能用别的东西来温，比如干姜，它守而不走，透散的作用没有草果那么好。草果芳香下行，能温中焦，又能透散。

后面几味就是调和的药。

知母清阳明的热。"脾为湿土，得温则运"，脾得不到温的时候，它是寒的，但这并不代表胃也是寒的，胃这时候可能还有热。"胃为燥土，得凉则安"，现在是脾要温得不到温，胃要凉却得不到凉。所以，草果知母要并用，草果温脾阳，知母清胃热，让脾和胃各得其所，中焦就能运转起来了。如果脾得不到温，湿就会越来越多，胃得不到凉，热就会越来越多，中焦湿热就会越来越多，继而导致胸脘痞闷。达原饮是要把脾胃的关系调理好，然后再把因脾胃之间关系不好而产生的一些不好的东西驱逐出去，这就是槟榔、厚朴的作用。

一个方子，我们可以通过多角度去理解。达原饮这个方子，我们就是从两个不同的角度去理解的：第一个就是说，槟榔、厚朴、草果这三味药是君药，其他药是调和之品。从另一个角度，我们也可以说，草果、知母是君药，一个温脾一个清胃，调其寒热，槟榔、厚朴驱邪，芍药、黄芩和甘草都是调和之品。

Chapter 7   Fuzi(radix aconiti carmichaeli) and Herbs Related to Deer

Now let us come to the medicines of Fuzi and herbs related to deer. Fuzi is a low-grade medicine, while the herbs related to deer are the animal medicines.

Fuzi (radix aconiti carmichaeli)

Characteristics of Fuzi and its Family Members

Fuzi is a perennial herbaceous plant whose root can be used as medicine. In essence, Fuzi has many root tubers, somewhat like potatoes. However, potatoes grow piece by piece separately, while Fuzi grows with the new root tubers attached to the old one. That is why it is called Fuzi (which means "attaching sons" in Chinese). Normally, one monkshood plant will bear one or two Fuzi.

Monkshood plant grows out of atuber called Wutou (aconite), which has more heat and stronger medical effects, just like the spicy old ginger. Around the aconite grow the new root tubers, which are Fuzi. The new root tubers have less medical effects. Some root tubers do not have lateral roots, and all the medical efficacy will be accumulated in the sole root tubers called Tianxiong, which have the greatest potence dimension. However, the sole root tubers are all hypertoxic.

In fact, Fuzi, Wutou and Tianxiong are medicines of the same category, with the only differences being the location where the tubers grow or the way that the tubers grow.

Wutou and Toxic Liquor

Wutou is conical in shape and relatively small in size, while Fuzi is partially round. Of course, the best Fuzi has a flat bottom, and umbilicate protrusion on the cortex. Remove the cortex and umbilicus when processing it. Fuzi is a medicine with a strong scent and heavy taste. It goes faster and can pass through the whole body to each and every point. It is a medicine that moves freely but does not hold on to certain points.

Fuzi is highly toxic because of its great heat in property. There is often such a plot in TV play that an emperor gives a cup of poisoned liquor to one of his ministers. After drinking it, the minister immediately suffered abdominal pain and then bleeds from nose and mouth to death. It is always said that the poisoned liquor in ancient times was Zhen liquor that was made by stirring the liquor with the feather of Zhenniao (a legendary bird with poisonous feathers). In fact, this is a misinformation. The most commonly used poisonous liquor is brewed with Sheng Wutou (raw aconite), which is thicker in density. It is of great heat, and able to enter the blood system. Thus, with the help of liquor, its medical effects will become more powerful. He who drinks it will have the blood of his whole body activated and feel unable to endure it in his heart immediately. By then, the blood-heat will invade into the five internal organs with an outward manifestation of bleeding from the seven orifices (noses, ears, eyes and mouth) until death. The seven orifices are subsumed to Yang orifices from which Yang Qi is vented. It is said that "the life essence of the five internal organs and six hollow organs is all directed upwards at the eyes". In fact, it is not only directed at the eyes, but in fact directed upwards at all the seven orifices. When blood surges in the five internal organs, it often rises and flows out of the seven orifices. This is how poison works in the human body.

The Way to Detoxify Fuzi

Those who have drunk the toxic aconite liquor will not be saved normally, since the poison is too powerful to save the life. But if a person is just poisoned by Fuzi, there is still time to bring the person out of danger.

Fuzi is of great heat, so cold medicine can be used to counteract it, or licorice is used to alleviate its heat, since coldness can drive away heat, and the sweet taste can relieve urgency. Cold medicines, such as the bitter and cold Huanglian and Xijiao (rhinoceros' horn), are able to clear the heat of the Yangming meridian. The Yangming meridian involves the hollow organs with much Qi and blood. When Qi and blood start to surge, Yangming will be the first to be affected, so it must be protected with the first priority. Huanglian can clear the heart fire, and so can Xijiao. The two herbs used together can give protection to the heart since at the critical moment of a desperate situation, the first priority is to protect the heart. In the past, the three herbs of Huanglian, Xijiao and Sheng Gancao (raw liquorice) were boiled into a decoction for detoxifying Fuzi. Gancao can alleviate the toxicity of all kinds of medicines, and its sweet taste also has the relieving effect, slows down the toxicity and prevents it from toxicity attack so rapidly and severely.

In addition, loess soil-mixed water can also be effective for alleviating toxicity since soil is mild and all things on earth will finally return to soil, so loess is the best antidote. The herbal loess is rarely seen in the north of China, but primarily in the south. However, the topsoil in the south is dirty, black or grayish in color, which should be removed to dig out the loess in the deep layer. Mix it with water, and then let it settle down completely. The upper layer of water is called Dijiang Shui (soil seriflux), which can detoxify many things like poisonous mushrooms and leeches. Of course, it can detoxify Fuzi, too.

Processing of Fuzi

After understanding how to detoxify Fuzi, it will be easier to understand the processing of Fuzi.

There are many ways to process Fuzi: some people say it ought to be soaked in licorice water; some say to soak it in black soya bean water; some say to mix it with well salt; and even to marinate it...... and so on.

The standard way to process Fuzi is to soak it in licorice water. First, scrape off the cortex and umbilicus of Fuzi, then crosscut it into four pieces, and put into licorice water to soak it thoroughly. After these procedures, parch it with slow fire until it becomes yellow in color. Then, spread it out on the ground of wet land after rain——but there should be no mud.

The purpose of spreading over on the wet land for a night is to remove its pathogenic heat since raw Fuzi alone is a medicine of great heat, and now it is parched on fire, perhaps resulting in enough heat to cause pathogenic fire. The soil is always mild without severe cold or great heat, and it can help to detoxify the parched Fuzi. Meanwhile, Fuzi on the ground can gain the earth Qi so that Fuzi would become mild in its property.

Gancao is a sweet medicine. Its sweet taste can help relieve the heat of Fuzi and slow down the function of Fuzi efficacy without compromising its hot property.

Furthermore, some people boil Fuzi with the urine of little children (any healthy boys who are under 14 years old). This method on the one hand is to bring the great heat of Fuzi under control with the help of cold attributes of children's urine; and on the other hand, children's urine in any case is turbid fluid and tends to go downwards. Fuzi combined with children's urine will be more prone to going downwards so that its heat could warm the Lower Jiao but not float up. However, some people dislike processing Fuzi with children's urine, and they worry this may restrain the powerful and severe properties of Fuzi since the boys' urine is cold in property.

Another method is to slice Fuzi and put it in water and let it float over and again until it becomes extremely mild. In prescriptions, some doctors will write Fuzi as Danfupian (slices of mild radix aconiti carmichaeli), whose strength is weakened, not as strong as Fuzi prepared with licorice water. In Zhang Zhongjing 's formulas, whenever Fuzi was used, a large dosage of licorice root would also be used in order to counteract the power of Fuzi. By the way, in some cases, the formulas may need to use Sheng Fuzi (raw radix aconiti carmichaeli), and then, licorice root will be even more necessary.

As for the so-called preparation of Fuzi with well salt, this practice needs to be researched. Well salt is naturally salty and cold, and if it is used for processing Fuzi, it will damage the hot attribute of the medicine. A medicine has its own attributes, just as a man has his temperament and personality, which the HR (human resource) officers may focus on when choosing employees. As far as medicines are concerned, more attention to the attributes and quality is required to pay in medication practice. The attribute of Fuzi is the great heat, and it should not be rubbed down by way of mixing it with the medicine of great coldness.

Those doctors who are expert at using Fuzi will not take counteraction with large dosages of cold and cool medicines, but they will only process Fuzi with a proper dosage of licorice water.

Fuzi for Treatment of Wind-Cold-Damp Related Arthralgia

Danfupian (slices of mild radix aconiti carmichaeli) mentioned above are often used in prescriptions. Fuzi, as a hot medicine, can go through the whole body. In case the cold-dampness is trapped in the body, can Fuzi be used to eliminate it? Definitely yes. However, for such a case, Danfupian should be used since it is more inclined to go into the meridians and collaterals to dispel pathogenic wind and eliminate coldness, curing the diseases like pains, arthritis, and rheumatism. The nature of Danfupian is, none the less, relatively hot; thus, a dosage of about 5g will work well, but sometimes, more (at most 15g) will be needed for the cases of more severe wind-cold-damp type of arthralgia. This is certainly a heavy dose for warming and activating meridians.

For such a case, Wutou can be used, too. Generally, the processed Wutou must be used instead in order to avoid its heavy toxicity. The addition of Wutou will have a stronger carminative effect. In case the coldness and dampness are strong, Fuzi can work effectively. Some middle-aged and elderly people (about 50 years old) in rural areas often suffer from severe arthralgia due to wind, coldness and dampness since they have to work outside in the wind and rain in many occasions, causing accumulation of the pathogenic wind, coldness and dampness in their bodies, which obstructs the meridians and collaterals. Therefore, many of them suffer from cervical spondylosis, lumbar spondylosis, ischialgia or pains in arms and legs. For a quick cure, either Fuzi or the processed Wutou may be used.

Fuzi Warms and Activates the Five Internal Organs

Even for warming and activating the internal organs, the processed Fuzi may also be used, but the raw Fuzi is rarely used. For rescuing patients from collapse, restoring Yang and bringing the dying back to life, Fuzi is indeed a very effective medicine with a function similar to hormone. Fuzi can activate the five internal organs and make them strong in an instant.

Fuzi and Renshen together make a formula called **Shenfu Tang**, which can strengthen the heart. For some cases, in order to achieve its potence, raw Fuzi is used for bringing the dying back to life. When a patient is dying, Renshen can function to "restore the primordial Qi from where nothing really exists" and Fuzi can restore the withering Yang.

Fuzi and Baizhu together make another formula called **Zhufu Tang** for invigorating the spleen. Fuzi and Baizhu are also used in many other formulas like **Lizhong Tang**. Baizhu is for tonifying the spleen. When used together with Fuzi for invigorating the spleen, they can rapidly restore the spleen Yang or the functions of the spleen itself.

Fuzi and Mahuang together can strengthen the functions of lungs. For example, **Mahuang Fuzi Xixin Tang**, in which Mahuang can purge the lung Qi. Mahuang and Fuzi used together not only can purge the lung Qi but also restore the lung Yang; Mahuang and Xixin used together can strengthen the functions of kidneys. Of course, for the purpose of strengthening the lungs and kidneys, Fuzi not only can be used together with Muhuang and Xixin, but also with Maidong. In fact, Maidong is a heavy medicine for nourishing the lungs, tending to moisten and clear the lungs. As a cold and cool medicine, Maidong used together with the hot medicine of Fuzi can cooperate to bring out the best of each other.

In addition, Fuzi and Rougui used together can strengthen the functions of the kidneys, too; Fuzi and Baishao used together can strengthen the functions of liver.

Uses of Fuzi and Rehabilitative Measures

All in all, Fuzi is a low-grade medicine according to **Sheng Nong's herbal classic**. It is a medicine of great heat and should not be misused or used long. Or otherwise, it may cause disorder in the blood and impairment of Qi, then resulting in blood stasis and inducing phlegm. In terms of Qi-blood phlegm stagnation, Qi and blood refer to the physiological state, and phlegm and stagnation, as a pathological consequence, occur due to the failure of Qi and blood circulation. Therefore, Fuzi may be effective for curing a disease for the time being, but will bring no end of trouble for the future. Fuzi, when used, can be perfectly effective at the very beginning and can bring the dying back to life, or make the listless patient become energetic immediately. However, this does not mean Fuzi will be effective on that patient forever, but on the contrary, it may and will bring many potential troubles. While Fuzi is used, many other cold and moist medicines have to be used for rehabilitative purposes. It is like a battle, after which a series of rehabilitative measures must be taken for the battlefield needs to recover and people need to be appeased. Similarly, some rehabilitative measures are also necessary for curing diseases.

Many books demonstrate that such and such formulas should be used for such and such diseases, but what rehabilitative measures should be taken is not mentioned? While learning TCM, one should carefully study how a disease is cured step by step from the very beginning, including what rehabilitative measures are to be taken after the disease has been cured. After that, the doctor may be able to link up what he has learnt with what have been described in TCM books. That is to say he has to apprentice himself to a medical expert who is willing to teach him the skills of curing procedures that might not be worth mentioning in books. Medical books all tell how to treat a symptom while a medical expert always teaches how to cure a disease or how to nurse a patient to the best condition of health.

He who is suffering from the wind-cold-dampness type arthralgia, such as ischialgia, may recover after taking the decoction of a prescription that contains Fuzi and Wutou, but looking at his tongue, the coating of the tongue may be a little yellow, and the tongue body may also be reddish, and the pulse is relatively rapid, all of which indicate that there is still endogenous heat. However, such endogenous heat mostly arises from Fuzi and Wutou that function in his body. What should be done then? The only way is to recover the "battlefield", that is, to use cold and moist medicines to clear up the aftermath.

Abuses of Fuzi and Remedies

A few years ago, I met with a girl who graduated from a TCM university. While in school, one of her teachers told her, "your hands are cold, which indicates Yang deficiency. " The teacher felt her pulse and told her it was tight due to coldness. She was given a prescription of modified **Fuzi Lizhong Tang** with some modifications. After she took it, she felt energetic. However, some troubles followed one after another: pimples developed on the arms. So, she again went to the teacher, who said, "well, the coldness is being dispersed now. " Then, she continued to use **Fuzi Lizhong Tang** with some modifications including a larger dosage of Fuzi as well. After taking it, she looked dim on the face. By this moment, the teacher said, "Dimness means fluid governing coldness, indicating that coldness is permeating outwards. After the coldness completely permeates out, you will be fine. " Thereupon, she continued to take medicine prescribed by her teacher. And soon, she found herself nearsighted, for which she had to wear glasses; before that, her eyes were very bright; she also had a sore throat after that; and her voice became raucous rather than the ringing voice as she had before. Only at that moment did she begin to have concerns about Fuzi medication that she had been taking for several months.

Later, she returned to Beijing in very poor health condition, with pimples on the arms all the time, and her face was still very dim. She looked older than her real age, and she suffered from a lot of phlegm and sore throat, often felt stuck up by phlegm with some terrible syndromes she did not have before she took Fuzi. All those consequences were actually the side effects of misusing Fuzi. All pains, sores and skin and external diseases are subsumed to pathogenic fire of heart, which in her case is reflected by the pimples on the arms

Although the dimness of face indicates it governs the kidney, which is subsumed to water/fluid, the dimness of face can also occur, to a certain degree, due to heat. Let us see the bottom of the pan over fire. It is black rather than white. Although fire flame is red in color, it will blacken a thing in case it is baked over fire for a long time. That is why long use of Fuzi will result in strong pathogenic fire, making the face dim. Of course, such a dim color of the face is different from the kind that comes from coldness since it arises from the endogenous fire.

Too much phlegm in her case is also due to the fire, that is to say, the body fluid is baked by the endogenous fire into thick substance, i. e. , phlegm, which is just like boiling for gel. Whenever there is heavily endogenous heat stemming from catching a cold, there will be an onset of phlegm like glue, accompanied by a sore throat (which also arises from fire rushing upwards). Throat is a critical gullet channel and it is very narrow. The fire in the other organs is dispersive, but once the fire reaches the throat, it will be concentrated and become severe. Therefore, the throat will get hurt, resulting in raucous voice.

The girl mentioned above is also a TCM university graduate. She told me that whenever she read the names of medicines like Maidong, Zhuli (bamboo juice), Shigao and Hanshuishi (gypsum rubrum), she would feel particularly comfortable in mind since she needs them in her body. Maidong, cold and sweet, can promote the secretion of saliva or body fluid; Shigao, cold and sweet, can clear the heat; Zhuli, sweet and cool, can reduce phlegm. All these medicines are suitable for her.

Her phlegm must be reduced with Zhuli, which is the juice extracted from bamboo through baking it over fire. One may take a piece of green bamboo and bake it on fire, and the green will start to sweat. In the ancient time, the ancient people baked bamboo slips and let them sweat out some juice. Then, they cut chinese characters on the sweating green bamboo slips called Hanqing (sweating green bamboo strips), which would not be damaged easily by worms. Bamboo juice, as a medicine, is cool and moist, and it can reduce phlegm. Those who take too much Fuzi will need to nourish Yin to promote the secretion of saliva or body fluid, and for remedies, Maidong and Zhuli should be frequently used. Of course, in case Yin is seriously impaired, some other Yin nourishing medicines may also be taken into consideration like Gualou (trichosanthes kirilowii maxim), Zhebei (thunberg fritillary bulb), Chenpi (pericarpium citri reticulatae), and Banxia (pinellia ternate). However, Banxia is a warm and dry medicine that should not be overused.

Rational Uses of Fuzi

My teacher often said: "Fuzi must be rationally used but not abused. " What does rational use of Fuzi refer to? Rational use means to use it right to the point, which has nothing to do with more or less use of it. It does not mean that those who are brave enough to use Fuzi can make rational use of it. Sometimes making little use or even no use of it can also be taken as the rational use.

Once my teacher wrote a prescription of **Bawei Dihuang Pill**, in which he used 3g of Fuzi and 2g of Rougui. I asked why these two medicines were used in such small dosages. He said, "It is like igniting a lamp. How much fire do you need to ignite a lamp?" I answered, "Just a match." He said: "That is right. 3g of Fuzi and 2g of Rougui are equivalent to a match that is enough to ignite a prairie." Therefore, it is unnecessary to use so much of it. This is also called rational use of Fuzi.

Chinese culture has constantly been talking about *Tao* (Way) and technique, which are two different things. *Tao* refers to a boundless thing, but technique refers to one or two unique skills. Fuzi is equivalent to a technique, and it must be used rationally. However, it should be considered in the circle of *Tao*. Moreover, Fuzi is of a low-grade medicine like a base person who should not be put in an important position. In a word, when Fuzi is used, one must draw on its advantages and avoid its disadvantages.

Deer

Characteristics of Deer

There area variety of deer, including elk, sika deer, red deer, giraffe and so on. Besides giraffes, which cannot be used as medicines (at least, I have never heard of it), all the others can be used as medicines, but the extent of efficacy is somewhat different.

The sika deer lives on the mountain while the elk lives in the marshland. The deer on the mountain will have slightly more Yang, while the deer in the marshland will tend to be slightly Yin-nourishing. But on the whole, they are all Yang-nourishing as medicines. No matter what kind of deer, they all run very speedily, so the property of deer tends to be warmer.

The properties of animal meat as medicine mainly depend on whether the animal can run fast or not. Pigs cannot run so fast, so pork is mild in property; cattle and sheep can run a little faster, so their meat is warm; dogs run much faster, so dog meat is hot; deer can run faster than dogs, so the venison (deer meat) is hotter. The other animals can also be analyzed in such a way. Therefore, careful observation in life can help learn many things.

Let us look at deer closely. The eyes are large, even bulging. The ears are large too, and they keep on moving all the time. Eyes and ears are Yang orifices.

The eyes are subsumed to the liver, and ears are subsumed to the kidneys. The Yang orifices are big, showing that the liver and kidneys function well, and also Yang is especially sufficient.

Male deer have large horns on the heads, but some deer have long necks and smaller horns. Deer with short necks usually have larger horns. Long neck or large horns are the signs of vigorous Yang. Of all animals, deer horns are linked with the governor meridian, and large horns signify that the governor meridian is very vigorous, so the products related to deer can tonify the governor meridian and Yang.

When deer browse on grassland, their heads always direct towards the sun, which helps them gain Yang from the sun and the sky.

The deer is a"leching" animal. A male deer needs a large herd of female deer to meet its lust. One "Yang" can match so many "Yin", indicating deer has very vigorous Yang and sufficient kidney Qi. Meanwhile, it can be seen that deer 's Qi is quite inclined to Yang. Any male animals that can mate with many females, or vice versa, will be more inclined to one side. Human being prefers monogamy, so Yin and Yang are relatively balanced.

Many parts on a deer's body can be used as medicine, and even the whole deer can be used as medicine called **Quanlu Pill**, which can strongly tonify both Yin and Yang, but cannot be taken without restriction. Here are the three parts from deer as medicines: Lurong (pilose antler), Lujiao (deer horn) and Lujin (deer's sinew).

Lurong(Pilose Antler)

In the spring of every year, when the new horn on the head of male deer is about to grow out, there will grow a purple-brown nodular lump with hair on the top. It is soft and very warm with blood inside, like a sarcoma, which would be the top-grade Lurong since its Qi has not been discharged yet. At that time, if it is cut off together with skull, that would be very cruel.

Now, Lurong will not be sawed off until it grows big enough with a second bar or larger so that the deer can survive. This is called Ju Lurong (sawed pilose antler), which is sawed off from the deer's head. Ju Lurong is also quite good in quality.

As Lurong continues to grow, deer will feel very uncomfortable. They will start to grind their antler on the trunks of trees or stones, resulting in fur being ground off with fresh blood dripping until the real, bone-like horns come into being. Deer horns grow very fast. In fact, of all animal organs, Lujiao grows fastest, which means that it has sufficient Yang and vital Qi, so it can tonify Yang. On the other hand, Lujiao belongs to the substance of flesh and blood, so it can nourish Yin, too. In short, Lujiao can tonify both Yin and Yang, and it is relatively more inclined to tonifying Yang, promoting hematogenesis of blood simultaneously.

Lujiao (Deer Horn)

Lujiao shares some common properties as Lurong, and simply it is not as pure and powerful as Lurong since the life essence of deer is all concentrated on Lurong. After Lurong grows into Lujiao, some of its life essence will be dispersed, though it still can warm Yang. Generally, Lujiao is not used directly for warming Yang and it is processed into two medicines: Lujiao Jiao (deer-horn gel) and Lujiao Shuang (cornu cervi degelatinatum).

Cut Lujiao into small pieces, soak them in running water for a few days, then simmer them over soft fire of mulberry wood. In this way, the gelatine inside Lujiao is boiled into water. Then, take out Lujiao, boil the broth into paste, and finally make it into Lujiao Jiao, which is a little greasy, and mainly used to tonify Yang. Lujiao Jiao is warm but not dry, and it is often used together with Guiban Jiao (tortoise plastron gel).

Guiban Jiao mixed with Lujiao Jiao, Renshen, and Gouqizi (fructus lycii) makes a formula called **Guilu Erxian Jiao**. some people may directly boil Guiban Jiao and Lujiao Jiao together into **Guilu Erxian Jiao**. **Guilu Erxian Jiao** is a very effective formula for those who suffer from Yin-Yang deficiency with just a little pathogenic influence. **Lujiao Jiao** can activate the governor meridian and Guiban Jiao can activate the Renmai meridian. From the perspective of the Eight Extra-Meridians theory of TCM, Lujiao Jiao and Guiban Jiao together can nourish the two meridians, which is equivalent to nourishing Yin and Yang.

Of course, those who suffer from only Yang deficiency, and who are unwilling or unable to use greasy medicines for nourishing purpose, may use Lujiao Shuang, which, in essence, is the left-over material after Lujiao Jiao is boiled into gel. Lujiao Shuang looks like pieces of dried bones, and they can be scraped into powder with a scraper. It has no greasy effect at all, but it can warm Yang with weak potence.

Some people, however, do need to warm Yang in such a mild way, especially the elderly people who cannot stand severe heat. The elderly people have relatively heavy endogenous heat and Yang deficiency at the same time since their primordial Yang (kidney-Yang) is not converged but changed into endogenous heat. The primordial Yang warms the human body, and the pathogenic heat makes troubles at every corner to set endogenous fires, which then induce phlegm. In such a case, due to the existence of the endogenous fire, Lurong cannot be used for tonifying purpose; due to phlegm, the greasy thing like Lujiao Jiao cannot be used, either, or otherwise, it will induce more phlegm. Hence, only Lujiao Shuang can be used to warm it up so that the old man will have less urination at night. In short, Lujiao Shuang and Lurong are suitable for different people.

Lujin (Deer's Sinew)

Deer can run very fast since it has many sinews with much strength. Pigs cannot run very fast, and they have very few tendons in the legs. Lujin is processed by pulling it out first, soaking in water and then drying in the air.

As it has been discussed in the above, the grass of Xianmao (rhizoma curculiginis) will be transformed into tendons in the bodies of sheep after they eat it. For the human being, Xianmao can warm Yang and nourish the muscle and tendon. All the organs of deer are quite similar in efficacies, but only some of them have stronger effects; some have milder effects; some are partial to nourishing muscle and tendon; some are partial to tonifying Yang; some are able to activate human muscles and bones; and some are able to activate the human governor meridian. The only difference is that they go in different directions with different degrees of potence. Lujin can nourish muscles and bones and cure strain, and make people strong. In the late stage of rheumatism, Lujin can be used for coping with the aftermath since some dry and severe medicines have been used to dispel the pathogenic wind, remove dampness and warm the blood vessels. Finally, under the condition that there is no pathogenic influence in between the skin, meridians and collaterals, Lujin can be used to consolidate and rehabilitate the health

Deer are gentle and warm in character. So, Lujin can warm anadesma, after which the pathogenic factors will be driven out by the vital Qi. Especially, those who undertake intensive physical work such as factory workers and farmers may suffer from some internal impairment, like the strain of lumbar muscles, pains from constant overwork in their bodies when they are getting older. Such internal impairment may be related to blood stasis or phlegm. When phlegm and blood stasis are almost removed, Lujin can be used for nourishing, which will help them feel energetic. But different from energy arising from the **Fuzi Lizhong Pill** is that the energy arising from eating Lujin can last long to make one feel comfortable.

Nourishing muscles and bones can help nourish the liver and kidneys. The dried deer sinew needs soaking in water for a long time before use. Just like sea cucumber and shark fin, the dried deer sinew is like collagen, and it requires soaking for a few days. In the soaking process, water must be changed frequently, after which it will become soft. Then, it can be stewed as food. In fact, Lujin is more used for food now.

Lujin is very similar to beef tendon. Those who are going to buy deer's sinew should buy the deer hooves. That can tell the deer species from the shape of the hooves.

While stewing deer's sinew, one should not stew it with the bones of other animals. Otherwise, some of the essential substance will get into the bones. Generally, it is cooked together with some lean pork. Deer's sinew is mild in property and light in taste, while pork is sweet and mild in property. Deer are subsumed to Yang and pigs are subsumed to Yin. When deer's sinew and pork are stewed together, they can balance Yin and Yang, and will not cause fire either after eating.

第七章 附子与鹿类

我们今天继续讲桂之属火部的方药：附子和鹿。一个是下品药，我们要放在花名册的最后；另一个是动物药，更要放在最后。

附子

附子性状及家族成员

附子是一种多年生的草本植物，根部入药，它有很多块根，有点像马铃薯，只不过，马铃薯是一个一个独立的，而附子则是新生的块根附着在老块根上，所以叫附子。标准的附子是一两一个。

附子这种植物，是通过块根繁殖的，种下去一个附子，上面长出植株，这个种下去的附子就成了乌头，热性更足，药力更大，就像作种的那块老姜，姜是老的辣嘛。乌头周围附着生长出新的块根，这就是附子，药力小一些。有的根，边上没有长出侧根，那所有的药力都在主根上了，孤家寡人，药力最大，就叫天雄。它们都是剧毒的。

其实，附子、乌头、天雄都是一类药，只是长根的部位或方式不一样。它们有相似之处，也有不一样的地方。

乌头与毒酒

乌头是锥形的，个头比较小。附子更偏圆一点，当然最好是平底，而且上面的皮上有脐状的东西，在炮制的时候把皮和脐去掉。附子是一味气味俱厚的药，跑得比较快，能通行全身，无处不到，走而不守。

附子是有剧毒的，因为其性大热。我们看电视里经常看到这样的情节，皇帝赐给某爱卿一杯毒酒，喝掉了以后马上腹痛，然后七窍流血而死。人们都说古代的毒酒是鸩酒，把鸩鸟的羽毛放在酒里搅一下，一杯鸩酒就做成了。其实这是一种误传。最常用的毒酒，都是用生乌头泡的，泡得比较浓。因为它大热走窜的，又能入血分，借着酒性，药力更猛。喝下去以后，人全身的血液都被鼓动起来，心脏马上就受不了，然后血热攻入五脏，外在表现就是七窍流血而死。七窍都是属于阳窍，是阳气发泄的地方。"五脏六腑之精气皆上注于目"，其实不仅仅上注于目，而是上注于七窍，当你五脏之中血液沸腾，往往往上涌，从七窍流出来。这是毒药发生作用的原理。

如何解附子的毒

喝了乌头毒酒，基本上人就完了，药力太快太猛，来不及救了。如果中了附子的毒，还有救治的余地。

附子大热，我们用寒药来平它，或者用甘草来缓它，因为寒就可以清热，甘就能缓急。寒药如黄连、犀角，黄连大苦大寒，犀角是灵物，最能清阳明的热，阳明为多气多血之腑，当气血涌动的时候，阳明首当其冲，必先保住。黄连能清心火，犀角也能清心热，二味同用，对心脏是一种保护。这时候情形十分危急了，先保心脏。过去，解附子毒的方子就三味药：黄连、犀角、生甘草，煎汤。甘草能解百药之毒，还有甘缓之用，能让毒性发作别那么迅猛急速。

还有，用黄土水也可以，因为土性平和，万物归土，黄土最能解毒。黄土，北方很少见到，南方才有。南方的土，在表的一层是脏的，发黑或者发灰，往里面一挖就是黄土了，取出来，用水搅和匀了，然后让它沉淀，等它完全沉淀以后，上面的那一层水也叫地浆水，能解很多毒，比如说毒蘑菇的毒、水蛭的毒，也可以用它来解附子的毒。

附子的炮制

我们知道了怎么解附子的毒，再去理解附子的炮制，就比较容易了。

炮制附子也有很多的方法：有人说用甘草水来浸，有人说用黑豆水来浸，有的说用井盐来拌它，甚至把它腌一腌……说法很多。

炮制附子的正规的方法就是用甘草水来浸泡。先把附子的皮、脐刮掉，然后一横一竖切把附子剖成四片，再把它放到甘草水中泡，要让甘草水把整个的附子泡透，再把它弄出来，用慢火炒黄，然后摊在泥地上。泥地在现在不是太常见，就是雨后的地，很潮，但并没有泥。

在泥地上摊一个晚上，是为了让它出火毒。因为附子本身就是一味大热的药，现在又放在火上炒，热性就太大了，形成火毒，所以把它摊在地上，因为土能够解火毒，而且土永远都是很平和的，没有大寒，也没有大热，把附子放在地上让它得地气，使附子性质也变得平和。

附子是一味热药，甘草是一味甘药，甘就能缓，能够在不损伤附子热性的情况下，让附子的热力发挥得缓慢一些。

也有加童便来煮附子的。童便就是小孩的小便，健康的小男孩（十四岁以下的小男孩都可以）的小便。用童便来煮，一方面是用童便的寒凉之性制伏附子的大热，另一方面，因为童便是一种浊水，偏于往下走，附子跟着童便在一起也更容易往下走，使其热力温下而不浮越。但因为童便是寒凉的东西，有人嫌用童便来制附子就抑制了附子的阳刚之气。

还有一种方法，把附子切成片，放在水里漂了又漂，漂得很淡很淡再来用，开方子的时候有的大夫会写"淡附片"，就是这个。它的烈性就要缓一些，终归不如用甘草水来炮制的附子好。仲景方里，用到附子，往往同时用到甘草，而且甘草的用量还比较大，这也是用来反佐附子。还有的方子里边会用到生附子，这就更要用到甘草。

至于后来又有人说用井盐来炮制附子，这种做法我觉得需要商榷。井盐是咸的，性寒，用它来炮制附子就损伤了附子的大热之性。人有性情，药也有性情，用人是用人的性情，用药更是用药的性情。附子的性情是大热的，你用大寒的药就把它性情给磨平了。然后你再大量地用，自诩高明，这还是在用附子吗？这不是在折腾吗？真正用附子，没必要用这些寒凉的药去制它，用甘草水来炮制它就足够了，也没有必要用那么大的量，适可而止就行了。

然后你再大量地用，自诩高明，这还是在用附子吗？这不是在折腾吗？真正用附子，没必要用这些寒凉的药去制它，用甘草水来炮制它就足够了，也没有必要用那么大的量，适可而止就行了。

附子治风寒湿痹

刚才讲的淡附片，我们经常会用到。前面讲过附子能够通行全身，同时又是一味温药。如果身上有寒湿不容易去掉，能不能用附子来把它赶走？可以的，这时附子就要用淡附片，淡附片更倾向于走身体的经络，它们能够驱逐风寒邪气。一些痹症，身上的一些痛啊、关节炎啊、风湿啊，就会经常用到淡附片。淡附片性质依然是比较热的，用量不宜太大，5克左右就足够了，当然也有用量比较大的，一般不超过15克，当然这是在身上的风寒湿痹较重的情况下。它属于温通的重剂。

乌头在这种情况下也可以用。一般必须用制过的乌头，不然的话毒性太大了。加了乌头，驱风的力度就比较强。如果寒湿比较强那么用附子就够了。风寒湿痹比较重的情况，往往发生在农村中老年——大概五十岁左右的人身上。因为它们年轻时在外面干活，顶风冒雨的，日积月累的风寒湿邪在体内阻滞经络。他们很多人有颈椎病、腰椎病、坐骨神经痛，还有胳膊痛、腿痛，有时会为了治疗得快一点，就可以用附子和乌头。

附子温通五脏

温通五脏也是用炙过的附子，一般用生附子的情况比较少。用在回阳救逆，起死回生，附子确实是一味非常好的药，有类似于激素的作用，当然不能把附子等同于激素，但它们有相似之处。它能够兴奋五脏，让五脏在瞬间变得坚强。

附子跟人参一起能强心，这就是参附汤。有时候为了取它的力性，就用生附子，这是起死回生的一个方。人快要死的时候，用人参"回其元气于无何有之乡"，用附子回欲绝之阳，把那一丁点快要消失的阳气给拉回来。

附子同白术是强脾的，所以有术附汤，就是一味白术加一味附子。在很多其他的方子里也会有附子和白术，比如说理中汤。白术是健脾的，配附子则能强脾，能够让脾阳或者脾本身各方面的功能迅速增强。

附子同麻黄一起用就会强肺。我们以麻黄附子细辛汤为例来说说。麻黄开肺气，加上附子就能够开肺气、回肺阳，同细辛一起又能强肾。当然强肺强肾不仅仅是同麻黄、同细辛，同麦冬它也可以强肺呀。麦冬是一味补肺的重剂，它偏于润肺，清肺，是一味寒凉的药，跟附子这个热药在一起，寒归寒，热归热，这也是相得益彰的配合。

附子与肉桂同用也会强肾，同白芍一起又能强肝。

附子的运用与善后

但毕竟附子在《本经》的下品，它是一味大热的药，不能乱用，用错了或者用的太久都不好。大热伤血也伤气，伤血就会导致血瘀，伤气就会导致痰。我们经常讲气血痰瘀，气血是生理状态，而痰和瘀是气血不行所致，是病理产物。所以，用附子往往是这样的：当时有效，后患无穷。刚开始用的时候，真是非常有效，起死回生，或者让病蔫蔫的人马上精力无穷。但是当时有效并不意味着以后一直这么有效，而且以后还会产生很多隐患。用了附子以后，必然要用大量凉润的药来善后，就像打完一场仗，咱们要打扫战场，安抚百姓，要做一系列的善后工作，这也是治病的时候要注意的。

书里面讲，什么病用什么汤主之，主完了之后怎么办呢？它是不会和你讲的。你必须看着一个病是怎么从头到尾一步一步治的，病治好了以后又是怎么善后的，才能把书上的东西联系起来，这个只有通过跟师来学，师父会耐心给你讲，书里面一般不屑于讲。书都是教你怎么去治一个症，师门则是教你怎么去治一个病，或者说怎么去把这个人调到最佳的状态。

一个风寒湿痹的人，比如说坐骨神经痛，你方子里用了附子、乌头以后，他不痛了，但你一看它的舌头，舌苔有点发黄，舌质也偏红，脉偏数，这说明还有内热。这个内热，很大一部分是附子、乌头带来的，即使没有这些症状，你也得考虑到，用了大量的附子、乌头，还在他体内发生作用，怎么办呢？还要打扫战场，用凉润的药来善后。

附子的滥用与补救

我前几年遇到一个女孩子，是某省中医药大学毕业的。在学校期间，有个喜欢用附子的老师对她说："你这个小女孩小手冰凉的，阳虚啊。"一摸脉，就说脉紧，有寒，给她开了附子理中汤的加减。她吃了以后，感觉还不错，精力挺充沛的。但问题也接踵而至：胳膊上长了些痘痘，去找这个老师。这老师说，好啊，寒在出来了。然后继续附子理中汤加减，附子量更大。吃过以后脸色又有点发黑，老师说，黑属水主寒哪，这是寒在往外透，寒透出来，你身体就好了！于是她继续吃，她又发现眼睛近视了，要去配眼镜了，而她以前的眼睛是很亮的。最后，嗓子也痛了，说话的声音都变了，沙哑了，不脆不嫩了！这下，她才开始怀疑。但到这时候，她已经吃了好几个月的附子了。

后来，她到了北京，身体非常不好，胳膊一直长痘痘，脸依然很黑，显得比实际年龄苍老，痰多，喉咙痛，老感觉得有痰堵着。这些症状都是她吃附子以前没有的。其实这都是附子带来的后遗症。她当时问我这是怎么回事，我说：诸痛疮疡皆属于心，就是皆属于火。胳膊上都起痘了，是火啊！有这么排寒气的吗？

脸黑，黑虽然是主肾属水的，但物极必反，热到一定的程度也会发黑。不相信，你去摸一下锅底，是黑的还是白的。你不会说锅底是一直在很寒的环境中变黑的吧。火虽然是红的，但火烤久了就会让一个东西变黑。你喝了很多的附子，底下的邪火太旺了，把脸熏黑了。这种黑不是寒象的那种黑，而是熏黑，是被内火熏出来的。

痰为什么多呢，因为火炼液成痰，把你身体的津液烤干了、烤稠了，成了痰，就像熬胶一样。感冒内热比较重时，痰也会像胶似的，还伴随喉咙痛。喉咙痛也是火在往上冲，喉咙这个地方是人体咽喉要道，太窄了，其他的地方火比较分散，一到咽喉这儿火就比较集中，烤得就更厉害。所以，咽喉就痛，声音就会变。

这位女生也是学中医的，她跟我说她后来看到麦冬、竹沥、石膏、寒水石这类药名，心里都会特别舒服，因为她身体需要这些。麦冬甘寒生津，石膏甘寒清热，竹沥甘凉化痰，这些药都适合她。

她的痰，必须用竹沥来化。竹沥就是竹子里面烧出的水。把一根青竹棍放在火上一烤，上面就会出汗。把竹简烤一下，让它出一点竹沥，然后在竹子上写字就不会有虫蛀，这就叫汗青。竹沥很凉润，能够化痰。吃多了附子，需要养阴生津，麦冬、竹沥都要经常用。当然如果伤更多的话，什么瓜蒌、浙贝，甚至陈皮、半夏也要考虑。半夏也是一味温燥的药，不能过度的用。

善用附子

我的师父经常讲这么一句话："附子要善用不能滥用。"什么叫善用附子？善用就是用得恰到好处，和用多用少无关。并不是说你敢多用就是善用，有时用得非常少也是善用，或者不用也是善用。

我师父开八味地黄丸，附子用3克，肉桂用2克，我问怎么用这么少？他说："这就像点灯，点一盏灯你需要多大的火？"我说："需要一根火柴就可以了。"他说："对，3克附子2克肉桂就相当于一根火柴，足以把一个草原点着。"没有必要用那么多。这也是善用附子。

我们中国历来讲有道、有术，二者是不一样的，道是无边无际的一个东西，术是一两个绝技、绝活，附子就相当于一个术，需要善用它，要把它纳入到道中来。而且，附子属于下品药，相当于一个小人，我们更不能重用它，用它一定要趋利避害。

鹿

鹿的性状

鹿的种类非常多，有麋鹿、梅花鹿、马鹿、长颈鹿等。除了没听说长颈鹿可以入药，其他的都是可以入药的，只是药效的轻重程度有些不同。

梅花鹿是生活在山上的，麋鹿是生活在沼泽里的。山上的鹿，阳性会稍微强一些，而沼泽里的鹿则更偏于养阴，但在总体上讲，它们都是偏于养阳的药。不管哪种鹿，都跑得很快，所以它的性质是偏温热的。

我们区分一种动物的肉或者入药是偏温，偏热，还是偏平，主要看它会不会跑。猪最不会跑，所以猪肉是平性的；牛羊稍微跑得就快一点，它们的肉就是温性的；狗跑得更快，所以狗肉就是热性的；鹿跑得比狗还快，所以鹿肉就更偏温热。其他的动物，也可以这样来分析。因此我们不需要去背书，多观察生活，就可以得到很多东西。

鹿眼睛特别大，还有点鼓，耳朵也特别大，还能动。眼睛、耳朵都是阳窍，眼睛属肝，耳朵属肾，阳窍那么大，说明它肝肾的功能好，还说明它阳气特别的足。

公鹿头上长角，特别大。有的鹿脖子特别长，角就小一些；脖子短的鹿，角就会大一些。脖子长或者角大也是阳气旺的标志。在所有的动物中，鹿角是连着督脉的，角大意味着督脉非常的旺，因此鹿能补督脉、补阳。

鹿吃草的时候，头会一直朝着太阳，这也能得太阳的阳气、得天的阳气。

鹿是一种"好淫"的动物，一只公鹿要一大群母鹿才能满足它。一阳就能配那么多阴，鹿的阳气非常旺，肾气非常足；同时也可以看出，它的气是很偏的，偏阳。凡是一个雄性的动物配很多雌性的动物，或者一个雌性动物配很多雄性的动物，都是有偏的。人类偏于一夫一妻，所以阴阳相对平衡。

鹿能入药的部位有很多，甚至整只鹿都能入药，叫全鹿丸，能峻补阴阳，但这种药也不能乱吃。我们主要讲鹿身上的三种药：鹿茸、鹿角、鹿筋。

鹿茸

每年春天，公鹿头上就会长出新的鹿角。鹿角刚生的时候，在鹿的头上有一个紫褐色的瘤状的东西，上面还有毛，软软的还没有长硬，很温暖的，里面有血，像一个肉瘤似的，这时候，它的气还没有泻，是顶级的鹿茸。将其连着脑骨一起砍下来，叫砍茸。当然，这只鹿也死了，这非常残忍。现在一般都等鹿茸长成二杠或更大一点后，把它锯下来，这样能够把这只鹿保留下来，这叫锯茸，就是从鹿头上锯下来的茸，质量依然非常好。

现在一般都等鹿茸长成二杠或更大一点后，把它锯下来，这样能够把这只鹿保留下来，这叫锯茸，就是从鹿头上锯下来的茸，质量依然非常好。

当鹿茸继续长大，鹿就会很难受，就会在树干上或石头上磨它的角，磨得鲜血淋漓，皮毛全部磨掉了，里面像骨头那样的真角才生出来。鹿角长得特别快，在所有动物的器官中，鹿角长得是最快的，这意味着它有很足的阳气、生发之气，所以能补阳。另一方面，它也是血肉有情之品，也能补阴。它阴阳双补，只是更偏于补阳，也能带动阴血的生成。

鹿角

鹿角依然有鹿茸的某些性质，只是没有鹿茸那么纯正，没有鹿茸的力量那么大，因为鹿的精气都集中在鹿茸上，鹿茸长成鹿角后，它精气依然在，只是已经分散了。鹿角依然可以温阳，但一般不直接用，而是将其炮制成两种东西：鹿角胶和鹿角霜。

把鹿角截成小段，在长流水中浸泡几天，然后再用桑木火小火慢炖，鹿角里面的胶质都煮到水里了，然后把鹿角取出来，把汤汁熬干，收成膏，就做成了鹿角胶。鹿角胶有点滋腻，但它仍然是以补阳为主，它温而不燥，经常与龟胶一起用。

龟版胶加鹿角胶，再加人参、枸杞子，叫龟鹿二仙胶。也有人把龟版和鹿角放在一起直接熬成龟鹿二仙胶。如果阴阳两虚，邪气不盛的话，用龟鹿二仙胶是非常好的。鹿胶通督脉，龟版通任脉，它们一起能补养任督二脉，养了任督二脉也就相当于养了人的阴阳。这是从奇经八脉的角度立意。

当然，如果只是阳虚，不愿意或不能用滋腻的药去补，那就用鹿角霜。鹿角被熬完胶后，剩下来的部分就是鹿角霜，看上去就是一节节枯骨，用刀片刮一刮就可以变成粉，一点滋腻的作用也没有了，但它仍然有用，仍然可以温阳，只是此时它温阳的力度非常微弱。

但有的人就需要以这种微弱的方式去温阳，尤其是老年人，他受不了太快，只能用这种微弱的方式。老年人内热比较重，同时有阳虚，因为他真阳没有收敛住，成为热了。真阳是温煦人体的，邪热是到处放火的，内热又生痰，怎么温阳？有火就不能去补，不能用鹿茸了，有痰就不能用滋腻的东西，否则会更加生痰，也不能用鹿胶，只能用一点鹿角霜温补一下。这样，他晚上起夜都会变少。总之，鹿角霜和鹿茸分别适合不同的人群。

鹿筋

我们知道，鹿是非常能跑的，它筋非常多、非常强劲。猪最不会跑，猪蹄筋非常少。把鹿筋抽出来，放到水中浸泡，然后再晾干，这就是鹿筋。

前面我们讲，羊吃了仙茅就遍体化筋，身上筋会特别多，人吃了就能温阳、养筋。鹿筋也能温阳、养筋。鹿身上的东西，作用都比较相似，只是有的作用峻猛一些，有的作用缓和一些，有的偏于养筋、有的偏于补阳、有的通人的筋骨、有的通人的督脉，它们只是走向不一样，程度不一样而已。鹿筋也是这样的，它能养筋骨、治劳损，它能够使人有力气。在风湿病后期，可以用它来善后，因为我们用了一些燥烈的药来驱风化湿，来温煦血脉，最后，在确保肌肤经络之间没有邪气的情况下，再用鹿筋来巩固、修复一下。

鹿性温，以筋入筋，所以能温筋。筋得到了温煦，即使还残留着一些邪气，也会被这股正气驱赶出去。尤其是遇到体力劳动强度大的，比如工人、农民等，到了年纪比较大的时候，积劳成疾，身上就会有很多暗伤。体力劳动过久，很多人身上都有腰肌劳损，或者酸痛之类，可能与瘀血有关，可能与痰有关，在痰和瘀化得差不多的情况下，可以用点鹿筋来养一养，吃了浑身来劲。但是这种浑身来劲与吃附子理中丸的浑身来劲又不一样，这种浑身来劲很舒服、很长久的。

养筋骨，就能养肝肾。鹿筋的成品是干的，吃的时候需要长时间泡，就像海参、鱼翅那样，它也相当于胶原蛋白，需要泡很长时间，而且边泡边换水，几天以后，泡软了，才能炖着吃。与其说是用来入药的，不如说它是用来吃的。

鹿筋和牛蹄筋非常相似，甚至有的人用牛蹄筋来冒充鹿筋。所以，我们买鹿筋的时候，一定要买带蹄的，从蹄子的形状，可以分辨鹿的种类。

炖鹿筋的时候要注意，不能与其他的骨头一起炖，否则其中的一些精华物质就会钻到骨头里去。一般与猪瘦肉一起炖就行了。鹿筋是温淡之品，气温而味淡，猪肉则是甘平的。鹿属阳，猪属阴，所以与猪肉同炖会比较好，取阴阳平衡之义，吃了也不容易上火。

Volume 4
Gypsum of Genera—Metal-categorized Formulas and Medicines

Chapter 1   Introduction of Metal-categorized Formulas and Medicines

Analyses of Metal Characteristics

Metal-categorized formulas and medicines are mainly cool and cold in properties. In the four seasons of a year, spring is warm; summer is hot; autumn is cool; and winter is cold. Autumn corresponds to the metal and coldness. The TCM learners should always keep in mind the concept of **Wuxing Doctrine**.

The Characteristics of Metal and Stone

Metal is corresponding to the west. Let us look from Beijing towards the west, where there are the provinces of Shanxi, Shaanxi, Gansu, Qinghai, and Xinjiang autonomous region in the northwest, and the provinces of Sichuan, Yunnan, and Tibet Autonomous Region in the southwest. It is a vast length and breadth of land – a very broad and vast land. **Shan Hai Jing (The Classic of Mountains and Seas)** says "The west is the land of metals and stones", where there are lots of deserts. Sand is in the category of metals and stones, and it is essentially different from soil. The Hetian Jade from Xinjiang, the best of all jades, is also in the category of metals and stones.

Even the people who live in the western areas speak and sing with the pitch of metals in tones that tend to be clear and melodious, loud and sonorous, while the people in the eastern areas sing more gently, corresponding to the sound of-wood. The songs in the western areas, for example, the song named *"Tibetan Plateau"* and the folk songs in the northern area of Shaanxi province all feel like the sound of metal. From one's speech and singing, it may be easy to judge which category the area he or she comes from belongs to in terms of **Wuxing Doctrine.**

The folks from the western areas in China usually show the characteristics of the metal. The people with metal characteristics are more sprightly, doughty, loyal and faithful. Let us take a look at *"Qin-feng"* from the **the Book of Songs.** It is a sort of folk songs originated from the kingdom of Qin back in 11th to 6th centuries BC. The vassal state Qin was located around the area of Hangu Pass; Historically, people living around those areas were considered to be the westerners of China. There is an obvious contrast between Qin's music and the music from the central area, like the vassal states Zheng and Wei. Zheng and Wei were located in the central plain of China, and their music was often labeled as being licentious or decadent. Whereas in the western songs and poems, there are much fewer decadence, but much more vigor and firmness. The poem titled **"Wu Yi"**(literally means **No Clothes**) from **"Qin-feng"** is an example of a song on the battlefield:

Who said there was nothing to wear?
Let us share the same campaign wear.
The king sends troops to the battlefield,
Repair my dagger-axe and spear,
Let us take revenge for the bitter hatred we share.

Who said there was nothing to wear?
Let us share the same underwear.
The king sends troops to the battlefield,
Repair my halberd and spear,
Let us set off to the battle together.

Who said there was nothing to wear?
Let us share the same battle skirt.
The king sends troops to the battlefield,
Repair my armor and weaponry,

Let us defeat the enemy and march on all the way.

Zhu Xi (one of the most famous Confucians in the Song Dynasty, 1130—1200) annotated this poem as: "The culture of the vassal state Qin emphasizes heroism, courage and strength; undaunted by perils… all manifested in their poems. " Because of such heroic character of the western Chinese, King Wen of Zhou initiated his revolting troops from the west Qi Shan around the 11th century BC to dispatch an expedition against King Zhòu of the Shang dynasty. The unification of the six states by the vassal state Qin around the 3rd century BC also began in the western areas. Similarly, the Tang Dynasty united the country starting from Shanxi. Even the same for the Chinese Communist Party, as their early operational base was established and deeply rooted around Shaanxi, Gansu and Ningxia. There must be a high correlation between the culture of those places and the higher success rate of revolting from the west.

According to Zhu Xi, "Yong Zhou is endowed with fertile soil and rich water, and the folks there are characterized with honesty and uprightness. " Yong Zhou refers to the area covering parts of Shaanxi, Gansu, Qinghai and Ningxia of China, where the people are endowed with the personalities of good manners and the quality of metals. So, they are bold, fierce, and more aggressive. Metals have three characteristics: hardness, sharpness, and coolness, which define its properties when it is used as medicine.

Stones Subsumed to Metal According to Wuxing Doctrine

Stones are subsumed to metal in properties according ***Wuxing Doctrine***. Although stones/rocks could be transformed into soil after weathering, soils and rocks are essentially different. Both metal and stone are hard, while soil is hard only when it is dried and agglomerated. However, once it is waterish, soil will become crumbly and slimy. Meanwhile, plants can grow out of soils but few plants can grow on rocks. Hence, stones/rocks are subsumed to metal, while soil is subsumed to earth. TCM learners should not try to analyze the material composition in a microscopic way, but should try to understand the herbal properties in a macroscopic way, which is also the distinction between the Chinese and the Western learning.

About Traditional Chinese Medicine (TCM)

TCM is established on the land of China, so, it might be another story when it is studied in the other countries. King Yu, the legendary ancient saint, divided the land of China into nine states for administration.

Among hundreds of thousands of plants, animals and minerals, the Chinese ancestors spared no efforts to select a few hundreds of best natural herbs, and then, figured out the most suitable locations of producing the top class medicines, and the later generations give the credit to Shennong tasting hundreds of herbs. In fact, this tells how the Chinese ancestors experienced and thought deeply about the properties of hundreds of medicines, which is also the result of attempts by the generation after generation. Therefore, the essence of TCM can only be acquired in the Chinese traditional mode of thinking.

Years ago, I was contacted by an American research organization with a plan to explore the authentic herbs in America. For example, they agreed that Sanqi (notoginseng) produced in Yunnan and Tianlin of Guangxi in China is the best herb, so, they want to find out which areas in America could produce the same quality Sanqi. And similarly, some other herbs such as Baizhu (white atractylodes rhizome) and Aiye (folium artemisiae argyi), where can such authentic herbs be produced in America? Are there any geo-authentic herbs available in America? It is indeed a huge project, I thought. It was too difficult to put into reality since such a project requires explorations by generations to observe and study in the broad land with solid traditional Chinese medicine knowledge and skills in the traditional Chinese mode of thinking along with numerous clinical practices rather than in any lab in a short time.

Shigao (Gypsum) as the Core Herb of Metal-categorized Medicines

In this volume, Shigao will be taken as a typical example of metal and mineral medicines to illustrate a bunch of cold and cool herbs. Of course, not all metals and minerals are cool or cold in properties. Xionghuang (realgar) and Liuhuang (sulfur), for instance, are extremely hot. Similarly, not all animal medicinal products are warm and hot, for example, earthworms are salty and cold in nature, and pork is neutral in nature. Someone might claim that donkey meat is cold. In fact, it is neither cold nor cool, but warm. It is usually regarded as being partially cool since it has a stronger Yin nourishing function and can be used to clear heat in blood, which gives an illusional impression of its being cool. Donkey meat is warm in property, but it has a cooling medicinal function. In practice, it is proved that some herbs are warm in property, but cool in function; and some herbs are cool in property, but warm in function, to which the TCM learners should pay attention in clinical practices or researches on herbs.

Cold and Cool Medicines

Functions of Cold and Cool Medicines

Cold and cool medicines have lots of functions. Unfortunately, lots of Chinese medicine books criticize such herbs strongly since when they are mistakenly used, Yang Qi in human bodies will be constrained, and the patient who continuously use such medicines could become listless, showing weakness in talking or walking, and even worse, he could get erectile dysfunction or loss of vision. Misuse of cold and cool herbs can also cause Qi stagnation, which may disrupt transportation and transformation (T&T) of Qi and blood, leading to more serious diseases. Therefore, when cool and cold herbs are to be discussed, it is necessary to know the potential negative effects first, and then the favorable effects.

Neither should one neglect or negate the cool and cold herbs or even dislike them simply because they were misused or overused by someone to cause some bad consequence, nor criticize a doctor since he or she uses cool and cold herbs in the prescriptions. All diseases are related to fire, even the symptoms caused by cold factors since fire arises when the symptoms become chronic. Cold and cool herbs are used to eliminate the pathogenic fire, whereas the pathogenic fire may arise from various factors. A lot of theories involved will be explained in this volume.

There are lots of cold and cool herbal medicines, whose functions are extensive and complex. It indeed requires lots of efforts to master the skills in using the cold and cool medicines. As a matter of fact, Chinese medicine practitioners not only should be adept at using "fire" but also "water". In Buddhism, the human world is said to be a house on fire, where human being cannot stay even for a moment. And inside everyone's heart, there is irrepressible anger like fire, shown as worries and anxieties. Therefore, human beings need cooling down, which is one of the reasons that cool medicines are prescribed.

Definitely, warm herbs are also needed. The world itself is of cold-heat complication. On the one hand, it is a house on fire with everyone's mind filled with irrepressible anger (fire); on the other hand, the world is full of fickleness and inexorability (cold and cruelty), which also make a person feel cold sometimes. So, both cold/cool and hot/warm medicines are needed, where applicable. Sometimes, cold and warm medicines are used together.

Cold and cool medicines can be categorized in many different ways. But I think it might be easier to learn according to the five tastes. Cold (as one of the four properties) goes together with the five tastes, therefore, there are sweet-cold medicines, bitter-cold medicines, salty-cold medicines, sour-cold medicines, and pungent-cold medicines. But here, "coldness" also covers the meaning of coolness.

Sweet-cold Medicines

The term of "sweat-cold" means that a medicine is endowed with both the sweet taste and cold property. Shigao as a sweet-cold medicine is not so sweet as white sugar but only a slightly sweet. Lugen (rhizoma phragmitis) is also sweet and cold, yet it is quite sweet with slightly cool nature. In addition, Maogen (couchgrass root), Tiandong (asparagus cochinchinensis), Maidong (radix ophiopogonis), and Shihu (dendrobe) etc. are also sweet and cool medicines.

Sweet-cold medicines can enter the stomach to clear the Qi system. And meanwhile, the sweet taste can enter the spleen to provide energy that the human body needs. These medicines can nourish the human body in a way of clearing, that is, to nurse the human health with clear and fresh nutrient substance slowly, just like sprinkling a plant with clear water. While a patient is recovering from a severe disease, or he is in a state of deficiency with floating heat, he will definitely need clear nourishment that the sweet and cold medicines can give to clear the floating heat.

The sweet-cold medicines in fact are sweet and cool, and to be exact, they are just slightly cold, for example, Shigao. The medicines in this category are not so cold as Huangqin (scutellaria baicalensis), Huanglian (coptis chinensis), andHuangbai (phellodendron amurense). The sweet taste entering the spleen can promote the T&T functions. Once the spleen Yang is stirred up, the Yang Qi of the entire body will be subsequently mobilized. As such, the slightly cold medicines won't matter too much.

Sweet-cold medicines first enter the stomach to clear the Qi system. According to the TCM conception, "the stomach is like dry earth, which will calm down when it is cooled", which means the cold and cool medicine can make the stomach comfortable. Some people claim that the Chinese medicine can cause impairment of the stomach. That is not correct. To be exact, only when Chinese medicines are misused, they may cause impairment of the stomach. As a matter of fact, the Chinese medicines, for example, the sweet-cold medicines can nourish the stomach if they are properly used. An experienced Chinese medicine practitioner would first protect patients' stomach Qi when he or she starts to write a prescription, as the TCM concept says, "Life can go on with the presence of the stomach Qi; otherwise, death will follow up".

Among the salty-cold medicines, for example, Xijiao (rhinoceros horn) and Muli (concha ostreae), of which Muli tastes very salty when it is freshly picked up on the seashore. Even though its savoury taste is reduced after it is washed over and again in fresh water. The salty-cold medicines also enter the stomach, but they clear the blood system instead. As it is known from the TCM conception, the stomach is an organ with abundant Qi and blood. The heat in both Qi and blood systems can congregate in the stomach, and will be transformed into the stomach heat.

The sweet-cold medicines enter the stomach to clear the heat from Qi system, while the salty-cold medicines enter the stomach to clear the heat from blood system. Therefore, these two categories of medicines should be chosen in line with the symptoms of the pathogenic heat.

Bitter-cold Medicines

Bitter-cold medicines, such as Huangqin, Huanglian, Huangbai, Zhizi (fructus gardeniae), Zhimu (rhizoma anemarrhenae), and Longdancao (radix gentianae), have powerful cold properties than the sweet-cold or salty-cold medicines. Huangqin clears the lung heat in the Upper Jiao; Huanglian clears the heat in the Middle Jiao; Huangbai clears the heat in the Lower Jiao; Zhizi clears lingering heat across the Tri-jiao. For Zhimu, it depends on what medicines it goes with. If used together with Huanglian, it clears the stomach heat; If used together with Huangbai, it clears the heat in the Lower Jiao. Huanglian tastes bitter, but in fact, Longdancao tastes much more bitter than Huanglian. Longdancao is an extremely bitter herb that can clear the damp-heat in the liver meridian. All the bitter cold medicines mentioned above are very strong and are used for eliminating the excess heat. These medicines, like the fire fighting pumps, are used to extinguish a conflagration in buildings. However, these medicines should not be used in a long run since "bitter-cold medicines spoil the appetite." The sweet-cold medicines nourish the stomach, and the salty-cold medicines do not harm the stomach too much, yet the bitter-cold medicines can definitely impair the stomach, resulting in poor appetite. That is why many patients do not have appetite after a long use of **Longdan Xiegan Tang**.

Qingwei San can be prescribed for the case of typical excess stomach heat with the symptoms of halitosis, yellow and thick tongue coating, or even toothache, mouth-ulcers, or pimples on the forehead. But it is better to use this formula when the stomach heat is more than dampness. Once the stomach heat is cleared with **Qingwei San**, the patient will have a better appetite. However, if the patient uses this formula continuously for long, his appetite may become poor again since **Qingwei San** contains the ingredient herbs of Danggui (angelica sinensis), Shengdi (radix rehmanniae recen), Huanglian, Danpi (cortex moutan radices), and Shengma (rhizoma cimicifugae), among which Huanglian is bitter and cold and it can spoil the patient's appetite. To such an extent, it will become quite troublesome.

Zhibai Dihuang Pill is made by adding Huangbai and Zhimu based upon the formula of **Liuwei Dihuang Pill** for those patients who have heat at the Lower

Jiao, but long and continuous use of this formula will result in some bad consequence like the low sexual desire.

And also, **Longdan Xiegan Tang**, containing Longdancao and Zhizi etc. , are extremely bitter and cold to purge the liver of pathogenic fire. Some chiefs or directors in offices or companies, who may frequently engage themselves in many social activities and drink alcohol a lot, or even criticize the others, or get pissed off, often find themselves in trouble of erectile dysfunction. That is usually because the liver meridian is trapped by the the damp-heat pathogens. In that case, **Longdan Xiegan Tang** can be used to eliminate the damp heat, after which such symptoms can be alleviated quickly, and even their sexual life would come back to the normal condition again. However, it is not suggested to go too far about the use of **Longdan Xiegan Tang** since over use of Longdancao will get the liver Qi over purged. The liver, in fact, needs warming, as it is Yin in nature and Yang in functions. Damp-heat usually arises in the liver from disharmony between its Yin and Yang. Once those damp-heat pathogens are eliminated, and the liver functions normally again, stop the medicine immediately as soon as it strikes the disease. Otherwise, Longdancao will impair Yin and Yang of the liver, which is similar to a troop dispatched to defeat enemies, after accomplishing its mission, the troop must be withdrawn from the battlefield, otherwise, the soldiers will turn domineering and bully the local citizens.

Therefore, try to avoid using the bitter-cold medicines too much in order to protect the stomach from spoiling the appetite. Even the sweet-cold medicines cannot be used at wills. For example, as for a cold attack arising from autumn-dryness along with pathogens in the lung, the sweet-cold medicines will induce phlegm in particular. Because of the autumn-dryness symptoms, TCM doctors generally tend to prescribe some medicines like Maogen , Lugen, Tiandong, Maidong for moistening purposein order to reduce dryness. But it is hardly imagined that the dry pathogens affecting human body in autumn is related to the external coldness. When the external coldness starts to constrain itself, the lung will also start astringency accordingly, which will then result in disorder of the lung functions. As a matter of fact, this is just false manifestations of dryness. In such cases, cold and cool medicines, if used, would result in further astringency of the lung and more dryness symptoms, which then induces more phlegm. That is to say, for such cases, sweet-cold medicines should not be used recklessly.

For human resources, it is wise to judge persons and put them in proper positions according to their strength and weakness in order to let everybody fully display his talents. Similarly, medicines should be understood and used at the right time and for the right cases in order to bring out the best effects.

Other Cold and Cool Medicines

As to the sour-cold medicines, the most typical one is Baishao (radix paeoniae alba or white peony root) in this category. Generally, the sweet-cold medicines, salty-cold medicines and bitter-cold medicines are the three most common medicines in life. Baishao as one of the typical sour-cold medicines will be discussed in the section concerning Yin nourishing medicines. The pungent-cold medicines are in fact the pungent-cool medicines, such as Bohe (mint), Jingjie (schizonepeta), etc. , which have been covered in the section regarding the treatment of the exogenous cold diseases. This volume will focus on the sweet-cold, salty-cold, and bitter-cold medicines.

第四卷　石膏之属－金部方药

第一章　金部方药概论

金性解

金部方药以寒凉为主。看到金，我们就想到寒凉。春夏秋冬，春天温暖，夏天火热，秋天凉爽，冬天寒冷。秋天对应金，对应寒凉。我们在学习中医的过程中始终要有五行的思维。

金石之性

金，对应西方。西方在哪？咱们从北京一直往西看，有山西，再往西就是陕西、甘肃、青海、新疆，这是偏西北的；偏西南的，还有四川、云南、西藏等地方，这是很广袤的一片。《山海经》讲"西方为金石之域"：西北有很多沙漠，沙子属金石，它们跟土有本质的区别；新疆的和田玉，是玉中极品，也属金石。

就连西方人说话、唱歌，都有金石之声。他们说话的音调比较脆，唱歌比较高亢。东部的人歌声或戏曲要柔一些，是木声。西边的歌，比如《青藏高原》，还有陕北民歌那种感觉，就是金石之声。你听一个地方的人说话、唱歌，就可以去猜测他们在五行方面偏重于哪一行。

西方之民有金石之性。金性的人比较明快，彪悍，义气，也比较忠贞。咱们看看《诗经》的《秦风》，就是秦国那一带民歌，秦国位于函谷关以西，历史上看那里属于西方之民。秦风跟郑魏之音就不一样，郑卫在中原，《诗经》的一些研究性著作经常讲郑声淫，郑卫之音就是一些靡靡之音。西部的诗歌，靡靡之音就要少一些，而是一种刚健之气。《秦风》有一首《无衣》："岂曰无衣？与子同袍。王于兴师，修我戈矛，与子同仇。岂曰无衣？与子同泽。王于兴师，修我矛戟，与子偕作。岂曰无衣？与子同裳。王于兴师，修我甲兵，与子偕行。"

朱熹对这首诗有一个注解，说："秦人之俗，大抵尚气概，先勇力，忘生轻死，故见于诗如此。"正是因为西部的人有这种品质，周文王伐纣就是从西岐起兵的；秦国统一六国，其发源地也是在西边；唐朝也是在山西那边起兵统一的全国；还有我党，也是以陕甘宁为根据地，才站稳脚跟的。为什么从西边起兵，就更有可能席卷全国呢？与这个地方的民风有很大的关系。

朱熹讲："雍州土厚水深，其民厚重质直。"雍州就在西部，这个地方水土很厚重，老百姓也很厚重，有金的性质，是非常剽悍的，比较有进攻性，也可以说有势如破竹之势。金有三个特质：坚、利、凉。坚就是坚硬，金属是非常坚硬的；利就是锋利，金属很锋利，可以做刀；凉就是寒凉，金属我们摸上去要比木头摸上去凉一些。它们在入药的时候也有这个性质，坚利、寒凉。

石头在五行上属金

石头在五行属性上是属金的。石头经过风化可以成为土，但是土和石有本质的区别。金是坚硬的，石头也是坚硬的。土不一样，它干结了就是坚硬的，一旦得到水，它马上就开始粘腻、蓬松。土上能长出东西来，石头上则很难长出东西。所以，石头是属金的，土是属土的。我们不能从微观的物质成分上面来分析，而要从它宏观的属性上去认识。这也是我们中国的学问跟西方的学问不一样的地方。

论中医，先以中国为本

中医是立足于我们中国的，如果你要到其他国家去考察那就另当别论了。大禹定九州岛，把华夏大地定出九个州来治理。

还有，古人经过长期的努力，在成千上万的植物、动物、矿物中，渐渐摸索、遴选出数百种最佳的，又摸索出哪里的哪种草药最好，后人将此归到神农尝百草，其实也就是说体验百草，去思考它们的性质，这是一代又一代人努力的结果，也是中国传统思维方式的产物。只有在中国传统学问的思维方式中才能学好中医。

很多年前，有个号称来自美国的研究机构给我看了很多材料，讲他们有一个计划，要在整个美国探索地道药材，比如，三七，云南及广西田林为最好，那么，美国哪里种田三七最好呢？还有白术、艾叶等，种在美国的哪里才算地道？美国本土又有哪些地道药材？这是一个很大且很难实现的项目，因为这需要一代又一代人，在广阔的天地之间，去仰观俯察，在切实的中医医疗实践中去摸索，无法通过实验室完成。在这个过程中，这个团队需要强有力的领导者，需要大家都有纯中医的思维模式，有深厚的中国文化基础，还需要在当地有充足的纯中医临床机会。

以石膏为金石统领，辨温凉当知体用

在金部方药里，我们以石膏等金石药为核心，来统领一大批寒凉的药。当然，也不是所有的金石药都是寒凉的，比如雄黄、硫黄就是大热的。正如不是所有的动物药都是温热的一样。比如说蚯蚓就是咸寒的，猪肉是平性的。但有人会问，驴肉不是寒凉的吗？其实，驴肉本身并不寒凉，甚至偏温。为什么大家都说它偏凉呢？并不是说它本身寒凉，而是说它养阴的力度比较大，能清血热，养阴养血就能清热，给大家造成一种凉的感觉。其实，它是体温而用凉，本体是温的，但用途是凉的。有些药本身是温的，但它发挥作用的时候，是凉的；有的药本身是凉的，发挥其作用的时候又是温的。我们在用的时候，常常会遇到。

寒凉药

寒凉药的作用

寒凉药的作用非常多。但很多中医书里对寒凉药多有批评，因为当寒凉药用错了的时候，它克伐了人体的阳气，让人越吃越蔫，说话、走路的力气都没有了，也阳痿了，甚至眼睛都看不见了。误用寒凉药，还能阻闭气机，而人又以气为主，当气机阻闭住的时候，身体的气血运化不开，病也会越来越重。所以，我们讲寒凉药的时候，首先讲寒凉药可能导致的不利影响，再去了解它的有利的作用，这就比较顺畅了。

但也不能因为有人误用寒凉或者过用寒凉就一味否定寒凉药，甚至会产生一种憎恨心，看到寒凉药就讨厌，见到某医生方子里开了寒凉药就认为人家水平不行。所有的病都跟火有关，即使是寒症，病久了也会生火。寒凉药就是用来祛邪火的。火的来路非常多，所以在这一部分，我们要接触的理论会非常多。

寒凉药品类多，运用广而且复杂，要用好凉药是一大功夫。中医要善于用火，也要善于用水。佛家讲，人世间就是火宅，像一个着了火的宅子，在里面一刻也不能待。而我们的内心，也有无名业火，很多人天天着急上火。所以，人需要清凉，这也是我们用凉药的一个原因。

当然，温药也需要用。这个世界本身就是寒热夹杂。这里一面是三界火宅，人人都有无名业火；另一面这里又世态炎凉，人心冷酷，冻死你。所以既要清凉，又需要温暖，该清凉的时候清凉，该温暖的地方温暖，不可偏执，有时候还需寒温并用。

寒凉药有非常多的种类，分类的方法也很多，我觉得，从五味的角度来分，比较易于掌握。寒属四气之一，四气宜跟五味相配，所以有甘寒、苦寒、咸寒、酸寒、辛寒。这里的寒，包含凉的意思。

甘寒药

甘寒，就是既甘甜又寒凉。石膏就是一味甘寒的药，它不会甜得像白糖，但微微有点甘味。芦根也是甘寒的，但它很甜，寒凉之性小一些。还有茅根、天冬、麦冬、石斛……都是甘寒的。

甘寒入胃，能清气分，而且甘能入脾，能给人提供能量。它养人是清养，就是用很清的东西来慢慢养人，就像给一颗树浇一些很清的水。人在大病初愈或者身体比较虚又有浮游之热的时候需要清养，甘寒恰能清浮游之热。

甘寒的药，其实只不过是甘凉而已，它们并不像黄芩、黄连、黄柏那样寒，或者说，只是微寒，就连石膏都是微寒的。甘寒药为什么寒性不大呢？因为辛甘发散为阳，甘入脾，能让脾运化起来，脾阳一生发，人体都阳气生起来了，即使药寒凉一点，也不会太过分。

甘寒首先入胃而清气分，"胃为燥土，得凉则安"，甘寒药一入胃，胃就会很舒服。有人说喝中药会伤胃，这是不对的。有伤胃的中药，更有养胃的中药，甘寒药就能养胃。药用错了才会伤胃，用对了不但不会伤胃，反而非常养胃。好的中医首先考虑到给人保胃气，"有胃气则生，无胃气则死"。

咸寒的药，如犀角、牡蛎等。牡蛎刚从海边捡来的很咸，洗干净后，咸味就不太明显了，但你依然能从中感受到那种淡淡的咸。咸寒的药也是入胃的，入胃而清血分。我们知道，"胃为多气多血之府"，所以气分的热、血分的热都会集中到胃里，转化为胃热。

甘寒的药入胃而清气分，咸寒的药入胃而清血分。可以视热邪的深浅而选用。

苦寒药

苦寒的药寒性比甘寒、咸寒药大一些。苦寒药如黄芩、黄连、黄柏、栀子、知母、龙胆草等。黄芩泻上焦肺热，黄连泻中焦之热，黄柏泻下焦之热，栀子清整个三焦浮游之热。知母看跟谁跑，它跟黄连，就清胃热，跟黄柏，就清下焦之热。人们经常讲黄连苦，其实，还有比黄连还苦的药，那就是龙胆草。龙胆草是极苦的一味药，主要清肝经湿热。这几味苦寒药力度都很大，用于清实热。这些就好比强有力的水泵，当大楼着火的时候，就要用它去灭火，但是用得太久就不好了。"苦寒败胃"，咱们永远记住这四个字。甘寒养胃，咸寒对胃也不会有害处，而苦寒绝对败胃，吃久了就不想吃饭了，所以，龙胆泻肝汤，很多人喝得太久，饭量就减了。

有人有胃热，刚开始口臭，舌苔黄、腻，甚至还有牙痛、溃疡，额头上长好多痘痘，这是典型的胃中实热，可用清胃散。当然，在胃热，并且热大于湿的时候才能够用。用清胃散把胃热一清，饭量马上就变大了。要是你觉得这方子不错就继续吃，吃得太多了，饭量又变小了，因为清胃散是这么几个药：当归、生地、黄连、丹皮、升麻，其中黄连苦寒败胃，把胃吃坏了，就比较麻烦。

知柏地黄丸，是在六味地黄丸的基础上加黄柏和知母，下焦有热，吃了很舒服，但吃久了，连性欲都没有了。

还有龙胆泻肝汤，龙胆草配上黄芩、栀子等，大苦大寒，是大泻肝热的。有人应酬特别多，喝酒也特别多，每天的工作就是训人，又是生气，又是吃喝，最后就阳痿了，为什么呢？这往往是湿热困在肝经，龙胆泻肝汤就可以考虑用，把湿热清掉，他这些症状马上就减轻了，性生活也正常了。他觉得这方不错，继续吃，吃过头又不行了，因为龙胆草用过了，肝气泄得太厉害了。肝是需要温煦的，它体阴而用阳，因为体用不和造成了很湿热。你把湿热给清掉了，肝的功能就正常了，但是你继续用龙胆草之类，就伤了阴阳。好比一支军队，一开始是来杀敌人的，敌人杀完了后它还在这，就可能会欺压老百姓了。

所以，苦寒药要尽量少用，防止苦寒败胃。甚至，甘寒的药也并不是所有的时候都能用的。比如秋燥感冒，肺中有邪，如果用甘寒药，痰马上就会变得特别多。因为有燥像，大家往往想到用点茅根、芦根、天冬、麦冬之类的东西润一下。殊不知，秋天，人体初感燥邪，燥为次寒，跟秋天的外寒有关，外寒一收敛，肺也跟着收敛，它的一些功能就得不到舒展，人体就会出现燥的假象，这时候你继续用寒凉药它就更加收敛，燥象会越来越明显，同时出现大量的痰。甘寒药在这种场合下是不能乱用的。

用人要知人善用，根据各人的长处和短处，做到人尽其才，才尽其用，用药也是如此，一味药该放在哪就放在哪，不要乱放，学会知药善用。

其他寒凉药

至于酸寒药，最典型的就是白芍了。我们平时主要讲甘寒、咸寒、苦寒，酸寒之说，我们讲得不多。以后讲养阴药的时候，咱们还会讲到白芍。还有辛寒药，其实就是辛凉药。我们习惯上讲辛凉，不讲辛寒。辛凉药薄荷、荆芥等，我们在上次讲治外感病的时候已经讲过了。我们在这部分主要讲：甘寒、咸寒和苦寒三类药。

Chapter 2 Shigao (Gypsum)

Shigao is a commonly used medicine. It is said that the four medicines: Renshen (Ginseng), Dahuang (rheum officinale), Fuzi (radix aconiti carmichaeli) and Shigao can bring the dying back to life since death takes place in the four cases of severe excess syndrome (for which Dahuang is used for discharging), severe deficiency (for which Renshen is used for tonifying), severe cold (for which Fuzi is used for rescuing the patients from collapse by restoring Yang), or severe heat (for which Shigao is used for clearing the heat). Shigao is one of the most critical medicines, which can bring life back from death.

Detailed Annotation of Shigao in Shennong Bencao Jing

In the book of *Shennong Bencao Jing*, Shigao is classified as a middle-grade medicine. The top-grade medicines have the function of "making one feel energetic and prolonging life" if it is used for long, while the middle-grade medicines are not supposed to be taken for long. Nobody has ever been taking Shigao for no reason everyday since it is only used when heat arises, especially for the heat occurring in Qi system. It is only used for curing illness, but not for health preserving purposes, nor for bringing longevity.

Shennong Bencao Jing says, "Shigao is pungent in taste and slightly cold in property, mostly used for treating the heat due to wind-cold attack, the counter-flow of Qi below the heart, fear or pant, dry mouth with bitter taste or even burnt taste, shortness of breath, abdominal hardness with severe pain; expelling the evil spirit; promoting galactopoiesis; and healing metallic tools-induced wounds. It is mined from the valley. " Following this brief description, let us try to analyze the medical properties and functions of Shigao.

The classics are usually simple in wording but rich in contents, which involves Yin and Yang, exterior and interior. It is quite similar to the human body, that is, the exterior refers to the skin and the interior refers to the five internal organs and the six hollow organs. TCM practitioners diagnose the conditions of the internal organs by examining the five sense organs, skin color, complexion, and facial countenance, which is a process of diagnosis from the exterior to the interior.

The classics can be studied in a similar way for understanding the rich implication from the simple words. For example, **Huangdi Neijing,** from the exterior perspective, it is about the medical theories; and from the interior perspective, it is about the medical treatment methods. Another example, **Shanghan Lun,** from the exterior perspective, it is about the formulas, while the interior part regarding the underlying theories is not shown at all. For **Shennong Bencao Jing**, it tells us about the medicines, while the theories and methods of treatment are also implied behind. Therefore, in order to acquire the full knowledge about TCM, the learners cannot solely depend on reading medical books since even the medical classics may just show half of learning. The remaining half will have to be acquired by following the medical experts through clinical practice.

Let us analyse the descriptions on Shigao in *Shennong Bencao Jing* word by word.

Meaning of the Chinese character "石" (Shí)

The term of "Shigao" in Chinese is composed of two characters, i. e. , Shi (石, stone) and Gao (膏, paste). Shi signifies that Shigao is a type of stone that is heavy in quality. That means it can be used to suppress the floating or lingering fire in the body. Fire, in either physiological or pathological state, tends to go upwards. Shigao can suppress the fire, indicating that it has the function of clearing fire.

Either in the nature or in human body, the pathogenic fire always go upwards. When one is suffering from pathogenic fire in the body (literally called "getting fire" in Chinese), it always shows up at the upper body, especially on the head. It is rarely heard that there is pathogenic fire at the feet. Shigao enters the lung channel to clear the heat in the Qi system, especially the heat in the lung and stomach channels. The lungs are located at the highest position in the body among all the internal organs, so the lungs will have to withstand fire from all sources, i. e. , all the organs; while the stomach is like an ocean receiving various substances from all the organs, and it is an organ rich in Qi and blood. Therefore, the stomach is easy to generate pathogenic fire. All types of pathogenic fire from the internal organs will eventually influence the lungs and stomach. The Qi of the lungs and stomach tends to descend to find outlets for the pathogenic fire. The liver Qi ascends from the left, while the lung Qi descends from the right; the spleen uplifts the clear, while the stomach descends the turbid, which guarantees the normal ascending and descending circulation inside human body. For the lungs and the stomach, the normal flow of Qi is descending. When there is excessive pathogenic fire, the descending function of these two organs will be impaired, and heat symptoms will arise accordingly. Shigao can suppress fire to help the lung and the stomach Qi to flow downwards so that the pathogenic fire will descend accordingly. And that is the meaning of the word "Shi" (stone), i. e., to suppress the fire pathogen and accommodate the descending Qi in the lungs and stomach.

Meaning of the Chinese character "膏" (Gāo)

The word Gao (膏) literally means paste or cream, which gives us a feeling of moistening. For instance, in many Chinese Brand names of creams or medical pastes containing the same word **"Gao"** like **Runfu Gao** (skin cream or skin lotion), **Pipa Gao** (loquat leaf extract), etc. All of such products imply that they are "滋润" (zī rùn, which means moistening). "润" (rùn) means "engendering fluids" or "promoting the secretion of saliva or body fluid". Shigao contains a lot of crystallized water. As it is known in the chemistry, the chemical formula of Shigao is calcium sulphate ($CaSO_4 \cdot 2H_2O$) that shows two hydrones or water molecules. While calcium sulfate can only be slightly dissolved in water, the moistening effect is actually produced by the crystallized water in Shigao.

The raw Shigao is white in color, and crystal clear in appearance. Therefore, Shi (stone) that gives out pasty shiny reflection is considered to have the best quality. If Shigao turns yellow in color, it should not be used as medicine any more since it is not purely sweet and cold in properties any more, but mixed with damp-heat elements in the process of crystallization, which will induce stranguria troubles (with symptoms such as yellow, short urine, or calculus stone, etc.).

The Shigao commonly referred to is raw Shigao. If a piece of raw Shigao is put into a furnace and heated till it becomes red hot, it will get dried-up without any moistening feature after the water contained is completely evaporized. Up to that stage, those substances are no longer the same as raw Shigao that is sweet-cold in property, but changed into Shu Shigao(calcined gypsum) that is salty-bitter in nature. Usually, it is forbidden to take Shu Shigao orally since it intensively induces astringency.

Shigao Mostly Used for Treatment of Wind-Cold-Heat Attack

Shigao as a medicine has very thin scent and taste. It is pungent and slightly cold in properties. Pungency means Shigao can go to the exterior to disperse the pathogenic fire and ventilate the stagnated heat.

Human beings have pores all over the body, through which Qi can move in and out freely. When the exogenous wind-cold pathogen is too strong for the defensive Qi to guard against, the human body will deploy the secondary instinctive self-defensive measure, i. e. , to shut up the pores. But in this way, the ventilative function is disabled and the healthy Qi is suppressed inside the body, which eventually results in the formation of pathogenic heat.

Therefore, when suffering from the wind-cold pathogen, one will have a fever. In case the temperature is not so high, the common pungent and dispersing medicines will work well; in case the temperature goes very high, it will be necessary to add a little Shigao to clear the endogenous heat on the one hand, and open the exterior to disperse the heat on the other hand. In this sense, Shigao is a medicine that induces sweat.

Shigao is used for treatment of the pathogenic heat due to wind-cold attack. When one is attacked by the exogenous wind pathogen from the exterior of the body, he or she specially becomes aversive to cold, which is a superficial symptom, and has a fever, indicating that the healthy Qi is stagnated inside the body and the closed pores obstruct the heat to be ventilated out of the body. In such a case, Shigao needs to be used to clear the heat in the Qi system.

The book *Shennong Baocao Jing* says Shigao is slightly cold in nature, but many Chinese medicine practitioners of the later generations believed that Shigao is excessively cold in nature. However, it is pungent-sweet in tastes, creating Yang that can disperse the cold outwards. Actually, Shigao is very cold in property, but it plays a slightly cold function, which will not excessively restricts Yang of the body.

However, the coldness of Shigao is also conditional. When it is properly used, it is slightly cold or even not cold at all since its cooling function can be targeted at clearing the pathogenic heat. Once misused, it becomes severely cold, and can sweep off the Yang Qi in the body. Furthermore, it also depends on the herbal compatibility. For some herbs, they show cool properties when matched with the cool herbs, or show hot properties when matched with hot herbs.

Anyway, please keep in mind that the slightly cold often indicates sweet-cold property, which will go to the Qi system to clear the heat there, while the salty-cold will enter the blood system, which will be discussed in the following sections.

Counterflow of Qi, Fright and Pant

In the term of "counterflow of Qi, and fright and pant", the stomach Qi tends to be descending. Both the large and small intestines can push the turbid downwards in order to discharge the wastes. The spleen is responsible for uplifting the clear and transport the life essences absorbed from the fluid and food in the form of Qi to each and every part of the body through the heart and lungs. This is the basic physiological process of human being. In case there is pathogenic fire in the stomach, the stomach Qi will be ascending instead of descending, which is called "counterflow of Qi".

The stomach Qi counterflow may take on various forms, such as hiccup and vomiting.

"Fright" is a symptom related to the heart channel. The heart fire has to descend and communicate with the kidneys. When the pathogenic fire is too vigorous, it disturbs the descending move of the heart fire, causing the heart fire to float up. So the heart fails to calm the mind, as such one may be easily frightened.

Pant is a symptom related to the lung channel. As stated by **Huangdi Nei-jing,** "the lungs suffer a lot from counterflow of Qi". The lungs are endowed with purifying and descending functions, which help descend fluid and fire. The pathogenic fire can induce the counterflow of the lung Qi. In fact, behind the symptoms of counterflow of Qi, fright and pant is actually the pathogenic fire. Of course, Shigao cannot be used for treatment of all types of fright and pant, but only the fright and pant caused by the severe heat in the Qi system.

Dry Mouth with Bitter Taste

The symptoms of "dry mouth with bitter taste" also arises from fire, as fire impairs the body fluid, causing impairment of Yin, which will result in dry and bitter or even burnt tastes in the mouth. Bitter is the taste corresponding to fire, and bitter taste in the mouth is mostly due to the pathogenic fire. When food is overcooked, it is burnt in the pot, sending out a scorched smell. Fire can turn food into something charred and bitter, and similarly, it can also cause one feel bitter in his or her mouth. Therefore, when those bitter and charred tastes arise in the mouth, one should know it is resulted from too much fire. The smell in the mouth is surely different from the scorched smell of burnt food in the pot, but there is similarity between them, which is called synaesthesia. Similarly, in Chinese language, there is a phrase called "辛苦"(Xin Ku). It can be used to refer to "辛"(Xin in Pinyin, means pungent in English) and "苦"(Ku in Pinyin, means bitter), and it can also be used to refer to "painstaking" in life. In the different context, "Xin Ku"refers to different things. But it gives us the similar feeling, therefore, both conditions are named the same as "Xin Ku".

Short of Breath

One respiration is defined as a cycle of an exhalation and an inhalation. When talking about "taking a break", it is also related to respiration, which means to slow down or relax respiration. Zhuang-tzu (an antient Chinese philosopher, in the the pre-Qin period) said that "the immortal beings are able to breathe to the ankles; and the ordinary human beings just breathe to the throat."

The ordinary people usually have shallow breath, inhaling and exhaling breath only to the troat, while the immortal beings, or the stylite could inhale deeply down to the ankles. It is known that there are chest breathing and abdominal respiration. Those who keep in good health always try to have a deep breath.

The pathogenic fire could affect the depth of one's respiration. Fire always floats upwards, causing Qi to become superficial and then obstructing deep breath. The kidney is regarded as the driver of inhalation. When the kidney Qi initiates its action and pulls downwards, a normal inhalation of air will be triggered naturally. With the lung contractive function, one can then exhale a breath. The entire respiratory cycle does not solely depend on the lungs, but it is a collaborative work among the lungs, kidneys, spleen and stomach. Therefore, breathing is, indeed, an important work to maintain a good health.

There is a Chinese idiom "Xin Fu Qi Zao", which literally means "once the heart floats, Qi will become restless". That means when a person becomes fickle, the breathing will become shallow and less effective, with which the mind would become more likely to float up. Therefore, when feeling nervous or having great pressure, one needs to take a deep breath to calm down his or her mind.

Moreover, the flashy and meretricious lifestyle may also result in the heart floating, which then affects the normal respirtation, and even the physical health as well.

All in all, the shortness of breath may arise from two main reasons. One is Qi floating caused by the pathogenic fire and the other one is the floating state of mind. Therefore, the key health maintenance is to cultivate one's mind to calm down instead of floating up. It is also the core of one's self cultivation. Never think that cultivation means to give up and suffer losses. Only those who practise health cultivation would feel the true benefits physically and spiritually. Pursuing a flashy and meretricious life would do harm to the Qi circulation, the state of mind, and the breathing cycle. And the normal breathing cycle is so essential to the health.

Physiological conditions and psychological states are always strongly corelated. Never think some factors are only psychological effects, and then think they are illusory or visional. In fact, psychological impacts are tangible, and they can cause diseases. For example, if one admires a flashy and meretricious life, he or she would become restless, showing bad complexion, and even feeling stuck up all over the body. If one can keep calm and grounded all the time, he or she can always breathe naturally and deeply, and surely becomes healthier over time.

While accepting something, each and every one of us would experience four steps: belief, willingness, action, and proof. The four-step principle can benefit many activities from health maintenance to practicing Buddhism. The same principle can be applied to curing illness as well, especially for the treatment of chronic diseases. It is necessary for patients to have confidence in fighting against the diseases. There is a saying that "Doctors do not knock at the patient's door", which means the medical practitioners will not approach a patient by themselves to give treatment of diseases. Only when the patient himself goes to a doctor's proactively with his or her willingness for help, can it be proved that he or she has confidence in the medical skill of the doctor. As such, it will be easier for the doctor to give treatment and the patient will also closely cooperate with the doctor in taking medicines. As a matter of fact, that "Doctors do not knock at the patient's door" is to enhance the faith and confidence from the patients, which is embedded with the delicate psychological factors.

Abdominal Hardness with Severe Pain

Regarding "abdominal hardness with severe pain", this, in fact, is excess fire symptom since pathogenic fire can generate pathogenic Qi, causing obstruction of Qi circulation in the abdomen, which then results in pains. The abdomen feels hard by hand and pressing on the abdomen will worsen the pains. Generally, pains can be differentiated as excess and deficiency types. The deficiency type of pains enjoy pressure from outside of the abdomen, and pressing can relive such pains. Whilst the excess type of pains dislike pressing since pressing can worsen such pains. Before treatment, it also has to be confirmed the causes that the excess pains arise from: **Qi stagnation, or blood stasis, or dyspepsia/food indigestion**.

Generally speaking, most of the cases of abdominal pains arise from Qi stagnation. Put it simply, the abdominal hardness with severe pain is resulted from pathogenic fire. In case such a symptom lasts many years with pain all the time, it may be resulted from blood stasis or food dyspepsia, which then cannot be treated with Shigao.

Expelling the Evil Spirit

Another function of Shigao is to expel ghost and evil spirits. Ghost is an illusory thing. Yin and Yang co-exist in everything in this world. Some of the things in this world are visible and some are invisible; some exist substantially in solid forms while some others are only entirely imaginary. In any cases, they do exist regardless of solid forms or void forms.

A healthy person usually cannot see ghosts. But those who suffer from deficiency of healthy Qi or vigorous pathogenic Qi are more likely to see ghosts. When one gets sick, he or she will have a great possibility of seeing ghosts since his or her sensing functions are out of the normal standard range, just as some of his or her physiochemical examination results are out of the normal range. The so-called ghosts are the delusions or illusions arising from phlegm, blood stasis, or vigorous pathogenic fire, etc. Especially in the case of vigorous pathogenic fire, the patient may see ghosts that can be eliminated after the fire is cleared.

Moreover, Shigao is a kind of metal and stone with sweet taste and cold property, and it is heavy in texture. So, it has the functions of clearing the floating fire and relieving uneasiness of mind for achieving body tranquilization.

Promotion of Galactopoiesis

Can Shigao be used to promote lactation after delivery? Lack of lactation after child delivery may stem from many reasons, one of which is the stomach heat due to the postpartum blood deficiency, or too high temperature in the room for preventing the lying-in lady from the exogenous wind and cold pathogens, or too much nourishing food taken by the postpartum lady. Therefore, various sources of heat, especially the stomach heat, can lead to stagnation, which then obstructs lactation.

Breasts are subsumed to the liver and stomach channels. The mammary glands are on the stomach channel. When the stomach heat arises, the breasts are the first to be affected. Therefore, the tissues, tubules and orifices inside the breasts may be obstructed, resulting in less milk secretion. When and only when the heat stays in the Qi system under the above-mentioned circumstance, Shigao can be used for clearing. Otherwise, some other methods may have to be reconsidered for treatment of less milk secretion.

For example, the lady may feel depressed after delivery for various reasons that result in stagnation of the liver Qi, which can also lead to insufficient milk secretion. In such a case, Shigao cannot be used. In addition, if lack of lactation is resulted from the blood deficiency, sufficient tonification of Qi and blood will have to be done necessarily. In that case, Shigao should be avoided. No matter what causes lack of lactation, so long as it develops to the symptoms of intolerable breast distention pain, or even fever, ulcerations with pus, Shigao can be used in the formulas to clear the heat. Briefly speaking, Shigao has the function of promoting lactation, but it should be used based on the syndrome differentiation.

Metal-inflicted Wounds

Wounds caused by metallic tools, such as knives and axes, are difficult to heal up, and they may worsen to ulcers and pus. After clearing the ulcers and pus, doctors also hope to promote flesh regeneration as soon as possible.

According to **Huangdi Neijing**, "All pains, itching and wounds are associated with the heart. " Wounds that are hard to heal up are mostly attributed to the presence of pathogenic fire in the heart. Therefore, some measures must be taken to clear the pathogenic fire and astringe the wound in order to promote healing of the wound. Shigao is cold in nature, which is good for clearing the fire and converging the wound. For clearing the pathogenic fire of wounds, raw Shigao is suggested to be a better choice; while for healing up the wounds and promoting tissue regeneration, calcined Shigao would be better since it is processed by calcining the raw Shigao, after which the calcined Shigao will become slightly salty and have an effect of stronger astringency.

Shigao is also used in making beancurd for its cold and astringing characteristics since its cold property plays a condensing and astringing functions so that soy-bean milk can coagulate into beancurd or beancurdjelly. From the perspective of TCM, it follows the same principle as that for healing up the wounds with Shigao. Here is a very useful formula called **Ganshi Shengji San** that uses Shigao to treat metal-induced wounds.

Ganshi Shengji San is used for astringing wounds after ulcers and slough are removed. This formula contains the herbal ingredients: Zhenzhu Fen (pearl powder) 20, Duan Luganshi (calcined calamine) 50, calcined Shigao 200, Huangdan (yellow lead) 20.

This formula is recorded in many books. I heard from a senior that the effect of this formula could be modified and reinforced by adding dog bone powder or calcinated dog bone powder.

Baihu Tang

Related to Shigao, there are some other formulas, the first of which is **Baihu Tang**. It contains the herbal ingredients of Shigao (gypsum) 1 *liang*, Zhimu (rhizoma anemarrhenae) 3 *qian*, Zhi Gancao (honey-fried liquorice) 1 *qian*, Jingmi (japonica rice) 5 *qian*. (Note: *Jin, liang* and *qian* are Chinese weight measuring units)

Baihu Tang Clears the Excess Heat in the Yangming Meridian

The formula of **Baihu Tang** is taken from *Shanghan Lun*. It is used for clearing the excess heat in the Yangming meridian. Foot-Yangming is of the stomach meridian; and Hand-Yangming is of the large intestine channel.

Yangming Meridian is abundant in Qi and blood, just like a person who has a lot money. If one is rich enough, he or she will be very likely to get carried away. Similarly, Yangming meridian with more Qi and blood is apt to generate excessive heat. Therefore, symptoms of the stomach heat and large intestine heat are very common in clinical practice.

According to *Shanghan Lun*, when pathogenic Qi invades the exterior of the human body, it must be driven away immediately by inducing perspiration. Otherwise, pathogens will move from Taiyang meridian to Yangming meridian, resulting in the stomach heat and large intestine heat. Some doctors complain that it is hard to deal with the diseases related to Yangming meridian described in *Shang-*

han Lun. Actually, as the pathogens go to the interior and transform into heat, the stomach heat can be cleared with **Baihu Tang**; the large intestine heat should be purged with **Chengqi Tang** and the like.

Many annotations have been made with various names like Yangming Meridian symptom or Yangming Hollow Organ symptom, etc. , but I would like to make it simple, i. e. , one is the stomach heat and the other one is the large intestine heat.

Baihu Tang for Treatment of the Five Severe Symptoms

The stomach heat usually has five severe symptoms of high fever, hyperhidrosis, severe thirst, dysphoria and surging/bounding pulse, for which **Baihu Tang** can be used for treatment.

High fever in most cases originates from Yangming meridian. In TCM, sweat is taken as the fluid of the heart. Hyperhidrosis refers to excessive perspiration, which is also promoted by the Qi of Yangming meridian. Severe thirst is attributed to the fluid impairment by the pathogenic heat, so water will be needed to make up. Dysphoria also arises from the stomach heat since the heart and the stomach are closely interlinked. When the stomach heat is accumulated to a certain extent, the heart will be affected. The Chinese character "烦"(fán, dysphoria in English) is composed of "火"(huǒ, fire) in the left and "页"(yè, head) in the right. The fire running up to the head will surely make one feel annoyed (i. e. , dysphoria). Bounding pulse refers to the pulse beating at large amplitude rapidly and powerfully, which is also a symptom of fire.

When all these five symptoms arise, **Baihu Tang** can be used without any doubt; But if only one or two out of the five symptoms arise, **Baihu Tang** may be just one of the choices.

Analyses of Baihu Tang Formula and Its Decocting Method

Baihu Tang is rather simple, in which the primary herbs are Shigao and Zhimu; the rest of the herbs act as accessories. When Shigao is used individually, it is slightly cold in nature, but if it is used with Zhimu, it will become extremely cold.

Zhimu is a kind of plant root, white in color with hairs on the surface. When used as a herb, it should be sliced with the hair removed first. Zhimu is bitter in taste, slightly pungent, sweet-cold in nature, moist and slippery in texture. It mainly enters the lung, stomach and kidney channels to clear the fire and nourish Yin. Its white colour indicates that Zhimu enters the Qi system and can clear the kidney fire. Huangbai is often used together with Zhimu. For example, **Zhibai Dihuang pill**, it is made on the basis of **Liuwei Dihuang pill** by adding Huangbai and Zhimu to clear the kidney fire. In contrast, Shigao used with Zhimu is to clear the lung fire and the stomach fire.

Concerning the use of Zhimu, please keep in mind two points: one is that it is used together with Shigao; and another is that it is used with Huangbai. Shigao used with Zhimu clears the pathogenic fire in the lungs and stomach, mostly affecting the Upper Jiao, while Huangbai used with Zhimu clears the pathogenic fire in the kidneys, mainly affecting the Lower Jiao.

When Shigao and Zhimu are used to clear heat, they may impair the stomach Qi. Although it was said "the stomach is subsumed to the dry earth, and it will calm down by coolness", yet the severe coldness will impair the stomach functions, showing "too much is as bad as too little". Therefore, honey-fried Gancao (liquorice) can be used to harmonize the other herbs to reduce the coldness of Shigao and Zhimu by slowing down the effect in order to conciliate the stomach.

Japonica rice is a type of rice with its properties in between glutinous rice and polished indica rice. It is a bit sticky in texture with good tastes, and good for nourishing the stomach. Of course, Japonica rice, if not available, can be substituted with glutinous rice, or with the ordinary rice. Rice is used to nourish stomach Qi. Having been bathed in the rice-rinsed water, Cangzhu will become weaker in its dry property and will not damage the stomach. With the similar concept, one can add more water when cooking rice. Once the water is boiling, he or she may have the rice-cooked water by filtering the rice. Such kind of rice-cooked water is very helpful for a patient who does not have appetite when he or she is sick. Japonica rice (5 *qian*) used in **Baihu Tang** is to ensure that the decoction has the characteristics of rice-cooked water in order to help nourish the patient's stomach Qi.

The duration and extent of decocting **Baihu Tang** needs to be properly controlled. ***Shanghan Lun*** stated, "the decoction will be ready when rice is well-cooked". It should be drunk while it is warm. Nowadays, for decocting **Baihu Tang**, one always starts with decocting Shigao for 15 minutes before Zhimu, Gancao and Japonica rice are put in, since Shigao is mineral, and it is quite difficult to extract the medical compositions out of it.

The principle of curing illness in TCM is to foster the healthy Qi concurrently in the proess of defeating the pathogenic Qi, which is shown anytime, anywhere and in any formula in order to achieve a balance.

Using Baihu Tang with Caution

Shanghan Lun suggests to use **Baihu Tang** in a very cautious way. Why is that? In that era when Zhang Zhongjing lived, the coldness is very severe. Therefore, more warm herbs are used according to ***Shanghan Lun***, such as Guizhi, Fuzi and Ganjiang (rhizoma zingiberis). **Baihu Tang** is severely cold, and it constrains the Yang in the body. Thus, **Baihu Tang** should be used with cautions.

The name **Baihu Tang** (the white tiger decoction) can tell that it is a very cold formula. According to Chinese traditional culture, *Baihu* (white tiger) is one of the four images representing four holy beasts. Baihu resides in the west and it corresponds to coolness and coldness. The wind from the west makes people feel cool and cold. A nursery rhyme sings: "tigers do not eat humans", which means that if and when a tiger is not hungry or under no threat, it will not hurt human being. But the white tiger is said to be very savage. So, **Baihu Tang**, when used properly, will have curing effects; otherwise, it brings troubles. That is why the ancient TCM doctors were all very cautious in using **Baihu Tang**.

A legend story about Wang Shuhe (a renowned doctor in the West Jin dynasty, also an editor of ***Shanghan Lun***) says that once his mother was sick, possibly with symptoms of high fever, dysphoria and serious thirst, he gave her mother treatment in many different approaches but none of them was successful, and he became very anxious and worried. At night, his mother was on her deathbed, and Wang Shuhe was pacing restlessly in the yard and chattering, "if she were not my natural mother, I would have used **Baihu Tang**!" He did not dare to use **Baihu Tang** since the destiny of his own mother made him overcautious to take any action. His student heard what he said and immediately made a **Baihu Tang** for Wang's mother, and she recovered soon after. Wang Shuhe was shocked, and his student responded, "I dare use **Baihu Tang** since she is not my own mother."

Qingwei San

Another formula called **Qingwei San**, which is also used for clearing the stomach heat.

Qingwei San contains the herbal ingredients: Huanglian (coptis chinensis), Shengdi (radix rehmanniae recen), Shengma (rhizoma cimicifugae), Danpi (cortex moutan radicis), Danggui (angelica sinensis).

Both **Baihu Tang** and **Qingwei San** can clear stomach heat, but **Baihuang Tang** focuses on the excess heat arising from the exogenous pathogenic attack in Yangming meridian. Such heat is still in the Qi system. **Qingwei San** often concentrates on the stomach heat that has accumulated for a long time and has caused impairement of Yin. This type of heat usually lies in the blood system.

In the formula of **Qingwei San**, Huanglian, bitter-cold in properties, functions as the leading herb to move in both Qi and blood systems to purge the heat from the Middle Jiao. The stomach, with abundant Qi and blood, can easily generate heat. In case the heat stays there for an extended period of time, the blood will be affected. Therefore, Shengdi and Danpi are used to cool the blood. Meanwhile, the stomach is taken as dry earth in TCM, and it becomes calm under the influence of coolness. Shengdi, Danpi and Huanglian are all cold herbs with bitter taste, playing a descending function, corresponding to that of the stomach Qi, thus, fire will be purged along with the stomach Qi.

However, Qi should not blindly descend, as the spleen is in charge of uplifting the clear, indicating that the turbid will descend, for which Shengma is added. Moreover, Danggui, as a warm herb, is also used in this formula to keep balance with the cold herbs. Danggui can nourish and generate blood concurrently in the process of clearing heat, which are needed by the stomach.

Qingwei San is particularly effective for clearing the stomach heat that arises from the miscellaneous diseases since it clears heat through nourishing the stomach. Danggui and Shengdi in the formula are the herbs functioning for tonifying effects. For some people in the modern time, heat accumulates in the stomach due to extreme indulgence of their appetites, whose typical symptom is bad breath (halitosis). Such a condition may be sensed from face-to-face chatting with those people. Those who suffer from this kind of stomach heat will also suffer gingival atrophy. Their teeth will wear out rapidly, or they even have frequent toothache. Some people claim that these symptoms are resulted from decayed tooth. In fact, the decayed tooth and stomach fire are inter-related. When there is fire in the stomach, it pushes turbid Qi upwards to the mouth, and then easily cause tooth to be decayed. Therefore, the stomach heat should be cleared in order to protect teeth from decaying. **Qingwei San** is an excellent formula for such cases and is used quite frequently.

By the way, there is modified **Qingwei San**, in which Shigao is added on the basis of its five essential herbs to intensify its potence of clearing the heat in both Qi and blood systems. The dosage of Huanglian is small, three gram per decoction. Therefore, it does not matter too much if one drinks **Qingwei San** for certain extended time since it is able to nourish the stomach; but it cannot be used too long since Huanglian is bitter, Shengdi and Danpi are cold in nature. Bitter and coldness can impair the stomach.

Modifications of Baihu Tang

In case that **Baihu Tang** is not timely used for a treatment, body fluid and Qi will be impaired by the heat in the Yangming meridian, causing the patients to suffer from extreme thirst and even short of breath. In this case, Renshen should be added to **Baihu Tang** to form a **Renshen Baihu Tang**. In modern time, American ginseng is used instead. American ginseng is very close in properties to the ginseng used in the days of Zhang Zhongjing since both of them can tonify Qi and promote the secretion of saliva or body fluid. As to the quality, the first grade of American ginseng as medicine refers to the ginseng that has a size of an adult finger, with thin and yellow skin covered with dense cross striation. It tastes bitter first, and then sweet with a bit of garland chrysanthemum flavor included. Only a bit of such ginseng can help to produce enough fluid.

Apart from the five symptoms previously mentioned for **Baihu Tang** to cure, there are some annoyed pain at joints, especially the finger joints, for which Guizhi (cassia twig) must be added to **Baihu Tang** to make **Baihu Plus Guizhi Tang**. Guizhi goes to the four limbs and is used to harmonize Ying and Wei systems.

If any conspicuous heat symptoms appear at the finger joints, accompanied by dampness symptoms, Cangzhu should be added to **Baihu Tang** to make **Baihu Jiazhu Tang**, or another name of **Baihu Plus Cangzhu Tang** since Cangzhu can eliminate dampness.

Baihu Plus Guizhi Tang and **Baihu Plus Cangzhu Tang** are used for curing rheumatic arthritis. However, when the joints become red and hot, a few doses of either **Baihu Plus Guizhi Tang** or **Baihu Plus Cangzhu Tang** will do good since the heat inside the body has to be cleared in this way.

Other Classic Formulas Containing Shigao (Gypsum)

Zhuye Shigao Tang

Zhuye (bamboo leaf) 5*qian*, Shigao (gypsum) 8 *qian*, Renshen (ginseng) 2 *qian*, Banxia (pinellia ternate) 3 *qian*, Maidong (radix ophiopogonis) 3 *qian*, Gancao (liquorice) 1 *qian*, Japonica rice 5 qian.

Zhuye Shigao Tang, in fact, is a modification of **Baihu Tang**. This formula is mainly used at the later stage of exogenous pathogenic attack. Fever consumes Qi, blood and fluid of the body. Therefore, under the conditions that the serious fever is abated, residual heat is still lingering, and the body fluid is impaired, and then, it will be necessary to clear the residual heat on the one hand and make up fluid for the body on the other hand. At this moment, the heat is not so severe, so, Zhimu is taken out of the formula and only Shigao will work well. Zhuye clears the heart fire by giving an exit for pathogenic heat through the large intestine and urination. TCM often tries to expel the pathogens out of the body instead of fighting against them inside the body.

Renshen, Banxia, Maidong , Gancao and Japonica rice are the herbal ingredients of **Maimendong Tang** from *Jingui Yaolue (Synopsis of the Golden Chamber)* . Ginseng tonifies Qi and promotes the secretion of saliva or body fluid, tonifies the spleen, lungs, and the necessary body fluid. However, it is not powerful enough to make up fluid with ginseng alone, so, Maidong is added. Maidong is semitransparent in texture, sweet and cold in nature, and very strong in function to produce saliva.

In heat diseases, some of the fluid consumed is transformed into sweat, and some is dried by the pathogenic heat into phlegm. Thus, phlegm arises after heat diseases are cured. Banxia is added to reduce the phlegm. Gancao and Japonica rice still function to harmonize the stomach Qi. **Maimendong Tang**, in fact, is a formula that can reduce phlegm and produce fluid concurrently.

Zhuye Shigao Tang can be interpreted as a modification of **Baihu Tang** by adding Zhuye, Renshen, Banxia and Maidong after taking out Zhimu; or a modification of **Maimendong Tang** with Shigao and Zhuye added. Formulas have unlimited possibilities of modifications.

Renshen and Maidong always remind of the formula of **Shengmai Yin** that contains Renshen, Maidong and Wuweizi (fructus schisandrae chinensis). Why Wuweizi is not used in the formula of **Zhuye Shigao Tang**? Because Wuweizi tastes sour, bitter, sweet, pungent and salty, with sourness as the primary taste. It enters the five internal organs and astringes the vital life essence there. Although textbooks and ancient practitioners said it only converges the vital Qi, not the pathogenic Qi, yet sour, as the primary taste of Wuweizi, does have an astringing function. It is not used just for sake of safety since it is not quite sure whether it can astringe the pathogenic Qi or not.

It is very important for doctors to know the way of coping with the aftermath in the process of curing illness. **Zhuye Shigao Tang** is a formula that is often used at the later stage. It can be used at the later stage of heat disease treatment all the year round, especially for dealing with problems arising from heat stroke in summer.

Maxing Shigan Tang and Daqinglong Tang

The formula of **Maxing Shigan Tang** contains Mahuang (ephedra), Xingren (apricot kernel), Shigao (gypsum) and Gancao (liquorice). Mahuang opens the lung orifice; Xingren makes the lung Qi descend; Shigao clears the lung heat; and Gancao relaxes the lung. These 4 sentences briefly give the principles and functions of this formula. Pathogenic Qi at the exterior can cause disturbance to the lung Qi, causing heat to accumulate in the lung and stomach. Mahuang and Xingren are used to get through the lung Qi so that heat can be dispersed out easily; it may not be effective enough. Therefore, Shigao is used to clear the heat directly. Gancao in this formula functions to tackle the stress in the lungs and coordinate the herbal actions of this formula. In this way, both the endogenous and exogenous pathogens will be dispersed.

Daqinglong Tang actually is a modified formula based upon **Maxing Shigan Tang**, or **Guizhi Tang**. **Maxing Shigan Tang** plus Guizhi makes the formula of **Daqinglong Tang**, in which Guizhi can intensify the potence dimension of inducing sweat. In addition, ginger and jujube used in **Daqinglong Tang** can arouse the stomach Qi to further promote sweat. Nowadays, **Daqinglong Tang** is seldom used since **Maxing Shigan Tang** already works well. **Daqinglong Tang** is exceptionally severe, so, generally this formula is prescribed dose by dose to target at the specific case based on syndrome differentiation.

Yuquan San

Yuquan San has only a few ingredients, containing Shigao (gypsum), Huashi (talcum powder) and Gancao (liquorice).

Yuquan San is related to urination, as the Chinese character"泉"(quan, means spring in English) in its name implies, "泉"(quan) is a euphemistic way of describing urination. For instance, **Suoquan pill** (literally means "reducing spring pill) is used to reduce a patient's urination, especially at night. "玉"(Yu, means jade in English) symbolizes that **Yuquan San** is used to make urine become limpid as jade. In the summer time, due to the hot weather, a lot of people may become upset, and they may have dark yellow urine, or even the hospital test reports sometimes show occult blood in urine, for which **Yuquan San** is effective.

Yuquan San is a modified formula by adding raw Shigao into the formula of **Liuyi San** that contains Huashi and Gancao at a ratio of 6 to 1, specially targeting at damp stagnation in the summer hot days. Huashi is quite thin in taste, which means it can excrete dampness and open orifices; but it is heavy in texture, which means it can take the dampness down so that the dampness can be excreted through urination. Huashi has miraculous functions of excreting dampness and break through stagnation. Huashi also has some unique functions in the treatment of calculus/stone diseases, as its Chinese name "滑石" (Huashi, literally means "slipping stone") implies that it can help stone to slip out of the body.

Summer heat pathogen is, in fact, a combination of dampness and heat, and it prevails in summer, causing obstruction of orifices in human body and affecting the normal circulation of Qi and blood. Thus, heat will accumulate and affect urination. Under that condition, urine may turn yellow and even reddish. **Yuquan San** is effective for these symptoms. In this formula, Shigao clears heat from the Qi system; **Liuyi San** resolves dampness and opens orifices while clearing the Qi system. However, if combined with **Zhuye Shigao Tang**, this formula will become more effective.

Rational Use of Shigao

All in all, Shigao is a crucial herb, and it is easy to interpret its function since it targets at severe fever and miscellaneous diseases stemming from heat in the Qi system.

Many TCM experts are adept at using Shigao. Back in the past, one of the four renowned experts in Beijing was Kong Bohua, who had an legendary title as "Shigao Kong" due to his exceptionally rational utilisation of Shigao into almost all the formulas he prescribed. Many of his patients in Beijing enjoyed very good socio-economic conditions and often overate, causing vigorous heat inside their bodies, therefore, Shigao is suitable for them to clear the pathogenic heat.

Nowadays, there are a lot of diabetes cases involving severe endogenous heat among the patients in Beijing. There is no doubt that many ways can be adopted to clear heat, but in most cases, Shigao shall be usedfor diabetic patients. My teacher always says, "Large dosage of Shigao must be used if hyperglycaemic index does not decrease. " Blood sugar does not go down since heat in the Qi system affects the blood system, but the blood heat is still at its beginning stage. Shigao is used to clear heat out of the Qi system and the blood system concurrently, the blood sugar will go down naturally. Of course, treatment based on syndrome differentiation must be kept in mind.

第二章　石膏

石膏是比较常用的一味药。有一个说法，四大药能够起死回生：人参、大黄、附子、石膏。因为人死无非四种情况：大实、大虚、大寒、大热。若是大寒，就要用附子来回阳救逆；若是大热，就要用到石膏来清热；若是大虚，就得用人参来补；若是大实，则用大黄来泄。石膏就是这四大起死回生药之一。

石膏经文详解

石膏在《神农本草经》中被列为中品。上品的药都有久服轻身延年的功效，中品药则不可久服。没见过谁没事天天喝石膏的，石膏必须是有热才能用，尤其是气分有热才能用，喝了也不会让你延年益寿。它仅仅是治病的药，不是养生的药。

《神农本草经》是这样描述石膏的："石膏，味辛微寒，主中风寒热，心下逆气惊喘，口干苦焦，不能息，腹中坚痛，除鬼邪，产乳，金疮，生山谷。"咱们今天就根据《神农本草经》中这么简短的一段话，把握石膏的药性、把石膏的用途全部讲完。

经典往往文辞简略，但是它背后有着非常丰富的内容。经典有阴有阳，有表有里。就像人体，表是皮肤，里是五脏六腑。中医可以根据一个人的五官、肤色、气色、神采去推其五脏六腑，这是由表入里。

经典也是这样的，我们可以从经典这么寥寥几句话看到经典背后的深意。比如说，《黄帝内经》在表是理论，在里有方法。《伤寒论》表的是方剂，在里的则是理论，它没有写上来。《神农本草经》呈现给我们的是药性，背后则是理论和治病的方法。要获取完整的学问，不能光看书，因为即使是经典，都只讲一半。这就需要靠师承，去把书里的内容付诸实践。

我们来把《神农本草经》对石膏的论述逐字分析一下。

"石"字解

把"石膏"这两个字拆开，一个是"石"，一个是"膏"。"石"意味着石膏是一种石头，在质地上比较重，说明它能重镇，能往下镇压人的浮火。火性炎上，火邪往上走，石膏能把它给镇压下去，这就是石膏清火的性质的一个方面。

在自然界或人体，邪火都会往上走。比如人上火，总是在上半身，尤其在头上，很少听说有人脚上上火的。石膏是入肺经的，清气分实热，尤其清肺、胃二经的热。这二经的热从何而来？肺是脏腑中位置最高的，五脏六腑所有的火，肺都得在上面给它扛着。胃为五脏六腑之大海，兼收并蓄，是多气多血之腑，容易生火。五脏六腑的火都会影响肺胃，所以，肺胃之气是下降的，这样才能给火很好的出路。肝从左升，肺从右降；脾主升清，胃主降浊，构成人体升降浮沈的正常循环。肺气胃气都以下降为顺，一旦邪火过大，肺胃降之不及，肺胃二经的火象就明显了。石膏往下镇，能够帮助肺气和胃气往下降，火也会随之而降。这是石字的涵义：镇压火邪，顺应肺胃之气下降。

"膏"字解

"膏"字给人润泽的感觉。比如，润肤膏、枇杷膏，都是滋润的。润，就能生津。石膏里面含有大量的结晶水，学化学我们知道，生石膏就是每一个硫酸钙分子结晶两个水分子。硫酸钙只能微微融于水，石膏起滋润作用的是其中的结晶水。

生石膏是白色的，晶莹剔透，给人一种膏的感觉是最好的。生石膏如果发黄，就不能入药了，吃了以后就会导致淋症，就是一些小便短黄不利、结石之类的病。因为它就不再是纯正的甘寒之性了，它结晶时混进了湿热。

我们通常讲的石膏都是生石膏。如果把一块生石膏放到火里边烧，会烧得通红，冷却后，它就变得干枯，那种润泽的感觉没有了，因为石膏里边的结晶水被烧蒸发了。这时候的石膏就跟生石膏不一样了，叫熟石膏，或煅石膏。石膏是甘寒的，一旦变成熟石膏，就比较咸涩，药性完全变。熟石膏一般是不能内服的，因为它的收涩性太强了。

味辛微寒，主中风寒热

石膏的气和味都很薄，"味辛微寒"，辛就能走表散火，宣透郁热。

人全身上下有很多毛孔，气通过毛孔自由出入，人就感觉很通透。当外面有风寒之邪较强的时候，人体卫气不足以自卫，就开启第二套防护措施，这也是一种本能的自卫，毛孔闭上了，但这样一来，正气在人体内就被遏制住了，人就不通透了，正气一被遏制，就会成为邪热。

所以，咱们受了风寒之后就会发热，发热不明显，用普通辛通透表的药就可以了，如果热盛，就要加石膏，一方面直接清里热，另一方面达表散热。所以，石膏还是能够发汗的一个药。

石膏"主中风寒热"。"主"就是主治哪些病，"中风寒热"指的是中外风，人体肌表被外面的风邪所伤，导致了恶寒、发热。恶寒是因为有表证，发热是因为人体的正气被遏郁在体内了，人体的毛孔被闭合住了，该透出来的热不能很好的透出来，于是热就郁在肌肤之间，然后发热。这时候都要用到石膏，所以感冒发热，石膏是经常用的一个药，这时候热在气分。这是"味辛"的作用。

《神农本草经》说石膏微寒，后世很多医家说石膏大寒。那它到底是微寒还是大寒呢？石膏本身确实是大寒之药，但是它兼具辛甘之味，而辛甘发散为阳，它的寒性会往外散掉，所以给人的感觉只是微寒。它有大寒之体，微寒之用。它本身是大寒的，但在发挥作用的时候是微寒的，不会过多克伐人的阳气。

但这个话也不是绝对的。石膏用对了，是微寒，甚至感觉不到它的寒，它的寒性全用在清热上了；用错了，它就是大寒，一下把体内那点阳气给消灭了。而且，一味药，你还要看它跟谁配伍，有的药跟凉药一块走就是凉的，跟热药一块走就是热的。

我们要记住，微寒往往意味着甘寒。甘寒走气分，清气分的热，如果是咸寒那就得走血分了，咸寒的药我们在后面要讲到。

心下逆气惊喘

"心下逆气惊喘"，心下就是胃，胃是主下降的。胃气下降，则大肠、小肠能往下降浊，让糟粕往下走。脾主升清，把我们从食物里吸取来的水谷之精微往上输送，再通过肺朝百脉、奉心化赤，以气血的形式输布到全身。这是人最基本的生理过程。如果胃中有火，胃气就不往下降反往上升，这就叫"心下逆气"。

胃气逆，能造成各种逆证，比如呃逆、呕吐。胃里面的东西，不往下走反而往上走，就吐出来了。

"惊"是心经症状。心火是要下降的，下交于肾，当邪火太盛，心火受扰，不能下行而随邪火之势向上浮动，心不藏神，人就容易受惊。

"喘"是肺经症状，"肺苦气上逆"，而且肺有肃降作用，能降水，也能降火。邪火又能导致肺气上逆。"心下逆气惊喘"，背后都是一个"火"字。当然，并不是所有的惊和喘都得用石膏来治，石膏主要治因为气分的大热导致的惊和喘。

口干苦焦

"口干苦焦"，也是火导致的。火伤津液，继而伤阴，会导致口干、口苦、口焦。苦是火的本味，口苦也多因火。食物在锅里面煮糊了，就会有一股焦味。火能够让食物变得焦苦，也能够让人嘴里有焦苦的感觉。这两种焦苦不是一回事，但很相似。当你嘴里有焦苦感时，你就应该知道这可能是火太大导致的。当然你嘴里的气息，肯定不能和锅里烧糊的气息一样，但是它给你的感觉是一样的，都是焦苦。这就叫通感。再比如辛苦，生活的辛苦跟药物辛苦的味道是两回事，但它们给人的感觉是一样的，所以都叫辛苦。

不能息

"不能息"，一呼一吸为一息。我们讲"休息"，也跟呼吸有关，就是让呼吸缓一缓。庄子讲"真人之息以踵，众人之息以喉"，普通人吸气只能吸到喉咙这，然后就呼出来了；真人就是有修行的人，他一吸能吸到脚后跟。呼吸是胸腔呼吸和腹式呼吸。懂得养生的人，总是会让自己的呼吸变得深长。

邪火，会让一个人呼吸表浅。火是往上浮的，火浮则气浮，呼吸就不能深长，因为肾主纳气，吸气的动力在肾，肾气在下面一动，往下一拉，人就自然地吸气，肺再一合，气就呼出来了。人的呼吸不光是肺的事，而是肺、肾、脾、胃都在发挥作用。呼吸是养生很必要的功课。

有个成语叫"心浮气躁"，心一浮，气就躁，呼吸就不能深长；心一浮，呼吸就不得力，呼吸不得力，心也更容易浮。所以很多人慌张或者压力大的时候，需要深呼吸，以安定心神。

再者，一个人如果爱慕浮华，也会导致心浮。心一浮，也会影响到呼吸，影响到整个身体健康。

总而言之，"不得息"，有两个原因，一是邪火令气浮，二是心气浮。养生的关键在于修心。心不要浮，要沉下来，这是一个人的修养问题，不要以为有修养就会很吃亏，只有没有修养的人才会觉得有修养会很吃亏。你自己有修养会觉得身心安泰，非常受用，至少你在身体上会比别人好一些。追慕浮华会伤气，会伤神，还影响你的呼吸，而呼吸又是健康的一个重要环节。

生理和心理永远都是相通的，咱们不要以为有些东西是心理作用，然后再以为心理作用是虚幻的。其实，心理作用是实实在在的，有的病完完全全就是心理作用导致的，你心慕浮华，气就会浮躁，脸色就差了，甚至浑身气机都不顺了；你能沉得住气，呼吸就能深长一些，久而久之，你会更健康。

我们接受任何东西都有四个阶段：信、愿、行、证。小到养生，大到修佛，都要经历这四个步骤。我们在治病的过程中也是这样的，尤其是治疗一些慢性病，要讲究一些策略，让病人生起信心。有个说法叫"医不扣门"，医生是不会主动去扣门给你治病的，要看病你得去求医。只有病人去扣医生家的门，去求医，才说明他相信这个医生，愿意让他看病，这样医生治起来就相对容易了，病人会好好吃药，最后去证实疗效。"医不叩门"是为了坚定病人的信心，其中考虑到了很微妙的心理因素。

腹中坚痛

继续回到经文，下面是"腹中坚痛"。坚硬而且痛，这是一个实证，是因为有火，火能生气，邪火生邪气，导致腹中气机阻滞，不通则痛，外面摸上去还很坚硬，而且按着更痛。痛是因为是实证。痛分虚实：虚痛喜欢按，按上去就不痛了；实痛则怕按，一按就会痛得更厉害，治疗的时候，要看这个实是怎么来的，是因为气还是因为瘀血，还是因为有食积……

可以说，绝大部分痛都是气痛，气运行不顺导致痛。"腹中坚痛"，说白了还是因为火导致的。如果腹中坚痛很多年了，而且一直痛，那就不是石膏能治的了。可能是因为瘀血，也可能因为食积。

除鬼邪

石膏还有一个作用，"除鬼邪"。

鬼是一种虚幻的东西，世界上的东西，有阴就有阳，有看得到的就有看不到的，有实实在在存在的，就有虚无缥缈存在的。不管是实还是虚，它都是一种存在。

正常人是看不到鬼的。但正气虚的人、邪气旺的人能看到鬼。人一旦生病，有些化验指标就不在正常值范围之内，他的知觉也可能不在正常的范围之内，要么高要么低，他就容易看到鬼。也可以说，这是因为痰、瘀、火旺等导致的一些妄知妄觉。尤其是因为火太重，人会见鬼。如果我们把火撤掉，人就不会见鬼了。

而且，石膏是金石之品，甘寒去火，质重能镇，也有清除浮火、镇心安神的作用。

产乳

产后没有乳汁，也可以用石膏来催乳么？

产乳也要辨证论治，产妇生完孩子以后没有乳汁有很多原因，这里针对的是其中的一种：胃热。首先，产后血虚，血虚就生热；第二，为了防止产妇受风受寒，房间要非常温暖，这也可能导致产妇的热；第三，刚生了小孩，饮食往往非常丰盛，这又可能导致胃热。这么多热，尤其是胃热，容易导致壅滞，乳汁就不通了。

乳房属肝经和胃经，其中的乳腺，是属胃的。当有胃热的时候，乳房也首当其冲。乳房里面的一些组织、信道、孔窍被遏住了，所以乳汁不通。这个时候热在气分。只有在这种情况下才可以用石膏来清。如果是其他原因的乳汁不通，就要另行考虑了。

例如，生完孩子后，觉得家里照顾不周到，或者生了孩子自己不满意，很郁闷，或者在坐月子期间吵架，肝气都郁结了。肝气郁结，乳汁也会不通，这就不能用石膏了。还有的人是因为产后气血虚而没有乳汁，这就要大补气血，更不能用生石膏。当然，不管是什么类型的乳汁不通，只要到最后乳房胀痛不可忍，甚至发热、溃疡、化脓，方子都可以用配伍石膏来清热。所以，石膏催乳的作用是不可以一概而论。

金疮

金疮是因为被刀砍斧剁身体受的伤，往往这种受伤口不容易愈合，甚者会溃烂、化脓，当你把这些溃烂、脓血清除以后，还得想让它赶紧长肉。

"诸痛痒疮，皆属于心"，伤口老不愈合就是因为有火邪。所以要清火邪，还要收敛疮口，促进愈合。石膏寒凉，寒主收引，是可以清火、收敛。清疮口火邪，宜用生石膏，收口生肌，宜用煅石膏。煅石膏就是把这个石膏烧熟，它就变成微咸而涩的，收涩性更强。

做豆腐用石膏，这也是在利用石膏的寒性和收涩性，因为寒主凝，涩主敛，两者共同作用才能让豆浆凝结起来，成为豆腐或豆腐脑。从中医角度讲，这和石膏用来收口是一个道理。石膏治金疮有一个很有用的方子：甘石生肌散。

甘石生肌散：珍珠粉20，煅炉甘石50，熟石膏200，黄丹20。用于腐肉已去，收口生肌。

这个方子现在很多书上都有。听前辈讲，在此方基础之上加上一味狗骨头，药效更好。狗骨头要磨细或煅成灰入该方。

白虎汤

围绕石膏，我们来讲一些方剂，首先就是白虎汤。

白虎汤

石膏一斤（一两），知母六两（三钱），炙甘草二两（一钱），粳米六合（五钱）。

白虎汤清阳明实热

白虎汤方来自《伤寒论》，是用来清阳明实热的。足阳明是胃经，手阳明是大肠经。

阳明经是多气多血之经。气多血多就好比有钱，人一有钱就容易头脑发热，阳明多气多血，也容易生热，临床上胃热、大肠热相当常见。

按照张仲景《伤寒论》的思路，当邪气侵犯人的体表，要用发汗的方式把它撵走，如果没有及时撵走，它就会从太阳经传到阳明经，从而导致胃热、大肠热。有人说《伤寒论》描述的阳明病不好把握，其实我们可以把它简化，知道其入里化热，导致胃热或大肠热，就好把握了。如果是胃热就用白虎汤，如果是大肠热就要让它往下泻，用承气汤类。

历代注家往往会耍概念，说什么阳明经证、阳明腑证，我则习惯于把它转化成大家都听得懂的语言，一个是胃热，一个是大肠热。

白虎汤五大证

胃热有五大表现：大热、大汗、大渴、大烦、脉洪大，这也是使用白虎汤的五大证。

大热就是发高烧，发高烧往往源于阳明；大汗，就是出汗非常多，汗虽为心之液，但出汗还在于阳明之气的鼓动；大渴，是因为热伤了津液，需要喝水来补充。大烦，也是因为胃热，心和胃是相通的，胃热到一定程度，心就会受到影响，"烦"字是火字旁加一个页，页是头脑，火往头脑上冲，人就会大烦；脉洪大，就是脉跳的幅度、力度都特别大，速度特别快，这也是火象无疑。这就叫脉洪大。

这五大证，如果全部出现的话，得用白虎汤无疑；如果只出现一两个，我们也可以考虑用白虎汤。

白虎汤方义及熬法

白虎汤的构成比较简单，主药就是石膏和知母，后面的药都是配上去的。石膏单用的时候的确是微寒的，但是它一旦跟知母配合起来，就再也不是微寒了而是大寒了。

知母是一种植物的根，白色的，外面还长一些毛。入药则把毛洗掉，切成薄片，它可以清热养阴。知母是苦的，微辛甘寒，也比较润滑，主要入肺经、胃经，还入肾经，能够泻火止水。它是白色的，白色走气分，能泻肾火。与知母相配的药还有黄柏。知柏地黄丸是在六味地黄汤的基础上加黄柏、知母，是泻肾火的。石膏配知母则泻肺火、胃火。

关于知母的用法，我们可以抓要点来记：一个是石膏配知母，一个是黄柏配知母。石膏配知母清肺胃之热，主要在上焦；黄柏配知母清肾里边的邪火，主要在下焦。

石膏、知母清热，又可能会伤胃气。虽说"胃为燥土，得凉则安"，但大寒大凉也会伤胃，凡事过犹不及。所以，要给胃一些适当的安抚，那就用炙甘草，它是调和诸药的，能够减轻石膏、知母的寒性，让寒性缓缓地发挥作用，不那么猛烈。

粳米是介于籼米和糯米之间的一种米，有微弱的糯性，也很好吃，这是最养胃的。如果没有粳米，我们可以用糯米代替；如果连糯米也没有，也可以用普通的米。退而求其次。米，就是用来养胃气的。把苍术放在淘米水里漂一漂，它的燥性就减弱了，不会伤胃。米汤也是这样，在做饭时，先在米里加上很多水。煮开以后，过滤出来的米汤是非常养胃气的，生了病的人如果不想吃东西，喝米汤是最好的。白虎汤用了五钱粳米，也让药汁有米汤的性质，能够养人的胃气。

熬白虎汤要掌握火候，《伤寒论》讲的是"米熟汤成"，熬到米熟了，汤有米汤的感觉，就可以了，然后温服。我们现在熬白虎汤，可以先煎石膏十五分钟，因为石膏是一种矿物，比较难煎出汁的，然后再把知母、甘草、粳米倒进去，再熬，其他药熬的时间要比石膏短一些。

既要打击邪气，又要扶植正气，这是中医治病的一个原则，时时处处都要用到，几乎在每一个方子里面都有体现。有驱邪就有扶正，永远都是平衡的。

慎用白虎汤

《伤寒论》用白虎汤非常慎重，为什么呢？张仲景那个时代寒气是比较重的，所以《伤寒论》用温药也用得偏多：桂枝、附子、干姜等。白虎汤大寒，把身体的阳气克伐掉了，所以应该慎用。

从白虎汤这个方名，我们也可以看出这是一个寒凉的方剂。东青龙，西白虎，南朱雀，北玄武。白虎就意味着西边，西边对应的是寒凉、是秋天。秋天的西风，能让人很凉爽，也能把世界吹得一片肃杀。白虎据说是最凶残的老虎，有童谣讲"老虎不吃人"，一般的老虎，不饿的时候，没有受到人的侵犯和威胁的时候，是不会吃人的，但白虎不一样，它杀气最重。白虎汤当用得好的时候有作用，用得不好的时候就有杀气，所以古代的医家用白虎汤都非常慎重。

传说，《伤寒论》的编者，西晋名医王叔和，有一次他母亲病了，可能出现了大热、大烦、大渴之类的症状，王叔和用了很多方法治不好，非常着急。晚上，母亲在屋里奄奄一息，他一个人在院子里焦头烂额地踱步，还一边唠叨："若非亲生母，必用白虎汤！"他不敢用白虎汤，怕用了危险，因为是亲生母亲，所以他瞻前顾后。他的一位学生听了这话，就赶紧自作主张开了一剂白虎汤给老太太喝下去了，老太太喝了病就好了。王叔和非常惊诧，那位学生就说："我敢用白虎汤，因为不是我亲妈。"

清胃散

另外，还有一个清胃热的方剂，叫做清胃散。

黄连、生地、升麻、丹皮、当归。

白虎汤和清胃散都是清胃热的，那二者有什么区别呢？白虎汤主要针对的是外感引起的阳明实热，这种热还在气分；而清胃散往往针对那种积了很久，而且都伤了阴的胃热，这种热在往往血分。

清胃散中，黄连苦寒，泻中焦之热，它气分血分都走，这是主药。胃为多气多血之府，容易生热，热久了就会影响血，所以用生地和丹皮来凉血。"胃为燥土，得凉则安"，生地、丹皮、黄连都是寒凉药，且味苦能降，顺随了胃气的下降之性，火也会随胃气而降。

但不能一味往下降，再加升麻来兼顾一下脾，脾主升清，升麻能升清，清气往上升也就意味着浊气往下降。也不能一味用寒凉药，还得加一味温药来平衡一下，这便是当归，而且当归配生地能养血生血，养血又有助于清热，这都是胃所需要的。

清胃散对于杂病类的胃热非常有效果，它是通过养胃来清胃的，其中的当归、生地都是带补的药。现代人有的饮食过度，导致胃中积热，典型的症状就是口臭，你和他面对面说话都会感觉到；他的牙龈就会萎缩得特别快，牙齿也会烂得特别快，甚至还会经常牙痛。有人说，牙痛牙烂，是因为虫牙。其实，虫牙也跟胃火有关，当胃里有火的时候，就会有一股浊气往上冲，冲到嘴里，在这种污浊的气息中就容易生虫子。所以治虫牙依然要清胃热。清胃散对于这类人来说，是一个非常好的方剂，经常用的。

有的清胃散版本，在这五个药的基础上又加了一味石膏，这就加大了它清胃的力度，气血两清啊。清胃散中的黄连通常用量较少。一般每剂一钱，也就是3克，所以，清胃散即使稍微多喝一段时间也是不要紧的，极能养胃；但也不要喝太久，毕竟黄连是苦的，生地、丹皮是寒的，苦寒败胃，喝久了可能会对胃不好。

白虎汤的加减

如果白虎汤用得太迟了，阳明之热已经伤了津液，伤了气，人都渴得不行，甚至有点气短了，此时应该在白虎汤的基础上加人参，这个方子叫人参白虎汤。现在，我们经常用西洋参代替人参。西洋参跟张仲景时代的人参更为接近，能补气，又能生津。西洋参并不是个头越大越好，最好的西洋参，一般像手指那么大的，皮薄而黄，横纹致密，尝之先苦而甜，还夹杂着一点儿蒿子杆的味道。只需要尝一点点，马上就会觉得津液满口。

除了有之前说的白虎汤五大证，还出现了骨节烦痛，尤其是手的骨节烦痛，那么，白虎汤中还要加一点桂枝，这就是白虎加桂枝汤。桂枝是用来调和营卫的，能够往四肢走。

如果手指关节出现了很明显的热象，又出现了湿证，那么在白虎汤里要加上苍术，苍术是化湿的。这就叫白虎加术汤，或者叫白虎加苍术汤。

白虎加桂枝汤、白虎加苍术汤是在治疗风湿性关节炎的时候用的。痛到关节发红发热，就用几剂白虎汤加桂枝或加苍术都好。这是因为体内有热，就用这种方式来清。

用到石膏的其他经典方剂

竹叶石膏汤

竹叶五钱，石膏八钱，人参二钱，半夏三钱，麦冬三钱，甘草一钱，粳米五钱。

竹叶石膏汤其实就是白虎汤的加减。这个方子主要是用于外感病后期收尾的，所有的发热都要消耗人体的气血津液，在大热已退、余热未清、津液已伤的情况下，要清余热，还要赶紧给人体补水。因为热并不是很大，所以去掉知母，光用石膏就行了。竹叶清心火，通大肠，利小便，能把心火通过大肠、小便排出去，给邪热以出路。能致一服，不致一死，要尽量把邪气赶出去，不要闷在体内乱打。

后面的人参、半夏、麦冬、甘草、粳米，这又是《金匮要略》中的麦门冬汤。人参益气生津，补脾补肺，也补充必要的津液。但是，人参补水分的力量依然不够，还要加麦冬。麦冬是半透明的，甘寒生津，特别能给人体补充津液。

热病消耗的津液都上哪儿去了呢？一部分是作为汗液排掉了，另一部分是被热邪炼干了。津液炼干就是痰，所以，热病之后体内往往有痰，所以加半夏来化痰。甘草、粳米依然是调和胃气的。其实麦门冬汤也是个能化痰，又能生津的一剂药。

竹叶石膏汤，既可以理解为白虎汤去掉知母加竹叶、人参、半夏、麦冬，也可以把它理解成麦门冬汤加石膏、竹叶，方子是变化无穷的。

看到人参、麦冬，我们就会想到生脉饮。它是由人参、麦冬、五味子组成的。竹叶石膏汤为什么没有用五味子呢？因为五味子兼有酸苦甘辛咸五种味道，又以酸味为主，能够入五脏，收敛五脏精气的。虽然书上、古人都讲它只收敛正气，而不收敛邪气，但它毕竟是以酸为主，酸就能收，谁能保证它一丁点儿邪气都不收敛呢？所以慎重起见还是不要用。

治病都要懂得善后，竹叶石膏汤往往是一个善后方，一年四季发热病善后都可以用，尤其是夏天暑证善后，用竹叶石膏汤尤其好。

麻杏石甘汤与大青龙汤

用到石膏的还有麻杏石甘汤，由麻黄、杏仁、石膏、甘草这四味药组成：麻黄开肺窍，杏仁降肺气，石膏清肺热，甘草缓肺急，这四句话就概括了麻杏石甘汤的原理和作用。表有邪气，肺气不通，热在肺胃之中越积越多，用麻黄和杏仁来开肺气。肺气通达了，热就容易散去。光开肺散热还不够，同时还得用石膏直接清热。再加甘草，一则甘以缓之，缓和一下肺里紧张的局势，二则调和诸药。这样，在表的邪散掉了，在里的热也清掉了。

大青龙汤，是在麻杏石甘汤的基础上加减而来的，也有人说是在桂枝汤的基础上加减来的。大青龙汤在麻杏石甘汤的基础上加上桂枝，发汗的力度更大。而且还加了生姜和大枣，鼓动胃气，继续加大发汗的力度。现在大青龙汤一般的都不怎么用，我们用到麻杏石甘汤就够了，因为大青龙汤非常峻烈，一般也就是一剂一剂地开，对症而用。

玉泉散

玉泉散的组成非常简单，就是石膏、滑石、甘草。

玉泉散，可以顾名思义。泉，往往是小便的委婉说法。比如，缩泉丸，就是让人的小便变少，尤其是夜尿变少。玉泉散也跟小便有关，它能让人的小便解得像玉一样清澈。夏天，很多人受了点热，就会心烦，小便发黄，到医院一检查，里面甚至有潜血，一个玉泉散就能解决这个问题。

玉泉散其实就是在六一散的基础上加生石膏。六份重量的滑石和一份重量的甘草，组成六一散，专门针对暑天湿气阻滞。滑石的气味很淡，质地很重，淡就能渗湿，能通窍；重就能让湿往下带，最终通过淡渗，从小便排出去。滑石非常便宜，但作用却非常神奇。它能滑掉人体的湿，打通阻滞；在治各种结石方面也有非常独到的功效，顾名思义，它能把结石给滑了。

夏天暑邪当令，暑就是由湿热二气组成的，暑气导致人体的很多孔窍不通，阻碍气血运行，热就容易堆积起来，热一盛，就会影响到小便，让小便发黄发红，这时候用玉泉散。石膏清气分的热，六一散化湿开窍，同时也清气分，如果与竹叶石膏汤一块合用，效果也会非常好。

善用石膏

总之，石膏这味药，很重要，也很简单、好理解，它针对的就是大热，尤其是气分的热引起的各种疾病。

很多中医善用石膏。北京过去有四大名医，其中有一位叫孔伯华，他在北京就被称为"石膏孔"，因为他特别善于用石膏，在很多方子里面他都会加上一味石膏。他是在北京看病，找他看病的人社会地位也比较高，往往都是一些吃多了的，还有一些火气比较旺的，内热比较重，用石膏来给他们清清热，非常合适。

现在，在北京看到很多的糖尿病人都是内热非常重，清热会用到很多方法，大多会用到石膏。在治糖尿病的时候石膏是经常要用到的一味药。我师父常讲："血糖不降，重用石膏。"血糖不降是因为气分有热，影响到血，血分的热还不算太深重。通过石膏清气分，兼及血分，血糖就会降下来。当然，这样做的前提是辨证论治。

Chapter 3　Lugen (Rhizoma Phragmitis), Maogen (Couchgrass Root) and Tianhua Fen (Radices Trichosanthis)

There are varieties of sweet-cold medicines, and different uses of them as well. Some people claim that the cold and cool herbs can impair the stomach, Qi-blood and Yang. It is true indeed. However, if appropriately used, these medicines will not cause impairment as they are imagined. Therefore, it does require some efforts to master the skills of prescribing the sweet-cold medicines in clinical practice. In fact, many of the herbs in this category are mostly sweet in taste and weak in cold property, for example, Lugen, Maogen and Tianhua Fen.

Lugen(Rhizoma Phragmitis)

Lugen is the root of common reeds. Reeds usually grows around 3 meters tall in freshwater rivers and lakes, blossoming white catkins in autumn. It can be seen in most areas in China, and those that grow in Yangcheng Lake in Jiangsu province, Bohu Lake in Anhui province, Poyang Lake in Jiangxi province, Baiyangdian Lake in Hebei province of China are all extremely good in quality.

Alleviating Water Retention, Promoting Secretion of Saliva and Opening Orifices

There is one line from the ***The Book of Songs*** "Reeds grow vast, and dews change into frost ". Reeds wither in late autumn, and the entire lake and river looks vast and hazy. The weather is getting colder and colder and moisture condenses into frost on the reeds. This scene always makes people miss their families with strong tender feelings. This is the right moment for harvesting Lugen.

Although reed withers in autumn, its root is still alive. Since Lugen lives in water all year, it gains the Qi of water, which makes it characterized with nourishing Yin and promoting the secretion of saliva or body fluid; growing in water also means it tolerates water, therefore it can alleviate water retention.

Water is the source of life, but it has to be the fresh/flowing water. The stagnant water or pathogenic water does harm to the human body. Lugen can refuel sufficient fresh water to human body while it concurrently drains the stagnant and pathogenic water/fluid. Many herbs that nourish Yin and promote the secretion of saliva or body fluid may bring in dampness, such as Shengdi, Shudi, Tianmendong and Maidong. If without timely transportation and transformation being carried out, phlegm will be produced. Lugen is the only exception since it has two-way regulating functions. For those who are easily subject to phlegm, Lugen is the best choice to reduce the phlegm on the one hand, and to nourish Yin and promote the secretion of body fluid on the other hand.

Opening Orifices and Harmonizing the Stomach

In the human body, there are many pores and orifices that can open and close freely. However, in case they are obstructed by phlegm and damp pathogens, one may fall sick. Lugen is hollow inside with joints all over its length. Generally speaking, A plant that has joints indicates that it can break through obstruction. Bamboo is another example with joints, and Zhuli (bamboo juice) as a medicine can open orifices in the human body, too. Lugen is similar to, but also different from Bamboo since Lugen has lots of tiny pores around the wall surface, which means it has stronger potence of opening orifices, and is able to communicate up and down inside the human body. With this concept, it is imaginable that Shi Changpu (rhizoma acori graminei) is aromatic with joints and it has even more potence in opening orifices, but it is weaker in terms of excreting dampness compared to Lugen since Lugen has a light taste.

Lugen enters the Yangming Meridian, dredges the large intestine and stomach. It also goes to the lung, spleen and kidneys. Many Chinese materia medica textbook say Lugen has a function of relieving restlessness. Restlessness is always related to the fire that runs to the head, causing distraction, which is also due to the fire disturbance. Lugen can relieve restlessness since it can get through the heart Qi and clear the accumulated endogenous heat due to obstruction of orifices.

Lugen controls nausea and vomiting, too, since it calms down the Middle

Jiao by nourishing the stomach and soothing the Yangming meridian. Lugen grows by extending its root into the sludge, which means it has a descending function, in keeping with the descending action of the lung and stomach Qi. Therefore, it prevents or arrests vomiting. Similar to lotus root, Lugen has character of preserving its purity even though it is growing out of sludge. It can help the clear Qi in the human body to ascend. Thus, Lugen can clear up the Upper Jiao of the body, nourish the lung Yin and let the lung Qi descend. The lungs dislike counterflow of Qi upwards since that may make one feel rotten.

Qianjin Weijing Tang

There is a famous formula called **Qianjin Weijing Tang**, which takes Lugen as the main herb.

Qianjin Weijing Tang contains the herbal ingredients: Lugen (rhizoma phragmitis), Yimi (coix seed), Taoren (peach kernel), Dongguazi (seed of Chinese waxgourd).

Analysis of Qianjin Weijing Tang Formula

This formula originates from **Qianjin Yaofang (Thousand Golden Formulas)** written by Sun Simiao (medical scientist in the Tang Dynasty), and the original formula contains Weijing (reed stem), Guaban (melon petal), Yimi (coix seed), Taoren (peach kernel).

Weijing is the stem of reed, and it was clinically proved not so effective as Lugen. Therefore, Lugen is gradually substituted for Weijing by doctors.

As to Guaban, there has been a lot of debates about its real reference, but now, Dongguazi is used instead since it has a function of eliminating stagnation including various stagnation of Qi and blood stasis. Dongguazi can also remove the greasy and turbid wastes from the human body. Besides, Dongguazi enters the liver channel, purges the liver heat and assists detoxification of the liver.

Yimi is helpful for lowering Qi and alleviating water retention. Therefore, it is used to purge the pathogenic fire but it does not impair the vital Qi.

Taoren and safflower are often used in pair to promote the blood circulation to remove blood stasis. Taoren goes to the six hollow organs to help blood to circulate; Safflower goes to the exterior and the five internal organs. When these two herbs are used together, they can take care of both the interior and exterior, and go to both the internal five organs and the six hollow organs. In this formula, Taoren functions to clear the hollow viscera, and descend the blood-arthralgia. However, it is inadvisable to stir up the blood too much, therefore, safflower is not used here.

Treatment of the Pulmonary Abscess

Qianjin Yaofang states that **Qianjin Weijing Tang** is used to cure the lung abscess. Pulmonary abscess refers that the lungs are clogged up by either phlegm or blood stasis.

There are many orifices in the lungs of human being, and lung abscess occurs when these orifices are obstructed by phlegm and blood stasis. When the phlegm and blood accumulate, they will generate heat, and are even transformed into pus. Under such conditions, the patients may feel rotten. Therefore, **Qianjin Weijing Tang** can be used for tackling these symptoms.

Lugen promotes the Qi circulation; Taoren disperses blood stasis; Dongguanzi eliminates stagnation and clear away waste; and Yimi descends Qi and alleviates water retention. These four herbs used together can eliminate the lung abscess.

Formation and Treatment of the Cold Due to Pulmonary Abscess

Many medical practitioners often prescribe or inject anti-viral medicines and antibiotics for patients who catch a cold or flu. This practice will trap and suppress the pathogens inside rather than disperse them out of the body. Some western drugs do have dispersing functions, such as drugs for inducing sweat, but many doctors now simply prescribe medicines that are seemingly quick fix, for example, the anti-inflammatory drugs, the anti-fever medicines, or anti-biotics. However, all of these medicines are extremely cold in nature.

Another example is intravenous fluid, which can consume the Yang of human body and trap the pathogens inside, causing the lungs' failure to disperse the pathongens out of the body. That is why so many patients suffer from too much phlegm and chest stuffiness after catching a cold. That is often a cold or flu arising from the functional obstruction of the lungs (since the lung abscess has not taken shape, and there are no symptoms of the lung functional obstruction, but it is quite close to the lung abscess). The laboratory tests may show nothing serious, but from the perspective of TCM, it might actually be a light case of lung functional obstruction. For such a case of a cold, **Qianjin Weijing Tang** can be used.

Clearing and Reducing Phlegm-heat from the Upper Jiao

By a logical extension of this point, **Qianjin Weijing Tang** can be used whenever phlegm-heat arises in the Upper Jiao, or pus (that can be also taken as a type of phlegm) at the upper portion of body since pus is the by-product from Qi and blood transformation. The phlegm-heat in the Upper Jiao involves various diseases, and here I only give one or two examples. When there is nasitis with purulent nasal discharge, or pharyngitis with coughing out thick phlegm, modified **Qianjin Weijing Tang** has been proved very effective. For further understanding the uses of this formula, it needs to make analyses through clinical case studies.

Lusun (Sparrowgrass)

The roots of reeds in the season of spring start to give out small shoots called Lusun. Lusun referred here is different from that being sold as vegetable (that grows in the dry land and is said to have an antitumous effect) in the markets. The Lusun referred here for medical use actually grows in fresh water.

One may suffer from fish heat (pathogens) in case he or she eats too much fish, and the Lusun grows out of Lugen can relieve the fish heat. Therefore, fish is always stewed with Lusun into a tasty dish. Of course, Lugen may be used instead of Lusun to eliminate the fish heat.

Lotus roots, to some extent, can also eliminate the fish heat since they grow in water with fishes as similar things always attract each other.

Examples of Lugen (rhizoma phragmitis) Compatibility And Miscellaneous

Lugen Used with Qingdai (Indigo Naturalis)

There is a folk prescription that combines Lugen with Qingdai (indigo naturalis), called **Lugen Qingdai San** to cure gastric ulcer. Lugen is sweet-cold in property, nourishing Yin and promoting the secretion of saliva or body fluid. The stomach enjoys the sweet-cold materials. Qingdai is extracted from Banlangen (radix isatidis). Banlangen is good at clearing away heat and toxic materials, so is Qingdai, which is also good at curing ulcer. Qingdai is the main ingredient in the formula of **Bawei Xilei San**, used for curing various ulcers.

Lugen and Qingdai added in the formulas for ulcers based on syndrome differentiation usually give a remarkable effect for the treatment of gastric ulcers.

Lugen Used with Huashi (Talc)

Lugen can also be used to treat different types of calculus/stone due to its moistening effect. Water is essential to our life, and it has a lot of advantages and uses like dish-washing and cleaning purposes. Curing the diseases involving the internal organs in the human body is just like dish-washing. Lugen is added into the formulas for curing uses just like adding water for cleaning purposes. The calculi/stones are similar to the scales in the thermos or kettles, which should be cleaned with the help of vinegar, or hydrochloric acid, or solid acid, and water should be added as well. Huashi (talcum powder) is often used to treat stone-related diseases. Huashi can clear the damp-heat to eliminate the the source of calculi formation. However, Huashi by itself is insufficient since water is also essential. Therefore, Lugen is added, acting as the "water catalyst" to make the treatment effectively.

Furthermore, Haijinsha (lygodium japonicum), Jinqiancao (lysimachia christinae hance), Daji (euphorbia pekinensis), Xiaoji (herba cepbalanoplosis segeti) may also be added to tackle the kidney stone. For the gall-stone, Zhizi (fructus gardenia) may be added additionally since gallbladder is the organ subsumed to the Shaoyang meridian, which is semi-interior and semi-exterior. The formula recorded in *Shanghan Lun* for curing the diseases involving the Shaoy-ang meridian is **Xiaochaihu Tang**. So, for treatment of gall-stone, **Xiaochaihu Tang** can be used with addition of Huashi and Lugen; in case the liver Qi stag-nation is involved, **Xiaoyao San** can be used with addition of Huashi and Lugen. Without doubt, it definitely takes time to dissolve and transform those stones within the body.

Nodes and Hairs on Lugen Needs to be Removed

Here Lugen refers to the dried Lugen. However, in the Qing Dynasty, even before the year of 1949, doctors preferred to use the "flowing water Lugen" or "fresh Lugen", which means they liked to use the fresh Lugen that is growing in the flowing water (the newly dug-out Lugen is particularly preferred) since the fresh Lugen is full of vitality and clean in the flowing water.

Lugen has a lot of root hairs when it is just dug out, and the hairs must be removed. To be more particular, some formulas even require that the joints of Lu-gen have to be removed as well, similar to the use of Mahuang. Lugen, in this case, functions to open orifices. The joints usually indicate the possibility of ob-struction. Therefore, removal of joints can bring in a better effect for opening ori-fices. What's more, joints of plants are usually heavy in texture with mud and dirt included, which is also a critical reason for removing the joints.

Measurement of Chinese Medicines

The ancestors did not use weight but volume to measure the dosage of Lu-gen. For example, the formula of **Qianjin Weijing Tang** initially prescribed two litres of reed stem. It is the same as for *Shanghan Lun,* in which some herbs are measured in weight, and some others are measured in volume. Therefore, it is clear "weight" is not the only standard to measure the dosage of herbs in TCM.

In *Shanghan Lun,* many formulas stated "one piece of a large-sized Fuzi" will do when the herb of Fuzi is involved. If a piece of large-sized Fuzi weighs 15 grams, it is not the same story that three pieces Fuzi of 5 grams each. Therefore, both *Shanghan Lun* and *Qianjin Fang* are very particular about herbal dosage measurements.

Contraindications of Lugen

Lugen seems to be a mild herb, but there are many contraindications in fact. So, precautions must be taken in use of it.

Lugen should not be used when one suffers from deficiency-cold in the Middle Jiao, or at the early stage of wind symptoms since Lugen can moisturize the body. As a Chinese idiom says, "water goes up when wind starts blowing", which means that strong wind can cause water level to go up, and even lead to gigantic waves. Projecting this phenomenon back into the body, in case Yin nourishing herbs are added at the time of strong wind attack, it might eventually fail to nourish but generate much phlegm instead. Lugen does not cause phlegm, but it depends on the extent to which it is used.

Maogen(Couch Grass Root)

Maogen is frequently used together with Lugen.

Characteristics and Uses of Maogen

Maogen refers to the root of couchgrass, which can be seen around China, especially in the desolated and uncultivated land. Its white catkins blossom in autumn before getting withered. Maogen, with lots of joints, is white in color with hard core inside.

Maogen is sweet-cold in nature, and it can enter the blood system. Generally, it appears to be white when dug out from the earth, but some of them appear purple in color, signifying it enters the blood system. Maogen nourishes Yin, promotes the secretion of body fluid, cools the blood, and clears the floating heat in the body. When it comes to the functions in the blood system, Maogen can remove blood stasis and eliminate the heat in blood. From the perspective of Qi system, Maogen can quench thirst, alleviate water retention and purge heat from the upper portion of the body through urination. Maogen can be used for the treatment of some calculi cases as long as there are blood heat-induced symptoms like ulcerations, bleeding disorders or some types of jaundice.

Nourishing the Stomach with Its Sweet-cold Properties

Severe excess heat needs to be cleared with bitter-cold medicines since these medicines are the most efficient and effective in purging heat. However, for the deficiency-heat, or the heat that has penetrated into the blood system, or deeply and chronically rooted heat, bitter-cold medicines may become ineffective. Hence, the sweet-cold medicines such as Maogen should be used instead. The sweet-cold medicines, on the one hand, can nourish Yin and tonify the healthy Qi; on the other hand, it can purge the heat appropriately. As such, the stomach Qi will not be impaired. Both Lugen and Maogen are good for nourishing the stomach without causing impairment to it. The stomach is an organ that has abundant Qi and blood. Too much Qi accumulation will lead to heat in the Qi system, and too much blood accumulation will lead to heat in the blood system. Once disharmony occurs between Qi and blood, the stomach heat will arise accordingly. Lugen goes into the Qi system to nourish the stomach by clearing heat, while Maogen goes to the blood system to nourish the stomach by clearing heat, too. Therefore, these two herbs create synergistic effects. In addition, Maogen grows in soil, while Lugen grows in water. The two herbs work together to keep balance for nourishing the stomach from Qi and blood systems.

Those who claim Chinese medicine impairs the stomach may not understand the fundamentals of TCM. It is the first priority for a Chinese medicine practitioner to protect the stomach function. In fact, only when the stomach Qi is sufficient, one can properly digest food and consume decoction. When the stomach suffers from the vigorous pathogenic fire and fluid deficiency, the T&T functions of food nutrients will be inevitably affected, and the herbal decoction can not be well absorbed, either. Hence, it is required to use the sweet-cold medicines cleverly and try utmost to nourish the stomach simultaneously in the process of curing diseases.

Bitter-cold herbs impair the stomach, while sweet-cold herbs nourish the stomach. After bitter-cold herbs are used, the stomach Qi will have to be tonified in order to recover its function; sweet-cold herbs are used to nourish Yin when the stomach Yin deficiency arises; in case the stomach Yang deficiency occurs, the spleen should be tonified in order to help Yang to ascend. The stomach is "the sea of the Qi of all the internal organs". Modern people often eat too much, which makes their stomach overloaded, eventually leading to an accumulation of stomach heat. Therefore, sweet-cold herbs like Maogen are necessary in order to promote the secretion of body fluid to nourish the stomach. However, Maogen is not suitable for the case that the Middle Jiao is in a deficiency-cold condition.

Maogen Popularly Used in Folk Prescriptions

Maogen is often used in folk prescriptions. Some southerners in China would drink Maogen decoction to cure nephritis; some people drink corn stigma decoction to cure edema; and some people might have severe blood heat with the symptom of red dots on the tongue. Such symptoms involving blood heat may be cured by drinking Mogen decoction.

Some of these folk treatments are effective and some are ineffective because of lack of syndrome differentiation. In any case, the folk treatments are carried out with the use of traditional Chinese medicines, which actually follow some TCM principles, but only lack rational induction and generalization. The real TCM attaches great importance to syndrome differentiation treatment: four ways of diagnosis, i. e. , looking, listening, questioning and feeling the pulse.

Maozhen (Couch Grass Shoot) and Maohua (Couch Grass Catkins)

Mogen germinates in spring and breaks out into sharp shoots called Maozhen. Drinking Maozhen decoction can help to break the pustule since Maozhen on the one hand has a growing potence that can intensify the vitality in the body; and on the other hand, it is like a needle that can make a puncture. Therefore, Mozhen decoction can help to burst the pustule.

Maohua blossoms in a fluffy form in autumn, and it has the function of stopping bleeding in no time in case one cuts his or her finger.

Maogen, Maozhen and Maohua are the highly-accessible herbs when needed.

Tianhua Fen (Radices Trichosanthis)

Tianhua Fen

Tianhua Fen is another sweet-cold herb. It has an alternate name as "Hua Fen". Hua Fen here does not refer to pollen from flowers, but the root of Gualou (trichosanthes kirilowii Maxim).

Gualou is a rattan plant. The inside part (after the peel is removed) of its root is Tianhua Fen, which tastes sweet, slightly bitter and sour, and slightly cold in nature.

Tianhua Fen has functions of clearing the heat in the lungs and stomach, reducing phlegm, quenching thirst, producing fluids, relieving swellings and removing stasis. Stasis or stagnation is involved with pathogenic heat, which can induce phlegm. Many swelling and stasis stem from phlegm – once phlegm and heat are removed, the swelling and stasis will also disappear.

Tianhua Fen goes downwards, so the phlegm in the Lower Jiao can be removed with Tianhua Fen. Furthermore, Tianhua Fen is white in color, and enters the lungs to moisten the lungs. Since the lungs and large intestine are interrelated via Yin and Yang, the effects of Tianhua Fen will then descend from the lungs to the large intestine. It downbears Qi through the large intestine. As to the effect of reducing phlegm, it can make phlegm descend from the lungs to the large intestine and then drain out. Hence, the functions of Tianhua Fen can be concluded as moistening the lungs, descending Qi, removing phlegm and purging the intestines.

Gualou(trichosanthes kirilowii maxim) and Gualou Xiebai Tang

Most parts of Gualou can be used as medicines. The fruit of Gualou is a small pretty melon in golden yellow color and can be seen in different places around China. The fruit, if used as a whole, is termed as Quan Gualou (the whole trichosanthes kirilowii maxim); the fruit peel as medicine is called "Gualoupi", which tastes sweet, slightly cold in property, and tends to go to the exterior and the lungs. Hence, it cures diseases related to chest and the lungs.

There are two renowned formulas related to Gualou in *Shanghan Lun*: one is **Gualou Xiebai Baijiu Tang**, and another one is **Gualou Xiebai Banxia Tang**. The similarity between these two formulas is they both contain Gualou and Xiebai (allium macrostemon) as the leading herbs. As it is known that Gualou is used for reducing phlegm. It is believed in TCM theory that "spleen is the source of phlegm, and the lung is the organ that stores phlegm". Phlegm is induced in human body since the spleen fails to transpform and transport the fluid and dampness in the body, and the life essence of water and grain is not properly transformed.

The primary function of the spleen is to upbear the life essence of water and grain to the lungs. However, the spleen may also send the turbid phlegm to the lungs. If the substance that the spleen upbears is good, like the life essence of water and grain, the lungs will then rapidly transport and distribute it to all parts of the body via all vessels; but in case the spleen gives phlegm to the lungs, the lungs will not be able to distribute it, resulting in accumulation of more phlegm.

As such, the lungs may be obstructed. In that case, Gualou and Xiebai must be used since Gualou can reduce phlegm and make the phlegm go downwards. Xiebai can invigorate the heart Yang and the Yang in the chest. In addition, Xiebai has a dispersing function, and it can purge the stomach and large intestine. By invigorating the function of the lungs, Xiebai will assist Gualou to transport the resolved phlegm to the stomach, and then drain out through the large intestine. Xiebai also has a laxative function and helps bowel movement.

Xiebai can disperse blood stasis, too. Gualou and Xiebai are paired herbs that are commonly used for curing the chest tightness and obstruction of Qi in the chest. In case a patient suffers from serious Yang deficiency, add some liquor into this herbal pair (Gualou and Xiebai) (since liguor travels to the four limbs) so that it amplifies the effects of Gualou and Xiebai. In case the turbid phlegm is serious, add some Banxia to Gualou and Xiebai to make a new formula called **Gualou Xiebai Banxia Tang**.

As a matter of fact, regarding the formulas recorded in *Shanghan Lun*, it is unnecessary to memorise them completely. What is necessary to do is to remember the main herbs in the formulas and grasp the concept concerning their modifications. For example, many formulas are modified on the basis of the formula of

Guizhi Tang. As long as one keeps in mind the major herbal ingredients of **Guizhi Tang**, he or she can then make modifications by adding or taking out herbs based on the pathomechanism. This practice is closer to the original intention and concept of *Shanghan Lun*. Therefore, when Yang deficiency occurs, doctors may add some liquor in the formula; or when the stomach suffers from Qi counterflow accompanied by the obstruction of rising turbid phlegm, doctors may add Banxia in the formula.

Thoracic Obstruction and Medication

Thoracic obstruction (or obstruction of Qi in the chest) refers to feeling of chest pain that may extend from the chest to the back at every inhalation and exhalation. This is a quite popular symptom taking place in the intellectual and the white-collar class. Therefore, the **Gualou Xiebai Banxia Tang** is often used for them. In the clinical practice, some other herbs may also be added, like Zhe Beimu (thunberg fritillary bulb), which can intensify the effect of Gualou for reducing phlegm since Zhe Beimu can enter the lungs to clear heat-phlegm there.

If it is not clear whether a patient suffers from heat-phlegm or cold-phlegm or a mixture of both types, the four herbs of Gualou, Zhe Beimu, Chenpi (pericarpium citri reticulatae) and Banxia can be used together (Gualou plus Zhe Beimu for reducing heat-phlegm, and Chenpi and Banxia for reducing the cold-phlegm). These four herbs basically go to the Qi system. The herbs for the Qi system should be taken as the leading medicines in the process of treating thoracic obstruction. However, the herbs that go to the blood system like Honghua, Danggui and Chuanxiong and so on may also be added so that both the Qi and blood systems are taken care in order to achieve balance of medication.

Gualou Ren (Snakegourd Seeds)

Gualou Ren, similar to Gualou peel in property, is sweet and slightly cold in nature. However, seeds have high content of oil fat. Like all the other kinds of seeds, Gualou Ren has moistening effects and functions of reducing phlegm and relaxing the bowels. People in the modern time have a better quality of life and rich food to enjoy, which will easily result in more phlegm accumulated and serious damp-heat in the body. That may cause unsmooth bowel movement. Gualou Ren can be very helpful and effective for such symptoms. In brief, Gualou Ren can decrease the endogenous fire, descend Qi and reduce phlegm.

In case one suffers from the thin sloppy stool, Gualou peel should be used instead of Gualou Ren in the formula of **Gualou Xiebai Tang** since Gualou Ren will worsen the symptom; in case one suffers from dry stool, the entire Gualou fruit can be used including the peel and seeds in order to keep a balance of medication. These modifications tell us that all medications must be made based on the syndrome differentiation.

Xiao Xianxiong Tang

There is another formula containing Gualou called **Xiao Xianxiong Tang** recorded in **Shanghan Lun**. This formula contains Banxia, Huanglian and Gualou, among which Huanglian clears heat from the Middle Jiao; Banxia reduces phlegm from the Middle Jiao; and Gualou causes mild laxation and guides the phlegm to move from the Upper Jiao and Middle Jiao downwards.

This formula is used to tackle the mistreatment of the exogenous cold pathogens with the symptoms like phlegm heat lodged within the chest, and pain arising from the failure of descending. When the exogenous pathogen stays in the lungs, the correct way is to disperse the lungs to induce sweat. Or otherwise, the pathogens may still remain in the lungs even if the wastes below the lungs have been purged with medicines to induce bowel movement. In that case, the phlegm-heat stagnated in the lungs will become more difficult to be dispersed.

The accumulation and stagnation of phlegm and heat in the lungs will cause an excruciating pain that is even worse when pressed. For such a symptom, Huanglian should be used to clear the heat, and Banxia and Gualou to remove phlegm. Banxia reduces phlegm by its warming function, whereas Gualou is a cold herb. These two herbs are used together as a herbal pair to reflect the concept of "combining the cold and warm herbs to reduce phlegm". Phlegm heat needs to be cleared up with cool herbs. However, based on the principle of "reducing phlegm via warming function", Banxia (as warm herb), Gualou (cool herb) and Huanglian (bitter herb) together make a formula called **Xiao Xianx-**

iong Tang.

Xiao Xianxiong Tang is not limited to tackle the mistreatment of exogenous pathogenic attack through purging downwards. It can be used for any sharp pain induced by phlegm heat stagnation in the chest. The combination of Huanglian and Banxia is a formula of "**Xiexin Tang**". After Gualou is added, **Xiexin Tang** is then modified into **Xiao Xianxiong Tang**.

Other Uses of Herbs in Tianhua Fen Family Herbs

Gualou peel, seeds, the entire fruit and Tianhua Fen (the root of Gualou) have been mentioned above and also known that all of them as herbs have the similar functions, but different parts of Gualou will have a particular uses. Tianhua Fen and Gualou peels are often used together to reduce the phlegm effectively in both the Upper Jiao and Lower Jiao.

Sometimes, different parts of Gualou can be used separately. For example, in case there is abscess around the Lower Jiao, Tianhua Fen plus Huangqi (radix astragali) will work effectively. Furthermore, Tianhua Fen not only scores signal success in the treatment of gynaecological diseases, it is also frequently used to quench the symptom of "thirst" suffered by the diabetic patients. However, treatment in any case must be given based on syndrome differentiation. In spite of the effect of quenching thirst, it does not mean that Tianhua Fen can cure diabetes.

第三章 芦根、茅根、天花粉

甘寒药，种类和用法很多。有人说用寒凉药就会伤胃、伤气血、伤阳，确实如此。但如果运用得当，就不会了。所以，甘寒药在临床使用中颇费拿捏。但也有很多甘寒药，以甘为主，寒性其实很小，比如芦根、茅根、天花粉，这都是我们经常用的甘寒药。

芦根

芦根就是芦苇的根。芦苇长在淡水河流湖泊里，能高出水面一丈，秋天开白色的芦花。我国绝大多数地方都有，江苏的阳澄湖、安徽的泊湖、江西的鄱阳湖、河北的白洋淀，这些地方的芦根都是非常好的。

利水生津通窍

《诗经》有"蒹葭苍苍，白露为霜"之句。"蒹葭"就是芦苇。到了晚秋，芦苇枯萎的时节，整个水面上看上去是苍茫的一片。天气更冷了，白露为霜了。人在这时候就会更加思念亲人，渴望温情。此时，正是采挖芦根的季节。

秋天芦苇虽然枯萎，但它的根依然是活的。芦根一年四季都在水里，得水气，所以能养阴生津；长在水里，还意味着它对水有耐受力，所以有利水的作用。

水是生命的本源，但必须是活水，如果是死水、邪水，又会给身体带来害处。芦根能够养足人体的活水，同时排掉死水、邪水。很多养阴生津的药，在给人体补水的同时往往会生出湿，比如生地、熟地、天冬、麦冬等，没有能够及时运化就很容易生痰。唯独芦根不一样，它的作用是双向的。所以，尤其对于痰性体质的人，既要给他化痰，又要给他养阴生津，芦根就是最佳选择。

开窍和胃

人体也有很多孔窍，可开可合，如果被痰湿等邪气堵住了，这些窍开不了，人就会生病。芦根有节，中间是空的，凡是有节的就能通，比如竹子有节，入药的竹沥都是能够打开人体孔窍。芦根有点像竹子，但跟竹子不一样，在它的壁上还有很多小孔，这意味着它开窍的作用更强，以窍开窍，能通人的上下。由此我们还可以想到石菖蒲，芳香而有节，所以开窍的力度大一些，但渗湿的力度不如芦根，因为芦根味淡，淡能渗湿。

芦根入阳明经，通大肠、胃，走肺、脾、肾。很多本草书上说芦根能够除烦。烦，与火有关，而且火到脑袋上去了。心烦则意乱，也是由于火的扰动。芦根能除烦，是因为它能够通心气，除内热。而内热积累，也往往是因为体内孔窍不通。

芦根还能止呕，因为它养胃，通阳明，能安定中焦。芦根一直往淤泥里边扎，这说明它是往下走的。人体肺气和胃气都是往下走的，芦根能让胃气往下走，所以可以止呕。芦根出淤泥而不染，跟莲藕很相似，它能够让人体的清气上升，所以芦根能够肃清上焦，润肺阴，降肺气。"肺苦气上逆"，肺气往上逆，人就会非常难受，芦根恰好又是降的。

千金苇茎汤

用芦根为主药的，有一个很有名的方子，叫千金苇茎汤。

千金苇茎汤

芦根、薏米、桃仁、冬瓜子。

千金苇茎汤方解

这个方子来自孙思邈的《千金要方》，原方是苇茎、瓜瓣、薏米、桃仁。

苇茎本来是芦苇的杆，我们在临床上发现芦苇杆的作用没有芦根好，后来就改用芦根了。

瓜瓣是什么，历来有争议，我们现在用冬瓜子。它有散结的作用，能够治体内的各种气结、血凝，还能够消除垢腻，清掉体内一些污浊的东西。而且冬瓜子走肝经，可以泄肝热，对肝的解毒功能还有一定的辅助作用。

薏米是我们经常吃的，能够下气、利水，把肺里的邪火泻掉，又不伤正气。

桃仁与红花是对药，用来活血化瘀。桃仁通血，走六腑，红花通气走表，又走五脏，桃仁红花一起用就表里、五脏六腑都走，桃仁在这里是通腑而下肺中血痹的，但又不宜过于动血，所以不用红花。

治疗肺痈

《千金要方》说，千金苇茎汤是用来治肺痈的。肺痈，顾名思义就是肺被壅塞住了，而肺被壅塞住，无非就是痰或者瘀血。

人的肺里面也有很多的孔窍，孔窍被痰、瘀血塞起来了，就出现肺壅，顽痰死血在面越壅越厉害，就会发热，一发热里面又会化脓，人就会非常难受。此时就要用千金苇茎汤。

芦根通气，桃仁通血，冬瓜子散结、驱逐污垢，薏米下气利水，这四味药就一起达成清肺除痈的作用。

肺壅型感冒的形成及治疗

现在很多感冒，医院治疗往往服用或注射抗病毒药乃至抗生素之类，把邪气镇压下去，而没能透散出去。虽然西药也有透散的，比如一些发汗的药。但现在很多大夫在治感冒的时候为了省事，发烧就给你退烧，发炎就给你消炎，抗生素之类的用上去，都是非常寒凉的药。

或者输液，输液本身就是一瓶凉水往里注射，消耗人体的阳气不说，还把一些邪气往体内压。这些邪气在肺里透散不出来，就壅在肺里了。所以现在很多人感冒了一段时间，痰特别多，又感觉到胸闷，这往往是肺壅滞型感冒（因为还没有形成痈，也没有中医"肺痈"所列症状，所以我们称其为"肺壅"，就是肺气壅滞，它与肺痈仅一步之遥）。通过各种仪器和指针检查，可能觉得那并不是很严重，但从中医角度讲，它其实已经构成轻微的肺壅了。千金苇茎汤在治疗这种感冒的时候就可以用。

清化上焦热痰

我们还可以推而广之：凡是上焦有热痰，都可以用千金苇茎汤。上焦在心肺，这一带有热痰都可以用千金苇茎汤。人体的上部有脓，也可以用。脓也是一种痰，是气血所化。所以这个方子妙用无穷，因为上焦的热痰的范围太广了，涉及的病种非常多，在这里我也只能略表一二。比如，鼻炎到了流脓鼻涕的时候，咽炎到了咳吐浓痰的时候，都可以用千金苇茎汤的加减来治，效果非常好。要更深地了解它的应用还需要结合各种临床病例来分析。

芦笋

芦根到了春天的时候就要发芽，长出像笋子那样的东西，这就是芦笋。注意，这里说的芦笋，跟现在菜市场里卖的，据说有抗癌作用，甚至被做成芦笋片的那种芦笋不是一个东西。那个是旱地上培养出来的，这里讲的芦笋是水里面培养出来的。

人吃多了鱼就会中鱼毒，芦根里长出来的芦笋就可以解鱼毒，所以可以跟鱼一块炖，味道非常鲜美。当然，如果没有芦笋，直接用芦根来解鱼毒也可以。

藕在某种程度上也可以解鱼毒，它们和鱼都是长在水里的东西，是同气相求的。

芦根配伍举例及其他

芦根配青黛

芦根配青黛，本来是一个治疗胃溃疡的偏方，叫芦根青黛散。芦根甘寒，养阴生津，胃也非常喜欢甘寒的东西。青黛是用板蓝根的整株植物提炼的，板蓝根善于清热解毒，青黛也一样，而且善治溃疡。用于治各种溃疡的八味锡类散的主要的成分就是青黛。

在辨证论治的基础之上，在方子里面加芦根和青黛，对治疗胃溃疡效果非常好。

芦根配滑石

芦根还可以治疗各种结石，因为它可以补水。水的用处非常多，刷盘子、洗碗、拖地都要用水。治疗人体的五脏六腑，就像刷盘子洗碗，五脏六腑弄脏了要洗洗。在药里面加芦根，就好比刷盘子拖地要用水。体内的结石就是污垢。我们刷开水瓶里的水碱要加醋，或者加盐酸、固体酸，同时还要加水。治疗结石经常用的药比如滑石，它能够把结石滑掉，而且滑石还能清利湿热，把产生结石的源头拿掉。但单用滑石是没有用的，还得加水，这水就是芦根。

此外，肾结石可以再加上海金砂、金钱草、大蓟、小蓟，胆结石还可以加上栀子。胆为少阳，属半表半里，《伤寒论》治少阳的方子是小柴胡汤，胆结石可用小柴胡汤加上滑石、芦根；如果是肝郁，可以用逍遥散再加上滑石和芦根。当然要清除结石是需要时间的，需要慢慢化掉。

活水芦根，去须去节

这里我们讲的是干芦根。清朝以及民国的医家治病，往往喜欢写"活水芦根"或"鲜芦根"，也就是在活水里面养的新鲜的芦根，刚挖出来的更好。因为新鲜的芦根更有生生之气。生长在活水里面，又有灵性，而且干净，没有污垢。

芦根挖出来的时候，旁边有很多须，要把须去掉。更讲究一点的，有的方子开芦根还要求去节，就像用麻黄的时候也要把节去掉。芦根在这里也是一味开窍的药，而节意味着不通，去节，其通利作用更好。此外，节往往比较重，而且往往有泥，这也是用芦根去节的一个重要原因。

中药计量问题

所以，古人开芦根往往不用重量来衡量，而用体积来衡量。千金苇茎汤原方讲苇茎用二升，就是讲体积。《伤寒论》也是，有的药用重量单位去衡量，有的药用体积单位去衡量，因为重量并不是衡量药的唯一标准。

《伤寒论》中很多地方都用附子大者一枚，一枚大附子就行了。比如这枚大附子重15克，如果拿3枚重5克的小附子来代替它，这就不是一回事了。所以，《伤寒论》里面药的计量是非常讲究的。《千金方》也非常讲究。

芦根使用禁忌

芦根看上去是一味很平和的药，但用起来依然有很多禁忌。

比如，中焦虚寒就不要吃这味药了，风象比较明显的时候，刚开始也不要用芦根，因为芦根补水，风太大了就不要来太多的水。有一个成语叫"风生水起"，风太大的时候如果水再涨，那就可能波浪滔天。也就是说，当人体的风太大时还给他养阴，可能养不了阴就要生出很多痰来。之前我们说过，芦根不生痰，但这也是有一定限度的，你把它惹急了它还是会生痰的。

茅根

和芦根经常一块用的还有茅根。

茅根的性状与用途

茅根就是茅草的根。茅草在全国各地都很常见，尤其是人迹罕稀的荒地里，高的大概有半人高，秋天开出白色的茅花，然后枯萎。茅根色白有节，中间有一根很硬的芯。

茅根甘寒，入血分。通常挖出来的茅根是白色的，但有的会发紫，发紫就意味着它能入血分。茅根养阴生津凉血，能够清除人体的浮热。在血分，茅根能够化瘀、消血热；在气分，茅根能止渴、利水，把人体上方的热通过利水的方式从小便往下排。有些结石，只要有血热的症状，就可以用到茅根。一切的溃疡、一切的出血病，还有黄疸之类的，只要是因为有血热，都可以用茅根。

甘寒养胃

严重的实热，要用苦寒的药来清，苦寒的药是泻热泻得最快的。如果是虚热，或者热已经渗透到血分里去了，渗透得很深，扎根得很顽固，苦寒药就没用了，就得用甘寒的药，如茅根之类。一面养阴，补正气，另一面适当地泻热，这样就不伤胃气。芦根、茅根都是养胃的，而不是伤胃的。"胃为多气多血之府"，多气就会导致气热，多血就会导致血热，所以一旦气血不调，胃热就会出现。芦根走气分，清热养胃，茅根走血分，也清热养胃，所以两药共享。而且芦根生活在水里，茅根生活在土里，可以说是气血兼顾，水陆并进，用它来养胃是非常好的。

说"中药伤胃"的人，其实是连中医最基本原理都不懂了。中医都是首先要固护胃气，因为人只有胃气足，才能吃饭，能喝药。胃中邪火炽盛，津液不足，必然饮食不化，药物也不能很好吸收，这就要求我们善于用甘寒的药，善于在用药治病的过程中养胃。

苦寒败胃，甘寒养胃，用过苦寒的药以后，我们还要把胃气给养起来，胃阴不足就甘寒养阴，胃阳不足就健脾升阳。胃为五脏六腑之海，对于现代人来说，因为吃得多，胃每天都要超负荷地运转，导致的胃热也多，所以在治病的过程中，尤其需要茅根等甘寒之品来生津养胃。当然，如果是中焦虚寒，那就不宜用茅根了。

民间偏方，常用茅根

茅根在民间的很多土方中经常用到。南方有人得肾炎，就在家天天煎茅根汤喝，喝了一阵子病就好了。还有人用玉米须来调理身体，有些水肿得比较厉害的，用玉米须熬水喝，久而久之也能喝好了；如果是血热比较严重，舌头一伸出来，舌头发红，小红点特别多，就跟血热有关，也可以坚持熬茅根喝。

民间的这些疗法，有的有效，有的无效，因为缺少辨证。民间的一些土方法，用的是中药，其实也蕴藏着一定的中医原理，但毕竟缺少理性的归纳。真正的中医是要讲究望闻问切辨证论治的。

茅针和茅花

茅根在春天即将发芽的时候往往会长出一些尖锐的针来，这叫茅针。用茅针煎水喝，可溃脓。茅针有生发的力度，当脓透不出来的时候，说明身体的生发的机能不够，所以用茅针帮助它生发一下，这是一层意思；还有一层意思，茅针是一种针，针就能刺破，一刺破，脓自然就溃烂了。

秋天茅花开了，是白色绒状的，它可以止血。比如手割破了，用茅花揸在上面，很快就能止血。

茅根、茅针和茅花，是我们必要的时候可以随手拿来用的药。

天花粉

天花粉

甘寒类的药还有天花粉，也叫花粉。天花粉并不是某种花的粉，而是瓜蒌的根。

瓜蒌是一种长藤植物，挖出根刮去皮，里面就是花粉。花粉，性味甘、微苦、微酸、微寒，能清肺胃之热，能化痰、止渴、生津、消肿散结。结跟热有关，天花粉能清热散结，还能化痰，很多肿和结都是痰造成的。把痰和热化掉，肿和结自然就没有了。

能清肺胃之热，能化痰、止渴、生津、消肿散结。结跟热有关，天花粉能清热散结，还能化痰，很多肿和结都是痰造成的。把痰和热化掉，肿和结自然就没有了。

花粉是往下走的药，因为它是根，根通常往下走。所以，下焦有痰的时候，也往往用到花粉。花粉是白色的，白色能入肺。能润肺，它又从肺里面往下走，肺跟大肠相表里，花粉经过大肠，能降气，降气跟它往下降的功能相关；能化痰，能把肺里的痰浊一直往下降，最后让痰浊从大肠排出去，是化痰的一味好药。因此，花粉的作用可以总结为润肺、降气、化痰、清肠。

瓜蒌与瓜蒌薤白汤

瓜蒌这种植物，很多部位都能入药。瓜蒌的果实是一种金黄色小瓜，比较可爱，在很多地方都有。整个果实入药，叫全瓜蒌，果皮入药就叫瓜蒌皮。瓜蒌皮甘、微寒，偏于走表、走肺，主治胸部、肺部疾病。

《伤寒论》里有两个非常有名的方子，一个叫瓜蒌薤白白酒汤，还有一个是瓜蒌薤白半夏汤。这两个方子是有相同之处的，主药都是瓜蒌和薤白。瓜蒌我们知道它是化痰的。"脾为生痰之源，肺为贮痰之器"。人为什么会有痰呢？是因为"脾"运化水湿不利，没有把人体的水谷精微运化开，就生出痰来了。

脾主升清，脾把水谷精微往肺里输送，同样的道理，脾也会把痰往肺里输送。如果脾输送的是水谷精微，是一些好东西，那么肺朝百脉，会迅速把这些好东西分发下去，输配全身；如果脾输送的是痰，那么肺发不下去，肺里面的痰就会越积越多。

肺就被壅塞住了。这时候就要用瓜蒌、薤白。瓜蒌是化痰的，能够把痰化掉，还能让痰往下走。薤白呢，可以开心阳、通心阳，通胸中之阳。薤白既能振奋肺阳，又能振奋心阳，还能散气，通胃，通大肠。它能开肺，把瓜蒌化掉的痰先通到胃，再通到大肠，最后把它排了。薤白还是一味很滑利的药，如果大便不爽利，薤白在上面打开肺气，能够让大便变得更容易解下来。

薤白不仅能够化痰，还有散血的作用。瓜蒌、薤白开胸阳，是治疗胸闷胸痹经常用的一个对药。假如阳虚比较厉害，可以在瓜蒌、薤白里面加一点白酒，酒行四体，从而加大瓜蒌、薤白的作用。假如痰浊比较多，可以在瓜蒌、薤白里面加一味半夏，就是瓜蒌薤白半夏汤。

《伤寒论》里面的方子也没有必要一个一个的去记，我们要记主要的药，然后记它的加减。比如说很多方子就是在"桂枝汤"的基础上进行加减的，我们记住桂枝汤，然后根据什么样的病机加什么药，根据什么样的情况减什么药，记住加减，才更接近《伤寒论》的本意。遇到阳虚的，可以加白酒；遇到胃气上逆、痰浊上壅的，可以加半夏。

胸痹及其用药

胸痹就是感觉胸部疼，一动或者一吸气，疼痛从胸部牵引到后背。现在知识分子、白领得胸痹比较多，瓜蒌薤白半夏汤会经常用到。在具体临床使用的过程中，还可以再加一些药，比如说瓜蒌配浙贝母，瓜蒌是一味化痰的药，配上浙贝，化痰的力度会更大，浙贝也走肺，化热痰。

如果病人的痰不知道是热痰还是寒痰，也可能是寒痰、热痰夹杂的，那么就用瓜蒌、浙贝化热痰，用陈皮、半夏化寒痰，四味药一块用。瓜蒌、浙贝、陈皮、半夏基本上都是走气分的。在治"气"的时候要兼顾"血"，在治"血"的时候要兼顾"气"。在治胸痹的时候，以气分药为主，因为胸痹偏在气分一些，但可以加一些血分药，比如加一些红花、当归、川芎之类的。

瓜蒌仁

瓜蒌里面的子叫"瓜蒌仁"，瓜蒌仁也是甘、微寒的药，性质跟瓜蒌皮有点相似，所不同的是，凡是仁，里面就有油脂。瓜蒌仁很润，能化痰、润肠。现代人吃得比较好，体内痰比较多，肠里面的湿热就重，大便容易不通畅。瓜蒌子，通大便，化体内的痰。瓜蒌仁能降火、下气、化痰。

前面讲的瓜蒌薤白汤，如果这个人大便很稀，那么我们就要用瓜蒌皮，而不要用瓜蒌仁了。如果他大便稀的话你再用瓜蒌仁，大便就更稀了。如果他大便很干的话，那么我们可以全瓜蒌，既用了瓜蒌皮也用了瓜蒌仁，这个就是一个兼顾。其实一个方子它的用药有时候都是没有固定的。我们要根据具体的情况而定。

小陷胸汤

还有一个用到瓜蒌的方子：小陷胸汤，也是《伤寒论》里面很有名的一个方子。小陷胸汤就是半夏、黄连、瓜蒌三味药，非常好记。黄连清热、清中焦；半夏化痰、化中焦；瓜蒌润下，能把上焦中焦的痰往下引。

这个方子治疗伤寒误下，痰热壅滞胸中，不能下行而作痛。外感病，邪气还在肺里，如果治疗时不去宣肺发汗，而是让它往下走，拉一下肚子，或者用一些往下走的药，结果肺以下的东西虽然泄掉了，邪气依然在肺里，再也透不出去了，会导致痰热壅在胸中，壅在肺里。

痰和热全部壅在这里，会非常痛，一按会更痛。这时候就要用黄连清热，用半夏、瓜蒌化痰。半夏是温化痰饮的一味药，瓜蒌是一味寒凉药，体现了"寒温并用来化痰"的思想。热痰要用凉药来化，但是考虑到"温化痰饮"，所以用了温药半夏、凉药瓜蒌和苦寒的黄连，构成"小陷胸汤"。

其实不光是伤寒误下，只要是痰热壅滞在胸中导致剧痛，都可以用小陷胸汤。黄连、半夏其实就是"泻心汤"，在泻心汤的基础上加了导痰下行的瓜蒌。

天花粉家族药物的其他用处

瓜蒌果实外面的皮是瓜蒌皮，里面的仁是瓜蒌仁，一块用就是全瓜蒌，它的根叫天花粉，他们的作用都有相通之处，根据不同的部位和具体病症，用法不同。花粉、瓜蒌皮经常一起用，既化上焦的痰，又化下焦的痰，通身的痰都能化一遍，效果非常好。

有时也可以单用，比如脓在下焦，用天花粉配黄芪，效果非常好。天花粉不仅治疗妇科病屡建奇功，治疗糖尿病也经常用到。天花粉是一味止渴生津的药，当糖尿病人或者消渴病人出现"渴"的时候，花粉可以经常用，但是依然要辨证论治，并不是说用天花粉一味药就能解决糖尿病或者消渴。

Chapter 4　Other Sweet-cold Medicines

Here are about some other sweet-cold herbs like Maidong (radix ophiopogonis), Tiandong (asparagus cochinchinensis), and herbs related to bamboo including Zhuye (bamboo leaf), Zhuru (bamboo shavings), Zhuli (bamboo juice) and Tianzhuhuang (tabasheer).

Maidong (Radix Ophiopogonis)

Maidong is listed as a top-grade herb in the **Shennong Bencao Jing** with the following statement, "It tastes sweet with a neutral nature and it is non-toxic, mainly used for tackling the Qi stagnation in the heart and abdomen, impairment of stomach due to underfeeding and overfeeding, obstruction of stomach channels, marked emaciation and shortage of breath. Prolonged administration of Maidong can make one feel more energetic without sense of hunger. "

Definition of Maidong

The name of Maidong is composed of two Chinese characters. The first one is "麦" (Mai), referring to wheat, one of the five grains (rice, millet, broomcorn, wheat, and bean). Grains enters the stomach, and "麦" (Mai) reminds us that it enters the stomach channel. Furthermore, among the five grains, wheat corresponds to summer, given that wheat become ripe in the early summer-time. Therefore, wheat is also a herb that is able to nourish the heart.

Maidong is so named just because it is shaped like wheat, and the wild Maidong is similar to the granule of wheat in size.

Maidong is a type of grass with long root growing under ground horizontally. Along the root grow lots of tiny tubers about twelve, fourteen or fifteen pieces called Maidong, signifying they are co-related with meridians in the human body. According to TCM theory, there are twelve meridians including three Hand Yin meridians, three Hand Yang meridians, three Foot Yin meridians and three Foot Yang meridians in human body, plus Ren (Ren Channel) and Du (Governor Channel), making 14 meridians and channels; furthermore, there is a spleen channel, totally making fifteen meridians and channels. These three numbers (12, 14, 15) precisely match the number of Maidong on each horizon root.

In Chinese culture, it is believed that there is a set number for everything in the universe, which is called "定数" (Dingshu, literally means definite number in English, signifying destiny). The meridians in the human body are definite and equal for everyone. The number of Maidong on its horizontal root is also definite for each root. Such phenomena shows that the nature coincides with human, here specifically referring to coincidence of the nature of Maidong with the nature of human body in number. The numbers here are not merely numbers in mathematics, but also a definite number (destiny) in universe. Therefore, numbers are perceived differently in Chinese culture as compared in western culture. Westerners may look at the numbers as values for calculations; but the Chinese will look into the things behind the numbers from cultural perspective. So many pieces of Maidong are connected with each other through one piece of horizontal rood under ground. That does mean Maidong has a function of dredging meridians and collaterals.

The character "冬" (dong) means winter. In the nature, spring gives life; summer makes things grow; autumn brings in harvest; and winter requires storage. Winter is cold and cool, which signifies that Maidong is a cold and cool herb, therefore, it can induce diuresis from the kidneys. Meanwhile, the four seasons correspond to the five internal organs, i. e. spring to liver, summer to heart, autumn to lungs, and winter to kidneys. Thus, Maidong enters the kidney meridian.

Chuan Maidong and Hang Maidong

Initially, Maidongis growing in Sichuan and Shaanxi provinces, China. Later on, Hangzhou in Zhejiang province of China also produces Maidong that is named as Hang Maidong. Now in the drugstore, there are Chuan Maidong and Hang Maidong available.

The east corresponds to spring, dominating growth and implying warm temperature; The west corresponds to autumn, dominating astringency and implying cool temperature. Sichuan, geographically, is located in the western part of China, therefore, Chuan Maidong is partially colder and cooler in property, while Hang Maidong is partially more moistening in effect. Both of them are actually cool and moistening in effects.

It is effortless to identify Chuan Maidong from Hang Maidong. The former is larger and plumpy and whitish in color, without wood-like core; the latter is smaller and not so whitish in color, with a wood-like core that can be pulled out. Hence, it is often read that Maidong should be used with the core removed.

Sweet Taste, Mild and Non-toxic Properties

Shennong Bencao Jing describes that Maidong has sweet taste, and neutral nature, but in fact, it is partially cool.

On the whole, Maidong is a sweat-cold herb that can nourish the stomach to promote the secretion of saliva or body fluid. However, there are quite a lot of herbs that have the similar functions such as the previously mentioned Lugen. What are the differences between these herbs?

Lugen is hollow in the middle and is able to clear the stagnation in the hollow organs either in the Upper Jiao or the Lower Jiao, while Maidong enters the lung and heart meridians, which is different from Lugen in the aspect of channel tropism even though both herbs enter the stomach. Maidong can disperse and soothe the stomach Qi, extending its effect to the four limbs, while Lugen is weaker in this aspect.

For Treatment of the Heart and Abdominal Qi Stagnation

The heart and abdominal Qi stagnation refers to the obstruction of Qi circulation in the stomach below heart. As previously analyzed, Maidong has a main root growing horizontally under ground. The horizontal root is just like the stomach Qi inside the human body, and the Maidong tubers on the sides of the main root are like the limbs connecting to the stomach Qi in the body. Heart and abdominal Qi stagnation can be interpreted separately as cardiac functional stagnation and abdominal Qi obstruction.

The cardiac Qi stagnation actually attributes to the stagnation of the stomach

Qi. The Chinese ancestors said there are ten types of cardiac pains, nine of which in fact are stomachache since stomach and heart are interconnected. Anatomically, the stomach and heart are quite close to each other. Thus, cardiac functional stagnation in reality is the stomach Qi obstruction. While the abdominal Qi obstruction actually is the obstruction of Qi circulation in the Middle Jiao, that is, the Qi stagnation in the spleen and stomach.

The Chinese character "结" (Jie) means "knot" condensed or entangled. In TCM terminology, there is a clear distinction between "凝" (Ning, means condensation in English) and "结" (Jie, means knot). Coldness induces condensation, while heat induces knot (both condensation and knot refer to stagnation or obstruction here).

When stagnation arises in the body due to pathogenic heat, the cool and moistening herbs will have to be used to break the obstruction. "Heart and abdominal Qi stagnation" indicates there is heat in the Middle Jiao, i. e. , in the stomach, which signifies that Qi cannot circulate and distribute to the four limbs, and it is obstructed inside to become stagnation of Qi. Thus, the symptom of "heart and abdominal Qi stagnation" occurs. This symptom is also related to obstruction of channels and meridians. Therefore, Maidong is used to moisten and nourish the stomach in order to dredge the channels.

For Treatment of Underfeeding and Overfeeding Impairment

Maidong can be used to treat the impairment of the stomach due to underfeeding and overfeeding. Underfeeding refers to suffering from hunger. In the modern society, many young ladies seek to lose weight via skipping meals, which will impair the Middle Jiao. Overfeeding refers to eating too much, which will impair the functions of the spleen and stomach. So, food and drink must be controlled in moderation, neither too much nor too little in life since either of them will result in impairment of the stomach and disharmony of functions, eventually inducing stomach heat or stomach Yin deficiency. Maidong can be used for nourishing purpose since Maidong has a function of killing two birds with one stone, i. e. , clearing the stomach heat and nourishing stomach Yin simultaneously.

For Treatment of Failure of Gastric Collaterals to Meridian Vessels

The so-called "obstruction of stomach channels" in **Shennong Bencao Jing**, in fact, refers to failure of gastric collaterals going to meridian vessels.

The stomach is an organ with an abundance of Qi and blood. Histologically, the stomach is densely covered with a lot of capillaries, and the peristalsis of the stomach is going on all the time. The gastric collaterals are inter-connected with the meridian vessels of all the internal organs, limbs and bones. When and only when all the connections are running smoothly, the stomach can really function as the "sea of Qi from all internal organs". Stomach plays the central function among all organs, and all the other organs will have effects on the stomach while they are functioning and vice versa.

When there is "obstruction of stomach channels", the the stomach will become isolated. Thus, some Qi and blood will be encapsulated inside, leading to disharmony between the spleen and stomach, which then result in various stomach diseases. Some of these stomach diseases are attributed to the failure of heat dispersion to the four limbs. Therefore, many patients prefer cold food or drinks even though they are suffering the symptom of cold hands. In that case, Maidong may be added in the formula to cool and nourish the stomach in order to dredge the meridians and collaterals.

For Treatment of Marked Emaciation and Shortage of breath

Maidong can also be used for treatment of marked emaciation and shortage of breath. Some skinny persons may feel short of breath in each respiratory cycle. Why is it so? In fact, those who suffer from stomach deficiency may become skinny since the stomach deficiency will cause poor transportation and transformation of life essence of water and grain, as such, they will definitely become skinny; those who suffer from the kidney deficiency will run out of breath.

Generally, the respiratory cycle of human being should be easy, deep and lengthy. There is a Chinese term called "Number of Qi", which means there is a pre-destined amount of respiratory cycles for a person in his or her life. When we say one's Qi number has reached its designated limit, we mean he or she is going to pass away. The breathing cycle is going on consciously or unconsciously, but in most cases, the breathing is going unconsciously. Whether the unconscious breathing goes deep or not depends on the kidneys. In case one's kidney Qi is vigorous, he or she can then take a deeper breath and slowly breathe out; otherwise, he or she may have to increase the respiratory rate with a shallow breath. Therefore, it is very important to nourish the kidneys well in order to extend the fortune destiny by decreasing the "Number of Qi" via breathing slowly and deeply.

Maidong can also tackle the marked emaciation and shortage of breath since it is able to nourish the stomach and kidneys. Maidong nourishes the kidneys by going into the lungs since Maidong clears most of the heat in the lungs and stomach, and the lung Yin can assist in generating kidney Yin. Based on TCM theory of "the lung metal generating the kidney fluid" (since lung-metal is taken as the mother of kidney-fluid), to nourish the lung is, in fact, to nourish the kidneys, which is taken that "when one organ (analogically, a baby) is deficient, try to tonify its source organ (analogically, its mother)".

Prolonged Administration Makes One Feel More Energetic and Less Hungry

Shennong Bencao Jing says, "prolonged administration of Maidong makes one feel more energetic and less hungry", which implies that Maidong is of a top-grade herb and can be used for a long time.

For a patient, feeling light does not mean that he or she loses his or her weight after taking the medicine, but he feels energetic rather than top-heavy.

That prolonged administration makes one feel less hungry means one does not get so susceptible to hunger since sufficient stomach Qi makes one have a stronger tolerance to hunger. Those who suffer deficiency of spleen and stomach are susceptible to hunger. Therefore, when the spleen and stomach Qi-functions are weakened, one may feel susceptible to hunger. When in hunger, some people may become perturbed since the deficiency-heat rushes up immediately in case of deficiency of stomach Qi. And also, the stomach and heart are inter-related. Thus, the rising stomach heat will impose some impact on the pericardium collateral, causing disturbance in the mind.

Shengmai Yin

There is a famous formula related to Maidong called **Shengmai Yin** (literally means pulse-activating decoction).

Shengmai Yin contains the herbal ingredients: Renshen (ginseng), Maidong (radix ophiopogonis), Wuweizi (fructus schisandrae chinensis).

The formula of **Shengmai Yin**, also called **Shen Mai Yin** (Ginseng and Maidong decoction), is originally recorded in the book *Qianjin Yaofang* written by Sun Simiao. From the perspective of its origin, both Renshen and Maidong are the main herbs in this formula, so it is named as **Shen Mai Yin**. But this formula is effective for nourishing the heart, which then activates the pulse since the heart dominates the blood vessels in which the blood and Qi circulate. Therefore, this formula is also called **Shengmai Yin** (pulse-activating decoction)

While observing a subject, one needs to look into its origin, and its modification as well since the origin can provide a reference, however, the modification is more worthy of researching.

The formula of **Shengmai Yin** is quite simple, but it has various applications. In the formula, Renshen invigorates the heart functions; Wuweizi functions to astringe heart Yin; and Maidong clears heart fire. All the three herbs direct their effects on the heart, which means they are able to take effect on the pulses. It fully deserves the name of **Shengmai Yin**. However, from another perspective, Renshen tonifies lung Qi; Maidong clears lung fire; and Wuweizi astringes lung Yin. Therefore, **Shen Mai Yin** is given to the formula, which seems ambiguous. In fact, it exactly illustrates this formula has extensive application.

In the formula of **Shengmai Yin**, American ginseng is often substituted for ginseng since it is far closer to ginseng in property for nourishing heart Qi according to *Qianjin Yaofang*. During the summer time, more perspiration is induced, for which many people feel dizzy and giddy since Yang tends to go to the exterior and is excessively dispersed with sweating. **Shengmai Yin** is quite good for maintaining health in summer. One may prepare ginseng, Wuweizi and Maidong at 1:1:2 ratio indicated in *Qianjin Yaofang* to make tea if in need.

Tianmendong(Asparagus Cochinchinensis)

Definition of "Tianmendong"

Tianmendong is the full Chinese name of Tiandong (asparagus cochinchinensis). It is similar to Maidong (radix ophiopogonis), and is listed as a top-grade herb in **Shennong Bencao Jing** with the following descriptions: "it has bitter taste, neutral nature and non-toxic in property. It is mainly used for tackling various rheumatism and hemiplegia, strengthening the bone marrow, killing the three parasites (i. e. roundworm, threadworm, pinworm), and eliminating the Yin-toxins. Prolonged administration of Tianmendong can tonify Qi, prolong life and make one feel more energetic and less hungry."

Tianmendong is the abbreviated name of Tian Men Dong, in which "天" (Tian) literally means "sky", signifying this herb is growing on the high mountains and can receive Qi from the sky; "门" (Men), literally means "door" or "gate" that can be opened or closed; "冬" (Dong), literally means winter, taking charge of storage, which correlates with the kidneys and fluid. "门冬" (Mendong, literally means "Winter Gate") can be interpreted as storing something, or unpacking things that have been put in stock. In brief, this herb can release the the securely stored life essence in the body and send it to where it is needed to help Yang ascend from the fluid.

Properties of Tianmendong

Maidong (Chinese full name is Maimendong) has been discussed in the above section and is known that it is able to dredge channels and meridians, since "门" (Men, literally means "door" or "gate") can be opened or closed. Similarly, Tianmendong is also a sweet-cold herb that can nourish Yin-fluid, regenerate body fluid and clear stomach heat. Then what are the differences between Tianmendong and Maidong? As a matter of fact, they enter different meridian channels. Maidong enters the Yangming meridians, that is, the stomach and large intestine meridians mainly for removing heat to promote salivation; while Tianmendong is a sweet-cold and nourishing herb that enters the bladder meridian to guide its effect of transforming environment from Yin to Yang. This can be proved that it functions to tackle various rheumatism, killing the three parasites (i. e. round-worm, threadworm, pin-worm), and eliminating the concealed Yin-toxins from corpses.

To some extent, Tianmendong is similar to Baibu (radix stemonae) in their functions of killing parasites. The parasites are partially Yin microorganism. An herb that takes effect of transforming environment from Yin to Yang in most cases can wipe out the haze-like Yin environment, after which the parasites will not be able to survive. Furthermore, the the concealed corpse is also a sort of Yin-pathogen escaped from underground. It can be the source of some weird diseases, for which Tianmendong can work well.

Meanwhile, Tianmendong is often used together with Maidong. One of them utilizes the vital life essence of fluid to dredge the Yangming meridians to clear the stomach heat, while the other one utilizes the vital life essence of fluid to dredge the Taiyang meridians to wipe out the haze in the body. They nourish the body on the one hand, and clear away hazes on the other hand, which is quite similar to the heavy rain, after which the sky becomes much clearer and brighter.

Sancai Tang

There is a formula called **Sancai Tang** related to Tianmendong.

Sancai Tang contains the herbal ingredients: Tiandong (asparagus co-chinchinensis) 2 *qian*, Renshen (ginseng) 3 *qian*, Dihuang (rehmannia) 5 *qian*.

This formula comes from ***Wenbing Tiaobian*** (***Treatise on Differentiation and Treatment of Epidemic Febrile Diseases***) written by Wu Jutong in Qing dynasty. Tiandong and Tianmendong refer to the same herb "asparagus co-chinchinensis" with two names. The initials of these three herbs in Chinese are: "天" (Tian, means heaven/sky), "地" (Di, means earth) and "人" (Ren, means human).

The main function of this formula is to tonify Qi, nourish Yin and regenerate body fluid. It is often used at the later stage of treatment of the diseases arising from the exogenous pathogenic attacks or miscellaneous diseases that cause impairment to Qi or Yin. The formula is relatively simple, but it has more applications. The herbal combination can repair the microcosmic world - the human body, so that the patient can recover and stand up strongly with tripartite balance of forces of the sky-earth-human system.

It is sure that some other herbs may be added to this formula at the stage of coping with the aftermath of a disease. In case Yin is particularly needed to be tonified, add Wuweizi and Maidong (or, together with Tianmendong to astringe the vital life essence in the body) to the formula; in case Yang is needed to be tonified, add Fuling (poria cocos) and Gancao to tonify the spleen since Fuling removes dampness from the spleen, and the sweet Gancao enters the spleen to re- lax the tension inside, which is something the spleen prefers. Therefore, **Sancai Tang** is often prescribed for patients at the stage of recovering from illness.

The secret of **Sancai Tang** is the dosage for each herb in its formula, i. e. , 2 *qian* (equals to 6 grams today) of Tianmendong, 3 *qian* (approximately equals to 10 grams) of Rensen and 5 *qian* (approximately equals to 15 grams) of Di- huang. Among these three herbs, Tianmendong is on the top of the prescription with a dosage of only 2 *qian*, signifying that the clear and light substance floating up to the sky ("Tian") should be used in a smaller dosage.

In a similar way, the heavy and turbid substances are subsumed to the earth, so Dihuang is used in a largest dosage of 5*qian* among the three ingredi- ents. Human beings are living in between the Sky and the Earth, neither heavy nor light, therefore, 3 *qian* of Renshen (corresponding to "Ren", human being) is used in a medium dosage. Therefore, it can be seen that **Sancai Tang** is very particular about the dosage of each ingredient in this formula. If the dosage is im- properly prescribed, this formula will become much less effective.

Clinically, Tianmendong should not be used too much long time, or other- wise, Qi in the body may be impaired. Actually, Maidong and Wuweizi plus **Li- uwei Dihuang Tang** makes the well-known **Maiwei Dihuang Tang**, or in anoth- er form, **Maiwei Dihuang pill**, which has an alternative name called **Baxian Changshou pill** (*the Eight Immortals Pill*) for tonifying both the lungs and kid- neys simultaneously, suitable for use in a long run.

Bamboo Category

Bamboo-related herbs are also important sweet-cold medicines, including

Zhuye (bamboo leaf), Zhuru (bamboo shavings), Zhuli (bamboo juice) and Tianzhuhuang (tabasheer).

Zhuye (Bamboo Leaf)

Zhuye is listed as a medium-grade herb in **Shennong Bencao Jing**, saying Zhuye tastes bitter, which seems different from that used in the modern time. Therefore, what was written in **Shennong Bencao Jing** about Zhuye cannot be quoted here.

The Zhuye that is used in modern time refers to Dan Zhuye (lophatherum gracile) that grows on the ridges or under woods, extraordinarily small in size with slight sweet taste and slight coldness in property. Leaves are usually very light, and they tend to float upwards. As medicines, leaves go to the Upper Jiao (heart and lungs). Zhuye as a medicine, with no exception, enters both heart and lungs, but it is sweet and cold, tending to descend because of its cold property. Therefore, Zhuye will ascend to the heart and lungs first, and then go downwards in order to subdue the over-activity of heart and lungs (i. e. , to downbear the heart and lung fire).

Zhuye has a diuretic function, and clears the heart fire through urination – this is the most essential therapeutic effect of Zhuye. In the process of treating the febrile diseases arising from the exogenous pathogens, Zhuye is always used to drain the febrile pathogens through urination in order to prevent the febrile pathogens from propagating inversely to the pericardium. By the way, Zhuye is also used in **Yinqiao San** and **Zhuye Shigao Tang** for eliminating pathogens and heat.

Daochi San

There is another Zhuye-related formula called **Daochi San**.

Daochi San contains the herbal ingredients: Shengdi (radix rehmanniae recen), Zhuye (bamboo leaf), Mutong (akebiaquinata), Gancao Shao (ural liquorice root tip).

As the name implies, **Daochi San** is able to eliminate the fire from the heart and small intestine through urination. Generally speaking, whenever there is fire pathogen in the heart and small intestine channels, there will arise some symptoms like frequent micturition, urgent urination in reddish or yellow color, or with some difficulty even with pains due to damp-heat stagnation. **Daochi San** comes from the book *Xiao' er Yaozheng Zhijue (Formula for Pediatric Drug Syndrome)*, which says "this formula treats the dry heat trapped in the heart or transferred to the small intestine, or the heart fire blazing upwards through meridians". **Daochi San** can be used for the symptoms like burning heat sensation, blush in the cheeks, mouth or tongue ulceration, thirst, preference for cold drinks, and sufferings from scanty dark urine, accompanied with dysphoria. In fact, scanty dark urine shows that the urinary system is trying to eliminate the heat from the small intestine but fail to eliminate it completely. **Daochi San** can help to clear the heat pathogen thoroughly.

Shengdi, as an herb for nourishing Yin and generating body fluid, cools the blood and goes to the kidney channel and bladder meridian, moving in the Yin system; Zhuye cools the blood but goes to the heart channel of Hand-Shaoyin and small intestine channel, moving in the Qi system. Mutong (akebiaquinata) can induce urination, but can be substituted with Tongcao (tetrapanax papyriferus) or Fuling (poria cocos) if needed.

The last herb in the formula is Gancao Shao (ural liquorice root tip), which is also Gancao but specifically the endmost part of its toot. It has both the harmonizing and descending effects, and it can move to the limbs and the Lower Jiao. People in the modern time often suffer from damp-heat in the spleen and stomach, for which Gancao Shao is more suitable.

Daochi San, after use, can make urination become light in color and much easier. These four herbs are all highly linked with one another: Shengdi and Zhuye can cool the blood. Besides, Shengdi is sweet-cold in property and is able to generate body fluid, nourish Yin and clear heat; Zhuye can generate body fluid, too, but it is not so powerful as Shengdi. Both Zhuye and Mutong can induce urination; Gancao Shao can harmonize all herbs involved in the formula; and concurrently, Gancao Shao has a descending function, so does Zhuye. Each herb plays multiple functions in the formula.

Daochi San is used specially for treating the inexplicable perturbation and annoyance, which is also quite common among children, showing much impatience and crying without any reason. Such conditions are often involved with their parents. When parents are perturbed and annoyed, their children will be the same. The only differences are that adults have better self-control, yet kids are comparatively more vulnerable and less self-controlled.

When adults are perturbed and annoyed, they may not suffer too much impairment, which, however, may cause some negative effects on their children and immediately result in children's emotional or physiological reactions such as scanty dark urine, as children are more vulnerable. Each and every parent has to beware of this or her words, action or even eye-contact since such behaviors or manners will affect the children psychologically and physiologically, and even his or her future development.

Zhuru (Bamboo Shavings)

Zhuru is the collateral of bamboo. Shave off the most superficial fresh green layer of a green bamboo. Upon shaving that layer, one can see the semi-greenish layer with a lot of thread-like fiber, and then continue to shave until the remaining part of the bamboo turns entirely white. Those thread-like shaved fibers in between the most exterior and the most interior of bamboo are Zhuru that is used as medicine. Bamboo around 1-year-old, neither too old nor too young, is the most suitable for obtaining Zhuru.

Zhuru enters the stomach channel, relieving restlessness and controlling nausea and vomiting. Wang Ang, a well-known TCM expert in the early Qing Dynasty, said that Zhuru can stimulate the appetite, and clear away the lung-heat and the heat in the Upper Jiao. Zhuru is suitable for tackling the vomiting arising from the stomach heat, but it is not suitable for vomiting arising from the stomach-cold since it is a sweet-cold herb.

Wendan Tang

Regarding Zhuru, there is a very typical and famous formula called **Wendan tang**.

Wendan Tang contains the herbal ingredients: Zhuru (bamboo shavings),

Zhike (fructus aurantii), Chenpi (pericarpium citri reticulatae), Banxia (pinellia ternate), Fuling (poria cocos), Gancao (liquorice) and Shengjiang (fresh ginger).

Wendan Tang also comes from Sun Simiao's *Qianjin Yaofang*, from which many formulas have been discussed in the above sections like **Qianjin Weijing Tang**, **Shengmai Yin**; and **Wendan Tang** is another one.

Wendan Tang is modification of **Erchen Tang** plus Zhuru and Zhike. Modifications of formulas are quite common, for instance, **Wendan Tang** and **Erchen Tang**, they are mutually modified, and **Erchen Tang** is becoming far more well-known. According to *Qianjin Yaofang*, the original **Wendan Tang** does not contain Fuling, but a larger dosage of fresh ginger, which might be the reason that the formula is named as **Wendan Tang**. Or else, it would be better to be called **Qingdan Tang** (**Clearing the Gallbladder Decoction**) since the decoction of Zhike, Chenpi, Banxia, Fuling and Gancao can regulate the Qi flow and remove obstruction, reduce phlegm, harmonize the stomach functions, clear heat, and activate the gallbladder. Specifically, Zhike and Chenpi regulate Qi, Banxia and Zhuru reduce phlegm, and besides, Zhuru also clears heat.

Wendan Tang is particularly for treating the disharmony between gallbladder and stomach. Disharmony can take place between the liver and stomach, also between gallbladder and stomach. The physiological functions of gallbladder, stomach and lungs all tend to descend, and the "fire" follows them to go downwards. When disharmony occurs between gallbladder and stomach, they will not work as one team to conduct the descending functions. The gallbladder is in charge of the Shaoyang channel, where the ministerial fire starts ascending instead of descending, it will induce vomiting, or cause phlegm-heat disturbance, resulting in insomnia.

Insomnia usually stems from the rising fire disturbance to the mind. And also, the rising fire will affect the spleen and stomach functions and induce vomiting or hiccups. When the rising fire affects the state of mind, palpitation and unpeaceful mind may also occur. The rising fire pathogen can also condense and transform fluid into phlegm that, in case of staying within the pericardium, or in the brain over an extended period of time, will eventually result in epilepsy. As a matter of fact, epilepsy is a disease caused by obstinate phlegm. Therefore, **Wendan Tang** is frequently used for reducing the phlegm gradually in order to give a treatment of epilepsy. Meanwhile, **Wendan Tang** is also very effective for treatment of insomnia stemming from perturbation and disturbance due to phlegm-heat. Clinically, manifestations for phlegm-heat insomnia is the greasy yellow tongue coating.

Waitai Miyao (Medical Secrets of an Official) and **Qianjin Yaofang** recorded some other formulas for treating insomnia, most of which contain Zhuru (or even there is a formula containing only one herb, i. e. , Zhuru). That can also prove that Zhuru can clear heat but it is not cold; it also resolves and clear phlegm-heat so that the Qi of Shaoyang channel can become smooth.

Zhuli (Bamboo Juice)

Zhuli is bamboo juice extracted by baking bamboo over fire. It is an excellent sweet-cold herb. Clinically, fresh ginger juice may be added but not too much to neutralize its coldness. Ginger is warm in property, and it is beneficial to reduce the phlegm. However, if the phlegm arises from heat pathogen, ginger may worsen the heat symptoms. Therefore, a little bit of fresh ginger juice will be enough.

Zhuli enters the heart, stomach and large intestine channels. Its primary functions are to clear heat, reduce phlegm and dredge collaterals. Zhuli is like the blood of bamboo and it runs on along the entire bamboo. Therefore, when used as a medicine, it can run on the entire human body as it runs through the bamboo. Zhuli can remove various phlegm-heat underneath the skin or outside of membrane, inside the internal organs, or in the limbs or bones. Furthermore, it does not cause any impairment of Yin while reducing phlegm. Thus, it is very effective for those who suffer from a stroke with phlegm-heat.

Tianzhuhuang (Tabasheer)

Tianzhuhuang is produced from the king-sized bamboo that grows in the south of China. When bamboos are damaged by worms or nature, some juice leaks into the enclosed bamboo segments, and dries up to form into yellow-white pebble-shaped substance, which is called Tianzhuhuang. In fact, it is condensed from Zhuli. Nowadays, it is rare to find naturally formed Tianzhuhuang. Most of the Tianzhuhuang in the pharmacy is artificially extracted from Bamboo via modern technology.

Tianzhuhuang is quite similar to Zhuli in the therapeutic effect, but it enters the spleen, lung and liver Channels. Clinically, both Tianzhuhuang and Zhuli are sweet-cold herbs, and are often used together to remove phlegm-heat. In prescriptions, Zhuli is often written as "fresh Zhuli" since it is fresh and fluid. It can run to the four limbs and reduce the phlegm all over the body. Tianzhuhuang is formed with Zhuli agglomerated day by day. It mainly goes to the Middle Jiao-the spleen, stomach and liver Channels and tends to reduce phlegm in the Middle Jiao.

第四章　其他甘寒药

今天讲麦冬、天冬，还有竹子这一类的药，即竹叶、竹茹、竹沥、天竺黄，这些药都是甘寒的。

麦冬

麦冬，《神农本草经》列为上品。《神农本草经》是这样介绍麦冬的："气味甘平，无毒。主心腹结气，伤中，伤饱，胃络脉绝，羸瘦短气。久服轻身不老、不饥。"

药名释义

麦冬，第一是"麦"。"麦"就是麦子，是五谷之一，谷物是入中焦，入胃的。麦冬的"麦"字就提示它能入胃经。麦冬不仅入胃经，还能入别的经。入哪一经呢？麦子在五谷里面对应的是夏季，而且麦子也是在夏初的时候成熟，所以麦子也是一味通心气的药，它能养心。

"麦冬"这个药名，为什么它最初出现"麦"字呢？因为野生的麦冬颗粒，形状就跟麦粒似，所以叫麦冬。

麦冬这种植物其实就是一种草，它的根很长横在土里，边上结着很多麦冬，一颗颗连在一起，有的一个根上会结十二枚，有的一个根上会结十四枚或者十五枚，意味着它和人体的经脉是相关联的。人体有手三阴经、手三阳经、足三阴经、足三阳经，加起来人体一共十二条经脉，如果再加上任督二脉，就是十四条经脉，如果再加上脾之大络，就是十五条经脉，十二、十四、十五，这个数字正好对应了麦冬一个横的根上长的数目。

天地之间的一切东西都有定数，这就叫定数。人的经脉是有定数的，麦冬一条根上长麦冬的颗粒数目也是有定数的。这个就是叫物性之自然合于人身，就是说麦冬的自然属性跟人的自然属性在数上有相合的地方。这个数不但是数目的数，而且是天地之间的定数之数。所以中国人看数跟西方人是不一样的。西方人看这个数只是一个计算的数值，而中国人看这个数，其背后有更多的东西。这么多颗麦冬因为有一条横的根把它们全部联络在一起，这也意味着麦冬这味药能够通络脉。

还有个"冬"字，"冬"是指冬天。春生、夏长、秋收、冬藏，冬天主封藏。冬天是寒凉的，"冬"字，告诉我们麦冬是一味寒凉药，而且它通肾水。四季跟五脏是对应的。春对应于肝，夏对应于心，秋对应于肺，冬对应于肾。看到"冬"字会想到肾，麦冬还能够归肾经。

川麦冬与杭麦冬

麦冬本来产在四川、陕西一带，后来杭州也有了杭麦冬，麦冬就有了川麦冬和杭麦冬之分。

东主春主生发，对应的是温；西主秋主收敛，对应的是凉。四川在西部，所以川麦冬的性质在寒凉方面更加突出一些，而杭麦冬在滋润方面更加突出一些。川麦冬偏凉，杭麦冬偏润，不过也只是有所偏而已。不管是川麦冬还是杭麦冬，它们都是凉润的。

在药材市场上，川麦冬和杭麦冬也很容易辨认。川麦冬肥大一些，很肥很白，其中没有木质芯；杭麦冬个头稍小，没那么雪白，其中有木质芯，可以抽出来。所以我们经常可以在某些书上看到麦冬要求去芯使用。

气味甘平，无毒

《神农本草经》说麦冬甘平，其实它还是偏凉的。

麦冬，从整体上讲，就是一味甘寒的养胃生津的药，但是甘寒的养胃的生津的药有许许多多，比如前边讲过的芦根，那么麦冬跟它有什么区别呢？

芦根中空，能通上通下，是通腑气的。麦冬入肺经、心经，归经跟芦根不一样，但同样入胃。麦冬能够宣畅胃气，通达于四肢；芦根在这方面的力量要弱一些，通经脉的功能不如麦冬。

主心腹气结

"心腹气结"，就是心下、腹中的气结住了。麦冬为什么能主心腹气结？前面讲了它是一本横生，如果人体的胃气好比麦冬中间横着的那条主根，那么四肢就好比一粒一粒的麦冬，它们是往边上延伸的。人体的胃气跟四肢是相通的，如同一颗一颗的麦冬跟中间横生的那条根是相通的。"心腹气结"拆开来看，就是心气结和腹气结。

心气结其实是胃气结。古人讲心痛有十种心痛，九种其实是胃痛，胃跟心其实是相通的；另一方面胃跟心的位置也比较靠近。所以讲心气结其实是胃气结。腹气结其实也是中焦气结，也是脾胃气结。

"结"就是结在一起。中医对于"凝"和"结"是有严格区分的。凝是凝，结是结，寒凝热结。

热一结就需要用凉润的药来化它。"心腹气结"意味着中焦有热，也就是胃中有热，也意味着气不能通达到四旁。气就容易结在里边，这就叫"心腹气结"。

"心腹气结"也是跟经络不通有关，所以要用麦冬凉润养胃，又疏通经络。

主伤中、伤饱

麦冬主"伤中，伤饱"，饥饿是伤中，过食是伤饱。现在有很多女孩子为了减肥，就不吃饭，这样就会导致伤中。伤饱，就是吃多了，也会伤脾胃，所以饮食要有节，不多不少。不管是吃多了还是吃少了，都会伤胃，都能导致经脉不和，引起胃热或者胃阴虚，它们往往伴随而来，所以都需要用麦冬来养。麦冬能够清胃热，又能够养胃阴，正好把这两方面的问题都解决了。

主胃络脉绝

经文还讲麦冬主"胃络脉绝"，就是治疗胃络不能通于脉。

胃是多气多血之腑，其中的毛细血管特别多，而且胃也是一直在蠕动的。胃的络脉跟五脏六腑、四肢百骸所有经脉都是相通的。只有这样，胃才能成其为五脏六腑之大海。胃是一个中心，五脏六腑都能对它产生作用。胃的好坏也能够对五脏六腑产生影响，这是因为胃络跟全身的经脉都是相通的。

如果"胃络脉绝"，那么胃就被孤立起来了，一部分气血就瓮在里边了，这样脾胃就不平和了，容易导致各种胃病。有的胃热，是因为热瓮在里边散不出去，不能达于四肢。所以，很多人胃热，喜欢吃凉东西，手却是凉的。这种情况，方中就可以用麦冬，凉润养胃，疏经通络。

主羸瘦短气

麦冬还主"羸瘦短气"。太瘦，呼吸的时候感觉到气短，这怎么解释呢？胃虚则羸瘦，肾虚则气短。胃虚就不能很好地运化水谷，人必然就会瘦。这个很好理解。

人的呼吸以绵长舒缓为佳。有一个词叫"气数"，就是人一辈子呼吸的数量，这是一定的。说某人气数已尽，就是说他要死了。人的呼吸，有时候是有意识的，有时候是无意识的，无意识的时候为多。无意识的呼吸是深长还是浅短，取决于肾。当肾气旺的时候，吸气就会深，然后再舒缓地呼出来。当肾气不足的时候，呼吸频率就会快，吸气也会不深，甚至很急促地呼吸了一阵子还觉得不够，要长吸一口气才能够舒缓过来。肾养好了，呼吸才能舒缓绵长，我们才能把一辈子的气数省着点用，用得久一些，把气数已尽的那一天尽量地往后推迟。

麦冬治羸瘦是因为它养胃，治短气是因为它养肾。麦冬养肾是通过养肺实现的。当它把肺胃之热都清得差不多的时候，肺阴就会生肾阴，养肺就会养肾，肺金生肾水，这就叫"虚则补其母"。

久服轻身不老、不饥

本经讲麦冬"久服轻身不老、不饥"。中下品药是不能久服的，麦冬是上品药，可以久服。

病人身体轻盈，并不是说吃了药以后，体重就由160斤变成130斤，而是你自己感觉到自己的身体轻了。

久服"不饥"，即是说不容易饿。胃气足则耐饥，脾胃之气不足就会容易饿。有的人一饿就心烦，为什么？因为胃气不足，胃里还有虚热，胃一旦空虚，胃热马上就起来了，因为胃和心是相通的，胃热一起来就影响到心包络，产生心烦，这是很不好的现象。

生脉饮

跟麦冬相关的有一个很有名的方子，叫生脉饮。

生脉饮：人参、麦冬、五味子。

生脉饮出自孙思邈《千金方》，也有人说它叫"参麦饮"。从起源上看，人参麦冬是里面的主药，根据药物的组成来命名就是参麦饮。但是后来为什么叫生脉饮呢？因为它能够养心，而心主血脉，养了心就能够生血脉，所以又叫生脉饮。

我们考察事物既要考察它的源头，也要考察它的流变，源头对我们来说有参考意义，流变则更值得我们研究。

生脉饮的组成非常简单，但是用途非常多。人参强心气，五味子收敛心阴，麦冬清心火，这三味药都能够作用于心，作用于心就能作用于脉，就可以当之无愧地叫生脉饮。但从另外一个角度，我们也可以讲人参是补肺气的，麦冬是清肺火的，五味子是敛肺阴的，生脉饮这个方子从名字上就有这么多的歧义，恰恰说明用途广。

生脉饮中的人参经常用西洋参来代替，因为西洋参更接近孙思邈写《千金方》那时候的人参，它能够养心气。夏天出汗比较多，人的阳气走表，心神外越，人有时候会昏昏欲睡，或者感觉到身上没有力气，这是因为人体的阳气过于发散，汗流得过多，所以生脉饮是夏天经常用的一个养生方，可以准备一点经常泡着喝。人参和五味子各用一份，麦冬用两份，按这个比例就够了，这也是《千金方》里的原始比例。

天门冬

"天门冬"药名释义

和麦门冬类似的有一个天门冬。天门冬在《神农本草经》里也是被列为上品。《神农本草经》讲，天门冬，"气味苦、平、无毒，主诸暴风湿偏痹，强骨髓，杀三虫，祛伏尸，久服轻身益气，延年不饥。"

天：天门冬生长在高山之上，能接天气。门是可开可合的；冬，主封藏，跟肾有关，跟水有关；"门冬"意味着可以把东西封藏起来，也可以把封藏的东西打开。总体说来，它就能够把你藏得最紧的东西打开，往上通。所以，它能够于水中升阳而上达。

天门冬的性能

前面讲的麦冬，它的全名叫麦门冬。门是可开可合的，它能够疏通经络。天门冬也是一味甘寒的药，能够养阴生津清胃热。那么它跟麦门冬有什么区别呢？它们的归经不一样：麦门冬通阳明，也就是通胃经、大肠经，以清热生津为主；天门冬通足太阳膀胱经，是一味甘寒滋润的药，能够从阴达阳。其除风湿、杀虫、祛伏尸，都是从阴达阳的效果。

天门冬在某种程度上跟百部有点像。百部能杀虫，天门冬也能杀虫。

虫是偏阴的东西，一个从阴达阳的药，往往就能够扫除那些阴霾；这些阴霾扫被除掉了，虫子自然就无法生存了。伏尸也是一种阴毒，就是从尸体里出来的毒气，能让人生病，是一些怪病的源头。天门冬能够去掉这些东西。

天门冬和麦门冬经常一起用，它们一个是用水的精气通阳明胃经清胃热，一个是用水的精气通太阳经来扫除人体的一些阴霾。一方面滋润，一方面扫除阴霾，就好比下雨，雨越下天地间越明亮、越清朗。

三才汤

关于天门冬，有一个方剂叫三才汤。

三才汤：天冬二钱、人参三钱、地黄五钱。

这个方子来自吴鞠通的《温病条辨》。天冬就是天门冬。这三味药的第一个字加起来就是：天、地、人。

这个方子主要是补气 养阴生津的，它主要用于很多外感病和杂病的扫尾，伤了气、伤了阴都可以用三才汤，药味比较简单，但作用比较大。它有补天、补地、补人之功，能把人体的小宇宙修复好，让你的天地人能重新鼎立起来。

当然，在善后的方剂里我们还可以再加入别的药，不要仅局限于这三味药。如果偏重于补阴，可以加入麦冬、五味子，天冬和麦冬就一起用了，五味子可以收敛精气；如果偏重补阳，可以加茯苓和甘草，茯苓和甘草是补脾，茯苓渗脾里湿，甘草味甘入脾，缓脾之急，脾喜缓，甘草正好可以缓，所以三才汤是病后康复经常用的方剂。

有人从三才汤发现一个秘密。天冬二钱，相当于我们现在方子开的6克，人参三钱，相当于现在方子开的10克，地黄五钱，相当于15克。天冬在最上边，清轻上浮者为天，它要很轻，要往上浮，所以剂量用得轻，走天的药用得少，只用了二钱。

重浊下沉者为地，走地的药地黄用了五钱，是最重的；人是在中间，不轻不重，用的是三钱。所以在剂量上，三才汤也是很讲究的。如果把用药剂量倒过来，这个方子就没那么好用了。

天冬，从临床上讲，不要用得过久，过久会伤气。麦冬可以一直用，经常用。麦冬、五味子再加上六味地黄汤，这就是麦味地黄汤，做成丸药，就是麦味地黄丸，又叫八仙长寿丸，同补肺肾，也可以久服。

竹类

竹类也是重要的甘寒药。主要包括竹叶、竹茹、竹沥、天竺黄。

竹叶

竹叶在《神农本草经》中列为中品。《神农本草经》讲的竹叶是苦的，和我们现在用的竹叶应该是有区别的，所以我们在讲竹叶的时候就不引用《神农本草经》的说法了。

现在我们用的淡竹叶，是田埂下或树林间生长的那种特别小的竹子的叶，甘淡微寒。叶子都是很轻浮的东西，会往上走，走上焦心和肺。竹叶也不例外，走心肺；但是它甘寒，寒则会往下走，所以这味药是先往上走，走到心肺，再往下走，所以能把心和肺的火往下降。

竹叶有利小便的作用，能够利心火，让心火从小便排出去，这是竹叶最重要的作用。在治疗外感温病的时候，为了防止温邪逆传心包，经常会用竹叶将一部份温邪从小便排出去。银翘散、竹叶石膏汤都用竹叶，清透邪热。

导赤散

看到竹叶我们想到一个方剂：导赤散。

导赤散：生地、竹叶、木通、甘草梢。

顾名思义，导赤散就是把心经、小肠这一路的火，通过小便的方式排出去。一般来讲，当心经和小肠经有火的时候，会出现尿频尿急，小便特别短，发红发黄，而且特别涩，甚至解的时候热痛不适。湿热粘滞在那里了。导赤散来自《小儿药证直诀》。方解是这样讲的："治疗心经热胜或移于小肠，心火循经上炎。"出现像热、脸红、口舌生疮的症状，甚至口渴，喜欢喝凉的，小便短、赤、涩，可能伴随有心气烦躁之类，就可以用导赤散。其实小便短赤，就是在排小肠里的热，但是它排不尽，导赤散可以帮助人体把小便里面的邪热排尽。

生地是一味养阴生津的药，能凉血，走阴分；竹叶凉血而走气分，两者都是很凉的药；生地走肾经和膀胱经，竹叶走心经、和小肠经；木通利小便，现在有人发现木通被污染了，有毒。所以去药店抓木通比较难，我们就不用木通了，用通草来代替；如果没有通草，用茯苓也可以。

还有一味药甘草梢，其实也是甘草，只不过是甘草最末端的部分，特别细，它能够往下走，引上达下。所以甘草梢会走人体四肢，还会走下焦。如果你既想让甘草缓一缓，又希望它往下走，那么就用甘草梢。现在的人，脾胃湿热较常见，我们没必要用很粗大的甘草，就用甘草梢，会更适合。

导赤散喝下去以后，小便很快就不那么红了，就通畅了。这几味药是环环相扣的，生地和竹叶都能够凉血。生地甘寒生津，养阴清热；竹叶也生津，只不过力度没有生地那么大而已。竹叶和木通，它们都能够利小便，最后甘草梢调和诸药，同时它还是往下走的。竹叶和甘草梢都是往下走的。这样，每一个药都是身兼多任。

导赤散是治心烦气躁的。心烦气躁，小孩特别常见，比如他非常不耐烦，喜欢哭。小孩的心烦气躁都跟大人有关。母子连心，父子也是连心的。什么叫连心？就是他们的心态、想法能够相通。当大人心浮气躁的时候，小孩会跟着心浮气躁的。所不同的是大人坚强，能控制自己；小孩脆弱，不能控制自己。

大人心浮气躁，没有表现出来，在身体上也没造成什么不好的影响，但是这个能量传递给小孩子，小孩子马上就心烦气躁了，加之他抵抗力比较弱，他马上就在情绪上表现出来，或者在生理上表现出来，出现小便短赤的状况。所以，父母的每一个心念、每一个动作、每一个眼神对小孩的心理、生理，乃至他的未来都有很大的影响。

竹茹

竹茹是竹子的络脉。拿一根青竹，刮掉最外面那一层很薄的青，刮掉以后就剩下一些半青不青的，里面有很多丝，再把这个丝刮下来，一直刮，刮到发白就不要刮了，刮下来的丝就是竹茹。最表层的不要，最里层的也不要，处在里外中间这一层的才是竹茹。生长了一年的竹子，最适合取竹茹，太老或太嫩都不适合。

竹茹入胃经，除烦、止呕，安徽名医汪昂讲它能开胃土之郁，清肺经之燥，除上焦的烦热。竹茹适合治胃热呕吐；如果是胃寒呕吐就不要用竹茹了，因为竹茹是一味甘寒的药。

温胆汤

关于竹茹，有一个很典型、很有名的方剂叫温胆汤。

温胆汤：竹茹、枳壳，陈皮、半夏、茯苓、甘草，生姜。

温胆汤的来源又是孙思邈的《千金方》。现在我们提到《千金方》就会肃然起敬。前面我们讲了很多的方剂，比如千金苇茎汤、生脉饮，都是来自《千金方》，妙用无穷，温胆汤也不例外。

有人看到温胆汤或许会说，这不就是二陈汤加上竹茹、枳壳吗？确实如此。但有意思的是，从起源上讲，是先有温胆汤后有二陈汤，二陈汤是在温胆汤的基础上减去竹茹和枳壳形成的。所以方子有加减，你既要会加它，又要会减它。后来二陈汤反倒更有名了，不过在《千金方》的原方没有茯苓，生姜的量非常大，也许就是因为生姜的量非常大，所以它才叫温胆汤吧。不然的话，如果光是竹茹、枳壳、陈皮、半夏、茯苓、甘草，那还不如叫清胆汤。因为它能够理气、化痰、和胃、清热、利胆。枳壳、陈皮理气，半夏、竹茹化痰，同时竹茹还能清热。

温胆汤治疗的是胆胃不和。有肝胃不和，也有胆胃不和。胆、胃、肺都是往下降的，火随之往下走。当胆胃不和的时候，它们就不齐心协力地往下降了。胆主少阳，少阳有相火，当火往上走的时候，人就会吐，或者导致痰热内扰，引起失眠。

为什么会失眠呢？因为火往上走，就会熏着脑子，脑子安静不下来，就会失眠。火往上走，脾胃之气受到影响，就会呕吐，或者呃逆、打嗝等；火往上走影响到心神了，还会导致心悸不宁；火往上走，火炼液成痰，痰在心包之间，或者在脑子里边留久了，就会引发癫痫。癫痫其实就是一种很顽固的痰症。治疗癫痫就是要把这个痰慢慢地化掉，会经常用到温胆汤。因痰热引起的心烦失眠，用温胆汤效果非常好。痰热不眠的表现就是舌苔比较黄腻。

在《外台秘要》和《千金方》中还有一些别的治失眠的方子，很多都用到了竹茹，甚至有个方子只有一味竹茹，这也说明竹茹是清热但不寒凉的药，它能够清化热痰。把这种痰清掉了，少阳之气就能得以舒展。

竹沥

竹沥是竹子在火上所烤出来的汁液，它是非常好的甘寒类药。如果怕它太寒凉了，可以在里面加一点生姜汁，因为生姜汁是温的，它能够中和掉竹沥的一部分寒性。同时，它也是一味重要的化痰药，且痰更喜欢温化，要略微有点温度才能够把它化掉，所以加一点生姜到竹沥里边，化痰速度会更快一些。当然这个不要兑得太多，如果是热痰，生姜放太多了它又会助长热邪，所以生姜略微放一点就行了。

竹沥入心经、胃经、大肠经，它的主要作用是清热化痰、通络。竹沥相当于竹子的血液，它运行于整棵竹子，通竹子全身。能够通竹子的全身也就能通人的全身，所以皮里膜外，五脏六腑，四肢百骸的热痰、顽痰，用竹沥都可以化掉。用它化痰不伤阴，对于中风有热痰的，有非常好的化痰清热作用。

天竺黄

天竺黄产在南方那种特别大的竹子里。竹子中因虫蛀或自然损伤，会流出汁液，汁液流到全封闭式的竹节之间，干了就结成黄白色的东西，象小石块那样的，这就叫天竺黄或者就叫竹黄，它是竹沥结成的。现在这种天然的竹黄已经很少了。我们用的天竺黄价格很便宜，它是人工制造的，就是用现代科技从竹子中大量提取。

天竺黄的药用效果跟竹沥比较相似，但它归脾经、肺经、肝经。在临床上，竹沥和天竺黄都是甘寒的药，经常一起用来化热痰。竹沥在开方子的时候写"鲜竹沥"，因它是流动的、鲜活的，走四肢，能化全身的痰；天竺黄是竹沥日积月累结成的，主要走中焦，走脾胃经和肝经，偏重于化中焦的痰。

Chapter 5　Salty-cold Medicines

Concerning the sweet-cold herbs discussed above, sweet taste enters the spleen and cold property means the herb can clear heat. The "cold" property in the category of the sweet-cold herbs, in fact, refers to that of the "sweet-cool" herbs since these herbs generally are not so cold. By comparison, the salty-cold herbs are much colder in property. The sweet-cold herbs enter the spleen and stomach to treat the diseases in the Qi system. However, the salty-cold herbs enter the kidneys to the deepest point in the body. As it is known that human body can be classified into four layers, i. e. Wei (Defense system), Qi system, Ying system, and Blood system from the exterior surface to the inner organs. Blood is considered to be the innermost layer. Therefore, salty taste can be utilized for blood treatments, and the salty-cold herbs usually play a good effect in clearing blood heat.

Analytical Method for the Four Properties and Five Tastes

Learning Chinese Medicines in an Inference Way

For learning TCM, the most important thing to do is to observe every herb, attentively examine its shape, the four properties and five tastes in the way of studying the principles implied in the herbs instead of rote memorization of the herbs.

Matrix of the Four Properties and Five Tastes

According to TCM theory, the sweet-cold herbs enter the Qi system, and the salty-cold herbs enter the blood system. Why is it so?

TCM stress that Chinese medicines have four properties (cold, hot, warm, cool) and five tastes (sour, bitter, sweet, pungent, salty). Let us arrange them into the following matrix:

Taste / Properties	Sour	Bitter	Sweet	Pungent	Salty
Cold					
Hot					
Warm					
Cool					

For instance, the sour taste mentioned in the above table can be combined with different properties of the "cold, hot, warm, cool" to form the combinations of the sour-cold, sour-hot, sour-warm and sour-cold; the cold property can be combined with the sour, bitter, sweet, pungent and salty tastes to form the combinations of the sour-cold, bitter-cold, pungent-cold and salty-cold. All these combinations come to a sum of twenty properties. Where can they go in the human body? What are their functions in the body? What Chinese medicines can these properties correspond to?

Now, let us restructure the table:

Taste / Properties	Pungent	Sweet	Bitter	Sour	Salty
Hot					
Warm					
Cool					
Cold					

The pungent taste is put at the top of the list since it runs to the lungs. In addition, divergence of the pungent-sweet taste is subsumed to Yang since the pungent and sweet tastes among the five tastes tend to be Yang by nature. Bitterness is more inclined to Yin. Sour-bitter tastes are subsumed to Yin since they induce gush and purgation. Salty taste functions to descend. Therefore, the arrangement of pungent, sweet, bitter, sour, and salty tastes is a sequence orientation from Yang to Yin, and the arrangement of hot, warm, cool and cold properties is a sequence orientation from heat to coldness, which form a matrix of properties of traditional Chinese medicines.

In this matrix, one can realize the law of medication, uses and functioning direction of Chinese medicines. Let us say, if a herb is pungent, it indicates that this herb is more inclined to Yang, dispersing and ascending towards the lungs; if it is sweet in taste, it will go to the Middle Jiao; if it is bitter, it will go to the Middle and Lower Jiao; if it is sour, it will go to the liver and go downwards; and if it is salty, it will go down further. This is an open-ended array, leaving a room for thinking over in the process of TCM development.

There are lots of salty-cold herbs, mostly used for cooling the blood. However, there are some other factors that may also determine the uses of the herbs in this category since the herbs come from different sources: plants, minerals or animals. Some of these salty-cold herbs might be slightly sweet or sour, which determines their different functions and effects.

Overall, there are few salty-cold plant herbs, and Cheqianzi (semen plantaginis) is one of them. However, by comparison, there are more salty-cold mineral herbs such as Hanshuishi (gypsum rubrum) and Fuhaishi (costazia bone), and also salty-cold animal herbs like Muli (concha ostreae) and Xijiao (rhinoceros horn).

Cheqianzi (Semen Plantaginis)

Functions of Cheqianzi

Cheqianzi is the seed of plantain. As a medicine, it is lubricative, sweet, salty and cold in tastes and properties. It enters the liver, kidneys, small intestine and bladder Channels with functions of inducing urination, promoting fluid metabolism and nourish the liver.

As it is mentioned above, seeds of all plants have a descending function. Cheqianzi, as an herb, has the same function. It enters the liver channel to help soothe the liver, which is one of the reasons of its inducing urination since Cheqianzi goes to the small intestine and bladder channels, regulating the interactions between water and fire. When water and fire is well in harmony, urination and dampness will be induced and discharged easily from the body. Cheqianzi is salty in taste and cold in property, entering the blood system to cure blood disorders such as haematuria.

For gynaecological disorders, Cheqianzi is also effective. However, since it slides downwards and may cause habitual abortion, it should not be used for ladies in pregnancy. But when there is dystocia (or difficulty in delivery), it can be used if necessary.

The Principle of Cheqianzi Inducing Urination

Both Cheqianzi and Fuling can induce urination, but they function in different ways.

First of all, Fuling is tasteless; it enters the spleen and help to eliminate the damp out of the body through urination; Cheqianzi, salty-cold in property, enters the kidneys to induce urination with the help of the liver's catharsis function. Therefore, Cheqianzi does not cause impairment of Yin in the process of inducing urination.

Secondly, it is known that the kidneys have the attributes of water and fire, that is, the kidney Yin and kidney Yang. When one is in a healthy state, the kidney Yin and Yang are imperceptibly holding together in harmony. When the kidney Yin and Yang are working in a state of disharmony, which will form damp-heat in the kidneys to obstruct urination, or cause frequent micturition, urgent urination, or odynuria. Cheqianzi, salty-cold in property, enters the kidneys and clears heat symptoms so that urination will become smooth.

Regardless of gender, there are two orifices at the private parts: one is called **Life Essence Orifice,** functioning as a passage for sperm; another one is called **Water Orifice,** functioning as a passage for urination. The kidney water/fluid is classified into Yin water/fluid that is the life essence/seminal fluid, and Yang water/fluid that refers to urine. The kidneys have to manage these two types of water/fluid concurrently. **Life Essence Orifice** and **Water Orifice** shall not open at the same time. When one is open, the other passage will be closed. Otherwise, some white turbidity may occur, that is, urine with seminal fluid – a manifestation of disharmony of the kidney water and fire.

The water-orifice opens only under pneumatolysis influence, i. e., the urinary bladder "starts to pass urine by means of pneumatolysis". The life essence orifice opens to release seminal fluid only under the action of fire, which means the fire of desire should be stirred up from the heart. Cheqianzi is able to open the kidney Qi to induce pneumatolysis, and help discharge the damp-heat out of the urinary bladder.

When pneumatolysis is going on smoothly, a lot of heat in the body can be cleared through water/fluid channel, and pathogenic heat will be unlikely to stay in the Lower Jiao to cause disturbance in the kidneys so that both the life essence orifice and water orifice can be better controlled. In these processes, Cheqianzi functions to promote the circulation of the kidney Qi, accelerate pneumatolysis and regulate the kidney Yin and Yang.

Clinical Experiences in Using Cheqianzi

Formulas involving kidney tonification often contain Cheqianzi. It can be added into **Liuwei Dihuang Pill** or **Bawei Dihuang Pill** in order to tonify the kidneys on the one hand, and improve pneumatolysis on the other hand. **Bawei Dihuang Pill** is a modified formula of **Liuwei Dihuang Pill** by adding Fuzi (radix aconiti carmichaeli) and Rougui (cassia bark). **Liuwei Dihuang Pill** is used for tonifying kidney Yin, and Fuzi and Rougui are used for tonifying kidney Yang. If both kidney Yin and Yang are tonified at the same time, imbalance might occur between the kidney water and fire. Therefore, Cheqianzi is added to induce urination. However, the formula already contains Fuling (poria cocos) and Zexie (rhizoma alismatis) that work to induce urination. Therefore, for those patients who are suffering from Yin deficiency, only Cheqianzi added will be enough in the formula, and Fuling and Zexie should not be used. Besides, Cheqianzi can be added into **Zuogui Pill** or **Yougui Pill** to promote the circulation of the kidney Qi in order to help eliminate the pathogenic heat or damp-heat from the kidneys.

Damp-heat is a conflicting symptom since resolving dampness often causes impairment of Yin and intensifies the fire symptoms, while clearing heat easily causes impairment of Yang and intensifies the damp symptoms. This may cause some trouble of imbalance. Cheqianzi is a best choice for treating damp-heat symptom since it is able to clear heat and induce urination at the same time.

Cheqianzi has one more function of reducing UA (uric acid) that is actually formed in the Lower Jiao due to damp-heat. As it is known, liquor may become sour if the temperature is too high in the process of brewing liquor. Similarly, food becomes sour too when it is fermented under the damp and hot conditions. These show that UA is "brewed" out of the damp-heat pathogens in the Lower Jiao. UA can easily induce dysuria. Cheqianzi can clear the damp-heat in the Lower Jiao and function to resolve UA.

Attention to the Use of Cheqianzi

Cheqianzi should be used with caution. Those patients who suffer from difficult urination due to physical weakness should not use Cheqianzi since such patients may not endure it. Although Cheqianzi is characterized with the properties of inducing urination without impairing Yin, this is a relative concept. In fact, impairment of Yin is likely to occur for those patients who suffer from Yin-deficiency. And also, Cheqianzi must not be used either for those patients who suffer from Yang exhaustion and collapse since Cheqianzi is a descending herb. Otherwise, it will worsen the collapse and further induces exhaustion. What's more, those who suffer from copious urine should not use Cheqianzi because of its property of inducing urination.

Besides, in the process of decocting herbs, Cheqianzi has to be wrapped up with cotton cloth separately, otherwise, it will sink and stick to the bottom of the gallipot.

Mangxiao (Mirabilite)

Cheqianzi can induce urination, and Mangxiao can move the bowel. Both of them are salty-cold in nature and have descending functions.

Varieties of Mangxiao (Mirabilite)

Mangxiao grows out of the saline-alkaline soil. In reality, there are many different types of Mangxiao with multiple names and different grades of quality, of which the "crude saltpetre" with some foreign substances included is called Poxiao (Glauber's salt) that is seldom used as a herb because of its poor quality. Poxiao can be purified into Mangxiao, standing there like rows of horse teeth, so it is also named as "Horse Teeth saltpetre". Actually, Mangxiao is sodium sulfate containing a lot of crystal water. Mangxiao can be dehydrated through weathering in the dry air, after which pure sodium sulphate can be obtained.

Poxiao has a very strong potency and it is seldom used as herb; however, Mangxiao is quite often used as herb due to its proper level of potency. Mangxiao can be further refined into Xuanming Fen (compound of glauber-salt and liquorice).

Dissolve either Mangxiao or Poxiao into water and boil it with radish and Gancao. Radish will absorb the impurities and gradually become salty, but it does not absorb all the salt. Besides, the radish juice is boiled out and mixed with the solution. Then, those residues of radish and Gancao are filtered out. In accordance with specific conditions, the boiling procedure can be repeated over and again and crystalized into Xuanming Fen. Radish is pungent-sweet in tastes, and it can relax bowel and lower Qi. However, Xuanming Fen is much milder in property for relaxing bowel. As a matter of fact, Poxiao, Mangxiao and Xuanming Fen have the similar medical properties, but they have different level of intensity.

Dahuang (rheum officinale) and Mangxiao (Mirabilite)

Mangxiao tastes salty with cold property, entering the stomach, large intestine and Tri-jiao Channels. Salty taste is able to soften hard masses. When the faeces are getting quite hard and difficult to pass the bowel, some salty herbs may be used to help soften it. To be more specific, Mangxiao is salty, pungent and bitter in tastes, and cold in property. Therefore, Mangxiao can play a dispersing and descending functions to help relax bowel.

Dahuang is pungent-bitter too, but it is not salty in taste, so it cannot soften hard masses, but it has moistening effect. Therefore, Dahuang alone will not be so effective in relaxing bowel. When Dahuang and Mangxiao are used together, they will become more effective and bring out the best in each other. These two herbs are used together mainly for tackling the excess heat symptom of dry stool retention. **Dachengqi Tang, Xiaochengqi Tang, Tiaowei Chengqi Tang** are the formulas that contain Dahuang and Mangxiao for treatment based on syndrome differentiation.

Apart from targeting at dry and hard stool, Mangxiao also has the function of getting rid of the stale and bringing forth the fresh, and wiping out the phlegm-heat bonding in the stomach and intestines. There are many substances passing the digestive system where it is hard to be kept clean. Therefore, some wastes and phlegm-heat may be accumulated and stagnated inside, resulting in diseases. Therefore, some people might often drink or be advised to drink Xuanming Fen or Mangxiao for the purposes of maintaining health, but I do not think it is advisable.

Dahuang and Mangxiao used together would have a much stronger potency for relaxing bowel. However, such potency may be further reinforced by adding Houpo (Mangnolia officinalis) and Zhike (fructus aurantia) to make a formula called **Dachengqi Tang** since these two herbs enter the Qi system and have descending functions to intensify the purging effect. Dahuang and Mangxiao can purge out rather than hold on. Those who suffer a lot from the Yangming excess heat symptoms like dry hard stool in the bowel can use **Dachengqi Tang**, which can be very effective.

If the symptom is not that serious, or the patients cannot tolerate the drastic purging, take another formula called **Tiaowei Chengqi Tang** that is made by using Gancao with Dahuang and Mangxiao since the sweet taste of Gancao can slow down the effect of Dahuang and Mangxiao to relax bowel.

Comparing with Mangxiao, Xuanming Fen is more reliable. Xuanming Fen tastes salty with cold nature, and it is able to resolve hard lump and clear heat. In addition, Xuanming Fen is also characterized with pungent-bitter taste that is effective for emptying the bowel. The radish used in the preparation of Xuanming Fen is equivalent to the effect of Gancao used in**Tiaowei Chengqi Tang**.

Regarding the preparation of Xuanming Fen, there are different opinions, but generally speaking, radish and Gancao are used in the processing procedures. Radish is generally used first and followed by Gancao. However, if the radish to be used is somewhat sweet in taste, do not use Gancao again; if the radish to be used is too spicy and pungent, it is necessary to add some Gancao into it. For the specific processing method for Xuanming Fen, please read the book of **Yixue Zhongzhong Canxilu (Records of Traditional Chinese and Western Medicine in Combination) written by** Zhang Xichun.

Salty-cold Sea Medicines

Muli from the epeiric sea, as an herb, tastes salty with cold property. It has the functions of nourishing the Yin and subduing the Yang. Muli is a type of sea-shell with the characteristics of metals and stones. It not only sinks downwards, but also resolves hard lump. Muli enters the liver, gallbladder and kidney channels. Muli is differentiated into raw Muli (raw concha ostreae) and Duan Muli (calcined concha ostreae).

Raw Concha Ostreae

Raw ostreae concha refers to the oyster shell that is collected from the sea-shore and is used directly after it is crushed into small pieces. Its main function is to resolve hard lump, nourish Yin and subdue Yang, which means it sedates the excessive Yang that floats upwards. Oyster shell has a glossy surface, indicating that it has certain moistening effect and it can nourish Yin, but its main effect is to subdue Yang.

Raw ostreae concha can also reduce phlegm, especially the obstinate and chronic phlegm retention that arises from the failure of smooth circulation of Qi in the body. As it is known, blood stasis may occur under the condition of blood stagnation. The phlegm and blood stasis due to unsmooth circulation over a long period of time will result in many diseases, even some types of tumors. Therefore, some salty-cold herbs, such as Muli, Walengzi (concha arcae), Fuhaishi (costazia bone) may be used now and then to resolve hard lumps.

Raw concha arcae, if it has to be used, should be crushed into small pieces of finger nail size with many sharp edges left rather than powder in order to a-chieve a piercing effect on the phlegm and hard lumps since the powder will have different property from that of raw concha arcae.

Calcined Concha Ostreae

Calcined concha arcae refers to the oyster shell that is processed in the way of calcinating, frying or baking, after which it will have conspicuous astringency. Whenever a shell or a bone is cooled down after calcinating, it seems that it can attach to the tongue surface when it is licked --- that shows its astringency.

Those patients who suffer from the symptom of sweating excessively will need to induce astringency, for which calcined concha arcae can be used. One famous formula called **Longmu Guizhi Tang** that contains Longgu (ossa draconis), Muli (concha arcae), Guizhi (cassia twig), Baishao (radix paeoniae alba) is mainly used to regulate Ying (nutrient Qi) and Wei (defensive Qi), and reduce perspiration as well.

Muli is also frequently used for treatment of premature ejaculation, which implies two aspects: one is the premature ejaculation due to the inability to hold back seminal fluid, so the the astringing function of Muli can be employed to hold it back; another aspect is that the ejaculation takes places ince the fire of the liver and kidney is stirred up. As it is discussed in the above section, the kidney water/fluid is classified into Yin water/fluid that is the life essence/seminal fluid that will ejaculate via fire transformation, and Yang water/fluid that refers to urine that will discharge via pneumatolysis. The fire of sexual passion from the liver can stimulate ejaculation. Muli can subdue and astringe the liver fire, thus it keeps the seminal fluid from premature ejaculation.

Compatibility of Muli (Concha Ostreae)

Muli is neither metal nor stone, but it presents the characteristics of metal and stone. What are the characteristics of metals and stones? Muli has a terribly hard shell, which is eligible to be put into the metal category. That is why Muli shows severe and piercing characteristics, and it can be used for resolving the obstinate phlegm.

Muli is very particular about its compatibility. It can be used with Chaihu (radix bupleuri) since Chaihu soothes the liver. By working together, Muli and Chaihu can achieve the targets of soothing the liver and removing stagnation. For the pain and hardness below the costal side, Chaihu and Muli must be used to soothe the liver and resolve the hard lumps and deep-rooted phlegm. In case there are hard lumps in the upper body, Muli and tea leaves can be used together since tea is able to upbear the clear first and then downbear the turbid; and this herbal pair can help to resolve the hard lump in the upper body. In addition,

Dahuang goes downwards, so it can be used together with Muli to resolve the hard lumps in the lower portion of the body, especially indefinable lumps around the thigh.

For liver cirrhosis, turtle shell, Zhe Beimu (thunberg fritillary bulb), Muli, and even Chuanshanjia (pangolin scales) are often used for treatment. Cirrhosis means it is "hardening" with worsening trend. Muli is salty-cold in nature that can be used to resolve hard lump, but it may not be so effective that turtle shell (attention: not tortoise shell) should be added in order to reinforce the curing effect. Both turtle and pangolin prefer to drill in wherever they are. Therefore, TCM believes that turtle shell and Chuanshanjia have the potential to resolve the stagnation and hard lump in the body. Zhe Beimu enters the lung and reduces phlegm, functioning to assist metal (the lungs) and calm wood (the liver) according to the *Wuxing doctrine*. Therefore, in the process of treatment of the liver cirrhosis, it is not only necessary to reduce phlegm, but also essential to assist the lungs in order to soothe the liver. Thus, based on the theory of "metal restricting wood", it will be reasonable for the liver to be restricted of its vitality by assisting the lungs.

Zhe Beimu is used for the treatment of liver cirrhosis by means of its effect in the lungs in order to achieve balance and harmony among the five internal organs based on the *Wuxing doctrine* of restriction among the five elements (wood, metal, water, fire and earth). Clinically, herbs that can resolve hard lump usually have many applications since it is better to keep the internal organs in a soft and flexible state. Wherever there is a hard lump, there will be Qi and blood obstruction. Therefore, it will be necessary to take measures to resolve the hard lump. Meanwhile, treatment should be given based on syndrome differentiation on the the specific locations of the specific internal organs.

Fuhaishi (Costazia bone)

The literal meaning of "浮海石" (Fuhaishi) in Chinese is "the stone that floats on the sea". Regarding the formation of Fuhaishi, there are many explanations, one of which is that Fuhaishi is formed by condensation of magma foam. In the course of volcano eruption, magma goes into eruption and generates foam. After cooling down, the foam will condense into foamed stones, which will then undergo seawater erosion and float on the sea or to the seashore under the action of sea wave. Another explanation is that Fuhaishi is formed by sea waves that lash the shore and generate a lot of foam. More and more form accumulates and dries up to form Fuhaishi, for which some micro-organisms may get involved.

Various abdominal masses can be resolved with the help of Fuhaishi since it is salty in taste and cold in property. Saltiness can soften hard masses and resolve the long-lasting phlegm that is not easily resolved with the common herbs.

Fuhaishi resolves the long-lasting phlegm, especially the fire-induced phlegm in the Upper Jiao since it can float upwards in the lungs. Besides, Fuhaishi is used to eliminate the pyrophlegm. After all, Fuhaishi is a kind of stone, and it is able to descend. Also, due to its saltiness, it enters the kidney channel. In brief, Fuhaishi enjoys the characteristics of ascending and descending in sequence to soften hard masses and remove long-lasting phlegm.

Fuhaishi can be used for tackling eye pterygium, treating ecthyma, and resolve various lumps, goiter and tumor; it can also be used for treating cough, especially the cough caused by long-lasting phlegm in the lungs, but it is not suitable for the slight phlegm and retained fluid, or the cough arising from the common cold or flu. In addition, Fuhaishi should not be hastily used at the very early stage of diseases. Only when the disease is quite serious with phlegm and heat in the lungs and stomach, can it be used to clear the heat and resolve the phlegm. However, Fuhaishi cannot be used for too long time since it restricts Qi and functions of the lungs and stomach. In particular, it is not suitable for those who have spleen deficiency.

Walengzi (Concha Arcae)

There are various types of shells in the sea. They all have similar functions, and yet each of them has its own uniqueness.

Walengzi has ridged surface that looks like corrugated roof tiles, not as shiny as Muli but more dried-up. Walengzi is also salty-cold in nature, entering the lung and stomach channels, effective for resolving the long-lasting phlegm, blood stasis and hard lump as well. Because of its lack of shininess, it cannot nourish

Yin, but it is very effective for treating gastric acid disorder or stomachache. The dried-up Walengzi has alkaline properties, so it can neutralize the excessive gastric acid. From chemical perspectives, Walengzi is composed of calcium carbonate that reacts with acidic solution. Thus, it is often used to treat excess stomach acid condition.

Walengzi is often used together with Wuzhuyu (fructus evodiae) and Huanglian (coptis chinensis). When the patient is suffering from some other diseases accompanied with gastric acid problem, Walengzi, Wuzhuyu and Huanglian may be added to the main formula, which will bring a better effect.

Haigeqiao (Concha Meretricis Seu Cyclinae)

Haigeqiao is the shell of the round meretrix available in the vegetable markets.

Shells in the sea appear in many shapes, of which the round one is called clam, the long one is called mussel, and the longer one is called razor clam that is also a sub-type of mussel. Their functions are quite similar, but Haigeqiao looks glossier and moister than Walengzi. Haigeqiao functions to reduce phlegm and resolve the hard lumps all the same, but it can nourish Yin as well.

Haigeqiao is a common medicine, and it has two forms available in drug store: crushed pieces and powder; they have the same chemical compositions, but they have different properties. Haigeqiao powder becomes less effective for softening hard masses, but it has slight astringing effect.

There is a book called *Haiyao Bencao* (*Herbal Medicines from Sea*) that discusses all types of herbal medicines from the sea.

Xijiao (Rhinoceros Horn)

When Xijiao is used as medicine, the tip of the horn is the best part.

Miraculous Function of Xijiao

Xijiao is bitter and salty in tastes and cold in property, entering the heart, liver and stomach channels to clear blood-heat. It is a very crucial herb for dealing with disorder in the blood system. There is a Chinese poem line saying: "A bit of rhinoceros horn makes one become clear in mind", which is actually a medical description. When the pathogenic Qi invades the pericardium, the heart fire will mask one's consciousness and mentality, making the patient muddle-headed. Just a little bit of rhinoceros horn will be able to clear the fire and open the heart orifice, and the patient will come back to his sense. Rhinoceros horn is such a magic herb with remarkable and instant effect. That is what the poem really means.

Rhinoceros horns are magical. It is said that "Human Qi shatters rhinoceros horn". Fresh rhinoceros horn is hard to crush into pieces. However, if it is tucked into the bosom to receive the warmth from the human body, it turns fragile and can be shattered with just a light knock at it. Besides, rhinoceros horn should smell a puff of faint scent, while a counterfeit product usually smells stink.

The top-grade rhinoceros horn is the dark rhinoceros horn that is black in color, and its powder is just like tobacco or cigarette ash. A very small dosage of it, around 0.5g or 1g, will be enough whenever needed. Generally, rhinoceros horn powder should not be decocted but mixed with the ready boiled decoction directly for drinking since it is very valuable, and just a little bit of the horn powder is sufficient to bring in the effect as the poem line suggests.

Essential Medicine for Treatment of the Blood Heat in Ying System

The theory of epidemic febrile disease looks at the human body from Wei (defensive Qi), Qi, Ying and Blood systems. Impairment of Yin may occur when pathogens enters the Ying and blood systems, resulting in blood heat. In such a case, pathogens may run into the deepest points in the body, and it is quite hard to get rid of them out of the body. In that case, the formula of **Xijiao Dihuang Tang** will be the best solution, which was also frequently used in the past.

Leukemia andsepticaemia in modern medical terms in fact attribute to the factors that pathogens enter the Ying system with manifestation of skin maculae. The maculae of septicaemia are quite obvious and terribly red all over the body and may turn purple pretty quickly, which is the sign of blood heat and blood entering Ying system. This symptom can be improved quickly with a bit of rhinoceros horn. However, the maculae of leukemia look light red in color, which is more troublesome and much harder to treat.

Forbidden Use of Xijiao Does not Really Protect Rhinoceros

Now, Xijiao has been forbidden to use, and even the ancient Chinese medical books noted that substitutions are suggested in order to protect the endangered rhinoceros.

Back in the past, rhinoceros horns were not obtained through hunting but from the naturally dead rhinoceros. Chinese medicine practitioners always try to make the best use out of everything, and they usually use the left-over materials as medicine to save the patients' life after rhinoceros horns are made into handicrafts. Now, rhinoceros horns have been banned, but it is still available in the black markets with a higher price since the cost is going up. High price for rhinoceros horns result in more illegal rhinoceros-hunting. Thus, rhinoceros are not receiving real protection.

However, this is not caused by the Chinese medicine practitioners prescribing such a herb, as they just use the left-over materials with full respect, especially for the magical herbs like horns from the dead rhinoceros.

Regarding protection of rhinoceros, simple ban of rhinoceros horns does not resolve the problem once for all. It should be managed by those who understand Chinese medicine and traditional culture from a humanitarian perspective. Otherwise, the ban may lead to more rhinoceros slaughtering events.

Tao Te Ching(by **Lao Tseu**) said, "What is cheap and hard to get always keeps the people from stealing. " The more strict with banning, the higher the price will be since there is always a demand. The similar case is about tiger bone. Tiger bone has been banned from being used as medicine, and then, how are the bones to be handled when a tiger is dead? I heard from a friend that tiger bones are stored in freezers after the death of a tiger. As it is known in TCM, tiger bone is warm and hot in nature as medicine, so long-lasting storing in freezer will make it lose its original efficacy, and eventually, it will come to a waste.

Xijiao Dihuang Tang and Angong Niuhuang Pill

Xijiao Dihuang Tang might be needed at certain stage of leukaemia treatment, and rhinoceros horns having been banned from using, the leukaemia treatment is, to some extent, becoming less effective. The formula of **Xijiao Dihuang Tang** is recorded in *Qianjin Yaofang, Waitai Miyao (Medical Secrets of an Official)* and *Wenbing Tiaobian (Treatise on Differentiation and Dreatment of Epidemic Febrile Disease)*.

Xijiao Dihuang Tang contains the herbal ingredients: Shaoyao (paeonia lactiflora), Dihuang (rehmannia), Danpi (cortex moutan radicis), Xijiao (rhinoceros horn).

In this formula, Dihuang often refers to Sheng Dihuang (radix rehmanniae recen), Shaoyao is often substituted by Chishao (radix paeoniae rubra), or occasionally by Baishao (radix paeoniae alba), or a mixture of both, since Chishao goes to the blood system to remove heat and blood stasis. The intention of the formula can be explained according to the TCM theory about the four properties and five tastes.

All the four herbs in this formula are cold in nature. Shaoyao is sour-cold; Dihuang is sweet-cold; Danpi is bitter-cold; and rhinoceros horn is salty-cold. Out of the five tastes, sour, sweet, bitter and salty tastes are included, and only the pungent taste (pungent-cold and pungent-cool properties) is left out. Why is it so? It is because the pathogen has entered the blood system, which signifies that no external symptoms are available. Therefore, it is unnecessary to use the pungent-cool herbs to relieve the exterior symptoms, but only the four sour-cold, sweet-cold, bitter-cold and salty-cold herbs are needed to eliminate the fire in the five internal organs and blood-heat. The mixture of Sheng Dihuang, Danpi and Chishao is an important herbal combination for cooling blood, which is then further reinforced by adding about 1g of rhinoceros horn.

Xijiao Dihuang Tang has a very strong effect for clearing away heat and toxic materials, cooling blood and opening the orifices. For hepatitis or hepatic coma referred to by the western medicine in modern time, this formula can also be used for treatment when some terribly serious heat symptoms arise; For sure, this formula can also be used for treatment of anaphylactoid purpura, leukaemia and septicaemia.

The formula of **Angong Niuhuang Pill** also contains rhinoceros horn, but now buffalo horn is used instead. Even though the pill still functions to cool blood, open orifices, clear away heat and toxic materials, yet the buffalo horn is a serious dilution of the function of **Angong Niuhuang Pill**.

The substitute now for rhinoceros horn is buffalo horn since both buffalo and rhinoceros live in water, sharing many similarities. All the mammals living in water have certain cooling and moistening functions. However, buffalo horn as a substitute for rhinoceros horn will have to be used in a much larger dosage. Generally speaking, 60 grams of buffalo horn might be equivalent to 0.5 gram of rhinoceros horn in respect of the effect. Even so, their functions are not fully identical. From the appearance of both animals, rhinoceros has a horn projecting on the nose which is subsumed to the Yangming channel, therefore, rhinoceros horns clears the excess heat in the Yangming channel. Buffalo horns grow at the two sides where the Shaoyang channel dominates. Thus, the different locations of horns on the animal body determine that they would have medicinal effects on different portions of the human body. Thus, buffalo horn can be used to substitute for rhinoceros horn, but they do have clinical differences.

Renzhongbai (Depositum Urinae Hominis) and Qiushi(Processed Urine Deposit)

Little Boy Urine, Renzhongbai and Qiushi

When a urine pot is used for a certain time, at the interior wall of the pot there will be a layer of crystallized white frost called Renzhongbai, or Niaobing (urine ice), which can be scraped off.

Not everyone's Niaobing can be used as medicine. The ancient TCM books say "the best Niaobing is that from small boys or the old monks living in the mountains". The Niaobing from the others is useless since it contains fire. The immature children have clean urine since they do not suffer from too much emotional fluctuation, nor have sexual life, nor have omnivorous habits or complex mindset. Old monks have a good practice of their religion, and have clean body and tranquil mind.

Urine from different people shows great differences. Stool and urine are the excreted wastes with toxins included, but where do those toxins come from? They are originated from diet and emotion changes. Human sleeping at night is similar to closing the body for cleaning. When lying in bed, human being will have their blood return to the liver where blood will be filtrated, through which the toxins that were generated from food intake and emotion changes during the daytime will then be excreted out of the body the next morning. After that, one will feel refreshed.

The existence of human urine sediment also reminds that one should not hold urine for too long. Otherwise, some symptoms like stranguria or various stones may occur.

Renzhongbai is salty-cold in nature, which can be used to decrease the internal heat and direct stagnated heat downwards. Children's urine, as a medicine, is salty-cold too, which is used to decrease the internal heat and remove blood stasis. In the past, those who fell over to hurtthe internal organs used little boys' urine for treatment in case that **Yunnan Baiyao** was not available. This on the one hand can make up the body fluid, and on the other hand disperse the blood stasis without causing any impairment to the body.

Qiushi (processed urine deposit) is produced by refining children urine with Shigao with a very complicated craftmanship. This craft is more commonly followed in Huanggang city, Hubei province, and Anqing city, Anhui province, China, where there are still factories for processing Qiushi.

Little boys' urine, Qiushi and Renzhongbai both have the similar functions with only slight difference. Little boys' urine decreases the internal heat and removes stasis due to blood stagnation, injuries from falls, fractures, contusions and strains, or treat swooning-off due to excessive loss of blood during child delivery. Qiushi mainly functions to nourish Yin and brings down a fever. It is also good for curing cough due to consumptive disease or fever due to tuberculosis. Renzhongbai is used for eliminating stagnation, clearing heat and decreasing the internal heat.

Renzhonghuang (Rulvis Glycyrrhizae Extractionis Sedilis) and Jinzhi ("Golden Juice")

Human faeces can also be processed into salty-cold medicines, such as Renzhonghuang and Jinzhi.

Renzhonghuang is made in the following way:

Find a piece of moso bamboo with the joints at both ends; Scrape off the outermost crust (since it induces astringency, and the permeability of the bamboo tube will be reduced; but the layer of Zhuru should be reserved); Drill a hole in the bamboo tube and fill the tube with Gancao (liquorice) powder; Seal the hole in the bamboo tube with a petiole of Chinese banana leaf. As the petiole of the leaf expands in water, it will seal up the drilled hole tightly.

On the day of the winter solstice, immerse those prepared bamboo tubes into a feces pit for the whole winter since the stool in the cold weather is not so easy to get decomposed and grubby to generate maggots, and then take them out after the day of Beginning of Spring (one of the 24 solar terms), and the processed Gancao powder (dried up in a place with good ventilation) in such a way is called Renzhonghuang.

Renzhonghuang is sweet, salty and cold in nature, which, having gone through the five internal organs, is effective for eliminating heat pathogens. Gancao has the function of relieving the internal heat or fever while the human excrement and bamboo are both cold in nature. Besides, bamboo is densely structured in its texture, and it can filtrate most of the turbid waste in the excrement with only the life essence extracted and reserved.

Regarding Jinzhi, it is the excrement from a healthy boy, which is filtrated and sealed up in a jar. The sealed jar is then buried under a road on which many people come and go frequently. After many-year staying underground (the longer, the better), the jar is taken out, and the liquid in the jar becomes very clear with no foul smell at all.

As the TCM books say Jinzhi is bitter and salty in tastes and cold in property. After it is buried underground for an extremely long period of time, it will become sweet, bitter, salty and cold in properties, and thus, it can enter the heart to purge fire for removing toxin. When there occurs pandemic, the heat pathogens will become extremely vigorous, which then result in the heat pathogen attacking the pericardium to make the patients sick seriously. For such a case, Jinzhi and Renzhonghuang will have a quick effect for treatment. By the way, when in emergency, Jinzhi and Renzhonghuang can eliminate all types of fire and heat toxins. However, it must be noted that they are used for clearing the excess heat only in Yangming channel. For those who suffer from deficiency in the Yangming channel, it is not advisable to use Jinzhi and Renzhonghuang since they may cause some impairment to the body.

By the way, the reason that Jinzhi and Renzhonghuang have such functions is that they still have some turbid Qi running downwards very swiftly from the stomach to the large intestine, and thus, they can send the toxins and heat out of the body.

The principles implied in these herbs are quite clear, but such medicines are seldom used since it is hard for patients to accept these substances psychologically. Therefore, some other herbs with weaker potency and slower effect are usually substituted for these two medicines.

Summary of Salty-cold Medicines

In brief, the herbs in the salty-cold medicine category include plant herbs like Cheqianzi; mineral herbs like Mangxiao, Poxiao, Xuanming Fen and Fuhaishi; animal herbs like Muli, Walengzi, Haigeqiao and Xijiao; and the last type of medicines related to human, including Qiushi, Renzhongbai, Renzhonghuang, Jinzhi and little boy's urine.

第五章　咸寒药

上次讲的是甘寒类药。甘入脾，寒清热，甘寒实际就是甘凉，甘寒药一般不会太寒。咸寒药则会更寒一些。甘寒药走脾胃，治气分。咸寒药则走肾，能进入身体的最深处。我们知道，人体由浅入深分卫、气、营、血四个层次，血是最深处的一层，所以咸能够治血，咸寒药往往有很好的清血热的作用。

四气五味分析法

细推物理学中药

我们要仔细观察每味中药，仔细推究它的形状、四气五味。不要死记硬背，要通过体察物理的方式去研究。

四气五味方阵

比如，甘寒药走气分，咸寒药走血分，为什么呢？

中药讲四气五味，四气是寒、热、温、凉，五味是酸、苦、甘、辛、咸。我把它们这样排出来，排成一个方阵，排列组合起来：

	酸	苦	甘	辛	咸
寒					
热					
温					
凉					

比如：酸，包括酸寒、酸热、酸温、酸凉；寒，包括酸寒、苦寒、甘寒、辛寒、咸寒。四气五味这样一排，得到二十种性质，它们分别走哪里？有什么作用？对应哪些药？我们可以这样来想。

我们还可以把这个表格改造一下：

	辛	甘	苦	酸	咸
热					
温					
凉					
寒					

辛排在最前面，因为辛走肺，辛甘发散为阳，五味中辛、甘偏阳；苦偏阴，酸苦涌泻为阴；咸往下走。辛、甘、苦、酸、咸是从阳到阴的排列，热、温、凉、寒则是由热到寒的排列，构成一个药性方阵。

在这个方阵里，我们可以体会用药的规律，还有各种药物的用途和走向。比如这个药是辛的，辛甘发散为阳，往上走、往肺里走；如果是甘的呢，就往中焦走；苦往中焦和下焦走；酸入肝，往下走；咸走得更下。这是一个很开放的方阵，让我们一直去思考，是一个完善自己的过程。

咸寒药有很多，主要用来凉血。但咸寒之外又有其他性质，决定了它们各自的用途。比如咸寒药中，有植物，有矿物，有动物；咸寒药中，有的带一点甘，有的带一点酸，作用都不一样。

咸寒的植物药并不多，我们讲一个车前子。咸寒的矿物药多一些，比如寒水石、浮海石。咸寒药里矿物药有不少，动物药也有不少，比如说牡蛎、犀角，都是咸寒动物类药。

车前子

车前子的作用

车前子是车前草结的种子，有滑性，味甘咸寒。车前子利小便，归肝、肾、小肠、膀胱经，行水泻热，还有养肝的作用。

以前说过，只要是植物种子，一般都有往下降的作用，车前子也是这样。车前子入肝经，能助肝疏泄，这是它利水的原理之一；车前子入小肠经、膀胱经，具有调节水火的作用，水火调则气化利，小便易出，水湿易去；车前子性咸寒，入血分，能治很多血症，如尿血。

对于胎产之类病症，车前子也有很好的作用。但往下滑就能滑胎，怀孕期间不能用，但是生产困难的时候，如果有必要，可以用。

车前子利水的原理

车前子和茯苓都是利水道的药，利水道也就是利小便，但是二者不同。

首先，茯苓淡渗走脾，通过作用于脾，把水淡渗出来，从小便而出；车前子咸寒入肾，通过调动肝的疏泄功能，让人排小便，并不淡渗，所以车前子利小便而不伤阴。

其次，我们知道肾分水火，分肾阴、肾阳，人体健康时，肾阴肾阳交抱于无形，和谐统一；肾阴、肾阳不和谐时，交织在一起成了肾中的湿热，湿热会闭住小便，或导致尿频、尿急、尿痛。车前子咸寒入肾，能把邪热清掉，小便就容易解出。

不论男性还是女性，阴部都有两个窍：一窍通精，叫精窍，是精液出入的地方；一窍通水，叫水窍，是小便出入的地方。肾水也分两种，一种阴水，一种阳水，阴水为精，阳水就是小便，肾同时管这两种水。精窍和水窍是不会同时开，精窍开时，水道就要闭上，水窍开时，精窍就要闭上。如果闭合不好，则产生白浊，小便带精液，这也是肾中水火不调的一种表现。

水窍需要气化才能出来，所谓膀胱"气化则能出焉"。精窍得火才能泻，要得火，心就要动，要有欲火，精窍里边的精才能出来。车前子通气化，能疏利膀胱湿热，通肾气帮助气化。

气化得以顺利进行，体内很多热就能从水道排出，邪热就不至于留在下焦，在肾里扰动，精窍和水窍的开合就能得到很好地控制。所以车前子能起到通肾气、促进气化、调节肾阴肾阳的作用。

车前子的使用经验

补肾的方子经常用到车前子。把它加在六味地黄丸或者八味地黄丸中，一边补肾，一边促进肾的气化。八味地黄丸就是六味地黄丸加附子、肉桂。六味地黄丸补肾阴，附子、肉桂补肾阳，现在肾阴肾阳双补，会不会导致肾里水火失调呢？完全有可能。所以加一味车前子以利小便。方子本身已有的茯苓、泽泻也是利水的。如果病人阴虚，茯苓、泽泻可以不加，只加车前子就行。把它加在左归丸、右归丸里，能通肾气，能把肾里的邪热、湿热泄出去。

湿热是一个矛盾的病症，化湿往往伤阴助火，清热则容易伤阳助湿，在治疗上往往不能兼顾。用车前子则不然，既清热，又能利水，恰好治疗湿热。

车前子还有减尿酸的作用。尿酸其实也是下焦湿热形成的。酿酒的时候，温度过高，酒就酸了，食物通过湿热发酵也会变酸。尿酸也是下焦湿热酿出来的。尿酸高容易导致尿痛。车前子能清下焦湿热，有解尿酸的作用。

使用车前子需要注意之处

车前子在用的时候是有讲究的。体虚性的小便不利，不要用车前子，身体会受不了。虽是利而不伤阴，但这也是相对的，阴虚的人利水过多，还是会伤阴；阳气虚脱、阳气下陷也不要用车前子，车前子是往下利的药，阳气下陷再用车前子，继续下陷，人就可能产生虚脱。车前子利小便，尿多就没有必要用了，用了反而有坏处。

此外，在煎药的时候，要把车前子单独用布包起来。车前子很细碎而外表粘腻，如果不用布包起来，就会沉底粘在药罐子底下结起来，容易把药罐烧坏。

芒硝

车前子是利小便的药，芒硝则是通大便的药。它们都是咸寒的，咸寒就能往下走。

从朴硝到玄明粉

芒硝长在盐碱地里，有很多种，也有很多名字，或者说有很多等级。其中有杂质，很粗朴的叫朴硝。因为质量太差，现在药用一般不用朴硝。对朴硝进行提纯，让它结晶出像麦芒那样尖锐的东西，就是芒硝。有的没那么尖锐，一排一排像马牙，叫"马牙硝"。芒硝其实是硫酸钠，含的结晶水较多。把芒硝、马牙硝放在干燥的空气里经过风化，得到"风化硝"，就是是不带结晶水的硫酸钠。

朴硝力度大，一般不用；芒硝有一定力度，较为常用。在芒硝的基础上，可以进一步提炼出玄明粉。

把朴硝或芒硝溶解在水里，加萝卜、甘草一起煮，萝卜一面吸收杂质，逐渐变咸，但又不会把盐分全部吸收，另一面，它的汁也会出来一部分，进入溶液之中。最后把萝卜、甘草这些渣滓去掉。根据具体情况，可以继续放萝卜进去煮，反复几次，最后进行结晶，就得到玄明粉。萝卜辛甘，能润下降气。玄明粉通大便，性质更为平和。朴硝、芒硝、玄明粉药性类似，胆子小的可以用玄明粉。

大黄芒硝

芒硝咸寒，入胃经、大肠经和三焦经。咸能软坚，大便硬在里面解不下来，可以用咸味的东西软一软。芒硝性味咸辛苦寒，辛能发散，苦能往下走，既辛又苦一般就能往下走而通大便。

大黄也是辛苦的，但大黄不咸，不能软坚，只有滑利的作用，所以单用大黄，泻下的作用并不太大，只有大黄和芒硝一块用，两药相得益彰，作用才大。大黄、芒硝一起主要用于治疗大便干结的实热证。大承气汤、小承气汤、调胃承气汤都是根据不同情况使用大黄和芒硝的方子。

除了针对大便干结，芒硝还能推陈致新，涤荡肠胃的痰热互结。肠胃每天进出很多东西，很难保证干净，常常会有一些残渣、痰热结在里面动不了，积累太多就会生病，所以要经常清理。有人经常就喝玄明粉来涤荡肠胃，甚至有人鼓励大家喝芒硝来养生。我不提倡，虽然芒硝有涤荡的作用，但涤荡多了、久了也不好。

大黄、芒硝一起用，泻下的力度比较大。如果还嫌力度不大，可以加厚朴、枳壳，它们通气分，能降气，可以增强往下推的力度。这就是大承气汤。大黄、芒硝走而不守。对于阳明实热症，体内有燥屎，大便干结，实在解不出来，人很难受，就用大承气汤，在大黄、芒硝的基础上加厚朴、枳实，让它们走得更快一点，速战速决。

如果情况没那么严重，或者病人经不起泻，就用调胃承气汤，在大黄、芒硝的基础上加一味温柔缓和的甘草，甘就能缓，就能拖住大黄、芒硝，让它们走得慢一点，让大便缓缓泻下来。

相比芒硝，用玄明粉更稳妥。玄明粉咸寒，咸能软坚，寒能清热，玄明粉也有辛苦的性质，辛苦能使人拉肚子，炮制过程用到的萝卜相当于"调胃承气汤"里的甘草。

做玄明粉的方法，大家说法不一，大体就是加萝卜和甘草。做的时候先用萝卜，如果那个萝卜带甜味，甘草就不要用了。如果那个萝卜辣得不得了，就有必要用一些甘草。制备玄明粉的方法，张锡纯在《医学衷中参西录》里面讲得非常清楚，感兴趣的话可以看一下。

牡蛎等咸寒海药

作为浅海贝壳，牡蛎作为一味中药使用，性质咸寒，益阴潜阳，化痰软坚。牡蛎属于贝壳一类，贝壳有金石之性，不仅能往下重镇，也有化痰软坚的作用。牡蛎入肝、胆、肾三经。牡蛎有生牡蛎和煅牡蛎之分。

生牡蛎

生牡蛎就是从海边捡回来的捣成小块儿直接用，其主要作用是软坚散结、益阴潜阳，能把人体升浮的阳气往下潜镇。生牡蛎有一定的光泽，说明有一定的滋润作用，能养阴，但其主要的作用还是潜阳。

生牡蛎还有化痰的作用，专化顽固的老痰。人体的气不能顺利通行会导致痰，痰积累久了就成了顽痰、老痰。血运行不畅会成为瘀血，瘀血时间长了也会非常顽固。当气血形成痰、瘀后，时间久了，顽痰死血导致很多病，就连很多肿瘤都是顽痰死血造成的。所以可以经常用牡蛎、瓦楞子、浮海石等咸寒之品去软化它们。

用生牡蛎时，打碎就行，不能打成粉，为什么呢？如果打成细粉，牡蛎的性质就变了，有收涩性，就跟煅牡蛎有相似之处了。生牡蛎要打成手指甲那么大的块，形成有很多尖角，有刺破作用，能刺破顽痰和结块。

煅牡蛎

煅牡蛎就是将牡蛎煅、炒或烧过了来用，它有明显的收涩性。凡是贝壳或骨头，烧红冷却，舔的时候感觉吸舌头，这就是收涩性的表现。

什么时候需要收涩呢？比如汗流过多，就需要收涩，可以用煅牡蛎。有一个很有名的方子叫龙牡桂枝汤，用龙骨和牡蛎，加桂枝、白芍，主要调和营卫，还可以收汗。

再比如，精关不固、早泄也经常用牡蛎。这里有两重含义：第一，早泄是因为精液迫不及待要出来，我们要把它收涩住，牡蛎正好有收涩的作用。第二，精液出来是因为肝肾之火在动。我们前面讲了，肾有阴水阳水，阳水就是尿液，得气化才能出，阴水就是精液，得火化才能出。人动情欲之火，精液就能出，而情欲之火来自肝，牡蛎能潜镇肝火，把肝火往下潜镇、往里收敛，能让精液不至早泄。

牡蛎的配伍

牡蛎不是金石，但有金石之性。什么是金石之性呢？牡蛎是一种很硬的壳，中医里讲"从介化"，坚硬的外壳，就可以往属性"金"性上靠。所以牡蛎有峻削之气，能化顽痰。

用牡蛎要讲究配伍。牡蛎可跟柴胡配伍，柴胡疏肝，牡蛎配柴胡则疏肝散结。胁下硬痛，一般柴胡、牡蛎两味药是必加的，一边疏肝，一边软坚散结化顽痰，胁下就不硬了。上部有结块，可以用牡蛎、茶叶，茶叶升清降浊，先往上走，再把浊气往下带，牡蛎配伍茶叶能消身体上部结块。大黄往下走，牡蛎配大黄就能消身体下部结块，尤其是大腿上的无名肿块，常用大黄配牡蛎。

肝硬化常用鳖甲、浙贝、牡蛎，甚至穿山甲等。硬化，说明"硬"得越来越严重，牡蛎咸寒，软坚散结，但一味药作用有限，还得用鳖甲。"鳖"是王八，不是乌龟。鳖在哪都喜欢往里钻，所以鳖甲有穿透性，中医都是这样取象比类的。穿山甲也善钻，山都能钻过去，体内结块也能钻掉、化掉。浙贝化痰走肺，有佐金平木的作用。治肝硬化，要平木，不仅要化痰，还得帮助肺。肝有病，就要辅助肺，肝属木，肺属金，通过"金克木"的作用对肝进行合理限制，对肝也有好处。

治疗肝硬化的时候，之所以用浙贝帮助入肺，就是利用五行相克的作用达到平衡、调和五脏关系。在临床上，软坚散结药用途非常多，体内五脏柔软比较好，哪个地方硬了，说明这里气血不通了，就要考虑软坚散结。当然还得根据具体是哪一脏、什么部位再斟酌用药。

浮海石

浮海石，顾名思义，就是浮在海面的一种石头。关于它的说法很多。一种认为，浮海石是岩浆泡沫凝成的。火山喷发的时候，岩浆喷发，产生泡沫，泡沫凝结，定型成泡沫状的石头，经海水腐蚀，孔会变大，久而久之，被海浪打到海边或者浮在海上。还有一种说法，认为浮海石是海浪形成的，海浪拍击海岸产生泡沫，泡沫越积越多，干了形成浮海石，可能其间有一些微生物也起了一定的作用。

治疗各种症瘕积聚，需要软坚散结，就要用到浮海石。浮海石性咸寒，咸能软坚，善于消磨顽痰。顽痰就是积累了很多年的痰，一般的药化不掉，得用矿物类药。

浮海石消顽痰，尤其善于祛除上焦热痰。浮海石以除热痰为主，还能化痰火，浮海石还走肺，往上升浮，所以主治上焦。但是，浮海石毕竟是一种石头，还是会往下走；而且它是咸的，入肾。所以浮海石能先升后降，一路软坚散结，消除顽痰。

浮海石还能点目翳、敷疮痘、消各种积块、瘿瘤等；能治咳嗽，特别是肺里有顽痰的咳嗽。如果是很轻的痰饮，或感冒导致的咳嗽都不可以用浮海石。刚咳嗽没几天，也不要贸然用浮海石。浮海石必须在病比较沉重的时候用，肺胃有热的时候用它来清热、有痰的时候用它来化痰。但是这味药不能久用，因为它能够克伐肺胃之气，脾虚之人，尤其不适宜用。

瓦楞子

海里的贝壳有许多种，它们作用基本相似，也略微有些差别。

瓦楞是一楞一楞的，跟瓦相似，没有牡蛎那么有光泽，显得比较干枯。瓦楞也是咸寒的，入肺经、胃经，也善于消老痰和瘀血，能软坚散结。因为光泽度不好，它几乎没有养阴作用，但是治胃酸、胃痛作用很大。干巴巴的瓦楞，一看就偏碱性。胃酸过多，可以用偏碱性的药去中和。从化学的角度分析，瓦楞就是碳酸钙，遇酸发生反应，酸被消解，所以经常用它治胃酸。

瓦楞通常跟吴萸、黄连一起用。假如病人有别的问题，但同时胃酸，可以把这三味药加进去，效果会比较好。

海蛤壳

海蛤就是菜市场的那种圆的文蛤的贝壳。

海里的贝壳，圆的叫蛤，长的叫蚌，再长一点的叫蛏子，蛏子也属于蚌类，它们的作用比较相似。海蛤更加润泽，比瓦楞有光泽多了，其作用依然是化痰，软坚散结，同时有养阴作用。

海蛤壳是常用药，需要砸碎使用；如果将其打成海蛤粉，则软坚散结的作用小些，微有收涩作用。海蛤粉和海蛤壳，一种磨成细粉，一种只是砸碎，它们的作用是不一样的。从化学分析的角度看它们是一种东西，但在中药的药用上，它们的性质有所区别。

有一本书叫《海药本草》，很有意思，讲海里的各种药，想了解各种贝壳的细微差异，可以参考这本书。

犀角

犀角就是犀牛的角，入药，角尖是最好的。

心有灵犀一点通

犀角苦咸寒，入心经、肝经、胃经，治血热解毒，是清血分非常重要的一味药。我们常讲的"心有灵犀一点通"，这其实是医学上的一句话，灵犀就是犀牛角，病人邪气入了心包，心火令人神昏，人就会变胡涂。吃点犀牛角，把火气清掉，心通了，人也就清醒过来了。犀牛角是有灵气的一味药，效果奇且快，这就叫"心有灵犀一点通"。

犀牛有灵气，犀牛角也就有灵气。有一句话叫"人气粉犀"，人气能让犀角变成粉。刚拿出来的犀牛角，要把它弄碎有点难，把它揣在怀里，让它得到人的温度，然后拿出来轻轻一敲就碎了。得了人气，犀牛角就容易被打碎。闻一闻，如果有一股清香，这个犀牛角就是真的，如果有股臭味，这个犀牛角就是假的。

最好的犀角叫乌犀角，是黑的，打成粉跟烟灰一样，用量非常少，0.5克或1克就够。一般不入煎汤药，而是用药汁冲兑喝下。这药太珍贵，舍不得用多，用这点也够了。"心有灵犀一点通"，一点点就够了。

热入营血必备药

温病分卫气营血，当邪气入了营分、血分，就会伤阴，导致血热。这时，邪气在人体最深处，不容易清掉，要用到犀角地黄汤，这是过去经常用的一个方子。

现在的白血病、败血症，往往是邪气入了营分。败血症好治一些，白血病难治一些，两种病症都通常伴随着发斑。败血症的斑非常明显，红得吓人，全身都是红点，很快变成紫色，这是血热，血入营分的表现，用点犀角会好得特别快；白血病也发斑，斑是淡红色的，千万不要以为粉红、淡红的斑好治，其实这样更难医治。越是邪恶的人，表面越温柔，越是不张扬。所以这种暗暗的，略微有点粉红的斑越可怕。

禁用犀角并未保护犀牛

现在犀牛角已被禁用，连中医古籍中提到犀牛角都要注明"用替代品",目的是为了保护已经濒临灭绝的犀牛。

其实,过去用犀角的时候,并不是猎杀取角,而是等犀牛死后再用。中医非常注重物尽其用,通常是把制作犀角工艺品剩下的边角料打成粉来救命。现在犀牛角虽然禁用了,但在黑市上仍然可以买到,只不过更贵,因为成本更高了。犀牛角的价格涨上去了,偷猎犀牛的反而更多了,犀牛并没有得到保护。

这并不是中医用犀角导致的,中医对所用的任何东西都充满敬畏,尤其是犀角这一类东西,因为犀角是有灵气的。中医用犀角,首先要敬畏犀角。敬畏犀角,就不会残忍地去猎杀犀牛,而是等犀牛死后再用,而且只用一些边角料,这就是中医的姿态。

在保护犀牛的问题上,并不是单纯禁用犀角就可以解决的。而是要让懂中医、懂传统文化的,有人文情怀的人来管理,一味禁用只能导致被猎杀的犀牛越来越多。

《道德经》说:"不贵难得之货,使民不为盗。"越禁用,价格就越高,因为需求永远是在的。虎骨也相类似。虎骨禁用后,老虎死了,骨头怎么办呢?听一位朋友说,现在的老虎死后就把虎骨一直冻在冰库里。虎骨是温热药,一直冻在冰里,时间久了,它就失去虎骨的作用了,其实也是一种浪费。

犀角地黄汤和安宫牛黄丸

在治疗白血病的某些阶段,可能要用到犀角地黄汤。现在因为没有犀角,其治疗效果会差一些。"犀角地黄汤"是《千金方》里的方子,《外台秘要》里也有,《温病条辨》依然在用。

犀角地黄汤:

芍药、地黄、丹皮、犀角

地黄用的是生地黄。芍药往往用赤芍,当然有时也用白芍,或者赤白芍都用一些。为什么要用赤芍呢?因为赤芍走血分,能凉血散血。方义其实很简单,用药性的四气五味就可以解释。

四味都是寒凉药,芍药酸寒,地黄甘寒,丹皮苦寒,犀角咸寒。酸、甘、苦、咸都有了,还差辛寒、辛凉。为什么没有呢?因为这时邪气已入血分,意味着没有表症了,不用解表就不用辛凉药了。用酸寒、甘寒、苦寒、咸寒泻五脏之火,来清血热。生地、丹皮、赤芍是一组非常重要的凉血药，再加一味犀角，犀角只需 1 克左右就可以了。

犀角地黄汤清热解毒、凉血开窍的功效特别大。现在西医讲的肝炎，严重到肝昏迷，热象非常严重的时候可以用；尿毒症到了热象非常严重的时候也可以用；过敏性紫癜、白血病、败血症都可以用。

安宫牛黄丸也用到犀角。现在的安宫牛黄丸用水牛角代替犀角，作用就大打折扣了，但依然有凉血开窍、清热解毒的作用。

现在犀牛角的代用品就是水牛角。水牛跟犀牛很相似，它们都生在水中。凡是生在水中的哺乳动物都有一定的凉润性。用水牛角代替犀角，用量要大很多，一般来说 60 克水牛角才能代替 0.5 克犀角。即便这样，它们的作用还不能完全等同。为什么呢？从外形上也可以看出来。犀牛角长在鼻子上，鼻子属于阳明部位，所以犀角走阳明，清阳明实热。水牛角长在两侧，两侧属于少阳部位。两种角在动物身上所处部位不一样，入药后在人体行走的部位也不一样，功效就有所差异。所以，虽然可以用水牛角来代替犀角，但是它们之间的差异还是有的。

人中白和秋石

童便、人中白和秋石

尿壶用久了，里面结一层白霜，把它刮下来，就是人中白，有的地方叫尿冰。

并不是所有人的尿壶里的尿冰都有用，古书讲"蒙馆童子及山中老僧者为佳"。一般人的都不能用，为什么呢？因为带火。没有发育的小孩，他们的小便是干净的。他们没有多少情绪，没有男女之事，吃的不至于太杂乱，思想也不是太复杂。老和尚有修行，身体比较清静，年轻和尚的都不行。

同样是小便，不同人的差异也非常大。其实，大小便都是排出人体的废物和毒，毒从哪来？从饮食和情绪中来。所以晚上睡觉，相当于人体关门打扫，这时"人卧则血归肝"，肝把血过滤一遍，清洗一遍，把白天饮食和情绪产生的毒过滤出来，早上通过大小便排出体外，排便后，人又清清爽爽的了。大小便里有很多毒，入药时就不能用含毒比较多的。

人中白还提示我们，千万不要憋尿。尿壶里的尿放一宿能结出白霜，尿在膀胱里憋一宿也会结出不好的东西。憋尿最后导致淋证，就是结石等各种病。

人中白咸寒，可降火，把郁热往下引导。小便从尿道排出，它轻车熟路，作为药喝下去依然从尿道排出。所以童便是咸寒的药，用来降火行瘀的。过去人摔到内脏了，用云南白药治。没有就用童便，一方面补充津液，另一方面可以化瘀，还不伤人。

把童便、石膏一起炼制，就成了秋石。炼秋石有一套很复杂的工艺，这里就不多讲了，因为我们没有这个设备。炼秋石在湖北黄冈、安徽安庆一带较多，安庆现在还有秋石厂。

童便、秋石、人中白的作用比较相似，只略微有差异。童便降火行瘀，治血症、跌打损伤、瘀血在里、产后血晕挺好。童便除了行瘀。秋石主要滋阴退热，因为经过炼制，治虚劳咳嗽、痨热比较有用。人中白的作用是行瘀、除热、降火。

人中黄与金汁

人的大便，也能做成咸寒的药，如人中黄和金汁。

人中黄怎么做呢？冬天用毛竹，两头都留节，刮掉最外面那层薄薄皮（为什么要把皮刮掉呢？竹子最外面的那层皮有收涩性，如果留着，竹筒的通透性就不好了，但是里面的竹茹要留着），然后在竹子外面钻个孔，用甘草细粉把竹筒装满。装满后，把芭蕉叶的叶柄削得跟竹筒的孔一样大小，塞进去封好口。芭蕉叶的叶柄见水膨胀，会把竹筒孔隙全部塞满，密封性好。

冬至那天，将竹筒浸到大粪池里，立春以后取出。为什么冬天浸泡呢？因为冬天大便寒凉，不容易腐烂，夏天则大便腐烂生蛆，秽浊不堪。取出后，把竹筒打开，将甘草末倒出，放在通风处阴干，这就是"人中黄"了。

人中黄甘、咸、寒，是大解热毒之品，通行五脏。甘草解毒，人的大便性寒。竹子性寒，非常洁净，也很致密，大粪通过竹子的过滤，相当于只有一部分的大粪汁渗透进甘草末中去了，所以污浊东西就不多了。这是一种萃取大粪精华的方法呀！所以人中黄能够大解热毒。

金汁是什么呢？取健康男孩的大便，滤汁装坛封好，埋到土里，而且必须埋到路底下，埋好后再把路填好，路上会有很多人走，经过很多年才能取出，时间隔得越久越好。取出后，你会发现，粪水变得清亮，没有臭味。

书上说，金汁苦、咸、寒，但如果埋得太久太久了，它就会变得甘、苦、咸、寒。入心泻火解毒。遇到瘟疫，热邪特别旺盛，邪热犯心包让人发狂，或者毒让人受不了，病势非常严重的时候，就用金汁或人中黄来解。喝下去就有效，速度特别快。用于急救，能降一切火，解一切毒。必须阳明有实热才能用，如果阳明没有实热，人虚虚的、蔫蔫的，用这个是会伤人的。

金汁、人中黄为什么会有这些作用是因为人中黄、金汁的重浊往下走，从胃到大肠，走得特别快，把毒和火都带下去。

这些药的原理我们都知道，但从来没用过，就是怕病人心理上难以接受，所以一般都会用别的药代替，就是效果差点、速度慢点。

咸寒类药小结

有关咸寒药，植物类有车前子；矿物类有药芒硝、朴硝、玄明粉、浮海石；动物类有牡蛎、瓦楞子、海蛤壳、犀牛角；最后与人相关：秋石、人中白、人中黄、金汁、童便。

Chapter 6 Bitter-cold Medicines

Huangqin, Huanglian and Huangbai are the representatives for the bitter-cold herbs. Huangqin clears heat in the Upper Jiao; Huanglian clears heat in the Middle Jiao; and Huangbai clears heat in the Lower Jiao. Briefly speaking, bitter-cold herbs target at severe heat symptoms. In case that the excess heat symptoms are extremely serious, bitter-cold herbs must be used to clear them away, which is called "bitter-cold medicines break heat straightforward" in TCM.

Analyses of Bitterness and Coldness

Tsun-ren Chen, an experienced TCM doctor from Hongkong, once met a maniac patient in Shanghai. The patient had rapid pulse, red facial color, crimson red tongue color with thick and greasy yellow tongue coating; and he was talking deliriously the whole day, "Please forgive me, Mr. Huang, I offended you before...". His family members even did not know which Mr Huang was the patient referring to and thought Mr. Huang was a ghost. Lots of doctors had tried various methods, but failed to cure the patient until one day Dr. Chen prescribed a formula containing the herbal ingredients of Huangqin (scutellaria baicalensis), Huanglian (coptis chinensis), Huangbai (phellodendron amurense), Huangzhizi (gardenia jasminoides), Sheng Dihuang (radix rehmanniae recen) and Sheng Dahuang (raw rheum officinale), etc.. After taking two to three doses, that patient ceased to scream "Mr Huang..." and recovered gradually.

Heat Causes Dizziness and Coldness Clears It up

Heat pathogens-related diseases can cause patients to become maniac and delirious. The primary symptom of fire pathogen can be simply summarized as "clear outside but confused inside", which means fire lights up the surroundings and sends out lights, but it will cause confusion and unconsciousness inside the body. From the perspective of personality, fire-character persons often show the personalities of "clear outside but confused inside", which means they seldom agree with or even often argue back with the others. Apparently, they seem to be sensible and clear-thinking, but actually the innermost being is a big mess.

Heat and fire can make one feel dizzy, while coldness can make one become clear and refreshed. Therefore, the fire-heat symptoms have to be treated with cold medicines.

Bitter-cold herbs generally have a function of eliminating dampness and clearing the heat including the excess heat and damp-heat. The bitter-cold herbs have another property, i. e. , a larger dosage has a larger potency dimension (the TCM principle of "bitterness purging heat"); a smaller dosage has a function of intensifying Yin (the TCM principle of "bitterness consolidating Yin").

Yin-consolidation with bitter taste is an important principle in TCM. Bitterness is able to make consolidation, which is the feature not only applicable to herbal effect, but also to human lives. Chinese people often use "bitter-cold" to describe a living status of a person (which means tough life). To some extent, "bitter-cold" conditions are good for a person since under the "bitter-cold" conditions one can always come to reason, while those who are living prosperous and wealthy life may tend to become cock-a-hoop. This is quite similar to a patient who recovers form dizziness and confusion due to heat pathogen after taking bitter-cold herbs.

One can survive and stand fast to keep his or her head in a "bitter-cold" condition, but the condition should not be overly tough since it may make one lose self-confidence and hope towards life. Similarly, too bitter herbs may cause impairment of Yang.

Restricting Hyperactivity to Keep Balance

Bitter-cold herbs are yellow in color, and generally their Chinese names often contain a Chinese character "黄"(Huang, means yellow). The yellow color is subsumed to the earth in the **Wuxing Doctrine**, corresponding to sweetness among the five tastes (sour, sweet, bitter, pungent and salty). It is unexplainable in modern science that the bitter-cold herbs are often yellow in color, but it is explainable according to **Huangdi Neijing**, which says " hyperactivity is harmful and should be restrained. " This means that if any one of the five elements in the **Wuxing Doctrine** is in excess, it will bring in harm, and then, another element will appear to impose some restriction on it, just as the saying goes, "too much water drowned the miller."

Zhang Yuansu in the Jin dynasty wrote a book named "*Yixue Qiyuan*" (*Medical Initiations and Sources*), saying, "The *Tao* of the **Wuxing Doctrine** (i. e., wood, metal, water, fire, earth) is that they behave as themselves when they are in small and proper dimension; however, they may behave like ghosts and thieves when they are in a state of excess, which means if they become too vigorous, the antagonistic element will start to take action." For instance, wood exists with its own attributes only when it is in the proper dimension; if it goes too far, it will change into a substance with other attributes.

And again, earth corresponds to dampness, while wood corresponds to wind, and wood restricts earth. When there occurs an unclear damp symptom, the manifestation is just dampness. At this stage, the patient's tongue usually is covered with thick and greasy coating and the tongue body becomes fat with teeth marks. Such a symptom is called "behaving as itself when it is in small and proper dimension". However, if the damp symptom turns very serious, the patient may start to tremble, which is a manifestation of wind. This is called "behaving as ghosts and thieves when it is in a state of excess." Damp pathogen is subsumed to earth; wind pathogen is subsumed to wood; and wood restricts earth, therefore, the wind symptom will occur when the damp pathogen becomes too vigorous.

Water droplets condensed on the window during winter time is an example of "too much coldness being transformed into dampness".

Similarly, breeze is considered as the wind; once the wind gets too strong, it will bring in some dryness since wind is subsumed to wood, and dryness is subsumed to metal. Too much wind will finally be transformed into dryness.

Extreme dryness will be transformed into fire since dryness is subsumed to metal and fire restricts metal. Too much dryness will be transformed into fire. That is why the dry substances catch fire easily.

This in TCM is a very important concept that is often used to analyze the transformation between the five pathogens (coldness, heat, dryness, dampness and wind) and the weather changes, including the six pathogens (wind, coldness, heat, dampness, dryness, fire) and the five elements (wood, metal, water, fire, earth). From the perspective of the **Wuxing Doctrine**, the fertile soil at a place means the Qi of earth is strong enough for trees to grow, which is actually the phenomenon of "too much earth will be transformed into wood."

A luxuriantly growing tree means it has so excessive Qi of wood that the wood will become harder in texture, which will be likely to bring in "disaster" of being chopped down by axes or saws. This phenomenon is called "extreme wood will be transformed into metal". The dead tree, if it still has excessive Qi of wood, may be fossilized into petrified wood (subsumed to metal category). This is called "too much wood will be transformed into metal."

In the battlefield, two warriors may fight face to face with cold weapons. The collisions of the two weapons often cause sparks. This phenomenon is called "too much metal will be transformed into fire".

The sores and ulcers on the skin are subsumed to fire, showing reddish color with a symptom of fire. When the fire is too vigorous, the sores and ulcers will no longer be red any more, but become festering and running ulcers. Similarly, meat gets rotted and decomposed into liquid more easily in summer. These are the phenomena called "too much fire is transformed into water".

The earth and sand always can run with flowing river, and settle down at the wide riverway to form a river delta. This is called "extreme water is transformed into earth". By the way, water in Chinese culture does not mean H_2O only but something larger in scale such as river, lake and sea.

Thorough understanding of the principle of "restricting hyperactivity to keep balance" can help one to comprehend why most of the bitter-cold herbs are yellow in color. The common cold herbs, such as Lugen (sweet-cold), generally do not appear to be yellow as Huanglian and Huangbai that are so bright yellow in color. Also, the cold herbs like Hanliancao (eclipta alba), Nuzhenzi (fructus ligustri lucidi) and Heshouwu (polygonum multiflorum) are black in their natural color, which are not too cold in nature. Only those herbs that are cold enough to certain degree will appear to be yellow-the color of earth.

Coldness is subsumed to water; earth restricts water; and extreme coldness is transformed into earth. Furthermore, in the **Wuxing doctrine**, the extremely bitter herbs correspond to the fire (hot in nature), but water restricts fire and extreme fire will be transformed into water (corresponding to coldness). Therefore, the extremely bitter taste must be cold in nature.

Huangqin (Scutellaria Baicalensis)

Huangqin enters the heart, lung, large intestine, small intestine, liver, gallbladder and the spleen channels, strong in taste but weak in Qi. The bitter taste is able to clear the heat out of the heart and lung. In addition, the bitter taste can also consolidate Yin, therefore, it can also intensify the Yin of the stomach and intestines. Heart and lungs are at the highest location among the five internal organs, enjoying the most abundant Yang, and these two organs may easily accumulate pathogenic heat, which tends to ascend. Thus, the heart and lungs are susceptible to the internal heat or fire. Huangqin enters the heart and lungs to clear heat, entering the stomach and intestines to clear heat and intensify Yin, and going into the liver and lung channels to remove damp-heat.

Huangqin clears the Upper Jiao while concurrently functioning in the Middle Jiao. Its effect can be intensified for ascending by processing it with liquor. The liquor-processed Huangqin can clear the heat above the diaphragm and resolve the long-lasting pathogenic heat accumulated in the lungs.

Huangqin has a good effect on clearing the lung heat, especially the excess heat. The lung is an organ where heat arises frequently, but some particulars must be taken for clearing the lung heat. The exogenous pathogen attack should be tackled by opening up the pores to disperse the pathogenic heat by the way of inducing sweat; the excess heat due to pathogenic attack on the lungs should be eliminated with Huangqin; the long-lasting pathogen attack accompanied with lung deficiency will have to be treated with Sangbaipi (cortex mori) and the like.

Withered Huangqin and Striped Huangqin

There are two types of Huangqin. One is the withered Huangqin that is an old and hollow root, appearing yellow outside and somewhat black inside. The withered Huangqin enters the lungs and moves along the exterior of the body to clear the long-lasting stagnated fire. In addition, it is similar to the large intestine, yellow and hollow in shape and color, therefore, it is able to clear the heat in the large intestine and treat all types of diarrhoea and dysentery.

Another type is striped Huangqin or alternatively named as "Ziqin", referring to the newly grown tender roots. Both withered and tender roots of Huangqin are harvested in August. The tender root is yellow with slightly greenish color. The green color means it enters the liver, therefore, the striped Huangqin is more inclined to go into the liver. Furthermore, the striped Huangqin also enters the lungs and performs a descending function; it is especially good at clearing the pathogenic fire in the liver and gallbladder. That is why striped Huangqin is used in the formula **Longdan Xiegan Tang** instead.

Some formulas use Huangqin in a poetic Chinese name "Qing Ziqin" (greenish Huangqin) to help the patients to relax themselves since many patients who have little knowledge about Chinese medicine always feel worried about the bitterness and coldness of Huangqin to cause Yang impairment.

Dahuang is another example. There is a saying, "Renshen (Ginseng) kills without fault, and Dahuang (rheum officinale) saves without merit", which means ginseng may also kill a patient if too much of it is used, but it will not be blamed at all since ginseng is a valuable herb; however, when Dahuang is used instead, even if it cures the illness, the patient may not believe it is Dahuang that does the work since Dahuang is not so valuable as ginseng.

Generally, most people are very cautious about Huangqin, Huanglian, Huangbai and Dahuang since they can impair the stomach due to their bitter and cold properties. Doctors often write Dahuang as "Jiang Jun" (means "general"). In formulas, "Shengjun" refers to raw Dahuang, "Chuanjun" refers to Sichuan Dahuang, "Jiujun" refers to liquor-processed Dahuang, which is just to help patients get relaxed.

Compatibility of Huangqin

The combination of Huangqin with Baizhu (white atractylodes rhizome) has the function of miscarriage prevention. Pregnant women usually suffer from poor T&T function in the Middle Jiao, resulting in heat stagnation. Furthermore, those who are in pregnancy have to be very cautious about use of herbs, especially, the bitter-cold herbs. Hence, Huangqin is used for clearing heat since Huangqin mostly goes to the Upper Jiao rather than to the Lower Jiao to disturb the fetus. In addition, Huangqin is able to get through the obstruction in the lungs, liver, large and small intestines, spleen and gallbladder. It is also mild in property and effective for clearing heat.

In such a combination, Huangqin is to clear stagnated heat and Baizhu to tonify spleen and to prevent miscarriage. Besides, Sharen (fructus amomi) may be added for upbearing purpose if necessary. In fact, for miscarriage prevention, Huangqin and Baizhu are the crucial herbs that are very effective for dealing with the threatened abortion caused by fetal heat. Therefore, The formula of **Taishan Panshi San** also contains Huangqin and Baizhu.

Huangqin and Baishao (radix paeoniae alba) are the common paired herbs to treat dysentery. The bitterness of Huangqin and sourness of Baishao functioning together can help discharge the damp-heat as quickly during dysentery. In addition, the sour taste of Baishao also plays an astringing role to preserve the life essence in body. Based on this herbal combination, Gancao may be added to slow down function of Huangqin and Baishao and tonify the spleen as well.

Chaihu and Huangqin are another important herbal pair. **Xiaochaihu Tang** contains the ingredients of Chaihu (radix bupleuri), Huangqin (scutellaria baicalensis), Dangshen (codonopsis pilosula), Banxia (pinellia ternate), Ginger and Dazao (jujube). Huangqin is one of the important herbs in this formula. Chaihu moves along the Shaoyang channel to reach the exterior, whereas Huangqin enters the Yangming channel to clear the internal heat. When pathogens stay at the half interior and half exterior stage to form stagnated heat, these two herbs may be used to clear it.

Another well-known formula is **Chaiqin Wendan Tang** that is a modified formula by adding Chaihu and Huangqin into the formula of **Wendan Tang** (recorded in *Qianjin Yaofang* by Sun Simiao). The formula of **Wendan Tang** contains the herbal ingredients of **Erchen Tang** plus Zhuru (bamboo shavings) and Zhike (fructus aurantia) or alternatively Zhishi (fructus aurantii immaturus) and Shengjiang (fresh ginger). The main function of **Wendan Tang** is to clear the phlegm-heat from the gallbladder channel.

In addition, **Longdan Xiegan Tang** also contains Chaihu and Huangqin for treating diseases related to the liver and gallbladder with their main functions of cooling the stagnated heat in the liver and gallbladder and eliminating the stagnated heat from the Shaoyang channel.

Bitterness and Coldness Impair Stomach and Contraindications of Huangqin

It is a biased opinion to say Chinese medicine impairs the stomach. Some of them do, but some do not. Therefore, it is not correct to treat different herbs as the same. In fact, any medicine, if used long, will bring in harms. Long-lasting use of bitter-cold herbs such as Huangqin, Huanglian, Huangbai and Longdancao does bring in impairment to the stomach functions, resulting in a poor appetite etc. .

However, Lugen and Tianhuafen (radices trichosanthis) nourish the stomach and does not bring in impairment to the stomach no matter how much they are taken. Those patients with Yin or Yang deficiency should not take bitter-cold herbs since frequent use of Huangqin does cause impairment to the stomach. Therefore, stop using Huangqin whenever there arise obvious impairment symptoms.

Huangqin can help clear the lung heat if it is used properly, but improper use may help the heat pathogens go further into or be trapped in the lungs. In that case, it may be very troublesome to eliminate the heat pathogens. With reference to the pulse conditions, the floating pulse means the pathogen is on the surface, for which Huangqin is not necessary; the weak pulse usually means blood deficiency, due to which the patients may not be able to tolerate the extreme bitterness and coldness. In such a case, the patients must be very cautious about the use of Huangqin.

Huanglian (Coptis Chinensis)

Characteristics and Functions of Huanglian

Huanglian is an extremely bitter, cold and dry medicine. It is well-known that Huanglian is bitter, but in reality, it is not the bitterest herb. In comparison, Longdancao (radix gentianae), Luhui (aloe) are much bitterer. Then why did our ancestors annotate Huanglian as a typical bitter herb? There is a Chinese saying, "Be the seventh and not the first", which signifies the seventh means to be relatively outstanding, while the first always means to be absolutely outstanding. In the real world, however, there is only relative excellence, and there is never absolute No. 1. Therefore, the Chinese people would rather be the seventh than the absolute first. Similarly, when it comes to the bitter herb, TCM takes Huanglian rather than the bitterest herb as an example to give illustration, which is to leave a room for life.

Huanglian enters the heart and spleen channels, clearing the fire, drying dampness and clearing damp-heat. However, it can only be used for clearing the excess heat and fire pathogens, or otherwise, Huanglian should not be used. Besides, bitterness and coldness often damages the Yang, which means Huanglian should not be used when a patient is suffering from Yang deficiency. Similarly, for the patients who are suffering from Yin deficiency, Huanglian should not be used, either, since bitter-cold herbs can impair the Yin resulting in dryness and fire; and eventually the fire symptoms become worse. As a matter of fact, for clearing Yin-deficiency fire, the most appropriate way is to use the sweet-cold herbs to nourish Yin.

For this reason, many people belittle the bitter-cold herbs like Huanglian. It is incorrect to have the idea of classifying herbal medicines into the good and the bad. In critical practices, the key is whether a doctor can use the herbs properly or not.

Han Mao and Jiaotai Pill

Han Mao, a TCM expert in the Ming dynasty, was famous for using Huanglian, saying "for the diseases involved with fire, Huanglian should be the first choice. " He wrote a book called *Hanshi Yitong" (Dr. Han's Medical Experiences)* with only thirty-seven pages, which is full of true love. Therefore, I prefer to call this book as **"The Classic of Filial Piety in TCM"**.

Han Mao's father was a general. Back in his time, there were endless wars and fights, and his father had to go out to battles, living a very tough life, which brought him a lot of diseases. Han Mao then put everything aside but devoted himself to learning TCM and took great care of his father in the battlefields. The book mainly recorded how he gave medical treatment to his father and other family members. His worries about the sickness of his family were all shown between the lines in the book, which also shows that he wrote the book with feelings of love. As it is always said, "absolute sincerity will move a heart of stone." With such a strong will, he acquired an extraordinary medical skill. *Hanshi Yitong* raises the concept that "Danggui cures illness in blood system; Xiangfu (rhizoma cyperi) cures illness in Qi system; Banxia (pinellia ternate) cures illness related to phlegm; Huanglian cures illness related to fire." All the other herbs may be used along with these four herbs, i. e. Danggui, Xiangfu, Banxia and Huanglian.

Han Mao is great since he made a lot of famous and effective formulas, such as **Sanzi Yangqin Tang**, and **Jiaotai Pill**. **Jiaotai Pill** contains only two herbs of Huanglian and Rougui (cassia bark), which is particularly used for curing insomnia, since Huanglian is for treatment of the fire-related diseases, to which insomnia is related as fire disturbs the mind. Therefore, a large dosage of Huanglian is used to clear the fire. Rougui is able to guide the fire back to its origin – the place where it is supposed to be. Meanwhile, Rougui is warm in property, so it can counteract the bitter-cold properties of Huanglian.

Huanglian is bitter-cold for nourishing Yin to clear the heart fire and Rougui is pungent-warm for nourishing the kidney Yang. They function together to mutually keep calm in order to cure the insomnia arising from imbalance between heart-Yang and kidney-Yin.

Zuojin Pill and Other Formulas for Gastric Acid Regurgitation

The formula of **Zuojin Pill** contains Huanglian and Wuzhuyu (fructus evodiae) at a ratio of 6:1. An important treatment principle in TCM is "**Zuojin Pingmu**", i. e., assisting the metal to soothe the wood". Metal in TCM refers to the lung while wood refers to the liver, so, "**Zuojin Pingmu**" means to assist the lung to soothe the liver. However, **Zuojin Pill** has nothing to do with the lung; actually, Zuojin should be named as **Pingmu Pill** (literally means soothing wood pill). The liver likes to be dispersed. In the case of depression of hepatic Qi, the liver stagnation can be easily transformed into fire to disturb the stomach, causing stomach disorder like acid regurgitation.

This formula uses a large dosage of Huanglian to purge the stomach fire for the purpose of clearing the liver fire. A small dosage of pungent-hot Wuzhuyu in the formula is also added for the purposes of descending the counterflow Qi and stopping vomiting due to the stomach fire on the one hand, and neutralizing the gastric acid and relieving stomach-ache on the other hand. Besides, Wuzhuyu can restrain the bitterness and coldness of Huanglian. Wuzhuyu can also direct the effect of Huanglian to the liver since its warm property is similar to the liver fire. Therefore, according to the TCM principle of "like attracting like", Wuzhuyu in this formula is acting as a "traitor" and leading Huanglian to the liver to eliminate the liver fire.

Wuzhuyu and Huanglian are the perfect match since Wuzhuyu and Huanglian are playing the warming and clearing functions respectively to soothe the liver and clear the fire, upbear the clear and descend the turbid in order to bring in a very good effect for treatment of gastric acid regurgitation. However, for the long-lasting acid reflux, Wuzhuyu and Huanglian may not work so effectively that the calcined Walengzi can be added since it also has the efficacy to control the gastric acid.

Xianglian Pill and Other Formulas for Dysentery

There is another formula called **Xianglian Pill** in which Huanglian is used. Regarding this formula, there are many versions, but the most classical one contains only two herbs of Huanglian and Muxiang (costustoot) for the treatment of dysentery, recorded in the book of *Taiping Huimin Hejiju Fang (Formulas of People's Welfare Pharmacy)* in the Song Dynasty.

Dysentery is usually caused by irregular meals or other exogenous attacks like wind, coldness, dampness or summer-heat pathogens, resulting in the damp-heat pathogens trapped in the stomach or intestines. Some of the pathogens may be discharged via dysentery but some still stay inside to grow continuously, which will then transform the ingested food and the substances retained in the stomach into sticky turbid toxins, causing diarrhoea again. Such a process is going on and keeping the patient going to stool over and again.

Dysentery is a foul disease that may kill the patient. **Xianglian Pill** is often used for curing dysentery with a very powerful function though it contains only two herbs. Huanglian is bitter and cold to dry dampness and clear the heat, while the symptoms of dysentery are dampness and heat, which are sourced at the heart and spleen. Huanglian is taken as the monarch herb in this formula since it can enter the large intestine to clear the damp-heat directly out of the heart and spleen channels, and eliminates the source of damp-heat. Wuzhuyu is not shown in the formula, but in reality, Huanglian is usually processed by the way of parching with Wuzhuyu-soaked water for reducing the coldness of Huanglian on the one hand, and sending down the turbid so that the turbidity of dysentery can be purged completely; on the other hand, the effects of Huanglian can be taken to the liver as well to clear the heat concurrently. Muxiang moves the Qi while it warms the spleen and stomach, ensuring the smooth circulation and functions of the Tri-jiao. And also, Muxiang purges the lung of pathogenic fire and soothes the liver in order to avoid the wood (i. e., the liver) restricting the earth (i. e., the spleen). Thus, the spleen and stomach will become peaceful and harmonious.

Shanghan Lun records a formula called **Baitouweng Tang** for curing dysentery. Actually, this formula can be used together with **Xianglian Pill**, which will bring in a pretty good effect.

In addition, there is another formula called **Qinlian Gegen Tang** for dysentery, which contains Huangqin, Huanglian and Gegen (radix puerariae). Essentially, the clear Qi is supposed to ascend while the turbid Qi is supposed to descend. Or otherwise, the turbid Qi moving upwards will induce vomiting; the clear Qi moving downwards will induce diarrhoea. Gegen is used to upbear the clear Qi, while Huangqin and Huanglian can clear heat and drive the turbid Qi and damp-heat pathogens to go downwards. Moreover, Gegen can also induce sweat to relieve the exterior symptoms to bring down fever.

Gancao may also be added in this formula since Gancao is able to reconcile the effects of the other herbs in order to harmonize the Tri-jiao and the stomach-intestine, after which the clear Qi will go upwards and the turbid Qi will go downwards normally. Thus, dysentery will be cured naturally.

Other Uses of Huanglian

Huanglian enjoys lots of functions, for instance, the single herb Huanglian decoction is able to wash away the eye diseases like red and swollen eyes arising from the excess fire. The washing effect may become much more effective if oral decoction is taken at the same time. How to distinguish the excess fire from the deficiency fire depends on the syndrome differentiation. The acute disease often develops very rapidly, which definitely arises from the excess fire. Such eye diseases can be washed away with Huanglian decoction.

Diseases with the symptoms of pain, itching and sores are all associated with the heart, and therefore, the formula containing Huanglian and Danggui as the monarch medicines, Gancao and Huangqin as assistant/adjuvant herbs can cure various sores and surgical diseases. That is the common herbal combination used by the TCM practitioners in the ancient time, and can still be used as a reference to date.

Huangbai (Phellodendron Amurense)

Huangbai is a tree cortex, bitter and cold in properties, entering bones, the kidneys and the bladder channel as well. It particularly goes downwards to clear pathogenic heat in the kidneys.

Zishen Tongguan Pill

Zishen Tongguan Pill contains three herbs: Huangbai (phellodendron amurense), Zhimu (rhizoma anemarrhenae) and Rougui (cassia bark). Damp-heat trapped in the Lower Jiao will cause disruption of pneumatolysis. Therefore, Huangbai and Zhimu are used in this formula for clearing the damp-heat in the Lower Jiao, followed by Rougui to guide the fire back to its origin to promote the process of pneumatolysis. This formula reflects the concept of simultaneous use of cold and hot medicines. Similar to this formula, there are many other formulas containing only two or three herbs to show the effectiveness of mutual restraints and simultaneous use of cold and hot medicines in order to achieve certain balance between medicines.

Zhibai Dihuang Pill

Zhibai Dihuang Pill is made based on the formula of **Liuwei Dihuang Pill** plus Huangbai and Zhimu. Huangbai enters the blood system, and Zhimu enters the Qi system. Therefore, **Zhibai Dihuang Pill** on the one hand tonifies the kidneys, and on the other hand Huangbai and Zhimu in the formula function to clear the damp-heat pathogens out of the kidneys.

In case the Kidney Yang needs warming up, Fuzi may be added to the formula of **Liuwei Dihuang Pill**, so that both Qi and blood can be warmed up with the help of Fuzi going to the Qi system and Rougui going to the blood system. Attention is called to the principle of using paired herbs, that is, both the herb for Qi system and the herb for blood system should be taken into consideration so that the effects of the herbs for both systems can bring out the best in each other, which will be far more effective than the two herbs used separately.

Sanmiao San

Sanmiao San contains Cangzhu (rhizoma atractylodis), Huangbai (phellodendron amurense) and Niuxi (radix achyranthis bidentatae), mainly for clearing the damp-heat from the Lower Jiao.

Huangbai itself functions to clear the damp-heat from the Lower Jiao, but in case the dampness is more serious than heat, Huangbai alone may not be sufficient for drying dampness, so Cangzhu is added to intensify the effect of drying dampness. Cangzhu is specialized in drying dampness, entering the spleen and the Middle Jiao, tonifying the spleen, after which the T&T function can be activated to further eliminate dampness from the Lower Jiao. Therefore, the synergistic effect of Cangzhu and Huangbai pair is exceptionally effective for clearing damp-heat from the Lower Jiao. Cangzhu and Huangbai used together make a formula called **Ermiao San**.

Niuxi is added to **Ermiao San** to direct the medicinal effect of Cangzhu and Huangbai further downwards. It is quite similar to the concept of targeted therapy so that the effect of clearing the damp-heat in the Lower Jiao can be intensified.

第六章　苦寒药

　　黄芩、黄连、黄柏都是苦寒药的代表，黄芩清上焦之热，黄连清中焦之热，黄柏清下焦之热，简而言之，苦寒药针对大热，如果实热非常严重，就必须用苦寒药去清，这在中医里叫"苦寒直折"，就是用苦寒药直接把热折掉截断。

苦寒解

　　香港老中医陈存仁，在上海行医时，看过一个病人，发了狂，脸红脉数，舌苔黄腻，舌质暗红，一天到晚说胡话："黄先生，你饶了我吧，以前我确实得罪了你。"他的家人也不知他到底得罪了哪个黄先生，都以为黄先生是个鬼。不少医生用了各种方法都没有治好，后来经过会诊，最后开了一个方子：黄芩、黄连、黄柏、黄栀子、生地黄、生大黄……，病人吃了两三剂便不再喊"黄先生"了，慢慢地好了。

火能令人昏，寒能令人清

　　病人发狂说胡话，是火症。火有一个明显的特征，叫做"外清明而内浊昧"。在外会照亮外围，给人光明；在体内则会让人头脑发昏。在性格上，火性格的人也是"外清明而内浊昧"的，这样的人总是看别人不顺眼，别人说一句，他会说十句反驳，好与人争短长，看似明白事理，思路清晰，内心却是一团糟。

　　火能令人昏，寒能令人清。火证就用寒凉药来治。

　　苦寒药一般都有燥湿清火的作用，不仅能清实热，还能清湿热。苦寒药还有一个特点，大剂量用时，清火力度大，所谓"苦以泻火"；小剂量用时，有坚阴作用，所谓"苦以坚阴"。

　　"苦以坚阴"是中医的重要原则，苦就能坚，不仅药具备这种性质，人也具备这种特性。中国人常用"苦寒"一词来形容人的一种生存状态。对于人来说，苦寒的环境有时反而是好的。比如大富大贵、得意洋洋的人，他的头脑往往是昏的，可能有时都不知道自己是谁了，但是一旦陷入苦寒的环境里，他的头脑会马上清醒过来，这就好比病人被热邪弄得头脑昏昏，喝了苦寒药就能清醒过来一样。

人在苦寒的环境中，会很冷静，也会有所坚守。但是环境也不能太苦，用药太苦就会伤阳气。生活环境太苦了，很多人就会失去自信，失去对生活的希望。

亢则害，承乃制

苦寒药一般都是黄色的，药名通常带个"黄"字。黄色属土，在五味上对应甘，为什么苦寒药都是黄色的呢？用现在的科学理论没法解释，但用《黄帝内经》的理论是可以解释的。《内经》有一句："亢则害，承乃制"，意思是说在五行中无论哪一行太过，都会有害处，接着就会出现制约它的那种属性。

金朝张元素的《医学启源》很有名，书中讲："五常之道，微则当其本化，甚则兼其鬼贼。"五常之道"就是五行之道，"微则当其本化"是说当五行每一行只有一点的时候，那么它就是它。假如太多，那么与之相克的属性就出来了。譬如说"木"，一点"木"是"木"，"木"太多就变得不像"木"了。

再举个具体点的例子：与土相对应的是湿，与木相对应的是风，木克土。当只有一点湿象的时候，它就是湿象。病人一般舌头舌苔滑腻，舌质胖大有齿痕，这叫"微则当其本化"。如果湿很严重，病人可能会颤抖，颤抖是风象，这叫"甚则兼其鬼贼"。因为湿邪属土，风邪属木，木克土，湿邪太过就会出现风象。

冬天外边冷，屋里窗上凝结出水珠，这就是"寒过极而兼湿化"。

小风那是风，风太大就会出现燥象。风属木，燥属金，风太过就会出现燥化。

燥过极则兼火化。燥属金，火克金，燥得太厉害就会着火，燥到了极点就会火化。

这种思想在中医里非常重要，要经常分析寒、热、燥、湿、风五种邪气、天气之间的转化。无论针对六淫还是整个五行而论都是这样。从五行的角度讲：某个地方土壤肥沃，就是土气过盛，就会长树木，这就叫"土过极则兼木化"。

木头长得太好，木气太旺，木质就会变硬，引来斧锯之灾，这就叫

"木过极则兼金化"。总之你太好了，克你的东西就来了。大树死后，如果未能充分腐烂，木气过旺不能运化掉，也会从金化，变成化石，所以有一种"木变石"，这都叫木过极则兼金化。

古人打仗，张三将军举刀便砍，李四元帅举起方天画戟相迎，两件兵器碰到一块火星直冒。金属碰撞摩擦时，金气最旺，就会着火，这就是"金过极则兼火化"。

身上生疮疡，诸痛疮疡皆属于火，只有一点火的时候它就会发红，一派火象。火太大的时候，它就不再发红，而会溃疡、流脓、流水；夏天肉容易腐烂，肉烂就会淌水。这些都是"火极则兼水化"。

土随水流，在河道的宽阔处沉淀下来，就会形成三角洲，这就是就"水过极而兼土化"。中国人眼中的水，不是水分子，而是指江河湖海。

知道了"亢则害，承乃制"的原理，就能理解苦寒药为什么多是黄色了。普通寒药，例如甘寒的芦根，它基本不发黄，不像黄连、黄柏黄得那么鲜艳；又如旱莲草、女贞子、何首乌，它们都是寒的，也都是黑的，黑是其本色，还不是太寒，只有寒到一定程度，才能成为黄色，呈现土的颜色，

因为寒属水，土克水，寒过极则兼土化。从另一个角度看，在五行里极苦的药对应的是火，应该是热的，但是水克火，火极则兼水化，水对应的是寒，药苦到极点则必然是寒的。

黄芩

黄芩归心经、肺经、大肠经、小肠经、肝经、胆经、脾经，味厚而气薄。味苦就能清心肺之热，苦以坚阴，能坚肠胃之阴。心肺在人体中位置最高，阳气最多，容易积累邪热，火性炎上，内火常往心肺走，所以是最容易热的。黄芩入心肺，能清热；能入肠胃，清热坚阴；走肝经、肺经，去除湿热。

黄芩清上焦，兼入中焦，可以通过用酒炮制来加强它往上走的作用。酒黄芩能清膈上之热，化肺中积累已久的邪热。

黄芩清肺热的效果比较好，不过要注意，肺有里热实热才能用它来清。肺最容易生热，清肺也有很多讲究。肺受外感，应该打开毛孔，通过出汗的方式把热往外透散；邪气入肺里，且是实热，才可以用黄芩；肺虚邪气深陷经久，则用桑白皮之类。

枯芩和条芩

黄芩有两种。一种叫枯黄芩，是黄芩的老根，中间部分烂空了，外面黄色，里面带一点黑色，走肺走表，清遏郁已久的火，它色黄中空，像大肠一样，能清大肠之热，治各种泻症和痢疾。

一种叫条芩，又叫子芩，一条一条的，是新发的嫩根，八月采收时，老根嫩根一起拔，然后分开。嫩根色黄，带一点青头，青色入肝，所以条芩入肝多些。条芩还能入肺，往下走，善除肝胆火邪，龙胆泻肝汤就要用条芩。

有的方子中写青子芩，名字很好听。过去病人也是懂一些中药的，很多人看到黄芩之类的药就会头疼，生怕苦寒药伤了阳气，有些医家就写成别的名字，让病人放松警惕。

就像大黄，过去讲"人参杀人无过，大黄救人无功"，就是说你给病人开了人参，即使把他吃死了，病人也不会怪你，毕竟你用了那么金贵的药。如果开了大黄，即便把病治好了，病人也不认为是大黄起了作用，可见这类药很冤枉。

大家普遍对黄芩、黄连、黄柏、大黄比较警惕，因为它们苦寒败胃。医家通常将大黄写作"将军"。生军就是生大黄，川军就是川大黄，酒军就是酒大黄。后来大家慢慢地都知道了，这些写法便又成了公开的秘密。

黄芩的配伍

黄芩配白术有安胎作用。孕妇通常中焦运化不好，郁积生热。怀孕期间不能乱用药，苦寒药尤其要慎用，故清热常用黄芩。因为黄芩以走上焦为主，不会去下焦伤胎。而且它能通肺、肝、大小肠、脾和胆，走的地方多，且比较平和，清热的作用又好。

用黄芩清郁热，用白术健脾、安胎，如果有下坠的感觉，还可以加砂仁往上升提。黄芩、白术是非常重要的安胎药，治胎热造成的胎动不安效果非常好，所以泰山盘石散里就有这两味药。

黄芩、白芍是治痢疾的常用对药。黄芩是苦的，白芍是酸的，酸苦涌泄为阴，痢疾时需要让湿热浊气尽快涌泄出去。用黄芩、白芍不仅能起到酸苦涌泄为阴的作用，还能酸收，把好东西收住，其中黄芩还能起到清湿热的作用。不要小看这两味药，他们都承载了很多功能。在此基础上还可加一味甘草，甘以缓之，且能健脾。

柴胡、黄芩也是一个重要的药对。小柴胡汤由柴胡、黄芩、党参、半夏、姜、枣组成，其中用了黄芩。黄芩、柴胡也是常见对药，一个走表，一个走里。柴胡，走少阳经达表；黄芩，走阳明经清里。当邪气半表半里形成郁热的时候，可以用柴胡、黄芩来凉解。

还有一个有名的方子叫柴芩温胆汤，由柴胡、黄芩加温胆汤组成。温胆汤是二陈汤加竹茹、枳壳，有的是加枳实、生姜，主要用于清胆经痰热。温胆汤出自孙思邈的《千金方》，当时的药方里面，生姜特别多，生姜多药就是温性的了，所以就叫温胆汤。

龙胆泻肝汤也用到了柴胡、黄芩。柴胡、黄芩常用来治疗肝胆疾病，其作用主要是降肝胆郁热，解少阳郁热。

苦寒败胃与黄芩禁忌

中药伤胃的说法，其实是一种偏见。有的中药伤胃，有的中药不伤胃，中药并非只有一种，不能一概而论。长期服用黄芩、黄连、黄柏、龙胆草等苦寒类药，多用久用往往会败胃，导致食欲减少等问题。

芦根、花粉等中药则是养胃的，喝多少也不会把胃喝坏。血虚的人，无论阴虚、阳虚，都不能用苦寒药。黄芩不要多用，用多了确实会伤胃；只有表症时也不要用黄芩。

黄芩，用对了能清肺热，用错了却又能把热往肺里拉，将热困在肺里，再想清掉会很麻烦。从脉像上看，脉浮，意味邪气在表，不要用黄芩；脉细，意味着血虚，人体承受不了黄芩的大苦大寒，则要慎用黄芩。

黄连

黄连性能

黄连是一味极苦、极寒、极燥的药。人们都知道黄连苦，其实黄连还不是最苦的药，更苦的药还有龙胆草、芦荟等。为什么古人只讲黄连苦，不讲龙胆草苦呢？中国有一句话，叫"只有第七，没有第一"。什么意思？第七意味着相对优秀，第一意味着绝对优秀，绝对的第一。世界上只有相对的优秀，没有绝对的第一。中国人宁可做第七，不愿做第一。所以中国人说药也是那样的，说到最苦的药不会把最苦最苦的药拿出来，只说黄连，不说那些更苦的，他要留一点余地。

黄连入心、脾经，能清火、燥湿、清湿热。但是必须有实热、实火才能用，否则不要轻易地用黄连。苦寒伤阳，阳虚也不能轻易用黄连。阴虚也不要轻易使用黄连，因为苦寒下夺，会伤阴，伤阴就会化燥、化火，然后火反而越来越大。清阴虚之火，宜甘寒养阴。

因此，有很多人就非议黄连等苦寒的药。实际上，药无优劣，关键在于人善不善用。

韩懋与交泰丸

明朝有一位医家叫韩懋，可谓善用黄连，他讲"火分之病，黄连为主"。他写了一本书，叫《韩氏医通》，只有三十七页，但是内容非常好，情真意切，我把这本书称作"医门孝经"。

他父亲是一位将军。在他生活的年代，战争不断，他父亲经常出征在外，很辛苦，落下了一身的病。韩懋就什么都不做，一心要把中医学好，跟着出征，给父亲治病，可以说是为父学医，书中记载的，也主要是为家人治病。当家里人生病了，他那种急切的心情是溢于言表的，这些病案也都是带着很深的感情去写的。精诚所至，他的技艺也很高。《韩氏医通》提出："当归主血分之病，香附主气分之病，半夏主痰分之病，黄连主火分之病"，其他的用药，可以围绕这几味药来。

韩懋这个人非常不简单，他自创的很多方子后来都成了名方，非常有效。比如三子养亲汤、交泰丸。三子养亲汤我们前面讲过。交泰丸是专治失眠的，只有两味药，黄连、肉桂。黄连的量大，肉桂的量少。黄连是主火分之病，失眠跟火有关，火扰心神，所以人睡不着，所以用大剂量的黄连清火。肉桂能引火归元，让火去它该去的地方，而且它性温，又能反佐黄连的苦寒。

黄连和肉桂，一苦寒一辛温，一阴一阳，一清心火一温肾阳，二者相互作用能让阴阳交泰，所以用于治疗心肾不交的失眠。

左金丸与治疗吐酸的方药

用到黄连的还有左金丸：吴萸用一份，黄连用六份。中医里面有一个重要的治疗原则，叫左金平木。金是肺、木是肝，左金平木，就是帮助肺来平肝。但左金丸跟肺毫无关系，其实应该就是平木丸。肝喜条达，当肝气不舒的时候，肝郁就会化火，肝火就会犯胃，表现出胃病，如吐酸等。

这个方子重用黄连，是用来泻胃火，通过泻胃火来泻肝火。加一点点辛热的吴萸，这是用来干什么的呢？因为一旦有胃火的时候，人就会呕，用了吴萸既可以降逆止呕，还可以制酸、止胃痛，还能约束黄连的苦寒之性。吴萸还能引黄连入肝，因为吴萸是温肝的，正好与肝火能够同气相求。吴萸在这里相当于一个叛徒，它带着黄连往肝里走，黄连就清了肝火。

吴萸和黄连是一对绝配，一温一清，能疏肝清火，升清降浊，治疗吐酸作用非常好，如果是那种顽固的、过久的吐酸，用吴茱、黄连还治不好，可以加上一味煅瓦楞，它也有制酸的作用。

香连丸与治疗痢疾的方药

用到黄连还有一个小方子叫香连丸。香连丸有很多种版本，最经典的版本是《太平惠民和剂局方》里的，就是两味药，黄连和木香，它是治痢疾的。

痢疾通常是因为饮食不节，饥一顿饱一顿导致的；要么是外感风寒暑湿，邪气内陷，湿热盘踞肠胃，它能够通过痢疾排出来一些，但还留着一些，继续增加，把一些吃下去的好的东西，或者肠胃里面本来就有的东西，蒸化成那种黏黏糊糊的恶浊之物，又往外拉，总是拉不尽，老感觉要上厕所，拉出一些浓浓的东西，这就是痢疾。

痢疾是一种恶疾，有时能拉死人的。治疗痢疾就经常会用到香连丸，虽然只有两味药，但它的作用很大。黄连，苦能燥湿，寒能清热，而痢疾就是湿热。湿热的源头在心脾，黄连能入大肠清湿热，又把湿热的源头给堵上，它是直接清心经和脾经的，因此用黄连作为君药。这里面没有写吴萸，其实黄连通常是用吴萸水炒一下，这样吴萸就能带着黄连去清肝，还能减轻黄连的寒性，还能降浊，让痢疾的浊气充分降干净。木香能够行气，同时还能温脾和胃，通利三焦，还能泻肺、平肝，让木不克土，保脾胃安和。

《伤寒论》治疗痢疾的还有一个方子叫白头翁汤，其实白头翁汤可以和香连丸一起用，效果也是蛮好的。

治疗泻痢的，还有芩连葛根汤，就是黄芩、黄连、葛根这三味药。我们知道，人体本来应该清气在上，浊气在下。当浊气在上，人就会吐；清气在下，人就会泻。葛根是升清气的，黄芩、黄连能够清热，让浊气、让湿热之气往下降。而且，葛根不但能够升清，还有一些发汗的作用，可以解表、退热。

当然这里边还可以加一味甘草，甘草是调和这些药的，它能够调和三焦，调和肠胃。肠胃调和，清气上升了，浊气向下降了，人的泻痢自然就没有了。

黄连的其他用途

黄连的用途很多，例如用一味黄连煎汤来洗眼睛，一切的因实火而起的眼病，如眼睛红肿，都可以用。如果配合内治，效果会更好。有人会问，怎么判断是虚火还是实火呢？很容易，如果眼病的时间太长，那就要仔细的去辨证了。如果是急性的，发展很快的，这肯定是实火，用黄连煮水洗，大胆地洗，没有问题。

诸痛疮痒，皆属于心，我们还可以用黄连、当归作为君药，甘草、黄芩作为佐药，治疗各种疮，乃至外科疾病，这是古人的常用配伍。我们现在仍可以作为参考。

黄柏

黄柏是一种树皮，它也是苦寒的，它能入骨、入肾，兼入膀胱经。它特别善于往下走，能清肾里的邪热。

滋肾通关丸

我们曾经讲过一个名方叫滋肾通关丸，它由三味药组成：黄柏、知母、肉桂。黄柏知母是清下焦湿热的；下焦被湿热困住，气化就会不利，用黄柏、知母把这些邪热清掉，然后再用肉桂，引火归元，促进气化，这也体现了寒热并用。所以很多这种两三味药的方子都体现了互相制约、寒热并用。黄柏知母是寒凉的药，肉桂是温药，它们之间就能达成一种平衡。

知柏地黄丸

知柏地黄丸是在六味地黄丸的基础上加知母和黄柏。知母走气分，黄柏走血分，要清肾里的湿热，就要在补肾的基础上加这两味清热的药。

如果要温肾阳的话，就是在六味地黄丸补肾的基础上，加附子走气分，肉桂走血分，那么就气血都温了。用对药有一个原则，往往是一个走气分，一个走血分，气血都兼顾了，它的作用就会相得益彰，就不是一加一等于二了，而是一加一远远大于二。

三妙散

三妙散由苍术、黄柏、牛膝三味药组成，主要用于清下焦的湿热。

黄柏本身就清下焦的湿热，如果湿重于热，那么黄柏燥湿的力度是远远不够了，所以加一味苍术，燥湿的力度就大了。苍术是专门燥湿的，还入脾经，入中焦，能健脾，一健脾就能化，能把下焦的湿进一步带走，所以苍术、黄柏清下焦湿热，效果比较好，这两味药在一起叫二妙散。

再加牛膝，引药下行，能让苍术、黄柏进一步往下走。这相当于靶向治疗，这样清下焦湿热的作用会更加明显。

Chapter 7　Bitter-Cold Medicines for Clearing Heat in the Liver

According to the **Wuxing Doctrine**, the liver is subsumed to the wood and wood is able to give rise to fire. Hence, much endogenous fire is originated from the liver and gallbladder, which means that clearing the fire must start with clearing the heat from the liver and gallbladder.

Longdancao (Radix Gentianae)

Longdancao is a type of grass with a very thin root. As a medicine, the root is usually picked in autumn and winter. It is mainly used for purging the damp-heat in the liver channel.

Longdancao in Chinese literally means "the Dragon's Gallbladder Grass". Dragon is a fierce animal, showing an image similar to a tornado (in Chinese Pinyin, it is "Long Juan Feng", which means the dragon rolls the wind) or waterspouts (in Chinese Pinyin, it is "Long Xi Shui", which means the dragon sucks water) in spring and summer seasons. Regardless of a natural phenomenon or an animal, it manifests that Yang Qi gives vent outwards violently under the sky. However, "dragon" (tornado and waterspout) will dive inside and hide up when obtaining Yin Qi, and that is why it is hard to see "dragons" in autumn and winter.

"Dragon" can also trigger up-and-down movements, poetically described as "leaping up and soaring into the spacious universe, or diving into and hiding up in surge billows". Such a phenomenon of the nature is quite similar to the liver fire, as it ascends to trigger the pericardium fire and descends to trigger the kidney Yang. As it is known, the kidney is subsumed to water, representing rivers, lakes and seas, and the heart and lungs are like the sky. When the liver fire floats in between the sky and water, it can trigger both the heart and kidney fire. Hence, once the liver fire burns up, it will put the heart and kidney in flame accordingly, so the liver fire is alternatively called "Fire of Dragon and Thunder". Gallbladder bile tastes bitter and has a descending function that can downbear fire and clear heat. So, the name of Longdancao suggests that it can clear liver fire and gallbladder heat.

Longdancao is bitter and acerb in tastes and severe cold in property. It enters the liver, gallbladder and stomach channels, functioning in the Qi system of the liver and gallbladder channels. As it is known, bitterness and coldness can eliminate fire; the bitter taste dries dampness; and coldness clears heat. Therefore, Longdancao can clear the damp-heat in the liver and gallbladder channels. And also, this herb goes to the Lower Jiao.

Treatment of Stranguria with Longdancao

Many diseases are involved with the liver fire, such as stranguria.

Regarding stranguria, it mainly includes five types: Qi stranguria, blood stranguria, stone stranguria, grease stranguria, and chronic stranguria. All types of stranguria primarily manifest frequent micturition and urgent urination, or the serious cases of odynuria, or yellow and reddish urine, or even urination occluded with sand or stone (called stone stranguria, which means urethral calculus). They are all attributed to damp-heat that arises from binge drinking, overeating, emotional disorder, or excessive sexual life, and so on. Damp-heat is the most terrible symptom to the liver.

When the liver and gallbladder damp-heat is trapped in the Lower Jiao, it will result in failure of Qi transformation, eventually bringing about stranguria. In the case of damp-heat stranguria, Longdancao should be used to clear the damp-heat with addition of some tasteless herbs that can induce diuresis such as Mutong (caulis akebiae), Tongcao (tetrapanax papyriferus), Zexie (rhizoma alismatis) and Fuling (poria cocos) and the like.

Besides, there is another type of stranguria called cold stranguria stemming from cold pathogens, with the manifestations of difficult urination and shivering before urination. For such cases, Longdancao should not be used. Even for the stranguria resulting from heat, in case the patient has already taken too much cold herbs, Longdancao should also be avoided. In general, Longdancao is only used for treatment of difficult urination or other similar symptoms triggered by damp-heat trapped in the Lower Jiao.

Treatment of Eye Diseases with Longdancao

Longdancao is often used for eye diseases, too.

The liver opens its orifices at the eyes. When damp-heat pathogens are trapped in the liver channel, and the heat is dominant over dampness, eye diseases will arise. The severity of ophthalmological disorders varies. A little gum in the eyes is normal at the time of waking up in the morning, while too much gum usually indicates liver heat; or some people may shed tears when lying down, which is also an indication of the liver heat, but these are just minor cases. In case the symptom becomes more serious, showing pathological changes at eyes, the first action to take is to clear the damp-heat in the liver, since the liver is an organ that is Yin in physique and Yang in function. Damp-heat usually occurs from disharmony between its Yin and Yang, for which Longdancao may have to be used. In addition, Longdancao is often paired with Chaihu for ophthalmologic diseases.

Killing Parasites with Longdancao

Longdancao is often used for killing parasites, too.

Similar to bugs and worms, parasites are born or transformed in/from the damp-heat environment. In the life, one may experience that insects grow out of the herbs kept at home in a particular year, especially in the first half of the year, but not in the other years, since in a particular year, the first half of the year is cold and dry; however, in some other years, the first half of the year is damp and hot, especially in the rain season (called plum rain), and under the severe damp-heat conditions. Likewise, when there is excess damp-heat in the human body, parasites will propagate terribly, which then results in diseases.

Longdancao itself does not kill the parasites directly, but it alters the environmental conditions where the parasites reside by clearing off the damp-heat so that parasites cannot survive. Therefore, it is the pathogens that lead to the growth of parasites, which then deteriorate the conditions of the disease. Thus, it is very important to transform the environment of the parasite growth and kill parasites as well.

TCM not only stresses the "killing" of pathogens, but it pays more attention to improving the health conditions under which the pathogens may not survive, as such, the parasites will be strictly controlled naturally.

Germs and parasites on the one hand need damp-heat environment, and on the other hand, they need wind for survival. Wind connects to the liver, so, when there is damp-heat in the liver channel, the pathogenic wind in the liver will function to assist the growth and reproduction of parasites and germs. Therefore, clearing damp-heat of the liver channel will indirectly come with pesticidal effect.

Treatment of Jaundice with Longdancao

Longdancao is used frequently for treating jaundice as well. Jaundice is classified into Yin or Yang types, and both types will manifest as yellow at the eye sclera, then yellow colors preads to the four limbs, eventually causing yellow color all over the body skin. These yellow manifestations are in fact caused by the excess damp-heat in the body.

There is a Chinese idiom saying "age coming with yellowish color at the eyes". Our eyes should have clear demarcation line between the black and white color. Black corresponds to the kidneys, hence the blacker the eyeball is at the iris, the more sufficient one's kidney Qi will be; the white color corresponds to the lungs, so, the whiter the sclera is, the more smoothly the overall body Qi circulation will become. That "age comes with yellowish color at the eyes" refers that both the black and the white of the eyes are turning yellow in color, which means damp-heat occurs in the lungs and the kidney Qi is not vigorous, either. That is to say one is getting old. Whenever there is damp-heat, there will appear yellow mark. The jaundice appears in the same way.

As for treatment of jaundice, there is a typical formula called **Yinchenhao Tang**, which, however, does not contain Longdancao. Generally speaking, it is unnecessary to use Longdancao to clear the damp-heat related to jaundice. However, there is one type called acute jaundice that is equivalent to acute hepatonecrosis named in the western medicine. It is an extremely quick developed symptom for which Longdancao must be used to snap the fire straight away with its bitterness and coldness.

Treatment of Skin Diseases with Longdancao

Longdancao often shows remarkable effect whenever there is damp-heat along the liver channel, including lots of dermatological disorders. From the channel and meridian map, it can be seen that many unknown pains tend to be along the liver channel since the liver is the "General-in-Chief" among the organs. Wherever the General gets in a trouble, it is often a serious trouble. Thus, Longdancao can be used for the treatment of all the diseases involved with the liver channel.

Once I met a patient who suffered from swelling pain below the knee and hepatitis B as well, characterized with a hot temper. As it is known, the diseases at this part of the body are involved with the liver channel. The oedema/swelling along the liver channel indicates dampness, and the pain often arises from heat pathogen. In fact, based on the syndrome differentiation and treatment in TCM, the swelling pain is called damp-heat. Therefore, I gave him the treatment of his swelling pain with Longdancao added in the formula, which was finally proved very effective.

Longdan Xiegan Tang

Longdan Xiegan Tang is a famous formula that uses Longdancao as the monarch herb. The formula has many versions, and here the version to be used is the one recorded in the book of *Yifang Jijie*" (*Collection of Formulas with Notes*).

Longdan Xiegan Tang contains the following herbal ingredients:

Longdancao (radix gentianae), Chaihu (radix bupleuri), Huangqin (scutellaria baicalensis), Zhizi (fructus gardeniae), Zexie (rhizoma alismatis), Mutong (akebiaquinata), Cheqianzi (semen plantaginis), Danggui (angelica sinensis), Sheng Dihuang (radix rehmanniae recen), Raw Gancao (raw liquorice).

Analyses of Longdan Xiegan Tang Formula

Longdancao is the monarch herb in this formula, going into the Jueyin liver-channel. The liver and gallbladder are interrelated organs with an exterior-interior relationship. Chaihu moves along the Shaoyang gallbladder Channel; Huangqin moves along the Yangming meridian. Chaihu and Huangqin are paired medicines that are frequently used to clear the liver heat and stagnation. Chaihu, Huangqin and Zhizi are all ministerial medicines for clearing the heat from the liver, gall-bladder and the Tri-jiao, intensifying the effect of Longdancao to purge the liver of pathogenic fire. Zexie, Mutong, Cheqianzi are bland-taste herbs used for inducing diuresis.

However, clearing damp-heat all the way will eventually cause impairment of the healthy Qi, especially impairing Yin. For nipping in the bud, some preventive measures must be taken, that is why Danggui and Sheng Dihuang as assistant herbs are added to enrich the blood and nourish Yin respectively.

In brief, **Longdan Xiegan Tang** functions to clear heat, induce diuresis and nourish Yin.

By the way, the combination of Danggui and Baishao are often used to nourish the liver and Yin. Baishao is sour with astringing effect, hence, it is not contained in **Longdan Xiegan Tang** in order to avoid the damp-heat being converged in the body.

In addition, Chaihu is used in **Longdan Xiegan Tang** instead of Chuanlian-zi (szechwan Chinaberry fruit). When the manifestation of liver Qi stagnation is not as conspicuous as the damp-heat, Chaihu should be used. The liver dislikes damp-heat the most, and it can function very smoothly once the damp-heat is cleared. Chuanlianzi can relieve stagnant Qi, but it does not take effect before damp-heat is cleared.

Uses and Contraindications of Longdan Xiegan Tang

Longdan Xiegan Tang is a very famous formula, and it can be used for treatment of many cases of excess liver Qi that generates the symptoms involved with gallbladder fire and damp-heat along the liver channel, such as bitter taste in the mouth, hypochondriac pain, epicophosis, swelling around the ears, itchiness at genitals, haematuria, or miscellaneous symptoms around the genitalia related to damp-heat along the liver channel.

Once a patient was suffering from poorly differentiated squamous-cell carcinoma at the penis, stemming from damp-heat accumulated along the liver channel due to his drinking the inferior quality liquor every day, for which my teacher prescribed him modified **Longdan Xiegan Tang** to clear the damp-heat.

After that, he was given **Gehua Xingjiu Tang** to eliminate the liquor toxins accumulated in his body. At last, the patient recovered from his long-lasting sufferings.

By the way, **Longdan Xiegan Tang** has some contraindications. It may induce vomiting for those who suffer from deficiency of stomach Qi; it induces diarrhoea for those who suffer from deficiency of spleen Qi; it also induces much urination or uroclepsia for those who are physically weak. It may even induce spermatorrhea for those who suffer from deficiency in the kidney or Lower Jiao. Therefore, **Longdan Xiegan Tang** should be used with much caution in order to avoid unexpected trouble.

Zhizi (Fructus Gardenia)

There are many types of gardenia, like domestically grown largehead cape jasmine that does not produce seeds, the wildly grown cape jasmine including mountain gardenia and water gardenia. Only the mountain gardenia can be used as medical herb. The water cape jasmine is large in size and thick in the cortex and flesh, and it cannot be used as medical herb but as dyestuff.

Ascending first and then Descending

Freshly collected Zhizi is red or reddish-brown in color, and it will gradually turn yellow during the sun-drying process. The ancient medical book says it enters the heart to clear the fire. Different from other seeds, Zhizi is very light in texture, and it can float upwards (for instance, the dry Zhizi can float on the water), which means it is able to enter the lungs. Zhizi is bitter-cold in property, so, it also has descending function. In brief, Zhizi has functions of clearing and descending the heart-lung fire.

After entering the human body, Zhizi will function to ascend first because of its light weight in texture, and then goes downwards because of its bitter-cold property. This herb moves downwards slowly in a roundabout way as the ancients said "it descends in a zigzag way". Because of that, it touches on a broad area to clear the stagnated fire and the lingering heat from the Tri-jiao in a thorough way, which is also the special effect of Zhizi.

Activating the Tri-jiao

All the lingering heat pathogens cleared by Zhizi will then be excreted through urination. Zhizi is taken as an herb that can induce diuresis. In fact, Zhizi itself does not induce diuresis but only regulates the urination channel through clearing the lungs and facilitating pneumatolysis within the Tri-jiao in order to achieve the target of inducing diuresis.

The Tri-jiao is known as the organ that is like "an official in charge of dredging the water passage". It can smooth the water passage in order to alleviate water retention and help eliminate the endogenous fire through urination.

Zhizi includes kernel and peel. The kernel is able to clear pathogenic fire out of the stomach, and the peel directs the effect to the exterior of the body to relieve the exterior heat. The charcoaled Zhizi can go into the blood system to clear the heat stagnation.

Zhizi Chi Tang

Zhizi Chi Tang is a famous formula recorded in **Shanghan Lun**, containing only Zhizi and Douchi (fermented soya beans). It should be prepared by decocting Zhizi first and then Douchi added in. This formula is used to clear the slight and shallow pathogenic factors in the Upper Jiao in order to cure the dysphoria and insomnia.

Zhizi can clear the heart fire and dysphoria, i. e. , the pathogenic fire in the upper part of the body since it has light and floating nature. Douchi is fermented beans that smells stale, which can help to drive the pathogens out of the body as one may feel sick to vomit when he or she smells the stinking odour or sees the nasty substance. Therefore, these two herbs used together can bring out the best in each other

When the pathogens stay in the Upper Jiao, **Zhizi Chi Tang** can induce vomiting to help eliminate the pathogens. Meanwhile, Zhizi functions to ascend first and then to descend, which will make the dysphoria go downwards from the Upper Jiao. Besides, this formula is very effective for clearing the pathogens out of the Upper Jiao in the process of treating a common cold/influenza.

Danpi (Cortex Moutan Radices)

Danpi is the cortex moutan radices. As an herb, it is often used together with Zhizi.

Peony flower is regarded as the king of flowers. Peony can blossom with that large, bright-colored and beautiful flowers, indicating that it has very vigorous wood Qi. Therefore, Danpi can soothe the liver and dredge the the channels and vessels.

Danpi is similar to Shaoyao (paeonia lactiflora) to some extent in that they are both bitter-cold in properties. But Shaoyao tastes sour and it plays a converging function to nourish the liver and Yin, while Danpi is pungent, bitter and cold in properties and it plays a dispersing function to disperse the liver and cool the blood.

Danpi for medical use is collected from the root bark of univalve red or white peony tree. Danpi enters the heart, liver, kidneys and pericardium channels to eliminate the blood-heat.

The formula of **Liuwei Dihuang Pill** for nourishing the kidneys also contains Danpi since it enters the heart channel. The ancient TCM doctors laid much emphasis on the interconnection between the heart and kidney while nourishing the kidneys. Danpi enters the heart and eliminates the heart-fire by directing the fire downwards. Dihuang nourishes the kidneys. In the process of nourishing the kidneys, it is necessary to clear the heart-fire simultaneously since the heart and the kidneys always keep close interconnection. Once the heart fire is stirred, the kidney fire will follow instantly.

Kulianzi (Szechwan Chinaberry Fruit)

Kulianzi, also called Jinlingzi, is very common around China. However, only those withlarge-sized fruits called Chuanlianzi produced in Sichuan province of China, can be used for medical purpose. It is bitter and cold with slight toxicity in nature, therefore, it can purge the heat, and goes into the liver to eliminate the stagnation.

Now, let us try to understand Chuanlianzi through their compatibility.

Jinlingzi San for Curing Pains

The first formula regarding Chuanlianzi is **Jinlingzi San**, which contains two herbs only: Chuanlianzi and Yanhusuo (rhizoma corydalis) (Yanhusuo is also known as Xuanhusuo) for treatment of pains stemming from Qi stagnation. Normally, out of ten cases of pain, there will be nine of them involving with Qi stagnation, i. e., the obstruction of Qi circulation. The Chinese characters "通" (tōng, means "get through") and "痛" (tòng, means "pain") are quite similar in structure for both of them are composed of the same component "甬" (yǒng, means "passage" or "pathway"). When a pathway gets through, there will be a smooth traffic on it. Similarly, when the passage or channel in the human body is clear without any obstruction, the stagnation or stasis will not occur, which then would not cause any pain. Furthermore, pains are often related to the liver Qi, therefore, soothing the liver will stop pains naturally.

In addition, some pains are attributed to blood stasis that is involved with the liver as well since the liver stores blood. Once the liver fails to promote the Qi circulation, it will induce blood stasis that has to be dispersed. TCM sticks to one principle for treating pains – if the pain just occurs, **Jinlingzi San** can work; but for the chronic pains that have been lasting for many years, say 7 or 8 years, **Shixiao San** will have to be used since the long-lasting pains must be rooted in the meridians due to stasis. The formula of **Shixiao San** contains two herbs: Wulingzhi (trogopterus dung) and Sheng Puhuang (raw cattail pollen).

By the way, there are heat-related pain and cold-related pain clinically. Fire always flames upwards. If the pain is originated from the lower part and conducts upwards, it must be a heat pain. For such a pain, Chuanlianzi may have to be used since it can snap the fire straight away and soothe the liver as well. If the pain is originated from the upper part and conducts downwards, it will be a cold pain. Hence warming treatment is needed.

Chuanlianzi Used with Xiaohuixiang (Fennel)

Chuanlianzi is often used together with Xiaohuixiang to treat hernia that certainly has to be treated based upon syndrome differentiation. However, Chuanlianzi and Xiaohuixiang are often put in the formula additionally.

Chuanlianzi is bitter-cold in nature while Xiaohuixiang is pungent-warm. The combination of these two herbs demonstrates the thinking model of utilizing both cold and warm herbs at the same time. Hernia usually is caused by cold-heat complication and the liver Qi stagnation. A common symptom of a chronic hernia is one side of the scrotum suddenly grows bigger – that is a manifestation of fire. Hence, a hernia often arises from the external restraint of the cold pathogens, and the internal stagnation of heat pathogen, causing stretching pain. Therefore, for such a disease, cooling and warming treatments have to be adopted simultaneously. The pungent-warm Xiaohuixiang is used to warm up the liver and regulate the flow of Qi; at the same time, the bitter-cold Chuanlianzi is used to regulate and clear the liver Qi stagnation. Attention is called that hernia takes place at the area along the liver channel, therefore, it is essential to regulate the liver Qi in order to cure hernia.

The Pesticidal Effect of Szechwan Chinaberry Tree

The root-bark of chinaberry tree can also be used as an herb for the pesticidal effect. Many trees suffer from insects or pests growing in them, but chinaberry tree is the only exception, even ants will not crawl on it, which gives us a clear and refreshing feeling.

The root bark of chinaberry tree can be used to kill various parasites in human body. It is often used together with Leiwan (omphalia), Shijunzi (quispualis indica) and Wumei (dark plum) to remove hookworm, pinworm, roundworm, or tapeworm. By the way, it is advisable to dig deeper into the earth for collecting the bark of the root underground. Similar to what has been discussed in the previous section about the root bark of white mulberry, the root bark of the chinaberry tree close to or exposed out of the ground is toxic, too.

Meanwhile, the coarse or freshly grown bark (in greenish or reddish color) of the newly collected roots must be removed for obtaining the part of the white bark since the red color goes to the blood system and the greenish color to the liver, disturbing the normal functions of the blood and the liver.

The flower and leaves of chinaberry trees are also useful. They can be spread on the bed to get rid of various bugs, insects or pests.

第七章　清肝类苦寒药

肝属木，木能生火，所以，火从肝胆起者甚多，清火就必须注意清肝胆。

龙胆草

龙胆草主要用来泄肝经的湿热。它是一种草，根部入药。它的根很细，在秋冬季节采。

为什么叫龙胆草？龙，是暴烈的，春夏季节，会有龙卷风，或者天上有龙吸水的现象。不管龙是一种自然现象还是一种动物，它都是天地间的阳气发泄于外，非常暴烈。但龙得阴则潜，秋冬季节，我们看不见龙。

龙还能上下引动，"升则飞腾于宇宙之间，隐则潜伏于波涛之内"，这与肝火也有很相似之处，肝火往上能引动心包络的火，往下能引动肾中之阳。肾属水，相当于江湖海洋，心肺就相当于天，肝火浮游于天与水之间，既能引动心火，又能引动肾火。所以肝火一旺，就导致心火旺，也导致肾火旺。因此我们把肝火叫做龙雷之火。胆，是苦的，是降的，能清热降火。龙胆草的名称，提示了它能清肝火、胆热。

龙胆草味苦 涩，性大寒，入肝、胆、胃经，是肝胆经的气分药。它苦寒泄火，苦以燥湿，寒以清热，所以能清肝胆经的湿热，而且它是走下焦的。

龙胆草治疗淋证

因为它能泄肝火，而跟肝火相关的病太多了，例如淋证。

什么是淋证呢，淋证有五：气淋、血淋、石淋、膏淋、劳淋，主要表现为尿频尿急，严重的还会尿痛，或者尿黄尿红，甚至里面有沙石。如果有沙石，那就是石淋了，相当于尿道结石。淋证都是因为湿热导致的，湿热的原因有很多，有可能因为喝酒、有可能因为暴饮暴食、也可能因为情绪不好、或者因为性生活过度，都有可能导致肝经的湿热。而肝是最怕湿热的。

肝胆的湿热盘踞在下焦，导致气化不利，产生淋证。在淋证以湿热为主的情况下，要用龙胆草来清它，再加上淡渗的药，如木通、通草、泽泻、茯苓之类。

另外还有一种冷淋，是因寒导致的淋证，除了小便不利之外，还表现为小便之前打寒战，这种就不能用龙胆草了。因热导致的淋证，如果吃多了寒凉的药，也不宜用龙胆草。一般是因为湿热盘踞在下焦导致的小便不利或者小便的各种问题，才可以用到龙胆草。

龙胆草治眼病

治疗眼病，也会经常用到龙胆草。

肝开窍于目，当湿热盘踞在肝经、热盛于湿的时候，经常会导致眼睛的一些疾病。眼病有轻有重，如果早晨起来略微有一点眼屎，这是正常的，眼屎太多了就是有肝热。还有人一躺下就流泪，这也是肝热。这是小问题，如果问题更大了，眼睛就要产生病变，我们首先要考虑到清肝的湿热。因为肝是一个体阴而用阳的脏器，当阴阳没有协调好的时候，就成了湿热，严重的话就可能要用到龙胆草。用龙胆草治眼病的时候经常配柴胡。

龙胆草杀虫

龙胆草还经常用来杀虫。

虫是湿热所生，湿热所化。要湿热的环境才会生虫。在我家里有一些中药材，有的年份就不会生虫，有的年份它就生虫，尤其是在上半年。比如2012年的上半年是太阳寒水司天，一般就会比较凉、比较燥，就不会生虫。2009年是太阴湿土司天，家里的药很多都生虫了，为什么呢？上半年尤其是入梅后，湿热比较重。当人体内湿热过多的时候，寄生虫也会繁殖的特别厉害，从而导致疾病。

龙胆草本身并不杀虫，但它能改变虫子生存的环境，虫子没法生存了，也就死了，龙胆草是通过清湿热来杀虫的。因此我们说，起先是病引起了虫，然后才是虫加剧了病。我们治病的时候如果光想着杀虫，而不改变虫子生存的环境，那么虫子是杀不尽的。

这也是中医的智慧，它并不仅仅是打打杀杀，而是把人体体内的环境调到最佳状态，病菌自然就没法生存了，寄生虫也就得到很好的控制了。

虫，一方面需要湿热的环境，另一方面，它得风则生。风气通于肝，当肝经湿热的时候，肝的邪风也会助长寄生虫或者病菌的滋生，通过清肝经的湿热，就可以间接地起到杀虫的作用。

龙胆草治黄疸

龙胆草还经常被用来治疗黄疸。黄疸分阴黄和阳黄，它首先是人的眼睛发黄，然后是四肢发黄，最后造成全身皮肤都发黄。为什么会发黄呢？也是因为人体湿热过重。

有个成语叫人老珠黄。眼珠应该是黑白分明，黑是代表肾，眼珠越黑，代表肾气越足；白是代表肺，白眼珠越白，说明全身的气机越顺畅。人老珠黄，就是白眼珠黑眼珠都发黄，白眼珠发黄意味着肺有湿热，黑眼珠不那么黑了，也发黄了，意味着肾气也不旺了，也就是人老了。湿热所过之处都会发黄，黄疸也是这样的。

治疗黄疸有一个很有名的代表方剂就是茵陈蒿汤，其中是没有龙胆草的。一般来说，黄疸也没必要用龙胆草来清。但是，有一种黄疸叫急黄，就相当于现在西医里讲的急性肝坏死，这种病来得特别急，势头非常猛，需要用苦寒直折其火，这时候需要用龙胆草。

皮肤病用龙胆草

凡是肝经的湿热，用龙胆草都特别有效，包括许多皮肤病。大家可以查一下经络图，看肝经在哪里。很多不知名的痛，通常是肝经上偏多。肝为将军之官，将军往往容易出点事，它不是那么太温柔，肝经上的病都可以用到龙胆草。

前几天我还看了一个病人，膝盖下边到脚又肿又痛，这怎么分析呢？首先这是在肝经的部位，而且这人还有乙肝，脾气也不好，在肝经的部位出现了水肿，一按下去，皮肤半天起不来，这说明有湿，痛就是因为有热。肿痛是一种现象，把它翻译成中医辨证论治的说法就是湿热，又因为痛的部位在肝经上，所以就是肝经湿热。在辨证论治的基础上，加了一味龙胆草，效果非常好。

龙胆泻肝汤

以龙胆草为君药的有一个著名的汤剂叫龙胆泻肝汤，龙胆泻肝汤有很多不同的版本，我们选取《医方集解》里面的。

龙胆泻肝汤：

龙胆草、柴胡、黄芩、山栀子、泽泻、木通、车前子、当归、生地、生甘草。

龙胆泻肝汤方义

这个方，毋庸置疑，龙胆草是君药，走厥阴肝经。肝和胆是相表里的，柴胡走少阳胆经，黄芩走阳明经，一个走表，一个走里，柴胡和黄芩是清肝热、解肝郁经常用的很有名的药对。柴胡黄芩是臣药，山栀子也是臣药，它既清肝胆之热，又清三焦邪浮之热，加强了龙胆草泻肝热的力度。后面，泽泻、木通、车前子这三味药都是淡渗利湿的药，能导热下行，从小便排出体外。

但是一直清利湿热，必然会耗伤人的正气，尤其是伤阴，所以要防患于未然，加当归、生地。当归补血，生地养阴清热。这是佐药。

所以龙肝泻肝汤的作用就是清热、利湿、养阴。

当归、白芍可以柔肝养阴，龙胆泻肝汤为什么不用白芍呢？因为白芍是酸的，酸能收敛，现在湿热这么重，就不要用酸药来收了，怕把湿热收敛住了。

为什么不用川楝子呢？因为这里肝气不舒的现象不明显，而湿热的现象明显，肝最怕的是湿热，先清掉了湿热，肝自然就运行起来了，肝气自然就顺了。而川楝子是破气的，如果在湿热还没有清掉的情况下就来破他的气，是破不动的，还会使人很难受。

龙胆泻肝汤的使用及禁忌

龙胆泻肝汤是一个很有名的方子，用的地方也特别多。凡是肝气有余，产生胆火、肝经湿热的症状，有些是口苦，有的是协痛、耳聋、耳朵肿、阴痒、尿血之类，还有生殖器周围有的很多病症，通常跟肝经的湿热有关，都可以考虑用龙肝泻肝汤。

大概是在 06 年，当时有个病人得了低分化性阴茎鳞癌，阴茎这个部位都烂掉了，医院说不好治，后来他就找到我师父，当时我师父给他开的方子就是龙胆泻肝汤。这人的阴茎鳞癌是因为喝酒导致的湿热，他一天起码要喝三两酒，而且喝的是那种劣质酒，酒的湿热沿着肝经，往下焦沉积。

下一步就用了葛花醒酒汤，继续清他体内多年沉积的酒毒，或者说修复酒毒多年来给他带来的伤害。这例癌症治疗的相当成功。

当胃气虚的时候，吃龙胆泻肝汤就可能会吐；当脾气虚的时候，服龙胆泻肝汤就可能会泻。如果空着肚子吃龙胆泻肝汤，小便会特别的多。当然要身体好才会觉得小便特别多，要是身体不好的话，有时候要尿失禁啦。肾虚、下焦空虚的人喝这个药，就会滑精，精液会不知不觉就出来了。所以，龙胆泻肝汤一定要慎用不要乱用，一旦用错了就很麻烦。

栀子

栀子花有很多种，家养的大栀子花是不结子的，野生结子的栀子又有山栀子和水栀子之分，入药用山栀子。水栀子个头大，皮肉稍厚，只能作为染料，不能入药。

先升后降，屈曲下行

栀子在刚采来的时候是红色或红褐色的，晾干慢慢就变黄了。古书里讲它色赤入心，能清火。栀子的子跟别的子不一样，别的子质地很重，栀子这很轻，轻则能浮，把干栀子扔到水里，它就能浮在水面上。轻浮就能入肺，但它又是一味苦寒的药，又能往下降，所以，它能清降心肺之火。

栀子进入人体以后，首先会因轻浮而往上走，后又会因苦寒而往下降。它往下降的速度并不快，而且不是直接往下走，而是拐着弯儿、绕着道儿往下走的，走得就慢，古人说它"屈曲下行"。这样，它涉及的面就广，就能把三焦的郁火、一些浮游之热，仔仔细细地清理掉。这是栀子的特殊作用之所在。

通利三焦

当栀子把这些浮游之热搜刮完了之后，会从小便里排出去。因此栀子又是一味利小便的药。其实，栀子并不利小便，而是通过清肺，通过促进三焦的气化，通过通调水道，达到利小便的目的。

我们知道，三焦是"决渎之官，水道出焉"。就是说，三焦能够通调水道，能够达到利水的目的，它让小便变得通畅，让身上的火从小便排出去。

栀子里边有仁，外面有皮，栀子仁能清胃中的火邪，栀子皮能够达表，能够解体表的一些热。把栀子炒黑，它就能入血分，清血分的郁热。

栀子豉汤

《伤寒论》有一个很有名的方子叫栀子豉汤，只有两味药：栀子和豆豉。煮的时候，先煮栀子，再把豆豉放进去。它用来清上焦的轻浅的邪气，治疗虚烦不眠等。

栀子能清心火、除烦，其性轻浮升越，能清在上之火。为什么要用豆豉呢？豆豉是用豆子发酵而成的，腐烂的气味，能帮助往外发。看到别人吐出来的东西，闻到那个气味也会想吐，它与生栀子轻浮升越之行一起，相得益彰。

如果上焦有邪气的话，那就吐吧；如果上焦没有邪气或者吐不出来，也没有关系，因为栀子是先升后降的。它能把上焦虚烦之邪给降下去。尤其在治疗感冒的时候，清上焦的邪是很好的。

丹皮

经常跟栀子一起使用的是丹皮，就是牡丹的根皮。

牡丹是花中之王，它的花为什么能开得那么大、那么鲜艳、那么好看呢？花是木气的喷发，牡丹花开得好，说明它得到的木气非常旺。得木之气，说明它是入肝的；它是春天开，也是入肝的，所以它能舒养肝气、通经脉。

丹皮跟芍药有点相似，但也有不一样的地方。它们都是苦寒的药，芍药是酸的，酸主收敛，丹皮是辛、苦、寒，辛则能散。白芍和丹皮常常一起用，一收一散，都是用来养肝的，一个柔肝养阴、一个散肝凉血。

用来入药的丹皮是取单瓣的红牡丹或者白牡丹的根皮。丹皮入心、肝、肾、心包四经，可以治血中的浮火，也就是清血热。

六味地黄丸里就用到了丹皮，取其入心经。六味地黄丸是养肾的，古人在养肾的时候非常注重交通心肾。丹皮入心，清心火，引心火下行。地黄是养肾的，在养肾的时候要注意清心火。因为心肾永远是要相交的，心火一动，肾火就跟着动。

苦楝子

苦楝子又叫金铃子。苦楝树大家都应该见过，全国基本都有，入药的是四川产的苦楝子，个头大，叫川楝子。它是苦寒有小毒的。苦寒就可泄热，还能入肝，破肝气。

我们可以通过两个配伍来认识川楝子。

金铃子散治痛

第一个配伍是金铃子散，只有两味药：川楝子和延胡索。这个方是治人体气痛的。十痛九气，十种痛有九种是跟气有关的，往往是因为气不通。"通"字和"痛"字是相似的，都有一个"甬"，甬是通道，路通了可以走，通则不痛；用病字头一压，通道坏了，不通则痛。我们要疏通道路，要通过疏理肝气。痛往往跟肝相关，通过疏理肝气可以止痛。

十痛九气，还有一种是瘀血导致的。其实瘀血导致的痛也是属肝的，因为肝藏血，肝不能疏通导致血瘀滞，就得化瘀了。因此中医治痛，有一个原则，初痛用金铃子散，久痛用失笑散。如果头痛、偏头痛都痛了七八年了，用金铃子散作用就不大了，因为久痛必瘀，久痛入络。这时候都得化瘀，要用失笑散。失笑散由五灵脂和生蒲黄两味药组成。

顺便说一下，痛还有热痛与寒痛的区别。火性炎上，如果感觉是从下往上痛，是从下往上牵引或从下往上传导，那么这必然是热痛，这时候肯定要用川楝子了，苦寒直折其火，而且通肝通气。如果痛是从上往下痛，从上往下传导、往下牵扯，那么这是寒痛，就要去温它。

川楝子配小茴香

川楝子还经常与小茴香一起，用来治疗疝气。当然，疝气也要辨证论治，在此基础上，经常加上苦楝子和小茴香。

苦楝子是苦寒的，而小茴香是辛温的，一寒一温，这也体现了寒温并用的思想，因为这种疝气往往寒热夹杂，因为肝气不通才会导致疝气，疝气郁久了，一个典型的表现就是一边阴囊忽然变大，这是一种火象。因此，疝气往往是寒束于外，热郁于中，牵扯作痛，所以在治疗的时候，要寒温并用。用辛温的小茴香来温肝理气，同时用苦寒的川楝子来理肝气、破肝气。为什么时时不忘理肝气呢？因为疝气的发病部位是在肝经上。

苦楝树的杀虫作用

苦楝树的根皮也能入药，有杀虫的作用。很多树上都有虫子，唯独苦楝树不长虫子，很干净，甚至蚂蚁都没有，给人以很清爽的感觉。

苦楝树的根皮可以杀体内的各种寄生虫，经常与雷丸、使君子、乌梅等一起用，不管是钩虫、蛲虫，还是蛔虫、绦虫，它都能清除掉。挖苦楝树根皮的时候，要挖深一些，千万不要用靠近地面的、或者长出地面的皮。前面我们讲桑白皮的时候也讲过，露出地面的桑树根是有毒的，同样，露出地面的苦楝树根皮也是有毒的，所以要挖深一点。

挖出后，还要把外面的粗皮、青皮去掉，要用最里面的白皮，千万不要用靠近外面的皮，也不要用发青和发红的皮，这样才不会伤人。为什么不能用发青和发红的皮呢？红色入血分，会动血，青色就入肝，所以不能用。

苦楝树的花和叶也都是很好的东西，可以用来铺床，可以杀虫，无论是看得见的虫还是看不见的虫，床上铺了苦楝树的花和叶，这些虫就都没有了。

Volume 5
Rehmannia of Genera-Water-associated Formulas and Medicines

Chapter 1 Introduction of Water-associated Formulas and Medicines

Inducing Astringency and Storing Effects

Water in the doctrine of five viscera corresponds to the kidney, which dominates the water/fluid. Water is the source of life.

As it is known, spring means birth; summer means growth; autumn means
harvest; and winter means storing. The east belongs to wood of genera, dominating birth; the south belongs to fire of genera, dominating growth; the west belongs to metal of genera, dominating harvest; and the north belongs to water,
dominating storing. All these fundamental principles included in the traditional
Chinese culture guide us to conduct ourselves in every respect in our life. Peking
University campus has gates respectively in the east, west and south, but has no
one in the north. Why? It is because the north dominates storing, so there should
be no gate in the north. The human body also has a north gate, that is, the kidney opens at the two lower orifices, i. e. , anus and urethra, besides, the female
vagina and the male seminal orifice are equivalently the northern gates of the human body. The kidney opens there, so these orifices should all be closed for storage. Of course, it does not mean they should never be opened, but just relatively
speaking, they should be closed up.

The kidney takes charge of both urinating and defecating, but whether one
can defecate and urinate smoothly is also related to the regulating function of the
liver. The liver dominates dispersing and regulating while the kidney dominates
astringency. Only when the liver and kidney coordinate and remain in harmony,

can one defecate and urinate naturally and normally in order to hold and evacuate the waste in a natural way.

In case the kidney fails in its functions of collecting and storing, there will arise the frequent defecation. Of course, the collecting and storing functions are not the duty of the kidneys only. The spleen and kidneys have to cooperate with each other closely. The spleen should exercise control overall and carry on T&T functions efficiently, and the kidneys should induce astringency, as such, defecation can then come into control and become normal. The urination depends on the cooperation between the liver and kidneys. In case they fail to cooperate well with each other, there will arise more urination, or frequent or even urgent urination.

In addition to inducing astringency, the kidney also dominates the function of storing. The book of *Four Essentials of Health Preservation in Wan's Family* says, "the top thing is to have fewer desires". First of all, emphasis is on abstinence, which means not to have excessive desires, including sexual and material desires etc. In the narrow sense, it refers to the sexual desire, which requires attention to abstinence on sexual life in the first place. Otherwise, the kidney storing function is nothing but an empty talk, and the abstinence on any other things will become groundless.

If the kidney is unable to play its storing function, it may impose some adverse influences upon the whole body. Those who think of sexual matter day and night, or lose control of defecation and urination and piss in the pants, or lose their self-control with uneasy mind and random thoughts, would be taken as being good for nothing. All of such states are related to the kidneys, which are resulted from that the kidney fails to conceal (store) their wills well. The kidney conceals the will and the spleen conceals the intention. In case the spleen fails to excise control over all and the kidney fails to induce astringency, one's aspiration will become frail, making him good for nothing. By the way, the will is also related to the five internal organs, not only influenced psychologically but also matched and interacted psychologically and physiologically.

As the foundation of life, the kidney mainly induces astringency and dominates storing. It not only induces astringency for defecations and urination, but also seals up one's desires, and conceals one's state of mind. The ancients went on abstinence and some eremites abstained themselves from the woman's charm, which is to cultivate their willpower, or to say, the concealing and storing ability of the kidney, through which the ancients managed to cultivate their mind and their willpower. So, the ancients stuck to the concept of "Following Precepts".

Nourishing Effects

In this world of the Five Turbidities (Buddhism term), human beings always care for nothing but lust. The desire is subsumed to fire, hence, a phrase of "the fire of desire" comes into being. Desire, if any, can never be satisfied fully since it can spread like fire. The more the desire is satisfied, the more inextinguishable the fire of desire will become. Water restricting fire is an unalterable principle, a natural thing, but fire in return may also impair water/fluid, which is called "reverse impairment" in TCM, a state of pathosis. If the fire of desire is too vigorous, it will definitely cause impairment of Yin, so nourishing becomes extremely important.

To nourish means to replenish water/fluid and nourish Yin. Nourishing involves tonifying Yin, Yang, Qi and blood. The reason why many people call replenishing as nourishing.is that nourishing takes a very large proportion in various replenishment. As for replenishing process, the top priority is to nourish Yin or blood, which are the material bases of life. For reviving the body, the first thing to do is not to prevent the body from getting withered. Otherwise, to nourish Qi and Yang will only become a disaster, so, the first thing to do is to treat Yin deficiency by replenishing body fluid, i. e. , to nourish Yin.

The five internal organs store essential life substances without discharging them, so nourishing should begin from the five internal organs. The Yin of the five internal organs is stored in the kidneys, so nourishing primarily starts with nourishing the kidneys. The water-associated prescribed medicines are all for nourishing herbs represented by Dihuang (rehmannia) for nourishing the kidneys.

Some medicines will also be discussed for nourishing the liver Yin like Danggui (angelica sinensis), Baishao (radix paeoniae alba), Shanyurou (common macrocarpium fruit) and Gouqizi (fructus lycii) etc.; and for nourishing heart Yin like wheat, Zaoren (jujube kernel), and Baiziren (platycladi seed) etc., and for nourishing the spleen Yin like Shanyao (Chinese yam) etc.; and for nourishing lung Yin like Yuzhu (radix polygonati officinalis), Shashen (radix adenophorae) etc. And last, some animal medicines for nourishing Yin will also be discussed like honey, Guiban (turtle plastron, or turtle shell), E-jiao (donkey-hide gelatin) and the like.

第五卷　地黄之属－水部方药

第一章　水部方药概论

固涩封藏之性

水，在五脏上对应肾，肾主水。水是生命之源。

我们知道，春生、夏长、秋收、冬藏，东方属木，主生；南方属火，主长；西方属金，主收；北方属水，主藏。中国传统文化的这些基本原理指导我们生活的每一个方面。北大有东门、西门、南门，没有北门，为什么呢？因为北方主封藏，不能开。人体也有北门，也就是肾开窍于二阴，肛门、尿道，还有女子的阴道，男子的精窍，都相当于人体的北门。肾开窍于这里，所以这些地方都得封藏得住，当然封藏并不是关着永远不开，它是相对的。

肾司二便。肾管着大便、小便。大便小便能出来，又跟肝的疏泄功能有关。肝主疏泄，肾主收摄，肝肾协调，大小便才能正常，想憋就憋，想排就排。

如果肾的收藏功能不行了，大小便就会多。当然，收摄也不光是肾的事。脾和肾还要合作。脾要统摄，要运化得力，肾要固涩，大便才能收得住。否则，要是脾肾出了问题，大便就容易多，一天好几次。小便则是肝和肾合作，如果它们之间没有协调好，小便就会多，或出现尿频、尿急的现象。

肾除了主收涩，还主封藏。《万氏家传养生四要》讲过"寡欲第一"。首先就强调节欲，这也属于肾的封藏。要把真精固涩起来，就要节欲，不要有过多的欲望。欲，包括性欲、物欲等各种各样的欲望；狭义上讲就是指性欲。节欲，首先就是性生活要注重节制，如果不节制，肾的封藏就是

— 627 —

一句空话了，其他的节制也无从说起。

肾没法封藏，对整个身体都不好。如果人一天到晚想着男女之事，我们就说他没出息；大便小便收涩不住，见到一点事就尿了裤子，也叫没出息；心神飞驰、浮想联翩，自控能力很差，都是肾没能很好地把志给藏住，也叫没出息，这些都跟肾有关。肾藏志，脾藏意，脾不能统摄，肾不能固涩，人意志就不坚定，这人就没出息。一个人的意志跟他的五脏也是有关系的，不仅仅是心理层面的东西，心理和生理都是相匹配的、相互影响的。

作为生命之本的肾，主固涩封藏。既要收涩大小便，又要封藏自己的欲望；还要收涩自己的心神。古人节欲，甚至有些修行人会以女色为戒，这是为了修定力，也是为了修肾的封藏能力，通过修肾的封藏来修心的定力，所以古人讲以戒为师。

滋补

五浊恶世历来都是人欲横流。欲望是属火的，所以有个词叫欲火。欲望是满足不了的，就像火一样越烧越大。欲望越得到满足，越不能熄灭。水克火是天经地义的，这属于生理，水本来就该克火；但火反过来又会伤水，这叫反侮，是一种病态。欲火太盛，势必伤阴，所以滋补就非常重要。

滋意味着补水、滋阴，补则有补阴、补阳、补气、补血。为什么很多人把补叫做滋补，那是因为滋补在各种补里面占的比重非常大，要补就要先补阴，或者说先补血，这些是生命的物质基础。要补身体，首先不能让身体枯槁了，如果身体都枯槁了，你补气、补阳，只能是祸害，所以先得滋阴，就是滋补。

五脏藏精而不泄，所以，滋补要从五脏入手。五脏之阴又藏于肾，所以，滋补又以滋肾为本。水部方药都是滋补类的，以滋肾的地黄为代表。

我们还会讲到滋养肝阴的药，如当归、白芍、山萸肉、枸杞子等；养心阴的药，如小麦、枣仁、柏子仁等；养脾阴的药，如山药等；养肺阴的药，如玉竹、沙参等。最后，我们还会提到养阴的动物药，如蜂蜜、龟板、阿胶之类。

Chapter 2　Dihuang (Rehmannia)

Introduction of Dihuang

Growing Environment of Dihuang

Dihuang is a quite common plant in the north of China, dark green in color, a little bit fluffy with purple flowers in spring. It is a perennial herbaceous plant, which is deeply rooted into soil to absorb the life quintessence from the earth with nutrient collected and stored to support it to grow tenaciously in the northern barren and dry land in China mainland. Its root is very big and can be used as medicine. Rehmannia in mandarin Chinese is named as Dihuang or Disui (means "the earth marrow") referring to the life quintessence or marrow of the earth, so Dihuang growing in the vigorous land often has better medical efficacy, and that growing along the waterside even has much better effects.

Dihuang produced in Huaiqing (now Jiaozuo city), Henan province of China is the best and pure herb when used as medicine since Huaiqing situates in the central area of China, where the land enjoys the strongest and purest earth Qi. Meanwhile, this area is in the north of China, where Dihuang absorbs the northern pure Yin. Dihuang produced in Jiangsu, Zhejiang, and Sichuang provinces of China usually have poorer effects of nourishing Yin-blood comparing with that produced in Huaiqing since the south is subsumed to fire, and Dihuang growing there absorbs the southern warm Qi in the growing process. Therefore, Dihuang produced in Jiangsu, Zhejiang, and Sichuang provinces is weaker for nourishing Yin, but is good for clearing heat.

Dihuang produced in Huaiqing is characterized with large size, many knots on the surface, and chrysanthemum pattern on the cross section. It can sink immediately when it is put in water. Such Dihuang is the best in quality. Of course, Dihuang produced in the areas around Huaiqing like Shanxi province, and Bozhou of Anhui province is also good but is inferior to that produced in Huaiqing.

Properties and Functionf of Dihuang

The fresh Dihuang is yellow in color. As a medicine, it is subsumed to the earth as its Chinese name "Dihuang" implies, i. e. , "Di" is subsumed to earth, and "Huang" is subsumed to earth, too. How does Dihuang go to the kidneys now that it is more subsumed to earth from the perspective of its earth properties? and why is it such an important medicine from the perspective of tonifying the kidneys.

According to the **Wuxing Doctrine**, earth restricts water. "Restrict", in essence, refers to a necessary abstinence. Water is very easy to run rampant and cause disaster, so earth has to be compacted to build up a dam in order to bridle water. And the kidney water/fluid also follows the same way. In order to accomplish necessary abstinence, the medicine like Dihuang, which has deeply absorbed the earth Qi, should be used. Only after the kidney-fluid is controlled in a reasonable way, can it then be better stored and the life essence of the kidneys be better preserved.

Each and every medicine has its own property and function. Dihuang contains rich juice with certain sugar content, which determines its properties of nourishing Yin, while some of its deuterogenic effects of helping T&T functions of the spleen and stomach determine its function to nourish Yin, too. However, it can induce phlegm dampness and stagnation while nourishing Yin, which may easily obstruct the T&T of the spleen and stomach, and then result in a poor appetite. This undesirable effect will only arise in the case of misusing Dihuang. Those doctors who are adept in the use of Dihuang can use it to help the patients have a good appetite rather than abdominal distension or indigestion, similar to those who are adept in the use of Fuzi will not make the patients have excessive internal heat.

Fresh Dihuang (rehmannia root), Dried Dihuang (Rehmannia) and Shu Dihuang (Radix Rehmanniae Praeparata)

Dihuang can be classified into fresh Dihuang, dried rehmannia andShu Dihuang (or abbreviated as Shudi) based on the different processing methods.

The newly dug-out rehmannia is called fresh Dihuang, or fresh Sheng Dihuang (radix rehmanniae recen) . After it is dried in the sun, it will be called dried rehmannia, which is also called Sheng Dihuang (radix rehmanniae recen) . After Sheng Dihuang is repeatedly steamed, or the best way is to steam and dry it in the sun for nine times repeatedly, it will become Shudi (radix rehmanniae praeparata) .

The fresh Sheng Dihuang may be used for dispersing blood since it has not experienced the treatment of fire. Anything, if without experiencing the treatment of fire, is taken as raw stuff, which has the characters of vivaciousness or activeness, and moves inside the body quickly with dispersing functions. Once having experienced the treatment of fire, it will become inactive, move a little more slowly, and function to keep neutralized and balanced, or even stay where it is without moving.

Dihuang is greasy in general. When it is used for nourishing Yin and clearing heat, it is not expected to remain at certain points, but to move as quickly. For such a purpose, Dihuang must be kept away from fire. Hence, if it is just for nourishing Yin and clearing heat, use fresh rehmannia, or at least, use dried rehmannia.

As for dried rehmannia, the thinner and smaller, the better it will be. Dihuang has a taproot, on which there are some small lateral roots. The dried rehmannia is prepared by cutting off the side roots and drying in the sun. The fibrous roots at the side of the taproot have more mobility with little stickiness or greasiness. The commonly used Sheng Dihuang is the thin and small Dihuang. The large Dihuang is always processed into Shudi. Hence, in prescriptions, Dihuang, whenever to be used, is often written as "thin Sheng Dihuang", "large Shudi".

Fresh Sheng Dihuang, dried Dihuang and Shudi share many similar effects like nourishing Yin and going to the kidneys, but they also have some differences: Fresh Sheng Dihuang functions to cool blood and clear heat with a stronger effect for dispersing blood; dried Dihuang for cooling and dispersing blood, but it is a little bit weaker in respect of dispersing blood, and the larger pieces of dried Dihuang is inclined to nourishing Yin. Compared with the fresh Dihuang, the dried Dihuang can be stored conveniently. Shudi is no longer cool any more but a warm medicine, which is mainly used for tonifying the kidneys and nourishing Yin.

Both fresh Dihuang and dried Dihuang belong to Sheng Dihuang, but now, the fresh Dihuang is rarely used, so the dried Dihuang is then simply called Sheng Dihuang. As to the name of Sheng Dihuang, in the medical records or formulas records, the ancients sometimes referred it to the fresh Sheng Dihuang and sometimes referred to the dried Dihuang.

Sheng Dihuang (Radix Rehmanniae Recen)

Nourishing Yin and Clearing the fire

The fresh Dihuang tastes sweet with slight bitterness and it is featured with severe coldness. Hearing about the slight bitter taste and severe coldness, one may immediately come up with the metal-associated formulas discussed previously involving many bitter-cold medicines but excluding Sheng Dihuang. The previously discussed bitter-cold medicines, for example, the bitter-cold and acerb medicine of Longdancao, the bitter-cold and pungent medicine ofDanpi, and the bitter-cold and light-floating medicine of Zhizi. Dihuang is a bitter-cold and sweet medicine. In the metal-associated formulas, the bitter-cold and sweet medicines have not been discussed yet since once a bitter-cold medicine has slightly sweet taste, it will suddenly change itself from a fire-discharging medicine into a medicine with the properties of not only discharging fire but also having nourishing effects since sweet taste itself has nourishing effect. Among all the previously discussed medicines like Zhizi, Longdancao, Huangqin, Huanglian, and Huangbai, none of them has nourishing efficacy, but once they are matched with slightly sweet taste, they suddenly will have nourishing effects and can then nourish Yin.

The fresh Sheng Dihuang can enter the spleen, stomach, heart, kidney and lung meridians, and can especially clear the stomach heat and nourish the stomach Yin. Generally, in the case of deficiency of kidney Yin, the stomach fire will become stronger. The kidney Yin and Yang, or to say the kidney fluid and fire, are intertwined together, so when the kidney Yin deficiency arises, part of the kidney fire on account of finding no place for settling down will spurt upwards to the stomach, resulting in too much heat in the stomach. But such heat cannot be cleared since for some stomach heat, the more one tries to clear it, the stronger it will become. If the source of the fire is not switched off, the deficiency of kidney still exists and the fire will continue to go upwards. The fire may be cleared away temporarily, but the fire may soon run up again. Such a fire is called deficiency fire which should be cleared when it is running upwards by means of nourishing Yin so that the fire in the kidney can find a place to settle down with the help of nourishing the kidney and tonifying the kidney Yin. With such a function, the fresh Sheng Dihuang can clear away the stomach heat on the one hand, and tonify the kidney fluid on the other hand.

Fresh Sheng Dihuang (Radix Rehmanniae Recen) Cooling and Dispersing Blood Stasis

Sheng Dihuang (radix rehmanniae recen) is an important medicine for cooling blood. In reality, the formula of **Xijiao Dihuang Tang** (Rhinoceros Horn and Rehmannia Decoction) is often used to cool down blood. The formula contains Sheng Dihuang (radix rehmanniae recen), Danpi (cortex moutan radices), Chishao (radix paeoniae rubra) and Xijiao (rhinoceros' horn). However, if the blood heat is not so serious and dangerous, try not to use Xijiao. Sheng Dihuang, Danpi, Chishao will be sufficient, or some Zhizi or Shigao can be added if necessary.

Yangming meridian is a channel with more Qi and blood, and the stomach is an organ of more Qi and blood. Sheng Dihuang is for cooling the stomach, which can be accomplished by means of clearing away the stomach heat, that is, to cool blood through Yangmiing meridian. Such an idea is exactly followed in **Xijiao Dihuang Tang**, in which the fresh Sheng Dihuang is preferred.

The fresh Sheng Dihuang also has the effects of dispersing blood stasis and relieving the physiological pressure. All blood stasis or swelling resulted from the bruises by falling or wounds or injuries by a heavy blow will vanish quickly after the smashed fresh Sheng Dihuang is applied to. Of course, for reinforcing its efficacy, take some Danggui, Sheng Dihuang, Chishao, Ruxiang (frankincense), Moyao (myrrh), and Rougui, and crush them together into fine particles, and wash it down with water, which can help eliminate various pain arising from blood stasis and traumatic injuries of falls, fractures, contusions and strains. In fact, there is another more complicated prescription for traumatic injuries, which in reality requires some specific addition or subtraction of medicines according to the specific injuries in the body.

As for the function of relieving the physiological pressure by the fresh Sheng Dihuang, it may be understood as under: the stomach heat may cause psychological pressure, and the fresh Sheng Dihuang can clear the stomach heat, so it can alleviate the physiological pressure; the blood heat can also cause psychological pressure, and the fresh Sheng Dihuang can cool blood, so it can alleviate the physiological pressure; blood stasis may result in the internal obstruction leading to the internal heat, causing psychological pressure too, and fresh Sheng Dihuang can disperse blood stasis, so it can also alleviate the physiological pressure. However, only such types of physiological pressure mentioned here can be relieved with the fresh Sheng Dihuang.

Sheng Dihuang together with Maidong (radix ophiopogonis) for Storing Energy and Hematogenesis

Sheng Dihuang and Maidong are paired medicines. Sheng Dihuang enters the spleen, kidney and liver, while Maidong enters the heart and lungs. When the two medicines are used together, they, by and large, go to all the five internal organs, and help for mental tranquility and hematogenesis. In case the blood deficiency arises, one may be in very low spirits. For instance, if excessive loss of blood takes place due to injury, the wounded would turn to his unusual lack of spirit and fail to fix attention to anything, which is called lack of spirits due to excessive loss of blood.

Impairment of Yin may also lead to low spirits. Typically, the students at high school are difficult to concentrate themselves. However, nobody should ask them since that is their privacy. In this period of time, they may suffer from masturbation, which may cause hurt to their life essence, that is, hurt to the kidneys. When talking about the spirits, we always refer to the life essence that makes a person become energetic and vital. The life essence here actually refers to the kidney essence, and the spirits refer to the state of mind.

The spirits of a person always involve two of the five internal organs: heart and kidney. The kidneys store the life essence and the heart stores the spirits.

When the life essence is sufficient, one will be in the high spirit, and he will also become vigorous and energetic; or otherwise, he will be inanimate and in the low spirit, who is then unable to control himself completely, or even fails to concentrate himself on anything he does, or fails in his learning. In fact, physiology and psychology are always interconnected, so Sheng Dihuang and Maidong are often used together for achieving mental tranquility and hematogenesis as well. Whenever seeing a patient, for example, a kid whose mother complains about his or her frequent failure to concentrate himself or herself, one should immediately understand what is going wrong and also know that Sheng Dihuang and Maidong will give him or her a better effect.

Zengye Tang

Sheng Dihuang and Maidong plus Xuanshen will make a formula called **Zengye Tang** (fluid-addition Decoction), which signifies to add blood and body fluid. Generally, **Zengye Tang** is used at the later stage of the warm disease (epidemic febrile disease). The warm disease refers to the febrile disease. In case it lasts too long, it may impair fluid, resulting in dry feces. In such a case, use **Zengye Tang** to make up some body fluid, which is just like transfusion, but the only difference is that transfusion is to transfuse medicine into the blood vessel while **Zengye Tang** is for drinking a decoction of some natural herbs into the stomach so that the vital life essence arising there will be transported to the spleen, and then to the lung from where it is transported to the whole body. This is a very mild, harmonious and natural transfusion process.

After the warm disease is cured, either dry feces or rough skin arising therefrom may be treated with **Zengye Tang**. But it has some drawbacks, that is, it can only add body fluid, but not lubricate to remove the accumulation of dry feces easily. So **Zengye Chengqi Tang** (literally, decoction for adding body fluid and upbearing Qi) is often used, i. e., Dahuang and Mangxiao are added on the basis of the formula of **Zengye Tang**, and even further add Zhike, Houpo, Gancao and the like when needed according to the specific conditions. **Zengye Chengqi Tang** on the one hand can make up some body fluid, and on the other hand, it can soften the feces and discharge the waste out of the body. This formula is often

used in clinical practices. The book **Shibing Lun (Treatise on Seasonal Disea-**
ses) *records such a way as* **Getting Trough with Pine and Cypress**, that is,
based on the formula of **Zengye Chengqi Tang**, pinenut kernel, Baiziren (platycladi seed) and apricot kernel are added, and they then produce an extremely
good effect for softening the feces and discharging wastes out of the body.

Shu Dihuang (Radix Rehmanniae Praeparata)

Processing of Shu Dihuang

As for Shu Dihuang (or called Shudi), the bigger in size, the better it will
be. For processing Shudi, it is better to use the larger Dihuang produced in Huaiqing city, Henan province of China. Cut it into small pieces with a bamboo
knife, soak it in the superior Huadiao-branded yellow rice wine produced in Sha-
oxing city, Zhejiang province of China, and mix some crushed Sharen (fructus
amomi) into it thoroughly, and then, put it in a wooden utensil to steam in an
earthen pot.

The wooden utensil is a barrel that is made of wood, usually used for steaming rice. This kind of utensil is still available now in some farmers' houses in the
south of China, and even some restaurants also use this kind of utensil for cooking. In the process of steaming Shudi, iron should not be used since Dihuang is
restricted by iron. In fact, all medicines for the kidneys dislike materials related
to iron. Once contacted with iron, medicines will cause impairment to the kidneys.

Shudi is usually processed in the following procedures:

Put the wooden utensil filled with Dihuang in an earthen pot for steaming,
after which the steamed Dihuang should be dried in the sun; then steam it and
dry it again in the same way; repeat the procedure for nine times. The extent to
which Dihuang is steamed and dried depends upon the real conditions in practice.

It must be processed in such a way over and again since steaming over fire
can help Dihuang to obtain the terrestrial fire, and drying in the sun can help it
to obtain the firmamental fire. The firmamental fire is different from the terrestrial
fire. The former is going downwards, equivalent to the heart fire, while the latter

is going upwards with the nature of fire being flaring up. When both the firmamental and terrestrial fires are perfused into Shudi to change the essentially cold and cool properties of Dihuang into sweet and warm properties, the original bitter-cold taste will then turn into sweet taste.

Sharen (fructus amomi) is mixed in that it can refresh the spleen aromatically, tonify the spleen and regulate the vital Qi and collect and guide Qi into the kidneys. Shudi is greasy but Sharen can both relieve the greasy influence of Shudi and guide it to regulate the five internal organs and finally go to the pubic region. As such, Shudi can better replenish life essence, enrich blood and seal up life quintessence without any side effects.

But some businessmen always process it in a rush, and few of them would like to take so much time in steaming and drying Dihuang in the sun over and again for nine times. So, doctors in different dynasties and eras in the history have been complaining about failure to find the top-grade Shudi. Actually, whoever deals with affairs must adjust measures to the local conditions, suit measures to the different persons and act according to specific circumstances. In case Sharen is not added in the processing of Shudi, doctors may add it when writing prescriptions, which will bring about the same effect. In case the businessmen do not steam and dry Dihuang for nine times, doctors could ask the patients to decoct the medicines for a longer time, or add some other warm medicines in the formulas, that is, try to adopt the good points and avoid the shortcomings for better effects in the process of treatment of diseases.

Zhang Jingyue's View on Shu Dihuang

Of all the ancient doctors, it was Zhang Jingyue, a well-known doctor in Ming dynasty who was most adept in using Shudi. He had a very precise discourse on Shudi: "Those who suffer from deficiency of the kidney Yin would have fever, or headache, or terrible thirst, or throat pharyngitis, or cough with phlegm, or panting, or spleen and kidney cold accompanied by vomiting, or deficiency fire with blood streak in mouth and nose, or fluid flooding on the skin, or deficiency of Yin and diarrhea, or mania due to Yang floating-up, or Yin exhaustion. For those who suffer from Yin deficiency and become absent-minded, Shudi can help them concentrate on themselves; for those who suffer from Yin deficiency and rising fire, Shudi can help to suppress the endogenous fire; for those who suffer from Yin deficiency and dysphoria, Shudi can help them calm down; for those who suffer from Yin deficiency and dysphoria, Shudi can help relax themselves; for those who suffer from Yin deficiency and fluid flooding, Shudi can help restrain themselves; for those who suffer from Yin deficiency and dissipation of primordial Qi (archaeus), Shudi can guide the primordial Qi to its source; for those who suffer from Yin deficiency and loss of both the life essence and blood and become thin and gaunt, Shudi can strengthen the stomach and intestines. And the most fantastic thing is Shudi plus dispersing medicine can induce sweat since sweat is transformed from blood, and Yin exhaustion will cause the patient to be sweatless. Shudi plus warm medicines can restore Yang since Yang rises from its foundation. If without strong foundation, Yang will not go up any further. However, Yang is characterized with rapidity, so, a little Renshen will do; but Yin is characterized with slowness, a small dosage of Shudi does not work at all. "

The primordial Yin deficiency may result in many diseases like fever, or headache, or thirst, or sore and choked-up throat, or cough with more phlegm, or asthma, or even vomiting due to the cold of the spleen and kidney, or mouth and nose bleeding due to deficiency fire inducing blood upwards, or edema due to fluid flooding on the skin, or diarrhea due to Yin deficiency, or mania due to Yang floating-up, or stroke (apoplexia) or falling down in a faint..., all of which can be treated with Shudi.

For those who suffer from Yin deficiency and absent-mindedness, Shudi can be used for treatment since it is characterized with the properties of greasiness and staying at a point, which can converge the life essence to help concentrate themselves without losing attention.

Shudi is heavy in its texture and can be used for treatment of the rising fire due to deficiency of Yin. Generally, a dosage of Shudi around 20 to 30g can help downbear the deficiency fire.

Shudi is featured with tranquility, and it can suppress mania. For those who suffer from Yin deficiency and dysphoria, Shudi can be used for treatment. Shudi is of a medicine with the feature of tranquility, and in contrast, the aromatic medicines can move here and there inside the human body. Houpo, Chenpi, Sharen, or Muxiang are added in a formula can cause stomach to rumble since the fragrance of these medicines function to activate Qi inside. Therefore, those who suffer from dysphoria or endogenous fire will not be advised to use the aromatic and Qi-stirring medicines but to use the tranquil medicine like Shudi to tranquilize dysphoria, which has similar functions to the suppressing medicines.

Deficiency of Yin can make the patient become irritable both physiologically and psychologically. Such irritability shows physiological stiffness and psychological tension. The elderly people, in particular, are easily subject to stroke (apoplexia) due to serious deficiency of primordial Yin (the kidney Yin). In case the stroke is going to take place, the patient will become very stubborn and ill-tempered, which is the manifestation of impatience due to Yin deficiency. Hence, whenever there are signs of emotion fluctuation of the elderly people at home, the family members should keep their eyes open since these might be the predictive signs of serious illness. The females may also become stubborn and impatient at the time of climacterium, so the family members should show understanding and sympathy for them rather than confrontation against them. Shudi is sweet in taste and can relieve the impatience, so it can be used to treat the stubbornness and impatience due to Yin deficiency.

As for the pathogenic fluid flooding due to Yin deficiency, Shudi may be used to tonify primordial Yin for treatment of fluid flooding and detumescence.

When dissipation of the primordial Qi arises from Yin deficiency, Shudi should be used to recover it; when impairment of life essence and blood arises from Yin deficiency, Shudi should be used for nourishing and strengthening the intestines and stomach. The more fantastic thing is Shudi plus dispersing medicines can induce sweat since sweat is transformed from blood. For those who suffer from serious deficiency of Yin, if only the sweating medicine (diaphoretic) is used without Shudi added at the same time, it will cause greater hurt, and not easily induce sweat, either.

Though Shudi is a medicine for tonifying Yin, yet it may also restore Yang when used together with warm medicines since Yang rises from Mingmen (the life gate, or the gate of vitality), so, if the primordial Yin were not to be tonified, it would not be easy to restore Yang, either.

Yang is rapid in property, so a little Renshen and the like will do for tonifying Yang and Qi; while Yin is slow in property, the medicine like Shudi and the like must be used in a large dosage, otherwise, it will not function effectively. Zhang Jingyue always used Shudi in a large dosage, about 2 to 3 *liang*, which is roughly equal to 60g to 100g. In the past, before visiting Anguo market of crude medicines in China, many people often had breakfast before day break, and three hours later, they would get hungry, and then they would go to medicine stores to find some Shudi for food like the dried sweet potato. Only a few pieces would make them feel full, causing no harm at all.

Zhang Jingyue was so good at using Shudi since most of those who visited him to seek for treatment were the high officials and noble lords who were intellectuals as well. The intellectuals often use their minds, i. e., the consumption of life essence and blood. In the past, when such people became dignitary, they usually had a few wives and concubines, which would consume a lot more life essence, so for them it was important to tonify Yin and replenish the life essence, after which they might feel physically comfortable. That was why Zhang Jingyue was able to achieve success one way or another. And however, in the modern time, when one is planning to use Shudi, he or she has to make judgement according to the specific conditions and should not indiscriminately imitate the ancients' experiences.

Selection and Use of Sheng Dihuang And Shu Dihuang

Sheng Dihuang and Shudi can be used in prescriptions according to the real circumstances. In many records of ancient formulas, the names of Sheng Dihuang or Shudi were not used in prescriptions but only the name of Dihuang was written instead. So, TCM doctors should make the decision by themselves to use Sheng Dihuang or Shudi according to the different syndromes of patients. For instance, in **Siwu Tang**, Sheng Dihuang is used in some cases, but in some other cases Shudi is used instead, or even for some other cases, both of them are to be used together.

When the patient needs more nourishing Yin and clearing heat, Sheng Dihuang should be used; if the patient has more serious phlegm, Shudi may make him or her have more phlegm because of the greasy property of Shudi, so in such a case, Sheng Dihuang should be used instead; if it is for reinforcing kidney to replenish life essence, Shudi should be used; if the patient suffers from Yin deficiency and blood-heat and the like, Sheng Dihuang and Shudi may be used together. For instance, **Liuwei Dihuang Pill**, it is not named as **Liuwei Sheng Dihuang Pill** or **Liuwei Shudi Pill**. This reminds us that both Sheng Dihuang and Shudi can be used alternatively. Generally, men often suffer from Yin deficiency, so Shudi is suitable, while women often suffer from blood heat, so Sheng Dihuang is suitable.

Guben Pill and Recuperation of Diseases

Sheng Dihuang has the efficacy of generating life essence and blood. It is so named not because it is crude. It is not processed through complex procedures, but just dried in the sun; it is still yellow in color inside with strong vitality in itself. For Shudi, after repeated (nine times) steaming and sun bathing, it becomes shiningly black with its natural properties being changed into artificial properties, so it is able to tonify the life essence and blood.

Sheng Dihuang used with Tiandong (asparagus cochinchinensis) is to generate life essence and blood; while Shudi used with Maidong (radix ophiopogonis) is to tonify life essence and blood. If for the purpose of both generating and tonifying life essence and blood, Sheng Dihuang, Shudi, Tiandong and Maidong can be used together. Sheng Dihuang and Shudi symbolize the earth while Tiandong and Maidong symbolize the sky and go to the lungs. Those medicines going to the lungs are subsumed to the sky. With availability of both sky and earth, when Renshen is added, it will go to the Middle Jiao, which is subsumed to human being. All Tiandong, Maidong, Sheng Dihuang and Shudi used in one formula will mean that the sky, earth and human being are all included, which makes a well-known formula called **Guben Pill** (literally means "root-securing pill") for the treatment of withered life essence and blood of the elderly people, or for recuperating purpose after illness. In essence, **Guben Pill** is a decoction of Tiandong plus Maidong, Sheng Dihuang and Shudi, commonly used for recuperation after illness.

After treatment of diseases, recuperation measures have to be taken. Reading about the medical cases of treatments by the doctors in the history, one can find the first and second diagnoses listed are actually the critical procedures for treatment. In fact, it is not an easy work to cure an illness completely. In the process of medical treatment, the ways for a common cold or for any other different syndromes are all different. The medicines will have to be changed according to different patients' conditions. After the patient recovers, some recuperation measures also have to be taken in order to tonify what have been consumed in the treatment of diseases. Just like a tree, if there are pests inside, the forest rangers will have to dig out the pests and then fill up the hole, after which they have to earth up the tree as well. To earth up is to reinforce the root of the tree. Similarly, after a disease is cured, it is also necessary to make reinforcement with **Guben Pill**. Attention is called that pill-type medicine is often used for recuperation after the disease is cured since decoction of medicines has a power to wash something away, while pills are slow and long lasting in their effects.

Liquored Sheng Dihuang and Gingered Shu Dihuang

Generally speaking, Sheng Dihuang can affect the stomach Qi, more of which will impair patients' appetite, so Sheng Dihuang is often parched with liquor. By the way, Shudi is often parched with ginger juice, after which it will not be greasy or sticky any more.

It may be asked that Shudi has been steamed and dried in the sun over and again for nine times and also added with some Sharen, and why is it still greasy? As a matter of fact, Shudi mentioned here refers to the radix rehmanniae praeparata which is not strictly prepared in the traditional way. It may have some side effects. In such a case, some remedies need to be taken. Ginger juice is warm, and Shudi, even if it is unqualified, will become warm after it is fried with the ginger juice. Meanwhile, ginger juice has a dispersing effect and it can stimulate the appetite, so after some ginger juice and Sharen are added, the radix rehmanniae praeparata, even if not processed through repeated steaming and drying in the sun, would have the similar effects to the qualified Shudi.

While reading the ancient books, readers should try to understand the sense implied in the characters. For instance, there is one ancient book, saying, "The Sheng Dihuang fried with liquor will not trouble the stomach, and Shudi fried with ginger juice will not be greasy anymore." This is to remind us how to deal with and improve Shudi if it is not processed in a qualified way. The quality stuff is of course fine, but for the things of poor quality, one also has to find a good and proper solution to make improvement and transform them into quality things. Shudi is now frequently used, but not all Shudi are processed in the traditional procedures since according to the traditional processing method, Shudi should be kept away from iron, but now Dihuang are all steamed in the iron pots and not cut with the required bamboo knives. In the industrial mass production, the stainless blade is being used instead of the bamboo knife, which in itself damages the medicine properties, and meanwhile, Dihuang has not been steamed and dried in the sun for nine times, either. One may have no choice but use the Dihuang from the drugstores, but it depends on how he or she will use it in a proper way. Those who always complain about the medicinal materials will finally be proved good for nothing.

Liuwei Dihuang Pill

Liuwei Dihuang Pill is probably produced in line with the most popular formula, and it is also the most well-known Chinese patent medicine, which contains the six herbal ingredients as the pithy formula says, "Di Ba Shan Shan four, Dan Ling Zexie three", that is, Dihuang (rehmannia) 8 *qian*, Shanyao (Chinese yam) 4 *qian*, Shanzhuyu (dogwood) 4 *qian*, Danpi (cortex moutan radices) 3 *qian*, Fuling (poria cocos) 3 *qian*, Zexie (rhizoma alismatis) 3 *qian*. Of course, the dosage for each herb here is for reference only, and can be increased or decreased according to the specific conditions.

Origin of Liuwei Dihuang Pill

Initially, **Liuwei Dihuang Pill** was not named as it is now, but named as **Bawei Dihuang Pill** since it originally contains 8 herbs, i. e., based on the present **Liuwei Dihuang Pill**, another two herbs Fuzi (radix aconiti carmichaeli) and Gui (cinnamomum cassia blume) are added. Gui sometimes refers to Guizhi (cassia twig), and sometimes refers to Rougui (cassia bark), i. e., **Guifu Dihuang Pill** for warming the kidney Yang.

If ED (erectile dysfunction) occurs due to the insufficiency of kidney-Yang, the herbs for warming the kidney-Yang like Yinyanghuo (herba epimedii), Buguzhi (fructus psoraleae) and Bajitian (morinda officinalis) are added on the basis of **Bawei Dihuang Pill**. By the way, in **Bawei Dihuang Pill**, Fuzi and Rougui can warm the kidney-Yang directly with severe intensity. When one uses medicines, he or she must take both the slowness and urgency into consideration, and exercise a combination of hardness and softness. The added herbs of Yinyanghuo, Buguzhi and Bajitian are a little milder but their effects can last long, so they will have a stronger intensity of warming the kidney-Yang. At the same time, these three herbs can go to the eight extra meridians as well to play an outstanding function.

If there arise dysfunction of pneumatolysis and edema of legs due to deficiency of the kidneys, **Bawei Dihuang Pill** can be used with addition of Niuxi (radix achyranthis bidentatae) and Cheqianzi (semen plantaginis). Niuxi can guide the medical effects downwards and function to break blood stasis, while Cheqianzi can alleviate fluid retention. The edema of legs is actually resulted from fluid retention; therefore, it is necessary to induce diuresis for removing edema. In case patients feel thirsty, add some Zhimu (rhizoma anemarrhenae) to clear heat. Besides, some Guiban (turtle plastron) may also be added in order to nourish Yin intensively. The function of Zhimu and Guiban is for nourishing Yin and purging the pathogenic fire. If patient feel dizzy and giddy or light in the head, add some Gouqizi (fructus lycii) and Tusizi (semen cuscutae) based on the formula of **Bawei Dihuang Pill**.

What have been listed above are some common additions based on **Bawei Dihuang Pill**. Well, there is also one well-known formula by way of subtraction from **Bawei Dihuang Pill**, that is, to take out Fuzi and Gui from the formula of **Bawei Dihuang Pill**. This subtraction was made by Qian Yi, a well-known pediatric doctor in Song dynasty in his book *Key to Children's Diseases*, a book specializing in pediatrics. As a matter of fact, **Liuwei Dihuang Pill** was initially prescribed for treating various pediatric diseases.

Children are generally immature physically. Just because of kidney deficiency, some children always utter in low, timid and weak voice or even become speechless sometimes; For some children, the fontanel does not close up due to the kidney deficiency; for some children, they always look listless due to kidney water/fluid deficiency; for some other children, the white of the eyes looks very big while the black of the eyes looks very small, and their complexion looks pale due to the kidney deficiency. So, whenever all the above symptoms appear, use **Liuwei Dihuang Pill**.

There are simply two reasons for Children's kidney deficiency. One is congenital deficiency, and the other is that children are subsumed to the category of wood and they are growing up with the help of the growing vitality of the liver. Children's liver-wood is always very vigorous, which can consume the kidney water/fluid since the liver wood grows depending on the kidney fluid. If the liver wood is too vigorous, it will consume the kidney fluid, and definitely the kidneys will have to work under great pressure, and thus, the kidney deficiency arises. Under this circumstance, **Liuwei Dihuang Pill** should be used for tonifying the kidneys.

When the liver-wood is too vigorous, it will restrict the spleen-earth, resulting in either diarrhea or poor appetite or the white of the eyes turning a little blue. The liver-Yang hyperactivity can also boost pathogenic heat to cause a fever. In that case, those who have a cold will suffer very serious fever. In order to keep the liver-wood mild without pathogenic fire, it will require to nourish and conserve the wood. As long as the kidney fluid is sufficient, the liver will be able to work normally, and the pathogenic fire will not stir up anymore. Hence, **Bawei Dihuang Pill** is modified into such a typical formula of **Liuwei Dihuang Pill** now. Normally, addition of herbs to a formula is relatively easy to make, but the subtraction of herbs from a formula is usually harder to make.

Forbidden Formula of Dragon Palace

The six herbs contained in **Liuwei Dihuang Pill** are perfectly matched, and it is even taken as one of the forbidden formulas of dragon palace.

In the medical circle, there is a legend that Sun Simiao, a medical expert in Tang dynasty cured the Dragon King of his illness, so the Dragon King was very grateful to him and gave him thirty forbidden formulas. The so-called forbidden formula refers to a simplified formula without any attached analyses, whose application is passed on from mouth to mouth without literal description. Those who did not hear of the formula were forbidden to use it, and that is why it is called a forbidden formula. Those who were handed down in a direct line from the master could then use such a formula miraculously.

Sun Simiao later on wrote a book called **Qianjin Yaofang** (**Thousand Golden Formulas**) precisely consisting of thirty volumes, each of which covers one of the thirty forbidden formulas of dragon palace. It was said that **Liuwei Dihuang Pill** is also a forbidden formula of the dragon palace, but I have checked **Qianjin Yaofang**, in which **Liuwei Dihuang Pill** is not covered in fact. **Qianjin Yaofang** is a book written in Tang dynasty, while the book **Key to Children's Diseases** was written in Song dynasty. By the way, the forbidden formulas of the Dragon Palace are probably not limited to thirty only, but it might be assumed that the Dragon King only gave Sun Simiao thirty formulas, and what we can guess is that the formula of **Liuwei Dihuang Pill** is beyond those thirty formulas.

In any case, the story of forbidden formulas of Dragon Palace is just a legend. That **Liuwei Dihuang Pill** was said to be a forbidden formula of Dragon Palace is merely to stress it is an excellent prescription. When **Qianjin Yaofang** was said to contain the forbidden formulas of Dragon Palace, it is also to stress that many precious "dragon pearls" contained in this book are worth researching. Of all the formulas contained in the book, what are the so-called thirty forbidden formulas of Dragon Palace really refer to is not quite sure, but this legend will definitely trigger our curiosity to study this medical work.

Qianjin Yaofang was written in Tang dynasty, which contains more formulas but less argument and analyses; The book of **Medical Secrets from the Royal Library** is also a formula-oriented medical classic, which recorded the important secret points shown in the form of medical prescriptions. Those who are interested in exploring into the significance of **Medical Secrets from the Royal Library** have to begin with **Huangdi Neijing (The Inner Classic of Huangdi)**, **Classic on**

Medical Problems (or **Classic on** 81 **Medical Problems**), **Treatise on Febrile and Miscellaneous Diseases**. By the way, *General Treatise on the Cause and Symptoms of Diseases* should not be neglected either since it is right on the contrary to **Qianjin Yaofang**, and **Medical Secrets from the Royal Library**. General Treatise on the Cause and Symptoms of Diseases contains argument and analyses but it does not contain the formulas that could be found in **Qianjin Yaofang**, and **Medical Secrets from the Royal Library**. And therefore, the three books of *Medical Secrets from the Royal Library, Thousand Golden Prescriptions,* and *General Treatise on the Cause and Symptoms of Diseases* should be put together for study.

Analyses of Liuwei Dihuang Pill Formula

Each and every character in the name of **Liuwei Dihuang Pill** is worth thinking over.

Regarding the Chinese character "六" (Liu, Six in English), the ancient Chinese mythological fictions Hetu ("River map" in English, in which there are ten numbers, from One to Ten, among which the five numbers of "One, Two, Three, Four, Five" represent "to creation", which are respectively corresponding to "Water, Fire, Wood, Metal, Earth" in the *Wuxing Doctrine*. The five numbers of "Six, Seven, Eight, Nine, Ten" represent "to shape".) and Luoshu ("Turtleshell Pattern" in English) tells that "One" produces water, but "Six" shapes it. " "生" (Sheng in Pinyin) means "to create", and "成" (Cheng in Pinyin) means "to shape". To create water refers to the number of "one" that represents the source. In order to transform the source into real water, in number it is corresponding to "Six" that refers to the number in image-numerology. This is a quite abstract theory, but when practiced on the human body, it will become much easier to understand. The lung is the source of water/fluid, which is so called that "One" produces water; The water/fluid in the human body is finally transformed into life essence and stored in the five internal organs, which is so called that "Six" shapes it. This is the way that water/fluid is produced and shaped in the human body as it is referred to. **Liuwei Dihuang Pill**, as a patent medicine, is to nourish Yin and tonify the kidney meridian, which means it is at

"Earth-Six-Shapes-It" stage. In image-numerology, it is numerated as 6, so it is named as **Liuwei Dihuan Pill**, signifying that it can nourish Yin and produce life essence.

Regarding taste, we have known the **Five Tastes** including the sour, bitter, sweet, pungent and salty. If the "tasteless" is included, they would make the six tastes. Let us see the medicine of **Liuwei Dihuang Pill**, in which Dihuang is bitter; Shanyurou (common macrocarpium fruit) is sour; Shanyao is sweet; Danpi is pungent; Zexie is salty; and Fuling is tasteless. All the six tastes are covered, which also means that **Liuwei Dihuang Pill** has six tastes and can go to the five internal organs, laying the foundation for its nourishing Yin. In TCM theory, Qi is subsumed to Yang, while taste is subsumed to Yin, so those who are physically weak should be warmed in the respect of Qi; those who are insufficient in the life essence should be tonified in the respect of tastes. " So, the six tastes tonify the life essence of the five internal organs in order to nourish the kidney life essence.

The formula of **Liuwei Dihuang Pill** can be divided into two parts: the first part includes Dihuang, Shanyurou and Shanyao for tonifying purposes, and the second part includes Danpi, Fuling and Zexie for discharging purposes. That is to say, **Liuwei Dihuang Pill** contains three tonifying herbs (generally called **Three Tonifications**) and three discharging herbs (generally called **Three Discharges**), but how do the three tonifying herbs carry out the tonifying process? The kidney is the place where the life essence is stored, and the life essence here refers to the water/fluid coming from the lungs, which is needed for the human body, and the white-colored Shanyao goes into the lungs to open the upper source of fluid. The lungs produce the kidney fluid, so the target of tonifying the kidney to produce the life essence is accomplished by the way of tonifying the lungs. Dihuang is to tonify the kidney fluid directly, which in turn can help to nourish the liver. The kidney fluid produced should be converged with the sour medicine, and so Shanzhuyu (which also goes to the liver) is used in this formula.

The three herbs of Shanyao, Dihuang, and Shanyurou are right in the chain of inter-promoting relation in the five elements of the **Wuxing Doctrine**, reflecting the lung metal producing the kidney fluid/water, which then grows the liver wood. Hence, both the source and its circulation are taken into consideration so that the kidneys are surely tonified. This also suggests a principle in clinical practice that both the source and the target should be taken good care of while an internal organ is to be tonified. This is process of **"Three Tonifications"**.

And then, how about the **"Three Discharges"**? Fuling and Zexie can clear water/fluid channels and activate the kidney Qi. If the kidney Qi fails to function properly, tonification will go down the drain. As discussed before, the kidney is involved with Yin and Yang, containing both Yin fluid and Yang fluid. Yin fluid refers to the life essence, and Yang fluid refers to urine. Yin fluid needs to be converged and stored and Yang fluid needs pneumatolysis for being discharged. Only when Yang fluid is discharged, Yin fluid can then be consolidated, which means the smooth Yang fluid discharge can guarantee Yin fluid consolidation. Furthermore, the smooth urine discharge can guarantee the seminal fluid to be consolidated. The urine is discharged only when pneumatolysis is going on smoothly; and the seminal fluid can come out when it is stimulated by the fire. Therefore, when the fire of desire is stirred up, the seminal fluid will then come out. And in a meantime, when there is pathogenic fire, it can also disturb the seminal fluid and Yin fluid, so, add Danpi——a cold herb to clear the pathogenic fire. Without the disturbance of the fire, Yin fluid can be consolidated naturally.

As a monarch medicine, Dihuang itself is for tonifying the kidney-Yin. When it is used in **Liuwei Dihuang Pill**, its effect for tonifying kidney-Yin can be multiplied with the assistance of so many other herbs.

In addition, this medicine is made into pills, which means it must be taken on a long-term basis. The kidney is located at the lower part, deeply inside the body. As such, it is very difficult to ensure that the symptoms can be lessened as the medicine takes effect. Therefore, this medicine must be taken on a long-term basis. On the one hand, it is more troublesome to prepare medical decoction every day; on the other hand, the pill-type medicine always takes effect slowly, but it is helpful for better absorption. By the way, pills are also convenient to take. Of course, The patent medicine of **Liuwei Dihuang Pill** is now also made into decoction called **Liuwei Dihuang Tang**, for which the dosage of the ingredients is as the above-mentioned: Dihuang (rehmannia) 8 *qian*, Shanyao (Chinese yam) 4 *qian*, Shanzhuyu (dogwood) 4 *qian*, Danpi (cortex moutan radices) 3 *qian*, Fuling (poria cocos) 3 *qian*, Zexie (rhizoma alismatis) 3 *qian*.

Dihuang Pill Family Members

In drugstores, many different Dihuang pills are available. As patent medicines, Dihuang pills have a large family in which the quite common member is **Guifu Dihuang Pill**, also called **Bawei Dihuang Pill**, which is for tonifying the kidney Yang, as discussed previously, and all the other Dihuang pills are derived by way of modification based upon the formula of **Liuwei Dihuang Pill**.

Zhibai Dihuang Pill

When Kidney-Yin deficiency arises, the pathogenic fire will appear in the kidney, for which **Zhibai Dihuang Pill**, made by adding Zhimu (rhizoma anemarrhenae) and Huangbai (phellodendron amurense) on the basis of **Liuwei Dihuang Pill**, can be used for treatment. Huangbai can clear both the fire in the kidneys, and dampness and heat in the Lower Jiao, but it should not be used for too long time since long-lasting use of it may result in erectile dysfunction (ED) or sexual apathy and so on. So, stop using Huangbai where it should stop after the pathogenic fire is cleared.

Guishao Dihuang Pill

Guishao Dihuang Pill is a patent medicine in which Danggui (angelica sinensis), Baishao (radix paeoniae alba) are added based on the formula of **Liuwei Dihuang Pill**. Danggui, Baishao are for enriching blood and nourishing the liver and Yin, which is for strengthening the liver function. In **Liuwei Dihuang Pill**, the ingredient of Shanyurou is for nourishing the liver, while Danggui and Baishao are used for guiding the kidney-tonifying effect of **Liuwei Dihuang Pill** to the liver for the purpose of hematogenesis by means of nourishing Yin and the liver simultaneously. Generally, **Guishao Dihuang Pill** is suitable for those who work with mind (resulting in blood consumption), or those who always stay up late. However, those who have greasy tongue coating or slippery pulse should not use this medicine. This medicine is merely suitable for those patients who only suffer from Yin deficiency due to too much consumption of the liver blood but with no obvious symptom of phlegm. In such a case, **Guishao Dihuang Pill** is used to nourish the liver and kidney simultaneously.

Qiju Dihuang Pill

Liver opens at eyes, so both the liver and kidney Yin deficiency may easily result in dim eyesight or blurred vision including nearsightedness (myopia). For such a case, use **Qiju Dihuang Pill**, which is made by adding Gouqizi (fructus lycii) and Juhua (chrysanthemum) based upon the formula of **Liuwei Dihuang Pill**. Both Gouqizi and Juhua are going to the eyes and they play functions of nourishing the liver and improving eyesight. Meanwhile, Gouqizi is a kind of seed/fruit that can descend, while Juhua is a flower that can ascend. As soon as the ascending and descending functions give their full play, the liver Qi will then be properly regulated.

All the life essence of the heart, liver, spleen, lung and kidneys will be infused into the eyes. Those who have vigorous internal organs would have bright eyes. Similarly, those who suffer from weak internal organs would have dim eyesight. Eyes are the windows of the soul and the five internal organs. The eyes, can tell the condition of the vital life essence in one's internal organs. In case that the liver and kidneys are weak, the eyes will be definitely affected. At the time of nourishing the liver and kidneys, special care of the eyes should be taken care as well, so Gouqizi (warm in property) and Juhua are added. To nourish the liver Yin with warm medicines can send the life essence of the liver and kidney Yin upwards. Juhua has ascending and dispersing effects, and it can disperse the bad factors out of the eyes, but also disperse the pathogenic wind and heat out of the liver meridians. Gouqizi and Juhua are paired medicines often used in ophthalmology.

Mingmu Dihuang Pill

Mingmu DihuangPill is derived from **Liuwei Dihuang Pill** by adding the herbal ingredients of Danggui (angelica sinensis) and Baishao (radix paeoniae alba), Gouqizi (fructus lycii), Juhua (chrysanthemum), Jili (tribulus terrestris) and Shijueming (concha haliotidis).

Jili here is for soothing the liver, of course, Chaihu (radix bupleuri) can also soothe the liver, but those who suffer the liver and kidney Yin deficiency should not use Chaihu since Chaihu may rob the liver of its Yin. Hence, Jili is used here instead. And Shijueming used here is for suppressing the liver-fire. The major efficacy of this formula is to tackle Yin deficiency of both the liver and kidney, and soothing of the liver and suppression of the liver fire are only accomplished incidentally. In brief, **Guishao Dihuang Pill** is primarily used for nourishing the liver and kidney Yin. After Yin of both the liver and kidney has been sufficiently nourished and replenished, Gouqizi and Juhua will play their functions of nourishing the eyes. And in the meantime, Jili and Shijueming are used to regulate the liver.

Those who suffer from serious liver and kidney Yin deficiency would be more susceptible to epiphora in wind. In such a case, **Mingmu Dihuang Pill** will be very effective for treatment. Those who are dim-sighted due to the old age may also take **Mingmu Dihuang Pill**. The medicines for nourishing the liver and kidney Yin used together with Shijueming not only would suppress the liver-wind and the liver fire but also reduce the blood pressure. Young people would be easier to become stubborn and irritable or even the eyesight is sharply worsened if they undertake too much work with their mind, or read and worry too much. For such cases, **Mingmu Dihuang Pill** may also be helpful for them.

All **Guishao Dihuang Pill**, **Qi Ju Dihuang Pill**, and **Mingmu Dihuang Pill** are made for the treatment of the liver and kidneys. All these pills are suitable for those who suffer from the syndromes of both liver and kidney Yin deficiency.

Qiwei Duqi Pill

Qiwei Duqi Pill is also derived from **Liuwei Dihuang Pill** by adding the ingredient of Wuweizi (fructus schisandrae chinensis). Wuweizi, sour in taste, is going into the five internal organs, and it can converge the lung Qi. Those who suffer from the influences of kidney deficiency may probably suffer from short and shallow breath. Chuang-tzu said: "An ordinary person may only breathe to throat, while the immortal is able to breathe to heels." That means the common people can only breathe a shallow breath to the throat, but the stylites can breathe deeply and let breath run to the heels, which of course is an exaggeration. In fact, what he really meant is that the common people breathe shallowly, while in breathing, their chests are moving up and down. However, the stylites are not the same, and while their chests move up and down, their lower abdomen can move up and down as well since they can breathe very deep breath. Is it necessary to breathe to the lower abdomen? Yes, it is. The kidney is in charge of storing Qi. When the kidney Qi is vigorous, there will be a force to pull Qi downwards. The more vigorous the kidneys are, the stronger the pulling-down force will be, and the more deeply a person can breathe. We often talk about deep breath, but actually the natural deep-breath depends on the kidneys. When the kidney Qi is vigorous and strong enough to store Qi, one will be able to take deep breath at every moment.

Each person has his "气数" (Qishu, literally means "Number of Qi", i. e., "destiny"). When a person is dying, it is called the "Number of Qi" has been running out, which means the number of his breath has been used up. He who can just breathe short and shallow breath may breathe many times per minute; He who are able to breathe deeply can breathe obviously fewer times per minute, and therefore, he will have more "Qishu" and the accumulated "Qishu" in his life will help to extend his life span, which tells us that deep breath is very important for us. What if one fails to take deep breath? Use **Qiwei Duqi Pill**, which can exercise control over Qi to some extent. Meanwhile, **Qiwei Duqi Pill** is also effective for treatment of Yin deficiency and night sweating arising from the kidney deficiency.

Maiwei Dihuang Pill

Maiwei Dihuang Pill is derived from the formula of Qiwei Duqi Pill by adding Maidong (radix ophiopogonis). Maidong here is for tonifying the lung Yin, and clearing heat as well. Besides, Maidong is commonly used in a pair with Wuweizi, and it can go into the heart and lung not only for dealing with the kidney's failure to take in Qi but also dealing with cough arising from the kidney deficiency, especially the dry cough of the old people due to kidney deficiency.

Maiwei Dihuang Pill has the same efficacy as **Qiwei Duqi Pill**, and it can nourish the lungs, too. Meanwhile, Maidong in this formula can also nourish the lungs. When the lung Yin is nourished sufficiently, which means the source of fluid is replenished sufficiently, the kidneys can then be well nourished. So, both **Qiwei Duqi Pill** and **Maiwei Dihuang Pill** are used for nourishing the lungs and kidneys. In addition, **Maiwei Dihuang Pill** has another name as **Baxian Changshou Pill** since it is often used by the old people to seek for longevity.

There are many other modifications of **Liuwei Dihuang Pill**. For instance, if the primordial Yin is insufficient, add some Guibanjiao (tortoise plastron gel) and Lujiao Jiao (deer-horn gel) to intensify the potency of Yin nourishing; if Yang is insufficient, add some Lurong (pilos antler) and Ziheche (placenta hominis) and the like.

Some patients may have poor appetite after taking **Liuwei Dihuang Pill**. This may result from that the spleen fails to transport and transform **Liuwei Dihuang Pill** due to much greasy Shudi and Shanyurou contained, so aromatic herbs like Muxiang (costustoot) and Sharen (fructus amomi) etc. can be added to help the spleen to carry on T&T functions. In this formula, Muxiang and Sharen are not for curing diseases but just for restraining the other medicines, which means this formula includes herbs for curing diseases and corrigent for counteraction effect, just like the army having soldiers for killing enemies and soldiers for supervising operations, too. Of course, the dosage of herbs is not fixed in this formula. As for the treatment of spermatorrhea and the like due to knockout of the vital life essence, Zexie should be reduced to a half, and Shanyurou may be increased in that it is sour and it can function for the purpose of astringency.

Regarding addition of herbs to **Liuwei Dihuang Pill**, there are too many cases to list, which needs considering carefully since it is used so widely in clinical practice. Water is the source of life; therefore, it will never go wrong to nourish the kidneys. Meanwhile, diseases are quite changeable, that's why **Liuwei Dihuang Pill** also needs modifying as needed.

Formulas of Zuogui and Yougui

The preceding section has discussed the addition of herbs to **Liuwei Di-huang Pill**. What about the subtraction of herbs from it? Those who suffer from Yin deficiency and become thin like a skeleton in skin should not use the medicines for alleviating fluid retention like Fuling and Zexie. In that case, Fuling and Zexie should be deleted from the formula. What if the kidney Qi is not to be activated? Take out Fuling and still keep Zexie in the formula. If cold symptoms arise without blood heat, it would be unnecessary to clear fire, and then Danpi should also be deleted from the formula. Even in some cases, only three of the six ingredient herbs will work, including Shudi, Shanyurou and Shanyao. For some other cases, the addition and subtraction of herbs may be made based upon the syndrome differentiation. Zhang Jingyue was very flexible with the modification of (addition and subtraction of herbs to/from) **Liuwei Dihuang Tang**, upon which he created four formulas: **Zuogui Pill**, **Yougui Pill**, **Zuogui Yin**, and **Yougui Yin**.

Zuogui Pill contains the herbal ingredients:

Shudi (radix rehmanniae praeparata) 8 *liang*, parched Shanyao (Chinese yam) 4 *liang*, Shanyurou (common macrocarpium fruit) 4 *liang*, Gouqizi (fructus lycii) 4 *liang*, liquor-steamed Chuan Niuxi (radix cyathulae) 3 l*iang* (Note: those who suffer from spermatorrhea should delete this herb), prepared Tusizi (semen cuscutae) 4 *liang*, Lujiao Jiao (deer-horn gel) 4 *liang*, Guijiao (tortoise plastron gel) 4 *liang*. First, steam Shudi and pestle it into paste, then refine it with honey and make it into pills as big as the phoenix tree seed. A hundred pills once, wash down with boiled water or light salt water before meals.

[Note: **Yougui Pill** can be derived from the formula of **Zuogui Pill** by deleting Guijiao (tortoise plastron gel), and adding Fuzi (radix aconiti carmichaeli), Rougui (cassia bark) and Duzhong (eucommia ulmoides)].

Zuogui Yin contains the herbal ingredients: Shudi (radix rehmanniae praeparata) 2 or 3 *qian* up to 1 or 2 *liang*, Shanyao (Chinese yam) 2 *qian*, Shanyurou (common macrocarpium fruit) 1 or 2 *qian* (Note: those who dislike sour taste may reduce the dosage), Gouqizi (fructus lycii) 2 *qian*, Fuling (poria cocos) 1. 5 *qian*, parched Gancao (liquorice) 1 qian. Take 2 cups of water to decoct the herbs for seven minutes, and then drink it before meals (when the stomach is empty).

[Note: **Yougui Yin** can be derived from this formula by deleting Fuling (poria cocos), and adding Duzhong (eucommia ulmoides), Fuzi (radix aconiti carmichaeli), and Rougui (cassia bark) for vigorous fire may impair Yin, and in that case, it is not suitable to clear dampness again].

As it is known, the left side is subsumed to water, and the right side is subsumed to fire. Both **Zuogui Pill** and **Zuogui Yin** are for nourishing the kidney-Yin, in which Shudi 8 *liang*, parched Shanyao 4 *liang*, and Shanyurou 4 liang are equivalent to the "**Three Tonifications**" in **Liuwei Dihuang Pill**. Gouqizi intensifies the nourishing effect of the liver. Lujiao Jiao is for nourishing Yang and Guijiao is for nourishing Yin. This formula takes care of both the kidney Yin and Yang. Tusizi is for warming the kidney Yang, and Chuan Niuxi goes downwards for dispersing blood stasis.

Yougui Pill can be derived from the formula of **Zuogui Pill**, by deleting Guijiao, and adding Fuzi, Rougui, and Duzhong. **Yougui Pill** is for nourishing Yang, and in the respect of its herbal ingredients, it is equivalent to **Liuwei Dihuang Pill** plus Fuzi and Rougui. Duzhong is for warming the kidneys, but it also clears the wind and dampness in the kidneys since the pathogenic wind and dampness often take advantage of the deficiency of the kidney to get in. Guijiao is deleted since it is a medicine for nourishing Yin. In the formula for Yang nourishing, excessive Yin nourishing will usurp the Yang nourishing role. Hence, deletion of Guijiao from the formula is for reducing the intensity of Yin nourishing but reinforce the function of **Yougui Pill**. As a medicine of pill, **Yougui Pill** can be taken on a long-term basis. By the way, **Zuogui Yin** and **Yougui Yin**, as drinks for daily use, contain very small dosage of herbal ingredients, so they are used with great flexibility. Fuling is deleted from the formula of **Yougui Yin** in that addition of Duzhong, Fuzi, and Rougui is for replenishing fire. If the fire is too vigorous, it will impair Yin, so, Fuling should not be used to eliminate dampness, or otherwise, it will impair Yin more severely.

Zuogui Pill, **Yougui Pill**, **Zuogui Yin**, and **Yougui Yin** are quite similar to **Liuwei Dihuang Pill** and **Bawei Dihuang Pill** in many aspects. They have many functions, but here we only discuss the principles behind the formulas rather than the treatment of specific diseases. Each formula has a variety of applications, after understanding the principles behind the formulas, TCM doctors will naturally feel easier to use them.

Siwu Tang

Principle of Development behind Siwu Tang

Originated from the book of *Welfare Pharmacy Prescriptions* compiled in Song dynasty, **Siwu Tang** contains four herbs only: Danggui (angelica sinensis), Chuanxiong (ligusticum wallichii), Baishao (radix paeoniae alba), and Dihuang (rehmannia).

There are many formulas composed of only four herbs, whose principle is often related to the law of spring birth, summer growth, autumn harvest, and winter storage. Danggui is a medicine for replenishing blood, and it is also able to tonify Qi (nourish the vitality). It is pungent and sweet in tastes, corresponding to the season of spring, so it is vital with the efficacy for hematogenesis. Chuanxiong is able to promote Qi to activate blood circulation and get through the blood channel in human body to let blood circulate smoothly, so Chuanxiong, corresponding to the season of summer, has the efficacy for activating the blood circulation. Baishao, sour in taste, goes into the liver, and it is able to converge the blood, corresponding to the season of autumn. Dihuang goes into the kidneys, and corresponding to the season of winter, it is able to store the blood. Therefore, the four herbs contained in **Siwu Tang** correspond to spring, summer, autumn and winter respectively. The blood is generated naturally through the process of birth, growth, harvest, and storage. If only one herb is used, it will be much harder to replenish the blood.

Of course, there are also many cases that only one herb can replenish the blood. Like Jixueteng (caulis spatholobi), mainly used for treatment of impairment of blood due to rheumatism, or for getting through the blood line in the meridians and collaterals in order to accomplish the purpose of nourishing blood. There is a saying, "Danshen can play the role of four different herbs. " In fact, Danshen is a medicine for dispersing blood stasis. As the saying goes like "If the blood stasis is not dispersed, the new blood will not be generated". Only after the blood stasis is dispersed will the new blood be generated naturally. All these herbs are inclined to eliminating the pathogens and intensifying the vital Qi. As for the nourishing and generating blood in a straightforward way, **Siwu Tang** could be the best choice.

Nourishing Blood Means to Nourish the Liver and Kidneys

Corresponding to **Siwu Tang** is **Sijunzi Tang** that contains Renshen (ginseng), Baizhu (white atractylodes rhizome), Fuling (poria cocos), and Gancao (liquorice). These herbs all go into the spleen, as we always say "to tonify Qi is to tonify the lungs and spleen, and to nourish blood is to nourish the liver and kidneys. " This saying can help and enlighten learners to understand principles in learning TCM. In fact, this statement is not precise, but TCM sometimes does need such a statement to reflect its vitality. Too much preciseness means inflexibility, which may not help cure the diseases of the living people. The relationship between the masters and apprentices in the field of TCM must be in harmony, otherwise it would be very difficult to articulate, or even sometimes argue for the sake of arguing. In the Analects of Confucius, there is a sentence saying that "A true gentleman gets along well with the others, but may not associate with them. A mean man associates with the others, but may not get along well with them. " A true gentleman is seeking for the harmony and mutual understanding and enlightening while discussing with each other about something; but the mean men will do in the different way that they always keep eyes on their personal interests in their mind. Once starting to articulate, they will argue with each other just for arguing. By the way, the mean men also have a converging idea. They always follow the suit, or will become annoyed whenever they see something different from what they insist on. In such a way, it is impossible for them to learn anything well. Chinese traditional culture is the study of gentleman, paying much attention to "harmony in diversity".

The beginners of TCM usually have two different states of mind: One is that they consider that they themselves are always right and look down upon all the others, which reflects a thought of "agreement in disharmony"; The other one is a different state of mind, that is, those with such a state of mind would like to take all the others' opinions into consideration and try to absorb what is valuable, which is actually the right state of mind.

Modifications of Siwu Tang

The composition of **Siwu Tang** is relatively simple. To put it simply, **Siwutang** is for nourishing blood, liver and kidneys; However, from the deeper sense, it is a fundamental formula for nourishing blood, and many additions and subtractions to/from it could be made on the basis of its formula. For example, the presence of pathogenic wind in blood often leads to some skin diseases, especially some very itchy rashes on skin, which can be treated by adding Jingjie (schizonepeta) and Fangfeng (radix sileris) to the formula of **Siwu Tang**; in case there is heat blood, add Danpi (cortex moutan radices) and Chishao (radix paeoniae rubra) to the formula of **Siwu Tang**; in case there is blood stasis, add Taoren (peach kernel) and Honghua (safflower carthamus) to the formula of **Siwu Tang**.

As to Dihuang in **Siwu Tang**, in case blood is slightly inclined to heat, Sheng Dihuang (radix rehmanniae recen) should be used; in case blood heat is not too serious, but Yin deficiency is more serious, use Shudi (radix rehmanniae praeparata); in case the blood stasis is more serious, use the tail of Danggui (angelica sinensis) instead of the main stem, and Chishao (radix paeoniae rubra) is used instead of Baishao (radix paeoniae alba); in case the liver Yin deficiency is more serious, the main part of Danggui should be used instead.

For any medicine, if it is used together with **Siwu Tang**, its medical effects will be guided into blood, and in such a case **Siwu Tang** just functions like an ingredient to enhance the effect of the medicine. But basically speaking, **Siwu Tang** is a tonic. If the exogenous pathogens are more serious, **Siwu Tang** should be used with caution, or otherwise, the pathogenic factors may get worse before they are cleared under the influence of nourishing, that is to say, the nourishing is not supplied to the human body but to the pathogenic factors, and then the disease will get worse because of the nourishing.

第二章　地黄

地黄概说

地黄的生长环境

地黄在北方很常见，就是那种深绿色的植物，有点毛茸茸的，春天还开出紫色的花儿，这就是地黄。地黄是多年生的草本植物，根部入药，它的根很大，深深扎进土里，去吸收大地的精华，同时收藏养分，以供自己在北方贫瘠而干旱的土地上顽强生长。地黄又叫地髓，是大地的精髓、骨髓。所以，在土气旺的地方生长的地黄，药力会更佳；长在水边的也会更好一些。

地黄的地道产地是河南怀庆，这里地处中原，中原是得地气最醇厚的地方；同时这里又属于北方，得北方的纯阴之气。江苏、浙江、四川等地产的地黄，养阴血的效果就不及怀地黄，因为南方属火，地黄生长过程中得了南方温暖的气息，所以它养阴的力度比较弱，但适合用来清热。

怀地黄的特点是，肥大，皮上有很多疙瘩，横切面上有菊花心，质地中，扔到水里马上下沉。这种地黄是最好的。在怀庆周边，比如山西、安徽亳州的地黄也不错，但跟怀地黄比还是逊色一筹。

地黄的体用

地黄在新鲜的时候，颜色是黄色的；从名字上看，地属土，黄也属土。这味药跟土太有缘了。有人问，地黄属土的属性有这么多，为什么还入肾呢？为什么还是一味如此重要的补肾药呢？

因为土克水。克，其实是一种很有必要的节制。水最容易泛滥成灾，所以要用土做成堤坝来挡着它，这样才能蓄水。这就是土克水。肾水也是这样的，要得到必要的节制，这就要用地黄这种得到土气特别重的药。肾水得到合理的制约才能更好的封藏，肾精才能得到更好的养护。

一味药有体用之别，地黄之体是滋阴的，它里面含有丰富的汁液，含糖；它的用也是滋阴的，靠的是它衍生的一些功能，也就是帮助脾胃的运化。地黄比较滋腻，容易妨碍脾胃，影响人的运化能力，让人吃不下饭，这是在用错的情况下，就会出现这种状况。而善用地黄的人，用了地黄不但不会让你吃完后感到肚子胀、不消化，反而能让你感到更有食欲，越来越能吃。就像善用附子就不会让人上火一样。

鲜生地、干地黄和熟地

地黄根据炮制的不同，可以分为鲜地黄、干地黄和熟地黄。

刚挖出来的地黄就叫鲜生地，或者鲜地黄，把这个生地直接晒干就是干地黄了，就是我们现在常说的生地。把生地反复蒸熟，最好经过九蒸九晒，就成了熟地。

鲜生地可以用来散血，因为它没有经过火。不管什么东西，没有经过火就是生的，性质活泼，能行能散，走得快。一旦经过火，就不活泼了，就走得慢一些，就能守中，甚至守而不走。

地黄总体来讲是滋腻的，当它用在养阴清热的时候，咱们不希望它守在那里，而是希望它赶紧走，所以就不能见火。因此，纯粹用来滋阴清热的时候，咱们用地黄就要用新鲜的，至少也得用干地黄。

干地黄是细的、小的好。地黄有一个主根，主根上有一些细小的旁根，取旁根晒干，就是干地黄了。旁根长在边上的，更有流动性，滋腻性小一些。我们经常用的生地黄就是这些细小的。肥大的地黄往往被做成熟地，所以，开方子经常写"细生地"、"大熟地"。

鲜生地、干地、熟地之间有很多相似的地方，都能滋阴，都能入肾。它们还有不一样的地方：鲜生地凉血清热，散血的作用强一些；干地黄依然是凉血、散血，但散血的力度较弱，如果是大片的干地黄，就偏于养阴。相对于鲜地黄，干地黄的优点在于方便保存。熟地不再是一个凉药了，而是一个温药，它主要用于补肾滋阴。

鲜地黄和干地黄都属于生地，现在鲜地黄用得少了，人们索性把干地黄叫生地。古人在医案或方书中提到的生地，有的是鲜生地，有的是干地黄。

生地

滋阴清火

鲜地黄味甘、微苦而大寒。一说微苦大寒，我们就会想到金部方药讲了很多苦寒的药，为什么当时没有讲生地呢？前面讲的苦寒的药，比如说苦寒兼涩的龙胆草，苦寒兼辛的丹皮，苦寒兼轻浮的栀子，那么苦寒兼甘的呢？这就是地黄了。金部方药没有讲苦寒兼甘的，因为苦寒一旦兼甘，就由一个泻火的药，摇身一变成了一个既能泻火，又有一定滋补作用的药了。因为甘味就有滋补的作用。前面的栀子、龙胆草、黄芩、黄连、黄柏都没有滋补的作用，而一带甘甜的味道马上就补了，就能养阴了。

鲜生地入脾、胃、心、肝、肺这五经，特别能清胃热、养胃阴。往往人在肾阴虚的情况下，胃火就会大，因为肾里边是肾阴肾阳，或者说肾水肾火，是交织在一起的，当肾阴虚的时候，会有一部分肾火因为得不到安顿而往上蹿，蹿到胃里边，导致胃热，所以很多胃热，不能光去清。有的胃热会越清越大，因为火源你没有关闭，这个人依然肾虚，火依然在往上走，你虽然当时清掉了，但是底下的火又来了，这种火叫虚火，虚火上炎的时候，应该滋阴清火，要养肾和补肾阴，让肾里边的火得到安顿，正好有这个作用，它一方面能够清胃热，另一方面能够补肾水。

鲜生地凉血散血

生地是一味特别重要的凉血药，我们经常用生地、丹皮、赤芍、犀角来凉血，这就是犀角地黄汤。如果不是那么严重和凶险的血热，我们就不用犀角了，何况现在犀角也不允许用。用生地、丹皮、赤芍就够了，必要时还可以加栀子或石膏。

阳明经为多气多血之经，胃为多气多血之腑。生地是凉胃的，通过清胃热来达到凉血的目的，从阳明经来凉血，犀角地黄汤就是这个思路，其中的生地，最好用鲜生地。

鲜生地还有散血的作用，能够化瘀，还能够解烦。凡是摔伤的，或者是被人打伤的，有瘀血肿胀，可以把鲜生地捣碎敷在患处，很快就能消掉。当然，如果要强化它的作用，可以用当归、生地、赤芍、乳香、没药、肉桂，放在一起捣成细末，喝下去，可以消一切的跌打损伤、瘀血作痛。治跌打损伤有专门的方子，这算一个简单的，还有更复杂的，要根据受伤的部位进行加减。

至于鲜生地解烦的作用，可以这样来理解：胃热能让人烦，鲜生地清胃，故可以解烦；血热能让人烦，鲜生地凉血，故能解烦；瘀血内阻，产生内热，也可能让人烦，鲜生地散血化瘀，也能解烦。只有这类的烦，才可以用鲜生地来解。

生地配麦冬，养神生血

生地和麦冬是经常一起用的药对。生地入脾、肾、肝，麦冬入心、肺。生地和麦冬这两味药加起来，基本上五脏都走遍了。它们能够养神而生血。人血虚了，神就会不足。比如，受伤失血过多，这个人就没有精神了，注意力也不容易集中，这就是失血过多导致神不足。

伤了阴也会无神。很典型的，有的小孩子到了高中阶段，注意力就不容易集中。为什么呢？你还不能问，这是他自己的事。这时候他可能误犯手淫，伤了精，伤了精也就等于伤了肾。精神精神，有精才有神，没有精就没有神。精就是肾精，神就是心神。

我们说一个人精神怎么样，就涉及两个脏，心和肾。肾藏精，心藏神。精足神就足，人就有神采，精不足神就不足，这个人就蔫头耷脑，自控能力差，精神不太容易集中，干什么都不利落，学习成绩肯定搞不上去的。生理和心理都是相互联系的，所以生地和麦冬经常在一起用，用来养神、生血。当我们看到这样的病人，家长带来说，孩子老是精神不集中。你心里应当知道可能会是怎么回事儿。这些药跟上去，效果肯定会好。

增液汤

生地、麦冬，再加一味玄参，就叫增液汤，就是给人体增加血液、津液的意思，它通常用在温病后期。温病就是发热的病，发热了很长时间，也就伤了津液，大便就会干燥。这时候用增液汤，给人体增加一些液体，就相当于给人体输液。只不过输液比较野蛮，直接给你灌到血脉里面去，咱们这个比较文明，用最自然的东西熬成汤喝下去，喝到胃里，游溢精气，转输于脾，然后脾再把这些东西升到肺里面，再由肺输布到全身。这个过程是一个很柔和、和谐、自然的输液过程。

温病好了以后的大便燥结，或者皮肤粗糙，都可以用增液汤。但是，它也有一个缺陷，就是只能够给人体增加液体，而不能够迅速润下通下，不能让燥结在体内的大便迅速通下来，所以经常用增液承气汤，就是在增液汤的基础上再增加上大黄、芒硝，有必要时再根据具体情况加点枳壳、厚朴、甘草之类。增液承气汤一面给人体增加液体，一面软化大便，把体内不好的东西排出去。这个方在临床上也会经常用到。在《时病论》中遇到这种情况，还用松柏通幽法，在这个基础上，加上松子仁、柏子仁、杏仁，效果也是特别好的。

熟地

熟地制法

熟地是越大的越好。制作熟地，最好是用河南怀庆府出产的大熟地，用竹刀切成片，加入上好的绍兴花雕酒泡上，再把砂仁捣成细末，拌进去。拌匀、浸透了以后，把它放到木甑里，再把木甑放在瓦锅上隔水蒸。

木甑是用木头做的一种桶，通常是用来蒸饭的。这个东西在南方农村还有，现在有些饭店做饭也是用这个。在蒸熟地的时候，不能象蒸饭那样放到铁锅里面蒸。地黄是最怕铁的，入肾的药都怕铁。一旦见铁，那么它入肾后就会对肾有一定的伤害。

把装有地黄的木甑放到瓦锅里面，蒸了以后，拿到外面去晒。晒得差不多了拿回来继续蒸，蒸得差不多了再拿到外面继续晒，然后再蒸。至于晒到什么程度，蒸到什么火候，都是有讲究的，这要在实践中才能知道。如此来回九次，熟地才算制成。

为什么要这么折腾呢？放在火上蒸，得的是人间的火；放在太阳下晒，得到的是天上的火。天上的火和人间的火是不一样的。天上的火是往下降的，相当于心火；人间的火是往上走的，火性炎上。天上人间的火同时灌注到熟地中，把本来寒凉的熟地变成甘温了，本来是苦寒的现在就不再苦，变成甘甜的了。

为什么要用砂仁拌呢？砂仁能芳香醒脾、健脾理气，还能纳气归肾。熟地滋腻，砂仁就会解除它滋腻的性质，还会让熟地通调五脏，最后纳入丹田，这样才能更好填精、补血、封髓。这样一来，熟地就没有副作用了。

但是商家总是很草率的，谁有工夫给你九蒸九晒啊！所以历代的医家都埋怨没有好的熟地，其实做事讲究因地制宜、因人制宜、因时制宜，咱们看病为什么不因药制宜呢？你不是不加砂仁么，我在开方子的时候就加进去砂仁，效果是一样的。你不是不九蒸九晒么？我让病人久煮一会儿，或者我再加点其他的温药进去，尽量想办法扬长避短，就可以了。

张景岳论熟地

古代的医家中，最善于用熟地的是明朝着名医家张景岳。他对熟地的论述非常到位："凡诸真阴亏损者，有为发热，为头痛，为焦渴，为喉痹，为嗽痰，为喘气，或脾肾寒逆为呕吐，或虚火载血于口鼻，或水泛于皮肤，或阴虚而泄利，或阳浮而狂躁，或阴脱而仆地。阴虚而神散者，非熟地之守不足以聚之；阴虚而火升者，非熟地之重而不足以降之；阴虚而躁动者，非熟地之静不足以镇之；阴虚而刚急者，非熟地之甘不足以缓之；阴虚而水邪泛滥者，舍熟地何以自制；阴虚而真气散失者，舍熟地何以归源；阴虚而精血俱损，脂膏残薄者，舍熟地何以厚肠胃。且犹有最玄妙者，则熟地兼散剂方能发汗，何也？以汗化于血，而无阴不作汗也。熟地兼温剂始能回阳，何也？以阳生于下，而无复不成乾也。然而阳性速，故人参少用亦可成功；阴性缓，熟地非多难以奏效。"

真阴大虚，可能导致很多病，有发热的，有头痛的，有口渴的，有喉咙不通且痛的，有咳嗽多痰的，有气喘的，有的会出现脾肾寒逆的呕吐的，有的则虚火把血往上引而口鼻出血，有的是水泛滥与皮肤而导致水肿，有的是因为阴虚而腹泻，有的是因为阳气浮越而狂躁，有的是因为阴血不足而中风昏倒在地……这些情况，都可以用熟地。

阴虚而神散，可以用熟地，熟地粘腻而性守，能聚精、聚神，使神不散。

阴虚而火升，可以用熟地，熟地质地重，一般二三十克熟地也就一小块，能往下沉降，可以降虚火。

阴虚而躁动，可以用熟地，熟地性静，能镇得住狂躁。那么还有不安静的药么？当然有，比如芳香的药，它会在人体各处走窜。在药里面加一点厚朴、陈皮、砂仁、木香之类的，肚子里面就会咕噜咕噜地响，因为药香窜通气。躁动的人，或者原本有火的人，就不宜用此类芳香走窜、动气的药了，要多一些文静的药，比如熟地，用来镇这个躁动，这和前面所讲的重镇有相同之处。

阴虚会令人变得急躁，这个"刚急"有两重含义：一个是生理上的，一个是心理上的。生理上就是僵硬，心理上就是性格上紧张。尤其是老年人，真阴大虚，容易中风，在临近中风的时候，他会变得特别倔，脾气特别大，这是阴虚而刚急。所以家里老人脾气变了，要注意可能是一种大病的征兆。女性在更年期也会因为阴虚而脾气变刚急，咱们一定要体谅，不要对着干。熟地味甘而能缓急，所以阴虚刚急，可以用熟地制之。

阴虚而水邪泛滥，可以用熟地，大补真阴，制水消肿。

阴虚而真气散失，要用熟地将其往回收；阴虚而精血受损，要用熟地补其脂膏，厚其肠胃。还有更妙的，熟地跟发散药一起用，就能帮助发汗，因为汗是血化的，真阴大虚的人若不用熟地，光用发汗药，伤害是很大的，汗也还不容易出。

熟地虽是阴药，但跟温热药一起用，又能回阳，因为阳生于下，来自命门，不补真阴，回阳不易。

阳性急速，所有用于补阳、补气的人参之类，用一点一点就可以了；阴性迟缓，所以像熟地这样的药，一定用量要大，否则难以奏效。张景岳用熟地往往一用就是二两、三两，也就是 60 克到 100 克这样大量的剂量。以前我们去安国药材市场的时候，往往天还没亮就吃完早饭就去了，三个小时后到了那就饿了，到卖药的人家到处找熟地当红薯干吃，吃几块就饱了，它是吃不坏人的。

张景岳何以这么善于用熟地呢？因为当时他的病人以达官贵人为主，又都是读书人。读书人耗心思，也就是精血内耗；等到发达显贵以后，又妻妾成群，耗精就会很多，所以给这些人治病要养他的阴，填他的精，这样才会舒服。所以，张景岳用熟地会如此左右逢源。我们在用熟地的时候，也要根据具体情况，不可照搬古人经验。

生地与熟地的选用

生地、熟地在一些方剂里都是可以酌情使用的，方书中的很多方子，不写生地、熟地，只写"地黄"，你可以根据病人的情况具体来用。该用生地用生地，该用熟地用熟地。比如四物汤中，有时候用生地，有时候用熟地，有时候则生熟地同用。

当更需要滋阴清热的时候，就用生地；如果病人痰象比较重，用熟地恐怕滋腻，让痰越补越多，这个时候也用生地；如果偏重于补肾填精的话，就用熟地；如果病人有阴虚又兼有血热之类的，还可以生地、熟地同用。比如说六味地黄丸，它为什么叫六味地黄丸，而不叫六味生地丸或六味熟地丸？也是提示你地黄可以用生地，也可以用熟地。往往，男子多阴虚，适合用熟地；女子多血热，适合用生地。

固本丸与疾病的善后

生地是生精血的，并不仅仅是说它是生的就叫生地，它没有经过那么多炮制，只是把地黄晒干了，里边还是黄的，它依然有生生之气，有生生之气就能够生精血。熟地，经过九蒸九晒，就不再是黄的了，而是黑得发亮，它已经改变了很多自然属性，变成人工的东西了，其作用主要是补精血。

生地配天冬，用来生精血；熟地配麦冬，用来补精血。如果既要生精血，又要补精血，我们可以生地、熟地，天冬、麦冬一块用。生地、熟地这是地，天冬、麦冬这是天，且天冬、麦冬都是走肺的，走肺的它就属天。天和地都有了，再加人参，入中焦，这是属人的。天麦冬、生熟地、人参，天地人都有了，这又成了一个很有名的方子叫固本丸，是用来治疗老年人的精血枯槁，或者是病后调养的。固本丸，其实就是三才汤再加两个药，在天冬的基础上加个麦冬，地黄则生地、熟地同用。这是在治病善后时，会经常用到的方子。

治病一定要善后。我们看前人的医案，列出的一诊、二诊，其实都是把关键的步骤给你讲出来了。但一个病真的有那么好治吗？没那么好治的。在治病的过程中，要是病人感冒了怎么办？病人出现了其他的一些变化，怎么办？病变则药变，病好了还要善后，需要把他治病期间消耗的一些东西补过来。好比一棵树，里边有虫子了，咱们把虫挖出来了以后，还要把以前那个口给堵上，然后再给这棵树培土。培土就是固本，把病治好了以后也要固本，用固本丸。这里用丸药，而丸药往往用于善后，在治病的过程中，往往用汤药的多，因为汤药有涤荡之势，而丸药的作用就缓而绵长。

酒生地和姜熟地

一般而言，生地会影响胃气，吃多了食欲就会不好，所以经常要用酒炒。熟地通常用姜汁炒，它就不再滋腻了。

有人说，熟地不是九蒸九晒了而且还加了砂仁了，到这儿你怎么还说它会滞腻啊？其实，在这里讲的熟地，就不一定是如法炮制的熟地了，它还是有一些副作用，你可以用其他办法去弥补。姜汁是温的，即使是不合格的熟地，你用姜汁一炒，它也变温了，而且姜汁能散，能够开胃，加点姜汁，加点砂仁，就算是本来没有经过九蒸九晒的熟地，也有跟九蒸九晒的熟地有差不多的作用。

我们读古书一定要看文字背后的东西。某一本书里边讲："生地酒炒则不烦胃，熟地姜汁炒则不泥膈。"这都是在提示我们，遇到没有如法炮制的熟地，应该怎么去驾驭它、调服它，把它变成可用的东西。好的东西固然好用，但不好的东西我们也要会用。用得好，它依然还是好东西。我们现在用熟地用得非常多，而且肯定不是按照古法炮制的。按照古法炮制，熟地是不能见铁的，但现在炮制过程中地黄是放在铁锅里蒸的，而且不是竹刀切，在机械化大生产中都是用不锈钢刀片来切的，对药材本身有损伤，然后又没有九蒸九晒，这样草草地弄出来就给你了，你难道就不用了？还是得用，就看你怎么用了。抱怨药材不好的中医，是最没出息的中医。

六味地黄丸

六味地黄丸可能是中医里知名度最高的一个方子或中成药。它的组成是六味药，有一个口诀，叫"地八山山四，丹苓泽泻三"，就是地黄八钱，山药和山萸肉都是四钱，丹皮、茯苓和泽泻都是三钱。当然这是一个参考剂量，在具体运用的时候可以酌情增减。

六味地黄丸的来源

六味地黄丸这个方剂，最初并不叫六味地黄丸，它有八味药，叫八味地黄丸，就是六味地黄丸方加上附子和桂。"桂"有时可以用桂枝，有时可以用肉桂，这就是桂附地黄丸。药店就能买到桂附地黄丸，是用来温肾阳的。

如果肾阳不足而阳痿，在八味地黄丸的基础上再加上淫羊藿、补骨脂、巴戟天等温肾阳的药，八味地黄丸里的附子、肉桂本身就可以直接温肾阳，而且力度峻猛，我们用药要缓急兼用，刚柔并济，加上淫羊藿、补骨脂、巴戟天这几味比较柔一点，但药力又比较长久一些的药，那么它温肾阳的力度会更大。而且这几味药又入奇经八脉，能建奇功。

因肾虚，气化不利而下肢水肿，可以在八味地黄丸的基础上加上牛膝和车前子。牛膝把药往下引，还有破血的作用，车前子是利水的。下肢是因为有水才肿的，所以要利水消肿。如果口渴比较明显，还可以加知母来清热；也可以加龟板，加大滋阴的力度。知母、龟板是用来滋阴泻火的。

如果遇到头晕，可以在八味地黄丸的基础上加上枸杞子、菟丝子。

上面是八味地黄丸一些常见的加法。八味地黄丸还有一个很有名的减法，就是去掉其中的附子和桂，把八味地黄丸减成六味地黄丸。这个减法是钱乙在《小儿药证直诀》中做的。《小儿药证直诀》是一本儿科的书，六味地黄丸最初是治儿科各种病的。

小孩身体稚嫩，往往出现肾虚，说话声音小小的、胆怯、弱弱的，甚至都说不出话，用六味地黄丸；小孩肾虚，囟门老合不上，用六味地黄丸；小孩没有精神，这往往也跟肾水不足有关，用六味地黄丸；如果眼睛里边白眼珠特别大，黑眼珠特别小，这也跟肾虚有关，依然用六味地黄丸；还有面色㿠白，也还是跟肾虚有关，还是用六味地黄丸。六味地黄丸也是儿科常用的一个方子。

小孩的肾虚无非两个来源，一个是先天不足；还有一个，小孩是属木的，因为他要生长，生长取决于肝，借助肝的生发之力来长，所以小孩的肝木就特别旺，肝木旺就会消耗肾水，因为肾水生肝木。肝木这么旺那就消耗肾水了，肾的压力就大了，就容易导致肾虚。此时就要用六味地黄丸来补。

肝木旺，克脾土，要么拉肚子，要么不爱吃东西，白眼珠发蓝。肝旺还能助长邪热，就会发热，一感冒发热就会非常的高。要让他的肝木平和，不生邪火，就应该滋水涵木。肾水足了肝就会趋于正常，邪火就不会妄动了。所以把八味地黄丸减成六味地黄丸，这是方剂的减法的代表作。我们经常讲一个方剂要加减，加法是很好做的；难的是减法。

龙宫禁方

六味地黄丸的六味药，搭配得天衣无缝的六味药。有人甚至认为这是龙宫禁方之一。

医界有这样一个传说，孙思邈治好了龙王的病，龙王非常感激他，就给了他龙宫的三十个禁方。所谓禁方，是光秃秃的一个方子，有方而无解，其用法都是口传心授的，不用文字表达出来，不得其传者禁用，所以叫禁方。而得其真传的人用这些方子，就会用得特别神。

孙思邈后来写了一部书叫《千金方》，正好有三十卷，每一卷里边就藏着龙宫的一个禁方。说六味地黄丸也是龙宫的禁方，但是我查了一下《千金方》，里边并没有六味地黄丸。《千金方》是唐朝的书，而《小儿药证直诀》是宋朝的书。当然，龙宫禁方可能不止三十个，可能龙王给孙思邈的就这三十个，六味地黄丸是这三十个以外的，我们只能这样解释。

当然，龙宫禁方只是一个传说，说六味地黄丸是龙宫禁方，只是在夸这个方子好而已。说《千金方》里藏有龙宫禁方，也是在强调这本书中有很多骊龙探珠的地方，但是这三十个方子到底是哪三十个，我们已经无法找出了。它只是动用我们的好奇心，让后世学医之人认真去读这本书。

《千金方》是唐朝的著作，方多论少；《外台秘要》也是以方子为主，作为一部经典，秘要就是秘传之要，它以方的形式体现。你要去探究《外台秘要》的意义，一定要以《内经》、《难经》、《伤寒杂病论》为基础，还有《诸病源候论》也不可忽视。《诸病源候论》正好跟《千金方》、《外台秘要》相反，它是有论无方。方子到哪里去找呢？到《外台秘要》和《千金方》里边去找，把《外台秘要》、《千金方》与《诸病源候论》结合起来看，就会有很多启发，有很多收获。

六味地黄丸的方义

六味地黄丸，这个方名的每一个字，都值得咱们琢磨。

六：《河图》、《洛书》讲"天一生水，地六成之"，"生"就是创造，"成"就是完成。生水在数上是"一"，这只是水的源头，这个水要成为真正的水，那么它在数上对应的是"六"，这个数是象数的数，比较抽象。但落实到人体，就容易理解了。肺为水之上源，这就是天一生水；水在我们体内，最后成为精，藏于五脏，这就叫地六成之。水在人体就是这样生，这样成的。六味地黄丸是一个滋阴养肾经的药，它在"地六成之"的阶段，所以它在象数上取的是六，所以叫六味地黄丸，意味着滋阴、生精。

味：我们知道四气五味，五味是酸苦甘辛咸，如果再加一个淡，正好是六味。我们看六味地黄丸的这几味药，地黄苦，山萸肉酸，山药甘，丹皮辛，泽泻咸，茯苓淡，六种味道都有了，这也意味着六味地黄丸兼具六味而能走五脏，这也是它能够滋阴的依据。气属于阳，味属于阴，"形不足者温之以气，精不足者补之以味"，六味补五脏之精以养肾精。

六味地黄丸这个方子可以分为两部分，地黄、山萸肉和山药这是上半部分，属于三补；丹皮、茯苓、泽泻是下半部分，属于三泻。大家都说六味地黄丸是三补三泻。三味药补，怎么补呢？肾是藏精的，精也是人体的水，它从肺来，山药白色入肺，开水之上源。肺金生肾水，通过养肺来达到养肾生精的目的。接着地黄直接补肾水，肾水又生肝木，而且肾水生出来之后要尽量把它收敛住，就要用一个酸药来收它，山萸肉是酸的，入肝。

山药、地黄、山萸肉这三味药正好是处在相生的链条上，体现了肺金生肾水、肾水生肝木，养肾要兼顾到它的源和流，这样才是真正的养肾。这也提示我们平时用药的一个原则，要补某一脏，既要顾其母，又要顾其子。这是三补。

三泻呢？茯苓、泽泻，泻水道，通利肾气，如果肾气不通，补了也是白补。我们前面讲过，肾分阴阳，有阴水和阳水。阴水是精，阳水就是小便。阴水要收敛、要封藏，阳水要气化、要往外泻。当阳水能往外泻的时候，阴水才能得到很好的巩固，这叫阳水通则阴水固，就是说小便通则精液固。小便得到气化就能出来；精液得到火就会出来，所以欲火一动，精液就能出来。邪火一动也能让精液不安，能让阴水不安，所以要加一味寒凉的丹皮来清火。火不扰动，阴水自然就能固。

地黄：地黄是君药，本身是补肾阴的，放到六味地黄丸方里面，它补肾阴的作用能成倍的放大，因为有了这么多味药的帮助，它不再是孤军奋战。

丸：为什么做成丸药呢？这意味着这个药必须长期服用，肾是人体最下方，也是最深处的脏器，药到病除很难，所以要长期服用。如果做成汤剂就比较麻烦，要天天熬药，这是一方面；另一方面，丸的作用会缓一些，也有助于吸收，服用起来会方便一些。当然现在也经常把六味地黄丸做成六味地黄汤，前面我们讲的"地八山山四，丹苓泽泻三"，也是做成汤剂的剂量。

地黄丸家族

我们在药店里可以看到很多的地黄丸，地黄丸作为中成药，有一个家族，经常见到的有桂附地黄丸，也叫八味地黄丸，是补肾阳的，前面已经介绍过了。其他的地黄丸，这是以六味地黄丸为基础，进行加减。

知柏地黄丸

当肾阴亏损的时候，肾里面就有邪火了，这时候用知柏地黄丸。知柏地黄丸是在六味地黄丸六味药的基础上，加知母、黄柏。黄柏清肾中之火，还能清下焦湿热；但是它不能久用，用多了人就阳痿了，或者说就容易性冷淡之类的。清火，要适可而止。

归芍地黄丸

归芍地黄丸，就是在六味地黄丸的基础上加上当归和白芍。当归、白芍是补血、柔肝养阴的，这是要加大养肝的力度。六味地黄丸中有一味山萸肉能养肝，加上当归、白芍，能把六味地黄丸补肾的功能往肝上引，是通过生阴来生血，同时养肝。一般劳心耗血、常熬夜的人适合用归芍地黄丸。但用这个药有一个前提，舌苔不腻，脉不滑，就是这人痰象不明显，纯粹的阴虚，而且是因为肝血耗得太多了，就可以用归芍地黄丸，肝肾同养。

杞菊地黄丸

肝开窍于目，肝肾阴虚，容易导致眼睛花，看不清，也包括近视。这时候可以用杞菊地黄丸，就是在六味地黄丸的基础上再加枸杞子和菊花。枸杞子和菊花都能走眼睛，养肝明目。枸杞子是一种子，能往下降；而菊花是一种花，它能往上升发。这一升一降，肝气就能调匀了。

心、肝、脾、肺、肾五脏的精气，都要灌注于眼睛。五脏旺的人，眼睛会炯炯有神，五脏弱的眼睛就没神了。眼睛是心灵的窗户，也是五脏的窗户。通过看眼睛，就可以看出这个人五脏的精气是强还是弱。当肝肾同虚的时候，眼睛就会受到影响。在滋养肝肾的同时，特别照顾一下眼睛，在里面加上枸杞子、菊花。枸杞子是温药，温养肝阴就能把肝肾之阴精气往上带；菊花是升散的，能把眼睛里面不好的东西散掉，还能散肝经的风热，所以，枸杞子和菊花是眼科经常用的一对药。

明目地黄丸

明目地黄丸，是在六味地黄丸的基础上，加上当归、白芍，加上枸杞子和菊花，再加上蒺藜和石决明，这个方子就比较大了。

加蒺藜是为了疏肝。柴胡也可以疏肝，但肝肾阴虚的人就不要用柴胡了，恐怕柴胡劫肝阴，所以改用白蒺藜来疏肝。加石决明是为了把肝火镇压下去。当然疏肝和镇压肝火是捎带着做的，主要还是治肝肾阴虚。所以依然是归芍地黄丸，大补肝肾之阴。肝肾之阴补足了，然后再用枸杞子、菊花养一养眼睛，同时用蒺藜、石决明来调一调肝。

好些人到了肝肾阴虚比较厉害的时候，容易迎风流泪，明目地黄丸也很管用。老眼昏花了，也可以用明目地黄丸。养肝肾之阴的药配上石决明，可以镇肝风、镇肝火，也有降血压的作用。年轻人如果劳心太过，读书、思考问题太多了，脾气易变得倔强暴躁，视力又急剧下降，也可以用明目地黄丸。

归芍地黄丸、杞菊地黄丸、明目地黄丸这三个地黄丸，都是从肝肾这两方面入手的。它们适合以肝肾阴虚为主要病症的人。

七味都气丸

七味都气丸是在六味地黄丸的基础上加五味子。五味子入五脏，味酸，能收敛肺气。有人因为肾虚影响到肺，呼吸就会变得短浅。庄子说过："平人之吸以喉，真人之吸以踵。"普通人呼吸只能呼吸到喉咙里，有修行的人呼吸可以一直呼吸到脚后跟。这是一种夸张的说法。其实他的本意是说平常的人呼吸比较浅，呼吸的时候胸部在起伏。有修行的人就不一样，胸部在起伏，小肚子也在起伏。因为气呼吸得很深长。呼吸到小肚子部位，应不应该呢？应该。因为肾主纳气，当人肾气旺的时候，就有一种力量把气往下拉。肾的力量越强，往下拉气的力度也越强，人的呼吸就会越深长。我们经常讲深呼吸，天然的深呼吸就取决于肾，当肾气旺的时候，肾纳气作用强的时候，我们每时每刻都是在深呼吸。

人都有气数，死的时候叫气数已尽，呼吸的次数已经用完了。当呼吸很短浅的时候，每分钟可能呼吸很多次；如果呼吸很深长，那么次数就会明显地变少，气数就够多用一段时间了，一生积累下来，会多用很多年，所以呼吸一定要深长。如果呼吸不深怎么办？用七味都气丸，它对气会有一定的统摄作用。同时，因为肾虚引起的阴虚、盗汗，七味都气丸也都是有作用的。

麦味地黄丸

在七味都气丸的基础上，再加麦冬，就是麦味地黄丸。麦冬是补肺阴的，还有清热的作用。麦冬和五味子是经常用的一个药对。它是入心、肺的，不但能够针对肾不纳气，而且能够针对肾虚型的咳嗽，尤其是老年人的肾虚型的干咳。

麦味地黄丸有七味都气丸的作用，它还能养肺。用了一味麦冬，它是用来养肺的。肺阴养足了，水之上源养足了，也能更好地养肾，所以七味都气丸和麦味地黄丸都是肺肾同养的方子。因为老年人经常用麦味地黄丸，所以麦味地黄丸还有一个名字叫八仙长寿丸。它是能让人长寿的。

六味地黄丸还有很多的加法，比如真阴不足，可以加强滋阴的力度，加上龟板胶、鹿角胶；如果是阳气不足，可以加上鹿茸、紫河车之类。

如果有的人吃了六味地黄丸以后不想吃饭。这是因为他的脾不能运化六味地黄丸。因为六味地黄丸里面的熟地、山萸肉都比较滋腻，这就要加上木香、砂仁等芳香的药来帮助它运化。木香、砂仁在这个方子里，并不是治病的药，而是治药的药。所以，方子里边既有治病的药，也要有治药的药，就像部队里有打敌人的，还有督战的。当然这个方剂的剂量不是固定的。如果治精气下脱导致的遗精之类，泽泻就少用一点，用一半；山萸肉是酸收的，可以多用一点来收一下。

关于六味地黄丸的加法，实在是太多了，要好好琢磨一下，因为它在临床上应用得太广。水是生命之源，养肾总不为错。病又变化多端，所以六味地黄丸也要跟着变。

左归和右归

前面讲的都是六味地黄丸的加法。那么，减法呢？

如果是阴虚的人，浑身都干巴巴的，就不能用茯苓、泽泻去给他利水了，可以去掉。如果他的肾气不通，怎么办呢？你可以只去掉茯苓，泽泻依然留着。如果一派寒象，没有血热，我们为什么还去清火呢？丹皮也可以去掉。甚至在有的情况下，你只在三补三泻这六种药中取三个就可以了，只用熟地、山萸肉、怀山药；其他的，你该怎么加，就怎么加。张景岳用六味地黄汤加减得非常灵活，他在六味地黄汤的基础上进行加减，创立了四个方子：左归丸、右归丸、左归饮、右归饮。

左归丸：大怀熟地八两，炒山药四两，山茱萸肉四两，枸杞四两，酒蒸川牛膝三两（精滑者，不用），制菟丝子四两，鹿胶四两，龟胶四两。先将熟地蒸烂杵膏，炼蜜为丸，如梧桐子大。每服百余丸，食前用滚汤或淡盐汤送下。（去龟板，加附子、肉桂、杜仲，为右归丸）

左归饮：熟地二三钱至一二两，山药二钱，山茱萸一二钱（畏酸者，少用之），枸杞二钱，茯苓一钱半，炙甘草一钱。水二盅，煎七分，空腹服。（去茯苓，加杜仲、附子、肉桂，为右归饮，火盛恐伤阴，不宜再渗利）

我们知道，左属水，右属火。左归丸和左归饮都是养肾阴的，大怀熟地八两，炒山药四两，山茱萸肉四两，这三个药就相当于是六味地黄丸的三补。枸杞加大养肝的力度；鹿胶是养阳的，龟胶是养阴的，这个既兼顾了肾阴又兼顾了肾阳；菟丝子是温肾阳的；川牛膝是往下走的，它能够化瘀。

在左归丸的基础上，去掉龟板，加附子、肉桂、杜仲，就成了右归丸。右归丸就成了补火的了，它也就相当于六味地黄丸加上附子、肉桂。杜仲也是温肾的，同时还能去肾中的风湿，因为肾一虚，风湿之邪往往就趁虚而入。去掉龟板是因为它是一个养阴的药，在养阳的药里如果过分养阴就会喧宾夺主，所以要去掉龟板，减少养阴的力度，体现右归。这是丸药，可以长期服用。左归饮和右归饮是作为日用的饮品，用量就小了，也灵活了。右归饮为什么要把茯苓去掉呢？因为你加了杜仲、附子、肉桂就等于是给它加了火了，火盛则伤阴，这样就不要再用茯苓来渗利它了，因为再利水就会伤阴伤得更厉害。

左归丸、右归丸、左归饮、右归饮跟六味地黄丸和八味地黄丸有很相似的地方。这样的方剂主治有很多，我们主要讲方子发挥作用的道理，具体治某个病我们讲的不多。每个方子的作用都是很广的，我们明白了道理以后，自然就会用了。

四物汤

四物汤中的生长收藏

四物汤出自《太平惠民和剂局方》，一共四味药：当归、川芎、白芍、地黄。

很多方子是由四味药组成的，其组方的原理往往跟一年四季的生长收藏有关。当归是一味补血的药，也能够补气，其味辛、甘，有生发之气，是生血的，对应的是春天。川芎能行气活血，能够把身上的血脉打通，让血迅速地长起来，所以说它是长血的，对应的是夏天。白芍是酸的，酸入肝，酸就能收，是收血的，对应的是秋天。地黄是入肾的，它是藏血的，对应的是冬天。所以，四物汤的四味药对应的是春、夏、秋、冬。血要经过生、长、收、藏这一个自然过程才能生出来，要是只用一味药补血就比较难。

当然，声称一味药就能补血的也有很多。像鸡血藤，它主要用于风湿伤血，或者用于通经络血脉，达到养血的目的。还有"一味丹参，功同四物"，其实丹参是一味化瘀药，"瘀血不去，新血不生"，把瘀化掉了，新血自然就生出来了。这些药偏于祛邪扶正，而真正要直接养血、生血，还是要用四物汤。

养血就是养肝肾

跟四物汤对应的还有一个四君子汤，由人参、白术、茯苓、甘草组成，都是入脾的药，可以说"补气就是补肺脾，养血就是养肝肾"。这话能够帮我们很好地理解中医，甚至能够帮我们开悟。其实，这话讲出来是不严谨的，但中医往往是需要这种不严谨的表述才能体现它的生动性。太严谨就死板了，死板的思想就治不好活人。中医的师徒关系一定要好，否则有些话都没法说，说出来你还会抬杠。《论语》有一句话，"君子和而不同，小人同而不和"，君子讨论一个问题的时候，追求和谐，相互理解，互相启发；小人就不一样，都是为了自己的那一点私利，头脑里都只有一些简单的思想，一说起话来都互相抬杠，喜欢争论。小人还有趋同的心理，看到大家都怎样他就也怎样，或是看到有人与自己不一样他就起烦恼。这样就学不好东西了。中国传统文化是君子之学，讲究的是"和而不同"。

初学中医，有两重境界，一重境界是，当你学了一些以后，就会自以为是，谁都瞧不起，这就是"同而不和"的思维在作怪。当你的境界提升，到了第二重境界就不一样了，这时候别人说的话你都会去考虑，去思考，去汲取里面有用的东西，这就对了。

四物汤的加减变化

四物汤的组成比较简单，它的意义浅显地讲就是养血，养肝肾；往深地讲，它是一个养血的基本方剂，在四物汤的基础上，我们也可以进行很多的加减。比如说血中有风，往往导致一些皮肤病，尤其是一些很痒的疹子，可以在四物汤的基础上加上荆芥、防风；如果血中有热，可以在四物汤的基础上再加上丹皮、赤芍；如果血中有瘀，可以在四物汤的基础上加上桃仁、红花。

　　四物汤中的地黄，如果略微偏血热的话，就用生地，如果血热不太明显，阴虚比较明显，可以用熟地；瘀血比较明显，当归可以用当归尾，白芍可以改成赤芍；肝阴虚比较明显的话，当归就用当归身，白芍就用白芍，这也是有很多的变化的。

　　任何一个药，跟着四物汤走，其药力就能很好地被带到血里面，四物汤在这里相当于一个药引子。但从根本上讲，四物汤是一个补药，如果是外邪比较重，四物汤就要慎用，否则在邪气没有被清掉之前，你就来补，可能就会导致邪气越补越厉害，你就没有补到身体上去，而补到病上去，把病越补越重了。

Chapter 3   Other Medicines for Nourishing the Kidney Yin

In accordance with TCM theory, the six hollow organs are subsumed to Yang and the five internal organs (i. e. , the five viscera) are subsumed to Yin. As for the six hollow organs, so long as they are kept unobstructed, they could remain healthy. As for the five internal organs, it is important to nourish Yin. In fact, nourishing is meant to nourish Yin of the five organs.

To nourish Yin of the five internal organs, the first thing is to nourish the kidney Yin. The kidney dominates water/fluid and storing the life essence, and water and life essence are the origin of life. "The bases of nourishment and defense against the pathogens lie in the quintessence of grains; and the firm foundation of longevity lies in the convergence of life essence. " And hence, regarding the principle of nourishment and defense, the most fundamental thing is to have a good appetite; Longevity or short life always depends upon how much life essence is accumulated inside the human body. The so-called accumulation of life essence is involved with two aspects: one is abstinence, and the other is nourishing.

The fundamental thing of nourishing Yin is to nourish the kidney-Yin since it is the kidneys that store the life essence. All the five internal organs can store the life essence, but finally, it is the kidneys that can store and seal up the life essence. If kidneys fail to store the life essence, there won't be much life essence to be stored by the five internal organs, either. So, the fundamental thing of nourishing Yin is to nourish the kidney-Yin. Dihuang is a representative herb for nourishing the kidney-Yin. Besides, Xuanshen (radix scrophulariae), Nuzhenzi (fructus ligustri lucidi), and Hanliancao (eclipta alba) can nourish the kidney Yin, too.

Xuanshen (Radix Scrophulariae)

In Chinese, radix scrophulariae isnamed as Xuan Shen, of which "Xuan" means "black". In Qing dynasty, the emperor Kangxi's real name was Xuanye, and in order to avoid the word "Xuan", Xuanshen (radix scrophulariae) was renamed as Yuanshen, which in some cases even now is still called by some people. It is bluish white in color, but will become black after it is dried, and it is very nutritious. Xuanshen produced in the North of China has better ascending and descending effects in medical practice. It is slightly bitter and salty in taste, and slightly cold in property, and fishy in smell.

Properties of Xuanshen

Basically speaking, the efficacy of a Chinese medicine can be known by its properties and smell. Xuanshen is bitter and salty in tastes. Its salty taste indicates it can go into the kidneys. It is slightly cold in property, which implies that it goes into kidneys to clear away the pathogenic heat. Among the five kinds of stink smells, the fishy smell goes into lungs, which means Xuanshen can also go into lungs. That is why Xuanshen enjoys both ascending and descending effects. When it ascends, it will rise to the lungs; and when it descends, it will fall to the kidneys. So, Xuanshen is a medicine for replenishing water/fluid and restraining fire.

Xuanshen is different from Huangbai and Zhimu in clearing away heat, and it mainly purges the floating fire in kidneys. Therefore, Zhang Yuansu, a doctor in the Jin and Yuan dynasties, said it is a cardinal medicine, which can command all kinds of Qi, and clear away all the turbid pathogens.

Why could the kidney Yin be in deficiency? The kidney Yin deficiency could be identified in some abnormal physical indicators shown in the examination result, so it is necessary to make clear of causes of such symptoms.

Indulgence in sexual pleasure, staying up late, and excessive worries all could result in kidney Yin losses. What consequences would the kidney fluid loss lead to? The kidneys are the place where the kidney Yin and Yang meet and interact. In case the kidney Yin is dificient, the kidney Yang will fail to find the place to go and will become a floating fire. "Yang stays outside as a manifestation of Yin; Yin lays foundation inside and Yang protects it from the outside." Just like a couple, if the wife at home keeps gentle and virtuous, the husband will surely come back home from the outside; If the wife is not alive, or the wife is not gentle and considerate enough, the husband may wander outside. That is to say, when the kidney Yin is deficient, the kidney Yang will find no home to return, and will become the floating fire that is very easy to go up. When the floating fire goes to the chest, it will make the patient irritable and feel annoyed, which is called "enshrouding fire in the chest" in ancient books; when this kind of fire continues to go up to the throat, it will cause sore throat; when it goes to the side of neck a little further, it may lead to scrofulosis, referring to many agglomerations at the neck like lymph nodes; and when it continues to rush up to the head, it will result in tinnitus and headache. This kind of floating fire can also go to the surface of the body to form some patches. However, such patches are actually not freckle but erythema on the body. Septicemia and leukemia can also cause some plaques. However, the plaques arising from septicemia are relatively deep-colored, and the plaques arising from leukemia are light pink, both of which are related to the floating fire in the kidneys. Anyone that suffers from these diseases mentioned above can use Xuanshen for treatment.

Comparison between the Uses of Xuangshen and Dihuang

Xuanshen has the effects of clearing up and purging downwards, so it can clear the upper floating heat and nourish the kidney Yin as well, but its role of nourishing the kidney Yin is far inferior to Dihuang. Then why does Xuanshen have to be used instead of Sheng Dihuang or Shudi for some cases?

Sheng Dihuang and Shudi are greasier. Those who suffer from pathogenic fire should take great caution about using the greasy medicines since pathogenic fire will be bonded together with the greasy medicine to transform into phlegm. The primordial Yin could be tonified only under the precondition that the pathogenic fire has been eliminated. Otherwise, to tonify Yin is like pouring oil into the burning hot pot, which will cause a fire all of a sudden. The hot pot must be cooled down slowly by the way of clearing the fire on the one hand, and considering Yin nourishing at the same time on the other hand. Only Xuanshen can accomplish such a task when there is the kidney Yin deficiency accompanied by the floating fire in the kidneys.

Comparison between Uses of Xuanshen, Huangbai and Zhimu

Huangbai (phellodendron amurense) and Zhimu (rhizoma anemarrhenae) could also clear the pathogenic fire in the kidneys. What is the difference between these two herbs and Xuanshen? When the pathogenic fire in the kidneys makes disturbance in the Lower Jiao, use Huangbai and Zhimu to clear the Lower Jiao; when this fire does not make any disturbance in the Lower Jiao and has been going upwards, Huangbai and Zhimu will become ineffective. Meanwhile, Huangbai is bitter and cold, which may spoil the stomach, so more Huangbai may cause trouble to the stomach. Just like a fight in the battle field, soldiers have to chase to beat the enemies wherever they flee. When they flee upwards, the soldiers should not chase downwards. Therefore, it is very important for doctors to get familiar with the diseases and the medical orientation in the process of treatment of diseases.

When the pathogenic fire is floating above, Xuanshen will be the best choice for nourishing Yin to lessen the fire. Of course, it is not advisable to use Xuanshen for too long time. Stop using Xuanshen after the fire is cleared. The kidney is subsumed to water and it is fond of warmth rather than coldness, so too much heat elimination may impair the kidney Yang or even restrict the primordial Qi.

Now, many patients are quite afraid of the cold medicines, and say they can restrict Yang. In fact, don't get feared since the disease, if there is any, will withstand it, and it won't do harm to the health of human body. However, when the disease is cured, stop using the medicine at the right time. No medicine is absolutely good or absolutely bad, and the key point is to use it right to the point.

Zengye Tang and Nourishing Yin and Clearing Fire at the Later Stage of Febrile Diseases

The febrile disease impairs Yin, so **Zengye Tang** may be used, which contains the ingredient herbs: Xuanshen (radix scrophulariae), Maidong (radix ophiopogonis), and Sheng Dihuang (radix rehmanniae recen).

This will further magnify the role of Xuanshen: the pathogenic fire in the chest is now cleared away with Xuanshen, which simultaneously nourishes the kidney Yin so that the kidneys can slowly put out the pathogenic fire. If and when the pathogenic fire is floating above, it would impair the lung Yin since fire restricts Yin. The lung is delicate and is unable to resist coldness and heat. So, when the kidney fire is floating upwards, the lung Yin will inevitably be impaired. Maidong is a strong tonic for tonifying the lungs, and it not only can clear away the pathogenic fire, but also nourish Yin. Maidong does not go downwards, and it can directly repair the impairment caused by the floating fire to the lungs. Sheng Dihuang also has the function of eliminating the pathogenic fire, and can nourish kidneys as well. But at the moment when there is still fire, Shudi is not used in order to avoid inducing phlegm. Meanwhile, Sheng Dihuang not being greasy, it has a stronger effect for clearing heat, and also, Sheng Dihuang is the lateral root, having a dispersing effect.

Two aspects should be paid to the treatment of febrile diseases: one is to nourish Yin, and the other is to properly handle permeability and dispersion. Medication should be light and flexible, but not sluggish. Shudi is more sluggish, and easy to converge the pathogenic factors. It has no permeating and dispersing effects. However, Sheng Dihuang is a little bit light and active, and it not only has the penetrating and dispersing effects, but also clears the pathogenic heat. Hence, when Sheng Dihuang is used together with Xuanshen, they can clear fire and nourish the kidney at the same time, and they are quite suitable for nourishing Yin fluid and clearing the floating pathogenic fire at the later stage of febrile diseases.

After the floating pathogenic fire is cleared away, stop using Xuanshen immediately, but Sheng Dihuang can be used continuously until the syndromes of phlegm and pathogenic fire disappear with only Yin deficiency remains. By this moment, substitute Sheng Dihuang with Shudi, and then, **Liuwei Dihuang Tang**, or **Maiwei Dihuang Tang** can be used boldly as necessary since by that stage there is no pathogenic factors existing at all and nourishing can be intensified.

At the late stage of the febrile diseases, some residual floating fire may remain in the chest, and the patients may suffer from annoyance, perturbation and sleeplessness etc. Therefore, Xuanshen can be used with Zhimu, Maidong and bamboo leaves and so on. Maidong can clear the lung fire and nourish the lungs as well; Bamboo leaves can clear the heart fire; Zhimu can clear the stomach fire; and Xuanshen can nourish the kidneys to lessen the floating fire. As such, the source of the floating fire is completely eradicated, and the enshrouding fire in the chest would naturally disappear.

Treatment of Sore Throat with Xuanshen

At the late stage of the febrile diseases, there will arise a sore throat accompanied with some macules. For such a case, there is a well-known formula called **Xuanshen Shengma Tang**, containing three herbs: Xuanshen (radix scrophulariae), Shengma (rhizoma cimicifugae), Gancao (liquorice), among which Xuanshen is for nourishing Yin and clearing the floating fire, and Shengma is for ascending to permeate outwards. It functions to bring up the medical effects to the throat and let the macules permeate outwards. By the way, Xuanshen is frequently used for curing the sore throat arising from Yin deficiency and the vigorous pathogenic fire.

There is another well-known medicine for curing the sore throat, i. e. , Niubangzi (fructus arctii), which is generally used for curing the sore throat arising from the exogenous cold diseases. The acute attack of sore throat, regardless of exogenous infection or endogenous diseases, can be cured with Xuanshen and Niubangzi. Of course, Niubangzi should be used in a large dose, preferably with half of the raw Niubangzi, and the other half of the parched Niubangzi, both of which should be crushed. As an herb of seed, Niubangzi goes downwards, lessens and disperses the endogenous heat. Due to its slippery nature, Niubangzi can help to thin and lubricate the feces so that the endogenous heat can be discharged with feces.

Xuanshen can clear fire, but also can thin and lubricate feces. So, in the case of thin feces, stop using Xuanshen. Otherwise, the physically weak person may have more serious diarrhea, even causing Yin depletion from diarrhea.

TCM often stresses that "the excessive perspiration results in Yang depletion, and the serious diarrhea results in Yin depletion. " Those who are seriously ill suddenly suffer from excessive oily and sticky perspiration must be extremely cautious. It might be Yang depletion due to excessive perspiration, and Yang escapes with sweating. The serious diarrhea resulting in Yin depletion refers that the anus seems to become a loose hole, and it cannot stop the feces discharging, so Yin fluid of the body will all go down to the drain. Both Yang depletion from the excessive perspiration and Yin depletion from the serious diarrhea could kill a person.

Xuanshen seems to be a very peaceful Yin-nourishing medicine, but if wrongly used, it could also kill a person, so, be careful!

Compatibility of Xuanshen for Improving Vision

Xuanshen (radix scrophulariae) used together with Dihuang (rehmannia), Juhua (chrysanthemum), Jili (tribulus terrestris), Gouqizi (fructus lycii) and Chaihu (radix bupleuri) can improve eyesight. Generally speaking, this formula is for the treatment of the dim eyesight arising from deficiency of the kidney and vigorous pathogenic fire. Because of Yin deficiency of the liver and kidney, the pathogenic fire of the liver and kidney will go upwards, making the patients feel dizzy and giddy, dim and faint in eyes, which are all of the manifestations of deficiency. Both Xuanshen and Dihuang could nourish the kidney-Yin; Gouqizi could nourish the liver-Yin; Juhua not only nourishes the liver-Yin, but also disperses the liver-heat; Jili could disperse the liver-heat; Chaihu could soothe the liver. When all these herbs are used together, they can disperse and soothe the liver, and nourish the liver and kidneys.

I keep on talking of nourishing liver all the time since the liver opens at the eyes, so actions must be taken on the liver for the sake of improving eyesight. In case the dim and faint eyesight arises from Yin deficiency of the liver and kidney, it may not be sufficient to nourish the liver and kidney Yin deficiency only, and it is also necessary to make clear the functions of the liver in order to take some remedies from different angles.

The kidney fluid helps the liver wood grow. Dihuang and Xuanshen are used to replenish the kidney fluid in order to nourish the liver wood. The liver likes to be smooth, so Jili and Chaihu are used to soothe the liver; The liver itself also needs nourishing with the tepid medicine, so Gouqizi, tepid in property, is just the right choice. Some wind-heat in the liver meridians can be dispersed with Juhua and Jili. The liver is nourished from different angles in order to guide the liver and kidney Yin to the eyes for the purpose of improving eyesight.

Treatment of Scrofulosis With Xuanshen

It has been discussed about the treatment of scrofulosis with Xuanshen in the previous section. Scrofulosis is greatly related to pyrophlegm. When the phlegm and fire are interweaved with each other to form mass, which will then become scrofulosis. It can be cured with Xuanshen used together with Beimu (fritillaria), Lianqiao (fructus forsythiae), Gancao (liquorice), Tianhua Fen (Radices Trichosanthis) and Bohe (mint) since the origin of the interties between phlegm and fire lie in loss of kidney fluid and the ascending pathogenic fire. Therefore, the critical way is to nourish the kidney fluid and clear the ascending pathogenic fire with Xuanshen, which, however, is not sufficient. It is necessary to exercise control over it fromsource to the flowline, i. e. , not only relieve the symptoms but also make permanent cure.

What should be done for relieving the symptoms? The phlegm and pathogenic fire have already interweaved with each other to form the stasis. In order to remove the stasis, generally speaking, a larger dosage of Zhe Beimu (thunberg fritillary bulb) should be used. By the way, Tianhua Fen (radices trichosanthis) can also nourish Yin, reduce phlegm and remove stasis as well; Lianqiao is used here to intensify the effect of clearing the pathogenic fire; Gancao should be used in a large dosage here, at least 10 grams, since its sweet taste moves slowly and functions to soften the stasis. Gancao can loosen the phlegm-fire interconnection so that all medicines can get in to play their medical effects.

In fact, it is not sufficient to use Xuanshen and Lianqiao only for clearing the pathogenic fire in the interweaved pyrophlegm, and it is also necessary to disperse the fire. Bohe is a cold medicine, which can function to open the exterior for dispersing fire. All the herbs used in this formula are frequently used for curing scrofulosis, but appropriate modifications of the formula need to be made according to the specific syndromes of different patients.

Treatment of Diabetes with Xuanshen

Xuanshen is one of the herbs frequently used in the treatment of diabetes, especially for treatment of the diabetes arising from Qi and Yin deficiency. Xuanshen has an effective function of quenching thirst, not only because it can nourish the kidney fluid and clear the floating fire, but the more critical point is that it can guide the kidney fluid to go upwards.

Those who suffer from diabetes are frequently thirsty because of the essentially dry nature of diabetes. The floating fire is continuously fuming inside the body, causing the body fluid to be dried up, and thus, the human body is also fumed to be dry consequently. Hence, Xuanshen is used for moistening purpose.

In the treatment of dryness, try to make little use of the seriously aromatic and dry medicines since the dryness inside the body and the dryness of medicines would make the situation worse. Consequently, the drier the medicine to be taken by the patients, the thirstier the patients would feel. Of course, "little use of the dry medicine" here does not mean "no use", but on the contrary, I mean a quite small dosage of dry medicine might have to be used since if only the Yin-nourishing and the cold moistening medicines are used, they may restrict the primordial Qi in the human body, or cause the body failure in the T&T functions. So, in the treatment of diabetes, a small dosage of Cangzhu (rhizoma atractylodis) can be used with Xuanshen. Cangzhu is a severely dry medicine, which can dry dampness and strengthen the spleen. When used together with Xuanshen, Cangzhu not only can function to moisten the body, but also converge the spleen fluid. Xuanshen can make feces become thin, but with the use of Cangzhu, the feces can be normal again. Cangzhu can further intensify the spleen of its T&T function, which would help to keep fluid from being discharged with the feces, and the fluid remained inside would also become the useful fluid for moistening the body. And therefore, the dry symptoms of diabetes will be relieved and improved, but certainly, this will take time and patience for moistening and nourishing effects.

Hanliancao (Eclipta Alba)

Similarities Between Hanliancao and Xuanshen

Hanliancao is a kind of grass in the south of China, and it likes to grow in wet places. When its leaves or stems are broken, some black juice, like ink, will outflow, so it is renamed as Mohanlian. It is sour and sweet in tastes and cold in property. The sour and sweet tastes can nourish Yin, so this herb used as medicine is for nourishing Yin. Meanwhile, the cold nature signifies that it can clear heat; the black color signifies it can go into the kidneys to nourish Yin and clear heat there. Over all, it has similar efficacies to Xuanshen.

Hanliancao goes into the meridians of the liver, kidneys, stomach, large intestine, small intestine to nourish Yin and blood. It has another similarity to Xuanshen, i. e., ascending effect. It is a relatively cold medicine, so those who suffer from Yang deficiency should use it with great caution, and especially those who suffer from Yang deficiency and slippery feces several times a day, should not use Hanliancao. Those who suffer from Yin deficiency with heat and dry feces could find an extremely good effect with the use of Hanliancao.

Of course, although Hanliancao has some similarities to Xuanshen, it is a different herb after all, and the natural properties of these two herbs are not quite the same. Xuanshen tends to clear the floating heat and penetrating downwards. Hanliancao is not that powerful, but it also has the effects of its own.

Blackening Hair and Consolidating Teeth

Hanliancao can blacken hair, similar to Heshouwu (polygonum multiflorum), but it is more powerful. The name "Heshouwu" ("He Shou Wu" in Chinese pinyin, of which "Wu" means "black") makes people fancy it could blacken hair, but in fact, the effect of blackening hair is not that striking. There are lots of requirements for processing it. If it is not well and properly processed, it would be toxic. After it is well-processed, Hanliancao is mild and more effective for medical use.

The hair of human being becomes yellow or grey in that there is heat inside the body, especially the blood heat. Hanliancao can nourish Yin and clear the blood heat. It is black itself, so, to take it orally can blacken hair, and also, to apply the juice of fresh Hanliancao to hair and beard for a certain period of time can also make hair and beard black.

Fresh Hanliancao can also help the loose teeth become consolidated gradually by rubbing the fresh Hanliancao on the teeth. In the past, many people used to put some medical powder called teeth powder on cloth to wipe their teeth. Such a teeth powder may be added with some Hanliancao too for consolidating the loose teeth. The ancients had their special way to wipe the teeth or rinse the mouth, which formed a lot of empirical formulas based upon the fundamentals of traditional Chinese medicine.

Treatment of Jiuchuang Fahong

Hanliancao has another good efficacy for treatment of Jiuchuang Fahong (post-moxibustion sore bleeding) .

There is a moxibustion called scar moxibustion. It is always said that "if you want to keep healthy, keep Zusanli acupoint wet. " That is to keep Zusanli acupoint in a state of ulcer all the time. When moxibustion is frequently done at Zusanli acupoint, the skin around the acupoint will be burned, which is called Jiuchuang (post-moxibustion sore) . Such a moxibustion sore is normal, but what is Fahong (sore bleeding) ? It does not mean it looks a little reddish, but like a flood. If moxibustion is frequently done, it will stir up the blood heat so that moxibustion sore point will start to bleed. Such a symptom is called Jiuchuang Fahong, indicating that the moxibustion was done wrongly, or moxibustion was overdone.

Moxibustion is not suitable for every person. If used improperly, it may consume Qi and blood in the dark even if the symptom of Jiuchuang Fahong might not arise. The moxibustion has a lot of obvious advantages, but it causes some risks in the dark, too.

When there arises the post-moxibustion sore bleeding, it might be that the blood heat does exist in the body of the patient. The moxibustion may just be the inducement that stirs up the pathogenic fire to result in blood failing to stay in the meridians and then starting to bleed. At this moment, application of some fresh or dried Hanliancao to the bleeding point, or taking some Hanliancao orally can stop the bleeding soon.

Nuzhenzi (Fructus ligustri lucidi)

Erzhi Pill

Hanliancao can remind us of another herb of Nuzhenzi (fructus ligustri lucidi), which is frequently used together with Hanliancao. The two herbs together will make a formula called Erzhi Pill (which means "Double Solstice Pill", the two herbs contained in the pill are collected at the winter solstice and summer solstice respectively).

Erzhi Pill (literally means Two-solstice Pill) is for tonifying the liver and kidney and is able to strengthen muscles and bones. Meanwhile, it also has the function of clearing heat. Nuzhenzi is mild, and Hanliancao is slightly cold with the effects of clearing heat, nourishing liver and kidneys, and strengthening muscles and bones. This formula is frequently used to nourish the kidney and Yin. Dongzhi (The winter solstice) is the most appropriate season for collecting Nuzhenzi, while Xiazhi (the summer solstice) is the most appropriate season for collecting Hanliancao. That is why this pill is called **Erzhi Pill**.

Implication of Nuzhenzi

Nuzhenzi bears on the privet tree, which is very tall with leaves all year round, not withered even in the winter season and looking like Dongqing (evergreen tree). The two trees are easy to be confused in appearance, but in fact, there is a slight difference between the two. The privet leaves are relatively longer and larger, approximately four or five inches long, and its seeds are purple black. There are varieties of Dongqing, and some of them have seeds, and some not. The leaves of Dongqing are much closer to round shape, and its seeds are red.

The privet tree (Chinese name "**Nü Zhen**") stands high slimly and very gracefully, neither withered in winter season, nor fearing the severe wind and snow. "**Nü**" ("female" in English) means this herb can nourish Yin, and "**Zhen**" (virginity) indicates this herb can go into the kidneys to play guarding and defending function, signifying that it holds fast to something.

According to Zhouyi (*Book of Changes*), the development of things always

— 689 —

experiences the process of "元" (Yuan), "亨" (Heng), "利" (Li), "贞" (Zhen), which correspond to spring, summer, autumn and winter respectively. Spring corresponds to "Yuan", referring to the beginning and birth; "Heng" means "very prosperous", referring to growth in summer; "利"(Li) has the lateral radical (刂), referring to "knife" in Chinese, which implies the meaning of "metal", as such "Li" signifies "gained" with an awful atmosphere; "Zhen" means "upright", corresponding to the season of winter, which signifies to store. "Zhen" also indicates the virtue of holding fast to something of "chastity". A privet(Chinese name "**Nü Zhen**") tree can bear a lot of seeds, so from this perspective, "**Zhen**" means more children, and more children, in the other way round, means "chastity".

Days ago, I read in microblog that "Chinese are shy of talking about sex, but they created a country of the largest population", which attempts to demonstrate a paradox. In essence, it is not as what he thinks. A large population does not mean a bad thing at all but actually means more human power.

Being shy of talking about sex means that everyone is abstinent about sex. Abstinence, to some extent, implies chastity, which means to give a good birth to and care of more children. Opposite to "**Zhen**" is lewdness, which, on the contrary, will result in infertility. And therefore, just because of "Zhen", a great country of the largest population is created. The lewdness will lead to childlessness, regardless of men or women.

Properties and Uses of Nuzhenzi

The privet tree starts to bear seeds in summer, and its fruits hang in the twigs and branches and slowly become reddish, purple and black until the winter solstice day. And then, Nuzhenzi will be picked and collected.

Nuzhenzi can be directly dried in the sun, or can also be steamed with liquor before drying. The liquor-steamed Nuzhenzi can dry faster. Nuzhenzi goes downwards, but after being steamed, it will be able to go upwards first to lungs, and then downwards to kidneys. As an herb, Nuzhenzi is a very mild medicine. From its Chinese name "Nü Zhen Zi", it can be known that it is as quiet as a virgin, that is to say, it is also inactive. But after it is steamed with liquor, it will become more active and much easier to digest and absorb.

Nuzhenzi tastes bitter, sweet and sour, and it is neither cold nor hot, but mild in property. It can nourish the kidney, reduce fever, and conserve/accumulate energy. Generally, those who suffer from Yin deficiency accompanied by pathogenic fire can use it; otherwise, it may result in stomachache and diarrhea.

Nuzhenzi also has the efficacy of improving eyesight and blackening hair. It is often used together with Juhua (chrysanthemum), Sheng Dihuang (radix rehmanniae recen), Jili (tribulus terrestris), Gouqizi (fructus lycii) for improving eyesight. Sheng Dihuang used together with Nuzhenzi can clear pathogenic heat and nourish the kidney. Of course, the medicine that can nourish the kidney will also be able to clear away pathogenic heat. As it is known, heat always makes one feel dizzy and giddy, and coolness can make one feel clear, which means "refreshed and clear-headed" on the one hand, and "clear eyesight" on the other hand. Jili is used to soothe the liver; Gouqizi is used to nourish Yin of the liver and kidneys; Juhua is used to calm the liver and disperse the pathogenic fire. This formula is similar to that related to the herbal combination of Xuanshen for improving eyesight in principle.

第三章　其他养肾阴药

我们知道，六腑为阳、五脏为阴。六腑以通为补，就是说要保持通畅，就是健康。五脏为阴，当养其阴，滋补就是围绕养五脏之阴来讲的。

养五脏之阴，首先就是养肾阴。肾主水，藏精，而水和精是生命的本源。"营卫之道，纳谷为宝；寿命之本，积精至刚"，营卫之道，能吃饭是最根本的；一个人长寿还是短寿，看他积累了多少精，所谓积精，一是节欲，二是滋补。

养阴的根本就是养肾阴，因为是肾藏精。五脏都藏精，最后要由肾来把精进一步封藏起来。如果肾藏精藏得比较坚固，那么五脏都能藏精。如果肾藏精藏不住，那么五脏也藏不了多少精。所以养阴的根本就是在养肾阴，而地黄是养肾阴的一个代表药。当然养肾阴不仅仅是地黄，还有我们将要讲到的玄参、女贞子、旱莲草。

玄参

玄就是黑的意思。康熙年间，因为康熙皇帝叫玄烨，为了避他的讳，玄参被改名叫元参，现在还有人这么叫。它的根是青白色的，晾干了以后是黑的，很有滋润性。北方产的玄参药效比较好。玄参味苦咸，性微寒，还有一股腥气，可升可降。

玄参的性能

一个中药，究其性味，基本就知道它有什么作用了。玄参味苦、咸，苦就能清火，咸就能入肾。性微寒，依然是清火，入肾而清火。它有股腥味，在五臭中，腥是入肺的，这意味着玄参还能入肺，所以它是一味可升可降的药。升就升到肺，降就降到肾。因此它是一味壮水制火的药。

玄参清火跟黄柏、知母有一些不同，它主要泻肾家无根浮游之火。所以张元素说它是一个枢机之药，能够统领诸气，上下清肃而不浊。

我们从头来看，肾阴之所以亏损，并不是因为某一项指标高了；相反，某一项指标高了是因为肾阴亏损导致的。要把这个因果搞清楚。任何化验结果都是病导致的，而不是说这个病是那个化验结果导致的。

纵欲、熬夜、思虑过度等，都能导致肾阴亏损，肾水亏了，又会导致什么后果呢？肾是肾阴肾阳相交抱的场所。如果肾阴亏了，肾阳就没有归宿了，它就成了浮游之火。"阳在外，阴之使也；阴在内，阳之守也。"就像一个家庭，有夫妻两人，妻子在家而且温柔贤惠，丈夫在外边就一定要回来；如果妻子没有了，或者妻子不够体贴，丈夫可能就会在外边游荡，所以肾阴亏损，肾阳就没有归宿，成了浮火，这种浮火很容易往上走，如果走到胸中就能让人烦躁，让人有心下懊恼的感觉，这个在古书中叫"氤氲于胸中"；这种火继续往上走，走到咽喉就导致咽痛；如果再往边上走一点，可能导致瘰疬，瘰疬就是脖子这个地方有很多的结块，像淋巴结那样的；如果继续往上冲，冲到头上就会导致耳鸣、头痛。这种浮火还会往体表走，形成斑。这个斑并不是雀斑，而是身上的红斑。败血症、白血病都会有斑。败血症的斑，颜色比较深；白血病的斑，颜色是浅粉红色的，这都跟肾中的浮游之火有关系。凡是遇到上边讲的这些病，都可以用玄参。

玄参与地黄的使用比较

玄参有清上彻下的作用，上能清浮游的热，下能养肾阴，但它养肾阴的作用远远不如生地、熟地。为什么在这时候非得用玄参而不要生地、熟地呢？

生地、熟地比较滋腻，当人体有火邪的时候，就要慎用滋腻的药，因为火通常会跟滋腻的药结在一起化成痰。要大补真阴，必须在清了火的前提下才能用。如果火没有清掉，你急于滋阴，就像锅被烧得滚烫，你再倒油下去，可能一下子就着火了。你得慢慢把锅凉下来，一方面要清火，一方面又要兼顾养阴，只有玄参能够同时担此重任，所以当肾阴虚，同时肾中浮游之火往上走的时候就得用玄参。

玄参与黄柏、知母的使用比较

黄柏、知母也是清肾中火邪的，它们跟玄参有什么区别呢？肾中火邪，如果在下焦扰动，就可以用知母、黄柏，来清下焦；如果这个火不在下焦扰动，已经往上走了，此时知母、黄柏就不管用了。何况黄柏是苦寒败胃的药，吃多了也不好。敌人往哪里走了，你就要朝哪里去追打，敌人现在往上走了，你就不要再往下进攻，因此，知道病和药的走向非常重要。

火浮游在上，应该滋阴降火，用玄参是最好的；当然玄参用的太久了也不好，当把火清掉以后，玄参就不要再用了。继续用下去，会导致什么后果呢？肾属水，喜温恶寒，清热过了头，就伤了肾阳。所以，只要火退掉了，就不要再用玄参了，不然的话，就克伐元气。

现在很多人见了寒凉药就非常害怕，说它克伐阳气。其实根本不用怕，有病则病受之，不会伤人的，中病即止就可以了。没有任何一个药绝对的好，也没有任何一个药绝对地不好，关键就是要用得恰到好处。

增液汤与温病后期的养阴清火

温病伤了阴，可用增液汤：玄参、麦冬、生地。

这就把玄参的作用进一步地放大了：火邪在胸中，现在用玄参来清火邪，同时来养肾阴，让肾慢慢地把火邪收下去。火邪在上边的时候，就会伤了肺阴，因火克金。肺为娇脏，不耐寒热，肾火浮游，肺阴必然受损。麦冬是一个补肺的重剂，能够清火，也能够养阴。麦冬不往下走，它直接在这里修复浮火对肺带来的损失。生地也是清火的，还能养肾。因为这时候依然有火，所以不要用熟地，恐生痰。生地不滋腻，它清热的作用要强一些，生地是地黄的旁根，旁根就有一定的散的作用。

治疗温病，一要注重养阴，二要注意透散，用药要轻灵，不宜呆滞。熟地比较呆滞，容易收敛邪气，不能透散。生地轻灵一些，能够透散，还能清热。生地跟玄参一起用，既能清火又能养肾，很适合在温病后期用来滋阴液、清浮火。

等浮火清掉了以后，就不要再用玄参了，生地依然可以用。到了没有痰象，也没有火象，仅仅是阴虚的时候，地黄就可以换成熟地。这时候六味地黄汤、麦味地黄汤等，就可以放心大胆地用了，因为这时候没有邪气啦，滋补的力度就可以加大。

温病后期，胸中容易残存一些氤氲浮游之火，人出现懊恼、心烦不眠等状况。怎么办呢？可用玄参配知母、麦冬、竹叶等。麦冬清肺火，还能养肺；竹叶清心火；知母清胃火。再加一个玄参，养肾以降浮游之火。把浮游之火的源头给杜绝了，胸中这种氤氲之火，自然就没有了。

玄参治咽痛

温病后期出现伴随着发斑的咽痛，那么有一个很著名的方子，叫玄参升麻汤，三味药：玄参、升麻、甘草。玄参依然滋阴，清浮游之火；升麻是升举的，往外透，一则把药力往咽喉上带，二则把斑透出去。玄参经常用来治疗阴虚火旺的咽痛。

治咽痛，还有一味很有名的药，就是牛蒡子。牛蒡子一般治外感病的咽痛。凡是急性发作的咽痛，不管是外感，还是内伤，都可以用玄参和牛蒡子。当然，牛蒡子要大量地用，最好用一半生的，一半炒的，把它捣碎。作为种子，牛蒡子是往下降的，能够降火，也有透散的作用，其性滑利，能够让大便变稀变滑，火更容易随着大便排出去。

玄参是清火的，也能够让大便很稀滑。假如大便稀就不要用它了，否则，身体好的人还能扛得住，身体不好的人可能就拉得更厉害了，甚至可能会导致洞泄亡阴。

中医经常讲"大汗亡阳，洞泄亡阴"。病重的人，忽然出很多的汗，而且跟油似的粘手，你要非常小心，可能是大汗亡阳，阳气随着汗就脱出去了。洞泄亡阴就是肛门好像成了一个洞，收不住了，大便一直往下泄，身体的阴液就全部下去了。大汗亡阳和洞泄亡阴，都会死人。

所以，玄参看起来是一个养阴的药，很平和，但是你用错了，也会把人治死，一定要注意。

玄参的明目配伍

玄参配地黄、菊花、蒺藜、枸杞子、柴胡这五味药，能够明目，一般是治疗因为肾虚火旺导致的眼睛昏花。因为肝肾阴虚，肝肾之火就会往上走，使人头脑昏昏、眼睛昏蒙，这都是属虚。玄参和地黄是养肾阴的；枸杞子是养肝阴的；菊花既养肝阴，又散肝热；蒺藜也能散肝热；柴胡能疏肝，它们一起合用，既能散肝，又能疏肝，能养肝，还养肾。

为什么总说要养肝呢？因为肝开窍于目，要明目就该在肝上多做文章。如果是肝肾阴虚导致眼睛看不太清的，只滋补肝肾阴虚还是不行的，我们还要把肝的一切性质弄清楚，从各个不同的角度来辅助它。

肾水生肝木，我们用地黄和玄参来滋肾水以养肝木；肝是喜欢条达、喜欢疏动的，所以用蒺藜、柴胡疏肝；肝本身也是要用微温的药来养的，枸杞子正好是一味微温的药；肝经上的一些风热，我们用菊花、蒺藜来散掉它，这就是从各个不同的角度养肝，使肝肾之阴上承于目，达到明目的目的。

玄参治瘰疬

上面我们讲过玄参治瘰疬。瘰疬跟痰火有很大的关系，痰火结成块就成了瘰疬了。玄参同贝母、连翘、甘草、花粉、薄荷合用，能治瘰疬，因为痰火互结的根源在肾水亏虚而浮火上行。用玄参滋养肾水、清上行之浮火，就管住了它的根本。光管住根本还不行，还要从源到流一直管住才行，既要治本也要治标。

用什么来治标呢？痰火已经互结了，就要散结，用贝母，一般用浙贝母，而且要用大剂量的浙贝母来化痰散结；花粉也是化痰散结的，就是栝楼的根，既养阴又化痰散结；连翘在这里是加大清火的力度；甘草在这里剂量要大，起码要用10克。甘就能缓，缓就能软。甘草可以让痰火互结变松一些，这样这些药的药力就能进去了。

痰火互结的火，我们用玄参、连翘来清还不够，治火还有个方法就是散火。薄荷是一味凉药，能开表、散火。这一组药是经常用来治瘰疬的，要根据病人的具体情况，进行适当的加减。

糖尿病中用玄参

玄参也是治疗糖尿病中经常用的一味药，尤其是气阴两虚型的糖尿病。玄参有很好的止渴作用，这不仅是因为它能够养肾水、清浮火；更重要的是因为它能引肾水往上走。

糖尿病病人通常会口渴，因为这个病从本质上讲是燥症。因为浮火老是在这里熏，津液被熏干了，机体被熏燥了。所以用玄参来滋润。

在治燥症时要注意，少用芳香燥烈的药。因为体内是燥的，药也是燥的，人吃了就会越吃越燥！说燥药要少用，但也不是一点燥药也不让用，相反还得略微的用一点燥药。如果一派的滋阴药与凉润药，可能会克伐人体的真气，或者让人体运化不动。糖尿病用玄参，同时往往还用一点苍术。苍术就是一个燥烈的药，能燥湿健脾。苍术配上玄参，它既能滋润，又能收敛脾津。玄参能让大便稀，但与苍术同用，大便就不稀了。因为苍术能够让脾的运化能力进一步加强，运化好了，很多水就不会随大便排出了，而变成有用的、滋润人体的津液了，人体得到了滋润，燥象就会缓解，作为燥证的糖尿病就会得到很好的改善。只不过是需要长时间坚持，慢慢地润养。

旱莲草

旱莲草与玄参的类似之处

旱莲草，南方的一种草，它喜欢长在潮湿的地方，叶子或者茎折断后，会流出黑色的汁液，像墨汁一样，所以又叫墨旱莲，其味酸甘、性寒。酸甘化阴，所以它是一味养阴的药；性寒能清热；它是黑色的，能入肾，能到肾里去养阴清热，与玄参有些类似。

旱莲草入肝、肾、胃、大肠、小肠五经，能够补阴养血。它跟玄参还有一个类似的地方，都是往下降，是比较寒凉的药，阳虚的人要慎用，尤其是阳虚、大便滑，一天有好几次大便的人，就不要用旱莲草。那种阴虚有热、大便干结的，用旱莲草就非常好。

当然，它虽然与玄参有相似的地方，但毕竟是不同的药物，它们的自然属性是不一样的。玄参倾向于清浮游之热，清上彻下。旱莲草没有那么神通广大，但它也有它的绝活。

乌须发、固齿

旱莲草能够乌须发，这有点像何首乌，但它比何首乌的作用还要强。何首乌的名字就让人觉得它能乌须发，但实际上，效果没那么好，而且对炮制的要求还很高，如果炮制不好，还会有毒。旱莲草则平和而有效。

人的头发之所以会发黄、发白，是因为体内有热，尤其是血热。旱莲草能养阴、清血热，而且它本身就是黑的，内服就可以乌须发，还可以用新鲜的旱莲草的汁往头发上、胡须上涂，涂一段时间也能让头发、胡子变黑。

如果牙齿动摇，可以用新鲜旱莲草来擦牙，可以让牙齿慢慢变得坚固起来。过去的人会把药粉放在布上来擦牙，这种药粉就叫牙粉。如果牙齿动摇，可以在牙粉里配入旱莲草。古人擦牙、漱口都有其特定的方式，这都是根据中医的基本原理来的，牙粉也有很多验方。

治灸疮发洪

旱莲草还有一个很好的作用是治疗灸疮发洪。

有一种艾灸叫疤痕灸，人们常讲"要想身体安，三里常不干"，就是让足三里经常处于一种溃疡的状态。经常灸足三里，那里的皮肤就被灼伤了，这就是灸疮，有一点灸疮是正常的。什么叫发洪？并不是看起来有点红，而是像发洪水一样，经常灸那个地方，把血热引动起来了，灸疮上血流不止，这就叫灸疮发洪。灸疮发洪意味着你灸错了，或者灸过头了。

艾灸不是所有的人都适合的，如果用错，即使不会灸疮发洪，可能也在暗中消耗你的气血，很多事情都是在暗中进行的，明着进行的事情也有，但是少。艾灸给人的好处可能是明着的，但是暗中也引发一些不好。

当艾灸发洪，血流不止的时候，你就要想到可能你本身就有血热，血热再被艾灸的火给引动起来，导致血不归经，于是流血不止。这时候就可以外用新鲜或干的旱莲草敷在上面，很快就能把血止住，或者内服旱莲草，也可以。

女贞子

二至丸

说到旱莲草，我们就会想到女贞子。女贞子、旱莲草等分放在一起用的，叫二至丸。

二至丸是补益肝肾且能强筋壮骨的，同时有清热的作用。女贞子是平性的，墨旱莲微寒，能够清热、补养肝肾、强筋壮骨。这是养肾养阴经常用的一个方子。为什么叫二至丸呢？因为女贞子是冬至时候采的最好，旱莲草是夏至时候采的最好，所以叫二至丸。

贞则多子

女贞子结在女贞树上，女贞树非常高大，一年四季都长叶子，冬天也不凋零，跟冬青有点像，二者容易混淆。其实，两者还是有细微差别的。女贞的叶子比较长、比较大，有四五寸长，结的子是紫黑色的；冬青树的种类很多，有的冬青结子，有的不结子。冬青树的叶子要圆一些，籽是红色的，再成熟也黑不了，不像女贞子又肥又黑。

女贞树亭亭玉立，经冬不凋，不畏风雪，非常坚贞。女意味着能养阴，贞意味着入肾，意味着能固能守。

《周易》讲，万事万物的发展过程，就是元、亨、利、贞，可以对应于春、夏、秋、冬四季。春对应元，意味着开始、生发；亨意味着很繁盛，就是夏天的长；利是一个立刀旁，就带有金字了，就意味着收了，有一股肃杀之气；贞就是正，跟正有关，对应于冬季，冬季要封藏。贞是坚守的美德。一棵女贞树上会结很多子，贞则多子，这是一个规律，反过来看，多子则贞。

前几天我在微博上看到一句话，说中国人羞于谈性，却制造了第一人口大国，他企图表明一种矛盾，可能想通过这个来说明中国人的虚伪，其实并不是这样的。正是因为羞于谈性，所以才会创造第一人口大国，而且创造第一人口大国也不是什么不光彩的事情，人多了也没有什么不好。

羞于谈性，说明在性问题上大家有节制。有节制就意味着贞，贞则多子，就能优生优育。跟贞对应的是淫，如果在这方面太过分了，反而生不出多少孩子，正因为贞才会创造第一人口大国。淫则无子，男女都是这样的。

女贞子的性能及用法

女贞子在夏天就已经结子了，它的果期特别长，会挂在枝头直到冬天慢慢变红，红得发紫，紫得发黑，等到冬至那一天，已经很冷了，把它采下来。

女贞子可以直接晒干，也可以用酒先蒸一下再晒干。用酒蒸了再晒会干得更快。女贞子是往下走的，用酒蒸一下，它就能够往上走，走到肺里面，先上后下，最终还是往肾里走。女贞子是一味很安静的药，看它的名字就知道，静如处子，是不活泼的，用酒来蒸一下，就会使女贞子变得更活泼一点，它就更容易消化、吸收。

女贞子味苦、甘、酸，它不寒不热，性平，能滋肾、退热、养精神，一般阴虚有火的人，用它会比较好；不是阴虚有火的人，用了可能就会肚子疼、拉肚子。

它也有明目、乌发的作用，经常跟着菊花、生地、蒺藜、枸杞子这些药一块用来明目。生地和女贞子一起是清热、养肾的，养肾就有清热的作用。热能令人昏，寒能令人清，用这些凉药，能够让人清，这个清，一方面是神清气爽，另一方面是让人的眼睛能看得更清。蒺藜是用来疏肝的，枸杞子是用来养肝肾之阴的，菊花是用来平肝散火的。这组药与玄参明目的那一组药，原理相同。

Chapter 4　Medicines for Nourishing the Liver Yin

According to the sequence of the kidney, liver, heart, spleen and lung, medicines of nourishing Yin of the five internal organs will be introduced in the following sections. The liver and kidney are in the Lower Jiao, so nourishing Yin of the liver and kidney will come the first. Comparatively speaking, there are more medicines for nourishing the liver and kidney.

Danggui (Angelica Sinensis)

Danggui is a very common medicine, and it is sweet, pungent, and slightly bitter in tastes, and slippery in nature. Danggui has a strong smell with both ascending and descending functions, and it can go into the three meridians of heart, liver and spleen with functions of nourishing blood and moistening dryness. It is an essential medicine for the heart meridian, and can be used in the formulas for nourishing the liver Yin or heart Yin.

Dominant Medicine for Inducing Blood into Meridians

The liver dislikes urgency, so the medicine of sweet taste should be used to relax it; the liver likes dispersing, so the medicine of pungent taste should be used to disperse it. The liver is subsumed to wood and wood dominates smoothness, so the liver most likes the pungent taste for dispersing. Danggui is pungent with a dispersing efficacy and sweet in taste, hence it can give the liver exactly what it wants.

The liver stores blood. Danggui can enter the liver, which is so beneficial to the liver that it helps the liver to generate blood. The liver storing blood signifies that blood does not circulate presumptuously. Let the blood return to where it should go, which is meant by its Chinese name "Danggui" (literally means "should return"), implying that it should return to the liver. If blood does not circulate in the blood vessel smoothly and quietly, it would not return to the meridians, resulting in many symptoms of bleeding. The blood that comes out of the vessels is called leaving-meridian blood that in fact should return to circulate in blood vessels and finally to the liver. This is what is meant it should go where it should go. So, Danggui is the main medicine that may or must be used for treatment of all diseases related to blood.

Consideration of Both Qi and Blood

Danggui, as a medicine for Qi in blood, is pungent in taste and it is able to disperse Qi and promote circulation of Qi as well. It is oily and lubricant, subsumed to Yin, but its pungent and sweet tastes and dispersing nature are subsumed to Yang, so Danggui is a medicine for both Yin and Yang, and good for both Qi and blood. That is why the ancients recorded Danggui as a medicine for Qi in blood, and it can tonify Qi and blood and promote circulation of Qi and blood as well.

"Qi is the general of blood, and blood is the mother of Qi". Qi and blood are interdependent, and neither Qi nor blood can go independently without the help of the other, so both Qi and blood should be given consideration at the same time. Danggui is just the right medicine that can give consideration to both Qi and blood. If blood only is to be replenished without tonifying Qi at the same time, the replenished blood may not circulate smoothly and would be easy to form blood stasis; On the other hand, if Qi only is to be tonified without replenishing blood at the same time, Qi will fail to find anything to depend upon and the surplus Qi will become the pathogenic fire. The blood failing to stay in the meridians will run wild because of Qi running about. If Qi stops running wild, the blood would not be easy to run about, so it is the general who should be blamed if his soldiers run wild. That's why Qi is metaphorically taken as a general of blood.

Subdivision of Danggui as Medicine

Danggui is subdivided into many different types, simply including Chuan Danggui (Sichuan angelica sinensis) and Qin Danggui (Qin angelica sinensis). The former one is produced in Sichuan province, China, with a very strong pungent and dispersing power, and it is good at promoting the circulation of Qi and blood and dispersing the blood stasis, while the latter one, produced in Shaanxi province, China, has a relatively weak pungent and dispersing power, but it has a stronger efficacy of nourishing Yin and replenishing blood. The root of Qin Danggui is featured with a round head and many tails, purple in color, heavy smell and quite moist in nature. Qin Danggui looks similar to horsetail in appearance, and it is also called horsetail angelica. Therefore, for promoting circulation of blood and dispersing blood stasis, it is better to use Chuan Danggui; and for replenishing blood, it is better to use Qin Danggui.

But now, in the pharmacy/drugstore, Danggui is not so subdivided, and it is merely cut and divided into three parts: angelica head, body and tail. The head of Danggui refers to the taproot; the body refers to the thick rootlets growing on the taproot; and the tail refers to the fibrous roots below the body of Danggui. Angelica head can break stasis, so it is used to disperse blood stasis; The angelica body can guard the Middle Jiao and nourish blood; And the angelica tail goes downwards, as the roots of all plants do, so it is able to promote the circulation of blood, that is, to disperse the blood stasis and guide it to go downwards. As a matter of fact, Danggui is often divided in such a way, but generally it is not cut and subdivided so strictly, but it is usually used as a whole including the head, body, and tails for breaking blood stasis, nourishing blood, and circulating blood. In the case of intensifying some specific efficacy, some other medicines may be added to support Danggui for that specific purpose.

Compatibility of Danggui

Danggui is a very vivacious medicine, and it is double-featured depending on the medicines with which it is to be matched. When it is used with tonic medicines, it will play the tonifying and nourishing functions; when used with laxative medicines, it will play a discharging function; when used with medicines of hot or warm nature, it will play a warming function; when used with cold medicines, it will play a cooling function. So, Danggui is a friendly medicine that is very easy to use.

Danggui used with Huangqi (radix astragali) makes a very well-known medical formula called **Danggui Huangqi Buxue Tang** (angelica sinensis and radix astragali blood replenishing decoction), also known as **Buxue Tang** (Blood Replenishing Decoction), which is able to generate blood. Danggui not only can tonify Qi but also enrich blood. Danggui generates blood by means of tonifying and circulating Qi, and with the addition of Huangqi, its efficacy of tonifying Qi can be intensified. As soon as Danggui helps to take the effect of Huangqi into the blood system, circulation of Qi will help promote the flow of blood, and the tonification of Qi will help generate blood as well. In case the tonification of Qi is not intensified enough, some Renshen may be added for assistance. The combination of Renshen, Danggui and Huangqi is just a variation of **Buxue Tang**.

Danggui is featured with pungent and aromatic tastes and moving property, which may consume Qi, so it is necessary to add some tonic medicines to tonify and circulate Qi yet without any impairment of Qi. Meanwhile, its pungent, aromatic and moving natures require a driving effect, which can be reinforced by tonifying Qi. Danggui combined with the medicines for tonifying Qi would have an intensified pungent, aromatic and moving effects but have no side effects. As such, Danggui will get stronger potency for generating and replenishing blood. And that is why Danggui can be more nourishing when used together with tonic medicines.

Danggui used with laxative medicines can function to discharge, for instance, to be used with Dahuang (rheum officinale), which in the formula acts like a general and moves yet without holding-fast. The angelica head can break blood stasis, and the angelica tails can promote circulation of blood, and however, the intensity of such effects is limited, so Dahuang is added in order to help reinforce the efficacy. Dahuang, as a laxative medicine, can go into the blood system to purge the blood heat out of the body with feces. But Dahuang is aromatic, too, characterized with the features of going to the large intestine and moving but not holding-fast. In spite of its going into the blood system, it is not strong enough. When Dahuang is used together with Danggui, it will have an intensified effect to go into the blood system, or to say, its effect of dispersing the blood stasis will be more powerful. Danggui used with Dahuang can very effectively disperse the blood stasis and relieve the pathogenic heat in blood. Suppose the dispersing effect is still not strong enough, I am afraid, in the case of fluid accumulation in the body, add some Qianniuzi (semen pharbitidis) to alleviate fluid retention. The three herbs Danggui, Dahuang and Qianniuzi used together have a very fierce intensity. In most cases, they should not be used in such a way, and only Danggui and Dahuang will do. By the way, both Dahuang and Danggui processed with liquor can be used instead since the liquor-processed Dahuang and Danggui can go upwards and to the limbs to clear away all the stasis and the pathogenic heat in the blood of the whole body.

Danggui is very oily and lubricant, so is Dahuang, both of which can then have the moistening function and go downwards. Danggui itself can thin feces, so before using it, doctors should get to know the real conditions of patients about the stool. In case the stool is dry, Danggui can be used in a larger dosage, like 5 *qian* or 1 *liang* if required. On the one hand, Danggui can directly moisten the feces, but on the other hand, Danggui can also indirectly moisten the feces in that it is good at managing and harmonizing the whole body and nourishing blood as well. And vice versa, in case the stool is thin, decrease the dosage or remove Danggui; in case the stool is in normal state, neither dry nor thin, 3 to 4 *qian* of Danggui will do.

Danggui Used for Symptoms of Arthralgia

Danggui is frequently used for the treatment of arthralgia. Bi (arthralgia) is involved with wind, coldness, and dampness. Wind arthralgia manifests the symptoms of moving pain, while cold arthralgia manifests the symptoms of pains in a specific position, and the damp arthralgia manifests the symptoms of feeling physically heavy. In fact, the three types of wind, cold, and damp arthralgia are interweaved, but not referred to a particular pathogenic factor only.

Danggui is often used for treatment of arthralgia. Generally, arthralgia is often accompanied by the pathogenic wind. The general principle for curing the pathogenic wind is to start with blood treatment, after which arthralgia will extinguish itself naturally. Danggui is also used for treatment of uarthritis. The generally matched medicines for treatment of arthralgia include Guizhi (cassia twig), Cangzhu (rhizoma atractylodis), Juhua (chrysanthemum), and Niuxi (radix achyranthis bidentatae). Guizhi can go into the four limbs, and it can also get through and activate Yang of the limbs, as such, the pathogenic wind, coldness, and dampness can be easily dispersed. Cangzhu is an aromatic medicine for eliminating the pathogenic dampness. The spleen dominates the four limbs, so all the diseases related to limbs can be cured through tonifying the spleen. Juhua can disperse the pathogenic wind and heat in the liver meridians. Niuxi can guide the medical effects to go downwards to legs, and Guizhi guides the effects upwards to the hands. When in urgency, the muscle will be deformed, which is related to the liver. And in that case, add some Baishao (radix paeoniae alba) to soothe the liver and nourish Yin, which could bring a very good effect on soothing muscles. In case fingers cannot be stretched straightly, the first thing to do is to eliminate all the pathogenic factors including wind, coldness, and dampness. And in such a case, try to use Baishao immediately in a large dosage to relieve and relax the muscles and bones.

In case there arise symptoms of heat like arthralgia and joint swelling, add some Shigao (gypsum); in case gypsum is still not strong enough, add **Baihu Tang**, for instance, **Guizhi Bahu Tang** or **Cangzhu Baihu Tang**.

There is another way, that is, for those diseases that are more serious at night, Danggui must be used. The normal reason why a disease is getting more serious at night is that the disease arises from Yin. For those diseases arising from Yin deficiency, Danggui must be used to regulate the blood conditions and nourish Yin. Of course, this is not an absolute case, but for reference only. As to the clinical treatment of diseases, it has to be done according to the specific symptoms.

Shenghua Tang

Danggui is often used in gynecology, especially after delivery of a baby. The woman just after delivery of a baby will be in a very special state: Qi and blood are in restless conditions, and lochia is not exhausted yet, and the bone joints are in a loose state, too. Under such conditions, Danggui can be used for appeasement and regulation, and the formula of **Shenghua Tang** (Decoction for Puerperal Blood Stasis) is then frequently used.

Shenghua Tang contains the herbal ingredients of: Danggui (angelica sinensis) 8 *qian*, Chuanxiong (ligusticum wallichii) 3 *qian*, baked ginger 5 *fen*,

Taoren (peach kernel) 2 *qian*, Gancao (liquorice) 5 *fen*, and Shudi (radix rehmanniae praeparata) 3 *qian* (added by Zhang Jingyue).

Danggui 8 *qian* in dosage is the monarch herb in the formula of **Shenghua Tang**, and all other herbs add up to less than 8 *qian*, which means Danggui is mainly to be used after the delivery of baby and all the other medicines are merely to help maximize the power of Danggui. Chuanxiong here is for better promoting circulation of blood. Danggui and Chuanxiong have some similarities in respect of promoting the circulation of Qi, by which flow of blood is promoted.

What is the baked ginger here for? It is appropriate to be cool before delivery and warm after delivery, which is a general principle to be adopted for delivery of babies. Since prenatal mother and child are held together, it is easy to generate heat. Hence, a little cool medicine can be used. After delivery of a baby, Qi and blood deficiency will arise, and it needs warming up. Meanwhile, in the process of promoting circulation of blood and dispersing the blood stasis, it is appropriate to use warm medicines too, in order to provide some energy for promoting Qi to activate blood. The dosage of baked ginger used here is only five *fen*, equivalent to 1.5 grams, which in fact is a very small dosage. Taoren 2 *qian* here is to disperse the blood stasis. Kernel usually is oily and lubricant, and it mainly goes to the six hollow organs. Since the maternal blood has just settled down after delivery of baby, Taoren should not be overused. Merely 2 *qian* will work, but some books mention to use 10 pieces of peach kernels. Gancao is used with a very small dosage of 5 *fen* in the formula.

Later on, Zhang Jingyue was most adept at using Shudi and he added Shudi 3 *qian* in the formula of **Shenghua Tang** to intensify the Yin nourishing effect. Shudi is used here in instead of Sheng Dihuang since Shudi is a warm medicine while Sheng Dihuang is inclined to have a property of coolness. The herbs used in **Shenghua Tang** are all inclined to be warm. **Shenghua Tang** is for regulating Qi and blood, and getting rid of blood stasis and bringing forth the refreshment. Only after the blood stasis is driven out of the body can the fresh things be generated and transformed, and that is why this formula is called **Shenghua Tang**——a decoction for generation and transformation.

By the way, as to the loose bone joints mentioned above, the pubis bone, i.

e. , the ossa pubis, is normally closed. At the time of giving birth to a baby, it "pops" open. In fact, not only the pubis bone opens, but also the bone joints in the whole body become loosened accordingly. After delivery, the pubis bone will close up again, and the bone joints of the whole body will close up, too, but it will take a relative longer time, at least, a hundred days to close up completely and perfectly. This means that within these hundred days the new mother must be very careful not to be exposed to rain or to pathogenic wind, i. e. , the unseasonal wind, for instance, the north wind in summer instead of the south wind, or the west wind in spring instead of the east wind. **Huangdi Neijing** (*the Internal Canon of Huangdi*) said "the pathogenic wind should be avoided at times". That is to say, try to avoid the harmful wind. Therefore, in the one-hundred-day period while the bone joints are still loose, those who even suffer from poor health and physical weakness can also become physically stronger if properly regulated and nourished. But if the pathogenic wind, coldness and dampness penetrate into the bone joints, it would become a hard nut to crack. Or, in this period, if those who keep on worrying all the time would suffer from some puerperal diseases. Of course, in this one-hundred-day period, the sexual life would also be bad for health.

Danggui can regulate and harmonize various Qi andblood disorder. Besides, irregular menstruation is in the scope of Qi and blood disorder. In TCM culture, the menstruation is named as "Yuexin" (monthly signal). It is said that "regularity of menstruation signals a good physical condition. " For the young ladies, so long as they have a regular menstruation, it will mean that they are physically healthy; Otherwise, it will mean some problems have arisen. The earlier or later or irregular menstruation all signal that Qi and blood are in disorder, and therefore, Danggui is usually the essential medicine for regulation of such a disorder.

Abuse of Danggui

Once it was popular to use Danggui powder among some people. After having taken the powder for some time, some ladies may suffer more leucorrhea due to two reasons: First, Danggui consumes Qi for its pungent and dispersing natures, making the spleen fail to exercise control over the leucorrhea dripping;

Second, Danggui is oily and lubricant, so, taking more of it will cause the leucorrhea to drip.

Therefore, only when the traditional Chinese medicine is used properly, will the side effect be avoided, otherwise, the side effects will result in some other troubles. Diseases can now be divided into two types: iatrogenic diseases and drug-induced diseases. Some diseases arise from the medical treatment, i. e. , the drug-induced diseases, such as the more leucorrhea, which is mostly due to eating too much Danggui powder. Therefore, in the prescriptions for such patients, don't use the herb of Danggui and try to make the body conditioning from the perspective of Qi and the spleen.

In TCM, only when the herbs are properly matched to suit the right cases of different symptoms, will there arise no side effects. Otherwise, more and long-lasting use of herbs may bring some bad effects. As for Danggui powder, in spite of its good function, it should not be abused or used for too long time.

Siwu Tang

Siwu Tang is a very famous formula containing Danggui (angelica sinensis), Baishao (radix paeoniae alba), Chuanxiong (ligusticum wallichii), Sheng Dihuang (radix rehmanniae recen), among which Danggui is the monarch herb and the other three herbs are for the purpose of intensifying the effects of Danggui. Danggui is used here to promote the circulation of Qi; Chuanxiong further intensifies the effects of Danggui to promote the circulation of Qi; Danggui replenishes blood, and Baishao used here is to soothe the liver and nourish Yin in order to help Danggui to enrich blood; Dihuang not only goes into the kidneys, but also intensifies the effects of Danggui to nourish Yin. As such, Danggui will be strong enough to have a greater potency for nourishing blood.

Development from Siwu Tang to Shiquan Dabu Tang

Blood is especially important for women, so **Siwu Tang** is very frequently used in gynecology. Many diseases can be treated with the modified **Siwu Tang** (i. e. , addition / subtraction of herbs to/from the formula), for example, for regulating menstruation, nourishing blood, or the treatment after delivery of babies.

Siwu Tang combined with Sijunzi Tang for tonifying Qi will form Bazhen Tang, which can tonify both Qi and blood. Bazhen Tang reminds us of Danggui Huangqi Buxue Tang. Danggui can tonify Qi, while Huangqi enriches blood. These two herbs used together can tonify both Qi and blood. Then, what is Bazhen Tang used for? In fact, Bazhen Tang is for intensifying the effects of Danggui Huangqi Buxue Tang. Both of them have the similar implication but only further intensify the effects of the two herbs of Danggui and Huangqi.

And then, on the basis of Bazhen Tang, add Rougui (cassia bark) and Huangqi (radix astragali) to form another formula called Shiquan Dabu Tang, which is a representative formula among tonic medicines.

Treatment of Physical Weakness in a Cold

Those who are at their senior ages or physically weak usually suffer from deficiency of both Qi and blood. In case they catch a cold, only relieving the exterior symptoms, clearing the internal heat and dispersing the pathogenic factors will not work well since all treatment must be carried out according to the patients' Qi and blood conditions. In such a case, try to select and add some tonic herbs into the formula of Bazhen Tang.

Shensu Yin is an example that follows such an idea. Take Renshen (ginseng) and Suye (perilla leaf) as the main herbs, and of course, according to the specific conditions, add Gegen (radix puerariae), Chaihu (radix bupleuri), Banxia (Pinellia ternata), Fuling (poria cocos), Zhike (fructus aurantii), Jiegeng (platycodon grandiflorum), Chenpi (pericarpium citri reticulatae), Gancao (liquorice) and the like.

The mistreatment of a common cold of patients who are physically weak will easily cause invasion of pathogen(s) into the interior of the body, resulting in endogenous heat due to Yin deficiency. The long-lasting low-temperature fever will cause one to feel rotten, and feel the heat erupting from inside the bone. In that case, the common medicines for relieving the exterior symptoms and clearing heat will not work well, so, add Chaihu, Biejia (turtle shell), Digupi (cortex lycii radicis), Zhimu (rhizoma anemarrhenae) and the like to the formula of Siwu

Tang to clear the deficiency heat and nourish blood as well at the same time.

Modifications of Siwu Tang

On the basis of **Siwu Tang**, add E-jiao (donkey-hide gelatin) and parched Aiye (folium artemisiae argyi) to form **Jiaoai Siwu Tang**. E-jiao is the refined life essence of the donkey flesh and blood, which can intensify blood nourishing; The parched Aiye is used to warm and activate the meridians all over the body and Mingmen (the gate of vitality). **Jiaoai Siwu Tang** can also tackle the coldness in the Lower Jiao and blood dripping like menstruation dripping, and prevent miscarriages and nourish fetus.

Jiaoai Siwu Tang is inclined to be warm, while **Qinlian Siwu Tang** is inclined to be cool. **Qinlian Siwu Tang** is formed by adding Huangqin (scutellaria baicalensis), Huanglian (coptis chinensis) and Danpi (cortex moutan radices) to the formula of **Siwu Tang**. **Qinlian Siwu Tang** is generally used for treatment of the premature menstruation that looks purple or black in color, which frequently arises from blood heat in most cases. Danpi is for clearing the blood heat. Huangqin and Huanglian are both for clearing heat too, but they clear the heat in the Upper and Middle Jiao. The heat in the Lower Jiao should not be cleared, or otherwise, the kidney Yang might be impaired.

If there exists blood stasis, add Taoren (peach kernel) and Honghua (safflower carthamus) in the formula of **Siwu Tang** to make **Taohong Siwu Tang** for promoting blood circulation to remove blood stasis. Wang Qingren, medical expert in the Qing dynasty, added the two herbs of Jiegeng (platycodon grandiflorum) and Niuxi (radix achyranthis bidentatae) to **Taohong Siwu Tang** to make the well-known **Xuefu Zhuyu Tang** to guide the medical efficacy upwards and downwards respectively in order to activate the whole body to remove stasis. In addition, **Gexia Zhuyu Tang**, **Shentong Zhuyu Tang** etc. are also available, which are formed by adding or subtracting herbs skillfully to/from the formula of **Siwu Tang**.

As soon as blood stasis is removed, the new blood will be replenished. So, **Siwu Tang** is suitable for all patients, fat or thin. In case the patient is fat, combine **Erchen Tang** with **Siwu Tang** since the fat people all suffer more phlegm.

In case the fat patient has more phlegm and Qi depression, put in Xiangfu (rhizoma cyperi), and Wuyao (lindera aggregate) and the like additionally.

In addition, please also note that in the postpartum period, the raw Baishao (cold and sour with astringing effect) used in **Siwu Tang** may impair the vitality and even discharge the liver Yang. In case that the patient has a poor appetite, stop using Dihuang for it is greasy and is able to cause the patients to have a worse appetite; in case that the patient has thin feces, try to reduce the dosage of Danggui; in case that the patient sweats a lot, stop using Chuanxiong since it is strong enough to run about inside the body. Sweating means too much moving factors are already available inside the body, which will get more serious if Chuanxiong is used. As it is known that sweat is the fluid of the heart, too much sweating will impair the heart Yin.

In fact, there are many modifications of **Siwu Tang**, which require practicing repeatedly in clinical practice.

Baishao (Radix Paeoniae Alba)

Converging the Liver Qi

The flower of Baishao looks like that of peony very much, but actually they are not the same. Peony is a woody plant, and Baishao is herbaceous plant. It is quite rare to see the herbaceous plants with large-sized flowers. There is a law in the nature, i. e., the size of the flowers of a plant is related to its germinal force. The larger the flower is, the stronger the germinal force will be, which means its root will have much stronger capacity to converge.

Plants are also particular about the balance of Yin and Yang. If the part of the plant above ground has stronger vitality, the underground roots of the plant will need stronger vigor for convergence, or otherwise, the plant will become top-heavy, especially those herbaceous plants. The bigger size of flowers signifies that the wood is full of vigor, requiring the roots of the plant to be able to converge the wood vitality, that is to say, to converge the wood Qi (energy), which in TCM means to converge the liver Qi and let it return to its origin to restrain the liver Qi from becoming too brutal.

In TCM theory, the liver is metaphorically taken as the organ of General Officer. What role can a general officer play? It is he who is needed to fight against the external evils, and to find solution to the internal contradiction among people, too. To defend against the exogenous pathogens needs the liver to provide power, and the endogenous pathogens inside the body also needs the liver to function properly in order to eliminate pathogens. That the liver controls dispersing implies the alexipharmic sense. But the "general officer" is also a hot-tempered organ that is easy to lose its temper and become brutal. So, Baishao, sour in taste, is used for converging purpose. The liver likes pungency and dispersion, and dislikes convergence, but Baishao definitely converges it a little in order to purge the liver of the pathogenic fire.

Nourishing and Purging the Liver

Baishao used together with Danggui can nourish the liver. Baishao functions to converge the liver Qi while Danggui functions to disperse it. These two herbs can give full play of their functions of nourishing liver Yin with their sour and sweet tastes, and in the meantime, the efficacy of Baishao can be reduced a little in the aspect of purging the liver.

Danggui and Baishao are frequently used to nourish the liver. But for purging the liver of pathogenic fire, Baishao should be used together with Chuanxiong since Chuanxiong can run about to intensify the effect of purging the pathogenic fire. As such, for nourishing the liver, use Danggui and Baishao; for purging the liver of pathogenic fire, use Baishao and Chuanxiong. It may be asked that Danggui, Baishao and Chuanxiong are just the three ingredient herbs contained in the formula of **Siwu Tang**, so, can **Siwu Tang** nourish the liver or purge the liver of pathogenic fire? In fact, it not only nourishes the liver but also purges the pathogenic fire. This formula reflects the Chinese way of thinking. Just like a leader, he often praises a person before he criticizes him. Similarly, a formula should be prepared for nourishing but also purging the liver so that the liver will be soothed, and function properly as it should do.

Six Functions of Baishao

Zhang Yuansu, a medical expert in Song and Jin dynasties, directly concluded the six functions of Baishao as: "to pacify spleen meridians; to cure the abdominal pain; to converge the stomach Qi; to stop diarrhea; to harmonize the blood systems, and to secure the grain of skin and the texture of the subcutaneous flesh. "

Baishao can pacify the spleen meridians since it can purge the liver of pathogenic fire. The spleen meridians become uneasy since the liver wood restricts the spleen earth. After it purges the liver of pathogenic fire, the spleen meridians will then be soothed.

It can cure the abdominal pain since pain often arises from Qi edginess. Zhang Zhongjing often used Shaoyao (paeonia lactiflora) and Gancao (liquorice) simultaneously to treat abdominal pain.

Shaoyao specially focuses on purging the liver of pathogenic fire. In fact, the edginess refers that the liver is in urgency, as the general officer may carry out the indiscriminate killing of the innocent people when he becomes impatient, so the abdominal pain arises. The acute pain in the abdomen is related to the liver. When the sour taste of Baishao functions to purge the liver of its pathogenic fire, the liver will become quiet. Regarding use of Gancao here, it is a "honey-lipped peace-maker". The combination of the gentle and the tough features will help the "General Officer" calm down, which means the liver calms down, and then the pain will disappear. In summer, a little Huangqin may be added, too. In case that the patient suffers aversion to cold, add a little Rougui or Guizhi to the formula.

Baishao can converge the liver and stomach Qi because of its sour taste. When the liver Qi is converged, the stomach Qi will then be astringed naturally.

Baishao can also stop diarrhea. When the catharsis force of the liver is too strong, patients will be susceptible to diarrhea. So Baishao can be used to purge the liver in order to weaken the catharsis force, and then diarrhea will be stopped. In addition, with the astringing function due to the sour taste, Baishao can help stop diarrhea, too.

Baishao can promote blood circulation. The liver is in charge of storing blood. When the liver Qi is smoothly regulated, the blood line will be harmonized naturally.

Besides, Baishao can secure the grain of skin and the texture of the subcutaneous flesh, which is also related to its astringing effect due to its sour taste.

The above-mentioned six functions are concluded on the basis of the properties of Baishao from the perspective of the sour-taste astringency and purging the liver of pathogenic fire. Therefore, it is very critical to know the properties of herbs in the process of learning TCM. Only after grasping the properties, can one conclude the efficacy of the herbs theoretically, and verify them in clinical practice.

Tongxie Yaofang

Shaoyao and Baizhu together can regulate the functions of the liver and spleen. There is a well-known formula named **Tongxie Yaofang** (Formula for Curing Abdominal Pain and Diarrhea) containing the ingredient herbs of Baizhu (white atractylodes rhizome), Baishao (radix paeoniae alba), Fangfeng (radix sileris) and Chenpi (pericarpium citri reticulatae), which can cure all kinds of abdominal pain and diarrhea.

Pain and diarrhea here refer that the abdominal pain arises first, and then diarrhea, after which the pain will disappear. But after a while, the pain arises again, so the pain and diarrhea repeat over and again. This symptom occurs due to what the **Wuxing Doctrine** calls "wood restricts earth". **Tongxie Yaofang** is very effective for the treatment of such a case. Later on, this formula was evolved into **Peizhong Xiemu Fa** in the book **Treatise on Seasonal Diseases** by adding a few herbs to intensify its effects.

Shanyurou (Common Macrocarpium Fruit)

Shanyurou is another important medicine for nourishing the liver Yin. Shanyurou, also called Shanzhuyu (cornus officinalis), is the fruit of a kind of frutex growing in Shandong, Shanxi, and Henan provinces of China. This kind of frutex blossoms in spring first, and then followed by germination-frondesce stage with long leaves. In winter, the leaves fall first, and the fruits keep on hanging on the twigs. The fruits, small in size, oval in shape and red in color, are usually picked and collected in October according to Chinese lunar calendar.

Many books list Shanyurou as an astringent medicine in the category of Yin-nourishing medicines. It is sour and acerb in tastes, and it can enter meridians of both the liver and kidneys with effects of securing the life essence, tonifying Qi, intensifying Yin, supporting Yang, warming the liver, and mildly tonifying Yin and Yang, which means it not only can tonify Yin but also tonify Yang in a mild way.

As a medicine, only the fruit pericarp and pulp of Shanyurou can be used with its kernel being removed. Generally speaking, its pulp is sour and its pericarp is acerb.

Dual Properties of Medicines

Regardless of barks or pericarps, all peels of plants or fruits are acerb in property, nothing else but only to the different degree of acerbity. The outside peel has to cover the fruit pulp inside, so it is bound to have acerbity, otherwise, it would not be able to exercise control over the whole plant or fruit; meanwhile, "peel" implies that it can run along the surface with permeability and dispersing property; or otherwise, the substance inside will get rotten. The peel should not only be astringent, but also permeable. However, astringency and permeability are of completely opposite functions of a medicine.

In nature, there often exists that one thing has two opposite properties, with only some particular partiality in line with their natural attributes. Some peels tend to be permeable and dispersing, for example, Wujiapi (cortex acanthopanacis) and Gualou (trichosanthes kirilowii maxim); And some tend to induce astringency, for example, Shiliupi (pomegranate peel). In fact, peels always combine both properties of permeability and astringency in nature. Of course, it also depends on how the herbs are to be matched, through which doctors are going to give play to the different properties of peels or to intensify some specific property.

The same is true of people. The sages and the devils always coexist side by side. He who is a man of virtue on one side might be a man of devil on the other side.

The same is true even for a Chinese character, for example, the character "乖" (guāi). When one tries to persuade a child, he/she always says to the child: "你要乖" (NǐYào Guāi), by which he/she means to tell the child to be persuasible. But there is another word "乖张" (Guāi zhāng), which means "eccentric and unreasonable". So, that is to say, the character "乖" (Guāi) has double meanings depending on its lexical collocation.

Here is another example "乱" (Luàn). It has a meaning of "putting in disorder". For instance, the Chinese idioms "乱臣贼子" (Luàn Chén Zéi Zǐ) (which means "treacherous ministers and traitors"), and "祸乱朝纲" (Huò Luàn Cháo Gāng, which means "to put the law of an imperial court in disorder"); But this character has another meaning of "putting an end to the chaos". For instance, King Wu of the Zhou dynasty said that he "有乱臣十人" ("Yǒu Luàn Chén Shí Rén") which does not mean he "has ten treacherous ministers and traitors, but means he "has ten ministers who can help to put an end to chaos".

Again, for the character "重" (Zhòng), for instance, "我们重教育，要安土重迁" (Wǒmen Zhòng Jiàoyù, Yàoāntǔ Zhòngqiān), which means "if we attach importance to education, we have to focus on settling down and taking caution to migration." So here the character "重" (Zhòng) in "重教育"("Zhòng Jiàoyù", which means to attach importance to education) is different from the character of "重" (zhòng) in meaning in the phrase "重迁徙" ("Zhòngqiānxi", which means "to take caution to migration"). "重教育"("Zhòng Jiàoyù") tells us to stress and attach great importance to education, while "重迁徙" ("Zhòngqiānxi") tells us to be cautious about the matter of migration, and try not to migrate at wills. The same character "重"(zhòng) has an opposite meaning in the two phrases.

Or again, the phrase"冤家" (yuān jiā, which means "enemy" in the idiom "冤家路窄" (Yuān Jiā Lù Zhǎi, which means the enemies run into each other), but when the lovers call their partners "冤家" (Yuān Jiā, which means "enemy") mutually, the phrase "冤家" (yuān jiā) would have the implied meaning of love.

These phenomena, in exegetical studies, are called counter-exegesis. Some things that do not make sense on the one side should be explained from the opposite side.

The Liver catharsis and the Kidney Storing

The acerb peel, if used with sour Shanyurou, will become particularly more astringent.

Shanyurou goes to the liver and kidney. The liver dominates dispersion and the kidney dominates storing, so, in this respect, the liver and the kidney are in an opposite position. Catharsis and dispersion are both related to the liver Qi. Only when the liver Qi is stirred up, can it then be dispersed. In case that the liver Qi is too vigorous and the kidney Qi is weak, it may be dispersed excessively, and then, the kidney may not be astringed and secured. In that case, Shanyurou can be used to converge the liver Qi.

All that go outwards is called dispersion. For example, urination and excrement signifies that the liver is playing its dispersing function. Those who are once in depression will suffer from constipation since depression will result in the liver stagnation, leading to malfunction of the liver dispersion. Similarly, in case that the liver is dispersed excessively, there will be too much or too many times of excrement, so, in the treatment of dysentery, pay much attention to the treatment of the liver and the regulation of liver catharsis.

Sweating is also associated with the liver dispersion. As it is known, sweat is the fluid of the heart, and the heart and liver cooperate to induce perspiration. So, only when the liver dispersion functions properly, can perspiration be induced in a normal way. Otherwise, the perspiration may not be induced. Or if the liver is dispersed excessively, the patient may sweat profusely all over.

The kidney fluid includes urine and semen. Semen is stored in kidneys, so only when liver Qi is stirred up, that is, when the erotic feeling/sexual passion is stimulated, the semen can then be released. But in case that the liver Qi is excessively vigorous and the kidney Qi is excessively weak, it may be excessively dispersed. Those who suffer from vigorous liver Qi and much weak kidney Qi will be susceptible to premature ejaculation, and the dispersing function of the liver may not be restricted by the storing function of the kidneys.

The liver and the kidney are contradictory at this moment. the kidney wants to secure the semen rather than to release it, but the liver insists on releasing it, and these two organs begin their severe competition. When the kidney Qi is vigorous, the liver wants to disperse, and the kidney does not let it disperse, then it will take a longer time to disperse; When the kidney Qi is weak, the liver wants to disperse, the kidney has no way to restrict it, and it will be immediately released. And therefore, when one wants to tonify the kidneys, he must converge the liver Qi by means of the astringing effect of Shanyurou.

Shanyurou, sourin taste, is for converging Qi of both the liver and kidney. It can disperse the liver Qi and restrict the vigor of the liver. Meanwhile, it can also nourish the liver to alleviate the dispersing function of the liver. In addition to its own inherent Yin nourishing and kidney consolidating function, Shanyurou is also effective for inducing astringency for the excessive dispersion of liver Qi, spermatorrhea due to the unsolidified kidney Qi, gatism of urine and feces, and abnormal sweating due to general debility.

Astringing the Vital Essence and Restraining the Mind

The liver controls dispersion, not only the physiological dispersion, but also the emotional dispersion. For example, he who wants to articulate dares to speak out, or he who wants to express himself can find a way to utter. This is also a case that the liver is dispersing. That's why those whose liver Qi is vigorous are always talkative since it needs to be dispersed. They not only need to release themselves physiologically, but also release their emotions and thoughts. However, the more they utter, the more vital life essence they will consume. Shanyurou in fact can not only astringe the tangible things, but also astringe the intangible things, that is, to astringe the vital life essence, but also to restrain the mind.

Therefore, Shanyurou can relieve uneasiness of mind. It is also quite effective for treatment of palpitation and absence of mind due to the heart Qi deficiency. This herb, of course, must be used together with some other herbs. Once the kidney deficiency arises, the absence of mind will arise accordingly. So Shanyurou is often used in the formula for tonifying kidneys, which is helpful for communication between the heart and kidneys, and for relieving uneasiness of mind in order to help collect the energy.

Prevention of Yin and Yang Breakaway

With such a strong astringent effect, Shanyurou can promote astringency for relieving depletion naturally.

What does "relieving depletion" mean? Normally, Yin and Yang in the body always hold together, that is, Yin and Yang contain each other. When one is dying, Yin and Yang in his body will be cut off. Yang runs upwards and Yin goes downwards. That Yang runs upwards shows the symptoms of sweating with only expiration but without inspiration; that Yin goes downwards shows the symptoms of Yin depletion due to continual diarrhea.

Therefore, Shanyurou is often used for relieving depletion in the first aid to make sure that Yang will be unlikely to escape upwards, and Yin will be unlikely to escape downwards so that Yin and Yang can still hold together. Shanyurou not only can relieve depletion, but also mildly nourish both Yin and Yang. Hence, at the critical moment of life or death, Shanyurou is frequently used with a larger dosage to turn the situation with vigorous efforts.

Zhang Xichun, one of the medical experts, often used Shanyurou for first-aid treatment. In the case of emergency, a large dosage of Dangshen (codonopsis pilosula) can be added for the poor people since the poor cannot afford to use Renshen, or **Shenfu Tang**, or **Dushen Tang,** but Shanyurou and Dangshen together would have the same effect actually. Definitely, Shanyurou will have to be used in a very large dosage around 2 to 3 *liang*, equivalent to 60 to 90 grams.

Promoting Smoothness of the Nine Orifices

Shanyurou also has the function of soothing the nine orifices including the seven orifices on the head (i. e. , two eyes, two nostrils, two ears, mouth) and the two lower orifices (i. e. , urethra and anus). All of these nine orifices may sometimes suffer from some unfavorable influences, like obstruction, or Qi depression. In that case, Shanyurou may be used to promote the smoothness of the nine orifices.

It may be asked that howan astringent medicine can promote smoothness of the orifices? The nine-orifice obstruction usually arises from the obstructed vital life essence. The vital life essence of human being has to go in and out of the nine orifices. In case that it is in deficiency, it will not be able to come in and go out of the nine orifices freely. Hence, the deficiency of the vital life essence will make the nine orifices obstructed. However, Promoting the smoothness seems to be contradictory to inducing the astringency, but in fact, they are unified with merely one step beyond.

Shanyurou Used in Liuwei Dihuang Pill

Shanyurou used in **Liuwei Dihuang Pill** actually implies a lot. Dihuang can tonify the kidney, but it is insufficient in inducing astringency and unable to help the kidneys for storing, so it is necessary to add the herb of Shanyurou. Shanyurou itself can nourish Yin of both the liver and the kidney, and at the same time, it can induce astringency of liver and kidneys, and astringe the Yin that is nourished by and with Dihuang. However, only inducing astringency is not enough, and then, the ingredient herbs of Fuling and Zexie can alleviate fluid retention and promote circulation of the kidney Qi. By means of inducing astringency and circulating Qi simultaneously, the vital life essence can then be astringed and the pathogenic factors are eliminated, too. This is the first function of Shanyurou in **Liuwei Dihuang Pill**.

Secondly, at the time of tonifying the kidneys, the liver should also be attended through nourishing. Shanyurou, sour in taste, can go into the liver, and it can nourish both the liver and the kidney simultaneously. It goes with Dihuang to reinforce the effects of nourishing both the liver and the kidney Yin. The kidney fluid/water generates the liver wood, so, when the liver Yin is sufficient, the consumption of the kidney Yin will be reduced.

Thirdly, Shanyurou, red in color, can go into the heart, and Diahuang, black in color, can go into the kidneys, so Diahuang and Shanyurou together can play the role of communication between the heart and the kidneys.

Shanzhuyu (Cornus Officinalis) and Wuzhuyu (Fructus Evodiae)

By the way, the last but not the least, it is hereby to remind readers that Shanzhuyu and Wuzhuyu are two different herbs though they have a similar name in Chinese. Wuzhuyu is a medicine of great heat for warming the liver Yang, while Shanzhuyu is just a small red fruit for nourishing the liver Yin.

For the sake of distinction, in prescriptions, Shanzhuyu is often written as Shanyurou, which will help patients know it is a medicine for nourishing Yin, while Wuzhuyu is just written as Wuyu (evodia), or Pao Wuyu (processed evodia) to show the differences.

Removal of Kernels of Shanyurou

In addition, in the use of Shanyurou, its kernel must be removed.

Now, Shanyurou bought from pharmacies occasionally have some kernels included, which must be picked out since the kernel of Shanzhuyu cannot be used as medicine due to its side-effect of spermatorrhea. The peel and pulp of Shanzhuyu are astringent but its kernel has no astringing effect, yet can cause spermatorrhea. Many herbs have such double and contradictory properties, for instance, Mahuang (ephedra) can induce sweat, but its root, on the contrary, can restrain sweating. And similarly, Gouqizi (fructus lycii) is warm in nature, but Digupi (cortex lycii radicis) is cold in nature. Such contradictory properties are often found in the same herb or plant.

Those doctors who are prepared to use Shanyurou in a prescription should have an overall vision about the effects of Shanyurou. Or otherwise, some critical effects about Shanyurou might be neglected.

As for a medicine, its efficacy should be considered comprehensively. For instance, when considering to use the Shanyurou for its astringency, one should not neglect the other effect like smoothening the nine orifices. Similarly, when talking about the homology of the liver and kidney, one should not forget some contradictory factors existing between the liver and kidneys. I have been emphasizing the open-mindedness and flexibility of thinking. While studying TCM, if one confines himself to certain disease itself, or to the pathophysiology only, he or she may get lost easily in some final verdicts, which then will keep him or her away from thinking freshly and alive. However, the human body is always fresh and alive, and diseases are always changing. Facing the changing diseases, those with an inflexible thinking will definitely fall into or cause troubles. Therefore, to learn how to think critically is very important.

Gouqi (Lycium)

Regarding Gouqi, it has been discussed in the section related to Digupi (cortex lycii radicis).

Gouqizi (Fructus Lycii)

Lycium plant is a frutex, generally 2 to 3 *Chi* in height, but it grows very high in Ningxia, China. Gouqizi (fructus lycii), as an herb, can warm up the liver and kidneys, and it can help promote the secretion of saliva or body fluid, support Yang, warm the body and blood, nourish the primordial Yin, relieve deficiency-heat and tonify the liver and kidneys. The top quality Gouqizi is ruddy in color, big in size, tight in grain density, and rich in pulp with less seeds. While the poor quality Gouqizi contains a lot of seeds with thin pulp. Ningxia is the authentic place of the origin of Gouqizi. In reality, Gouqizi produced in the whole region of the northwest of China are all extremely fine in quality.

Zhang Jingyue used Gouqizi in all his prescriptions of **Zuogui Yin**, **Yougui Yin**, **Zuogui Pill** and **Yougui Pill** to accomplish his goal of warming and nourishing the kidneys by means of nourishing the liver. Both the liver and the kidneys are in the Lower Jiao, where the life essence is stored up but also coldness is easily accumulated. The life essence needs warming for transformation, so in the process of nourishing Yin of both the liver and kidneys, some partially warm medicines are frequently used. However, it should not be too warm, otherwise, it will lead to pathogenic fire therefrom. In this respect, Gouqizi is a best choice for it is sweet and warm but not dry.

Bath with Lycium

Each and every part of Gouqi plant can be used as medicine. The lycium leaf, also called Tianjing grass (Sky Life-essence Grass), is edible when it is tender; it can be used for bath when it grows old. The root bark of Gouqi is called Digupi (cortex lycii radicis), which is also a medicine.

The ancient health care providers paid great attention to the Gouqi bath. *Compendium of Materia Medica* cited from *Dongtian Health Preserving Re-*

cord as: "On January 1, February 2, March 3, April 4, and even December 12 respectively in Chinese lunar year, a bath with lycium leaf boiled water can make one shiny and avoid catching diseases. "

Later in the Ming Dynasty, there was a health care provider named Gao Lian. In his *"Zunsheng Bajian"* (Eight Annotations on health Care), he highly advocated the Gouqi bath. He mentioned the Gouqi bath, but he did not make clear which part of lycium should be used, Gouqizi (fructus lycii), or lycium leaf, or Digupi (cortex lycii radicis) ? Different books give different descriptions, so one may make judgement by himself or herself. In fact, his original idea refers to all the parts of lyceum plant, including the lycium leaf and the root since taking a bath is to wash the whole body. It might be the most effective way to use the whole of lycium plant to nourish the whole body of human being.

The lycium leaf goes to the exterior surface, which is good for cleaning the skin in a bath. Gouqizi can nourish and moisten skin, from which skin absorbs the nutritious elements to tonify the liver and nourish the kidneys. Digupi (cortex lycii radicis) eliminates the deficiency heat, and it can permeate into the bones to clear away the deficiency heat from the whole body, so a certain dosage of Digupi should also be used. This is the formula quite commonly used for health care baths in the ancient time.

Favorable Conditions for Health Maintenance

It may be asked why to choose January 1, February 2, and March 3 in the lunar year. Health care and treatment of diseases are very particular about the favorable climatic, geographical and human conditions.

The human condition here refers that the effectiveness of a formula, to some extent, depends on a patient's mental state. When the patient has a good state of mind, the formula may function effectively even if it is not a best formula. In case that the patient is in a bad mood, even the best formula could not play its full efficacy in the treatment.

As to geographical conditions, lycium plants are quite popular in the north of China, but when used as medical herb, only the lycium plants grown in Ningxia is the best. This is about the geographical condition.

What is the most incredible is the favorable climatic condition, i. e. , on which day should the herb be used. The reason why we choose to use this formula on January 1, February 2, and March 3 in Chinese lunar year is, to a great extent, out of psychological consideration. Or even if one does not strictly follow this time requirement, but in the mind, such an idea about the favorable climatic condition should be established. In fact, this formula can also be used on January 2, February 3, or March 4 or any other days. In the past, it was required to use this formula for only 12 times a year, which was the minimum requirement since Gouqizi is produced in the northwest where transportation was underdeveloped in the ancient time. Besides, Gouqizi was always quite expensive, people in the midland even had fewer chances to eat Gouqizi in the past, much less chances they would have to take fructus lycii baths. So, the ancients tried to restrain themselves from taking fructus lycii bath. But now, of course, it is much more convenient to get Gouqizi wherever you are. The more you use, the more helpful it will be for the local economic development of the northwest of China.

第四章　养肝阴药

我们依照五行相生的顺序，也就是按肾、肝、心、脾、肺这个顺序，把养五脏之阴的药一一介绍一下。因为肝肾是处在下焦，在养阴方面是首当其冲的，所以养肝肾的药要多一些。下面我们学习养肝阴的药。

当归

当归是极其常用的一味药，味甘、辛、微苦，性滑，可升可降，有很浓烈的气味。当归入心、肝、脾三经，有养血润燥之功，是心经的本药。把当归放在养肝阴或养心阴的药中，都是可以的。

引血归经，血家主药

我们知道，肝苦急，以甘缓之；肝欲散，以辛散之。肝属木，木主条达，是喜欢辛散的，当归味辛能散；肝不喜欢急，所以用甘甜的来缓它，当归味甘。当归辛甘兼具，对于肝来说是投其所好了。

肝藏血，当归如此有益于肝，所以它能够入肝来助血海，能生血。肝能藏血，意味着血不妄行，让血回到它该去的地方，当归的意思就是应当归来。如果血不在血管里老老实实地走，就叫血不归经，会导致很多出血的病症。出来的血就叫离经之血，它是该回到血管里去的，回到肝脏里去的，也就是说，当归。所以当归是血家的主药，跟血相关的病，都可以用，甚至可以说是必用当归。

气血兼顾

当归，味辛，能散气、行气，是一个血中气药。它又有油性，能润滑，润滑为阴，辛甘发散为阳，它是一味阴阳皆备的药，也可以说它对气、血都有作用，能够益血中之气，所以古人说它是血中气药，能够补气补血，行气行血。

"气为血之帅，血为气之母。"气和血是相互依存的，不能够光有气没有血，也不能光有血没有气，气血要兼顾，当归正好是兼顾气血的药。光补血不补气，补的血行不动，就容易成为瘀血；光补气不补血，气就没有依附，气有余便是火。血不归经，就会乱跑，是因为气乱跑，血就跟着乱跑；当气不乱跑了，血也不容易乱跑，所以士兵乱跑怪元帅，元帅就是气。

当归入药时的细分

当归分很多种，简单地可以分成川当归和秦当归。川当归是四川产的，辛散的力度大，是比较刚猛的一味药，它善于行气，行血化瘀。秦当归产于陕西一带，辛散的力量要弱一些，养阴补血的作用要大一些。秦当归的头很圆，尾特别多，外表是紫色的，气味很厚而且很滋润。由于秦当归的性状挺像马尾，所以又叫马尾归。如果用来行血、化瘀就用川当归；如果用来养血，就用秦当归。

但现在药店里边不这样分，它把当归分为头、身、尾三个部分。当归头是主根，当归身是主根上长出的粗大的支根，当归尾则是当归身下面的须根。当归头是破血的，可以化瘀；当归身能守中焦而养血；当归尾则往下走，一切植物的根的末梢都是往下走的，所以它能够行血，也就是瘀化下行。在用当归的时候，经常会如此区分，但一般也不分得这么细，直接用全当归就行，头、身、尾都有了，同时破血、养血、行血。如果要强化它哪一方面的作用，我们可以再加其他的药来辅佐它。

当归的常用配伍

当归是一味非常活泼的药，能文能武，看它跟着谁配伍。跟着补药它就补，跟着泻药它就泻，跟着热药它就温，跟着寒凉药它也会凉，所以这味药非常好用。

当归配黄芪，就构成一个非常有名的方剂，叫当归黄芪补血汤，又叫补血汤，是能够生血的。当归既补气又补血，通过补气行气来生血，加上黄芪就强化了它补气的作用。当归把黄芪的药力往血分里边一带，气行则血行，益气则生血。如果嫌它益气的力度不够还可以加人参。人参、当归、黄芪照样是补血汤。

当归辛香走窜，这就要耗气，所以就要跟上补气的药，让它能够补气、行气而不伤气；同时，其辛香走窜的性质需要一个推动力，这也需要补气，气足了，推动力才强。所以当归跟着补气的药一块儿，它辛香走窜的力度会加大，同时又没有副作用，这样它养血、生血的作用就会更强，因此说，当归跟补药在一起就会更补。

当归跟泻药在一起则泻，它可以配大黄。大黄是将军，走而不守。当归头是破血的，当归尾是行血的，但毕竟破血、行血的力度都是有限的，加上大黄，力度就大了。大黄是一味泻药，是入血分的，能清血热，它能够把血热随着大便一起清出去。但大黄是芳香的，走大肠，走而不守，它虽然入血，但它入血的力度还不够。我们把当归和大黄一块用，那么大黄入血分的力度就更大了，或者说破瘀血的力度就更大了。用当归配大黄来化瘀、解血中之毒非常好，如果嫌不够，体内有积水，还可以加牵牛子，牵牛子是利水的。这三味药一起用，力度就比较猛了，一般不要用，用当归和大黄就够了，还可以用酒大黄、酒当归。用酒炒过后，它们就能往上走，往四肢走，就能够把全身的瘀血和血中之毒从上到下清一遍。

当归是很油润的，把当归切开以后，就会看到里面很油润，油润就有润下的作用，大黄也有润下的作用，它们都会往下走。当归本身就能让大便变稀，我们用当归的时候要注意，一定要问问病人的大便的情况。如果他大便干，那么你可以多用当归，可以用到五钱，必要时可以用到一两。当归可以润大便，让大便不那么干，这是直接的理由，间接的理由呢？当归善于管理、善于调和，它能够养血，血养足了大便也不会那么干。反过来，如果病人大便很稀，当归就要少用或者不用。如果大便干稀适度，可以用三四钱。

用于痹症

当归是治疗痹症常用的一味药。痹有风、寒、湿三种。风痹会有游走性的疼痛，寒痹会痛在一个地方，湿则肢体沉重。实际上，往往风、寒、湿这三痹往往是交织在一起的，只是有所偏重，并不是只有哪一种邪气。

治痹症经常会用到当归。痹症往往兼风，而治风先治血，血行风自灭，这是一个基本的原则。痛风也会用到当归。治痹症一般的配伍是当归配桂枝、苍术、菊花、牛膝。桂枝能走四肢，而且能通四肢的阳，把阳气鼓动起来，风、寒、湿邪就容易被驱散。苍术是芳香燥湿而且健脾的药，脾主四肢，通过健脾，能够治四肢的病。菊花能够散肝经的风热。用牛膝就可以把药往下引，往腿部引；在手部用桂枝把药往上引。如果说筋急，筋都变形了，这跟肝有关，可以加上白芍来柔肝养阴，疏筋的力度非常好。如果手指都伸不直了，当然先要兼顾到风、寒、湿，把邪气祛得差不多了，马上得来舒缓筋骨，这就要用大量的白芍。

如果有热象，比如关节肿痛，那么加石膏；如果石膏力度还不够，可以加白虎汤，例如桂枝白虎汤、苍术白虎汤。

还有一个技巧，凡是病在晚上更严重的，必用当归。为什么晚上病会严重呢？因为这个病在阴，病在阴，就要用当归来理血养阴。当然这并不是绝对的，我们知道有这么回事就行，临床灵活处理。

生化汤

妇科经常用当归，尤其是产后。女子生完孩子后，处在一个非常特殊的状态，气血不安，恶露未尽，全身的骨节都会松动。用什么来安抚调理？用当归。产妇会经常喝一个方子叫生化汤：

当归八钱，川芎三钱，炮姜五分，桃仁二钱，甘草五分，景岳加熟地三钱。

生化汤的君药就是当归，用了八钱，其他所有药加起来也没有八钱，这就是说，产后用当归，其他的药只是帮助当归，让当归的作用发挥到最大化而已。川芎是为了更好的行血，当归和川芎有相似的地方，都能行气，并通过行气来行血。

为什么加炮姜呢？产前宜凉，产后宜温，这是一个原则。因为产前母子交抱在一起，容易生热，既然容易生热，可以用点凉的。产后气血虚了，可以适当温一温，而且行血化瘀的时候，适当的用一点温药，也可以给这些行气活血的药提供能量。炮姜只用了五分，相当于现在的1.5克，非常少。桃仁用了二钱，是化瘀的，它是一种果仁，有油润性，主要走的是六腑，因为产妇气血刚刚安定下来，桃仁不要多用，用二钱就够了，有的地方说是用十枚。甘草用五分，也非常的少。

后来张景岳在生化汤的基础上，加了三钱熟地，加强养阴的力度。熟地是张景岳最擅长的一味药，为什么用熟地不用生地呢？因为熟地是温药，而生地偏寒凉。生化汤的这几味药都是偏温的，用生化汤的目的就是在调理气血、逐瘀生新，把瘀血逐了，新血才能生，才能化，所以叫生化汤。

顺便提一下，前面讲的骨节松动，是为什么呢？交骨，也就是耻骨，平时是合着的，生孩子的时候"啪"的一下开了，其实这时候并不只是交骨开了，全身的骨节都相应地要松动。产后交骨会合上，全身的骨节也会相应地合上，但要严丝合缝，也需要过程，要一百天才能完全合上。这就意味着这一百天要非常的注意，不要淋雨，不要吹了虚邪贼风。虚邪贼风就是不符合季节的风。比如夏天本该起南风却起了北风，春天本应起东风却起了西风。《内经》讲"虚邪贼风，避之有时"，就是要躲避这种风。所以，骨节松动再合上这百日期间，如果调养得很好，即使你以前有很多病，身体很弱，也能变强。如果有风、湿、寒入侵到骨节里面去了，就很麻烦了。或者说，在这期间你有很多烦恼忧思，也会落下很多月子病。在这百日期间，如果有性生活，也对身体不好。

凡是气血乱的，都可以用当归来调理。还有什么情况是气血乱呢？就是月经不调。中医把月经叫月信。"月信准，体自安。"只要月经准，说明身体好；月经不准，说明身体有问题。来得快、来得慢，或者不是按月来，这都是气血乱了，当归往往是必用的。

当归粉不可滥用

前不久，流行吃当归粉。有的人吃了以后，出了问题：白带多了。白带多，有两个原因，一是当归辛散耗气，对脾就会有一定的影响，导致脾不能统摄而带下淋漓。二是当归油性润滑，吃多了，白带就会往下滑。

所以，中药也得用对了才没有副作用，用错了同样会有副作用，同样会导致别的病。现在有医源性疾病，有药源性疾病，就是说，有的病是治出来的，这个叫药源性疾病，像这种白带多就是因为吃当归粉吃出来的，这种病人的方子里就不要加当归了，应该主要从气、从脾这方面来调。

中药只要用对了，也就是配伍精良、对症准确，就没有副作用，否则，用多了也是不好的。所以，哪怕是当归粉，也不能长期吃。

四物汤

四物汤是非常有名的一个方剂：当归、白芍、川芎、生地。其君药是当归，后面几味药都是强化当归作用的。当归行气，川芎进一步加强当归行气的力度；当归补血，用白芍是为了与当归一起柔肝养阴，使其补血；地黄既是入肾的，又是为了加强当归养阴的力度。这样一来，当归如虎添翼，养血的力度就更大了。

从四物汤到十全大补汤

女子以血为主，所以四物汤在妇科里边是使用率非常高的一个方子，很多病都可以用四物汤来加减治疗。例如调经、养血，在胎产里边都会用到这个方子。

四物汤合上补气的四君子汤，就是八珍汤，它就气血双补了。我们看到八珍汤就会想到当归黄芪补血汤。当归是补血的，黄芪是补气的，两个在一起，气血双补。那为什么还要用八珍汤呢？八珍汤是对当归黄芪汤作用的放大，它们的含义是相似的，只是在两味药的基础上，壮大了它们的队伍。

在八珍汤的基础上再加肉桂和黄芪，就叫十全大补汤，是补剂的代表方。

体虚感冒，且补且清

老人或体弱者，气血两虚，他们如果感冒了，纯用解表清里散邪的方法，还是不行的，因为这一切要以人体的气血为基础，那怎么办呢？可以在八珍汤中选一些补药，加进去。

参苏饮就是这个思路，以人参和苏叶两味药为主，当然还可以根据具体情况加葛根、柴胡、半夏、茯苓、枳壳、桔梗、陈皮、甘草之类。

体虚感冒误治，容易造成邪气内陷，造成骨蒸劳热，长期低热，人也非常难受，感觉热是骨头里边发出来的。在这种情况下，普通的解表清热药就不管用了，可在四物汤中加上银柴胡、鳖甲、地骨皮、知母之类，一边清虚热，一边养血。

常用的四物汤加减

在四物汤的基础上，加阿胶和炒艾叶，就是胶艾四物汤。阿胶是血肉有情之品，增强养血的力度；炒艾叶是温通的，温通全身、温通命门。胶艾四物汤还治疗下焦有寒、血收不住那样的月经淋沥不尽；还能固胎、养胎。

胶艾四物汤是偏温的，芩连四物汤则偏凉。芩连四物汤就是在四物汤的基础上，加上黄芩、黄连、丹皮。一般用于月经提前、颜色发紫、发黑，这往往是血热。丹皮清血热，黄芩、黄连也是清热的，但主要是清上焦和中焦的热，为什么不能清下焦呢？因为恐伤肾阳。

如果有瘀血，那么就在四物汤的基础上加桃仁和红花，活血化瘀，这叫桃红四物汤。王清任在桃红四物汤的基础上加桔梗向上提，加牛膝向下带，一上一下，通身去瘀，这就是著名的血府逐瘀汤，此外还有膈下逐瘀汤、身痛逐瘀汤等几个方剂，都是加减得非常妙的。

瘀血一去，新血就生，哪怕这个人很瘦，也可以用。如果是胖子，那么肥人多痰，可以在四物汤的基础上再加二陈汤。如果兼有气郁，可以再加香附、乌药之类。

另外，还要注意，在产后，四物汤里如果是用白芍的话，那么用生白芍性寒酸收，容易伤生生之气，把肝阳给泄掉了；如果吃不下饭，就不要用地黄了，因为地黄是滋腻的药，会让人更不想吃饭；如果大便稀，当归要少用；如果出汗多，川芎就不要用了，川芎走窜的力度很大，汗多说明身体中走窜的东西已经不少了，再用川芎，可能汗就更多了。汗多也不好，因为汗为心之液，汗出多了会伤心阴。

四物汤的加减非常多，而且灵活，我们在临床中要反复体会。

白芍

收敛木气

白芍花开得很像牡丹，但它跟牡丹不一样，牡丹是木本的植物，而白芍是草本的，草本植物能开那么大的花，是非常难得的。一般自然界的植物有个规律，开花的大小，与其生发之力有关。花开得大，生发之力就强，生发之力越强，说明它的根就越能收敛。

植物也讲究阴阳平衡，外面生发得厉害，下面就需要强有力的根来收敛，否则植物就变成头重脚轻了。尤其草本植物更是这样。开花大，意味着木气旺，就要求植物的根能够收敛木气，收敛木气就是收敛肝气，让肝气归根返本，这样就能够制约肝气，不让肝气太暴虐。

肝为将军之官。将军是个什么样的人物呢？抵御外邪需要他，解决人民内部矛盾也需要他。抵御外邪要肝提供动力，身体本身的毒也需要肝的疏泄作用来排解。肝主疏泄，就有解毒的意思在里面。但将军的脾气也很大，容易暴虐，所以用白芍来酸收，肝喜欢辛散，不喜欢收敛，白芍非要给它收一下，所以有泻肝的作用。

养肝与泻肝

白芍配当归，能养肝。白芍是收的，当归是辛散的，一收一散，就把酸甘养肝阴的作用发挥到极致，又把白芍酸收泄肝的作用给淡化了。

养肝时候经常用当归白芍。如果要泄肝，则用白芍配川芎。川芎走窜，就加大了泄肝的力度。所以养肝就用当归白芍，泄肝就用川芎白芍。有人问了，当归、白芍、川芎一起用不就是四物汤里的三个药吗？那么四物汤到底是要养肝还是泄肝呢？它既要养肝又要泄肝。这个组方就体现了中国人的思维方式。就像一个领导，批评一个人之前先表扬他，讲究一个平衡。开方也是这样的。一打一摸，既养肝又泄肝，肝就晕乎乎了，这样才能把它给调服。既有让你很舒服的地方，又有让你不舒服的地方，然后让你把该做的事情做好，不敢去做不该做的事情。

白芍的六大作用

张元素把白芍的作用归纳得非常直接："安脾经一也，治腹痛二也，收胃气三也，止泄利四也，和血脉五也，固腠理六也。"

为什么能够安脾经？因为它能够泄肝。脾经不安是因为肝木克脾土，泄了肝气，脾经就安了。

为什么能治腹疼呢？腹疼往往是因为腹中气急，急则疼。张仲景治腹疼常芍药和甘草并用。芍药专以泄肝。里急，其实是肝在急，好比将军一急起来就滥杀无辜，肚子里面就疼了。所以腹中急痛跟肝有关，酸以泄肝，肝就不急了。为什么又要用甘草呢？甘草是甜言蜜语的一个和事佬，这样一个软，一个硬，然后这将军就服了，不急了，也就不痛了。到了夏天，可以加一点黄芩；如果病人恶寒，可以加一点肉桂或者桂枝。

白芍为什么能收胃气呢？胃气不收，是因为肝气不收，酸就能收肝胃之气。

白芍还能止泻痢，也就是能够治拉肚子。当肝的疏泄力度太大的时候，人就会容易泻痢。用白芍泄肝，让肝的疏泄力度减少，泻痢就容易止住。此外，酸还能收。泻痢就是收不住，我就直接用酸味来给你收住。

白芍能利血脉，因为肝藏血，肝气和则血脉和。

白芍固腠理，也就是固皮肤肌表，这也跟它的酸收之性有关。

这六个作用都是围绕白芍酸收、泻肝的本性来展开的，所以我们认识一个药，要认识它的本性。抓住了本性，其他的作用我们可以在理论上推出来，再在实践中去验证。

痛泻要方

芍药跟白术一块能够调和肝脾的，有一个很有名的方子：白术、白芍、防风、陈皮，这就是痛泻要方，它就治疗所有的痛泻。

痛泻就是先有肚子痛，然后拉肚子，拉完就不痛了，但过一会儿又痛，这样痛一阵，泻一阵。这是木克土造成的。用痛泻要方，效果非常好。痛泻要方后来在《时病论》里面演化成了培中泻木法，加了几味药来强化它的作用。

山萸肉

养肝阴还有一个重要的药就是山萸肉。山萸肉也叫山茱萸，它是一种灌木的果实，产于山东、山西、河南一带。这种灌木春天先开花，后长叶，到冬天的时候，叶子先落，果实还会在枝头，一般都是在农历十月份去采，那是一种椭圆形的小红果。

山萸肉在很多书里并不是归在养阴的药中，而是归在收涩药里。山萸肉的味是酸、涩的，入肝、肾两经，它的作用是固精秘气、强阴助阳，它能够温肝，平补阴阳，就是说它既能补阴又能补阳，补得又不是太峻猛。用山萸肉要把核挤掉，光用外边的皮和肉。一般来说，它的肉偏酸，皮偏涩。

用山萸肉要把核挤掉，光用外边的皮和肉。一般来说，它的肉偏酸，皮偏涩。

双面属性

无论是树皮、果皮，凡是皮都有涩性，只是程度有轻有重而已。皮在外边，要把里面的东西包住，它必然有涩性，不然统摄不住；是皮，又能走表，有透散性，否则里面的东西就会烂掉。皮不但要收涩，还要透散，而收涩和透散是两种完全相反的作用。

大自然中，往往同一个东西上有两种截然相反的属性并存。只是根据自身的自然属性有所偏重。有的皮偏重于透散，比如五加皮、瓜蒌；有的皮偏于收涩，比如石榴皮。不管是偏于收涩还是偏于透散，它都是既透散又收涩的。当然也要看你怎么配伍，通过配伍发挥哪种属性，它的哪种性质就会得到强化。

人也是这样，有多少红就有多少黑，在这方面你是圣贤，可能在那方面你就是魔鬼。

就连字也是这样的。比如一个"乖"字，我们哄小孩说"你要乖"，这就是听话的意思。还有一个词叫"乖张"，就是不听话。所以"乖"既有听话的意思，又有不听话的意思，到底是哪个意思，要看它跟哪个字一起。

再比如说"乱"。有弄乱的意思，比如"乱臣贼子，祸乱朝纲"；还有治乱的意思，比如周武王说他"有乱臣十人"，就不是乱臣贼子了，而是能够治乱、平乱的得力臣子。

还比如"重"。我们重教育，要安土重迁，也就是重迁徙。"重教育"跟"重迁徙"是不一样的。重教育就是要加大教育的力度，重迁徙就是要在迁徙这个事情上比较谨慎，不能乱迁徙。正好又是相反的意思。

又比如"冤家"。"冤家路窄"是仇人见面，但在情侣之间互相称冤家，又充满了一种爱意在里边。

这些，在训诂学里叫做反训，有些东西正面讲不通，要从反面来讲他的意思。

肝的疏泄和肾的封藏

皮都有涩性，加上山萸肉是酸的，所以它的皮更偏于收涩。

山萸肉是走肝肾的。肝主疏泄，肾主封藏，肝和肾在这方面的功能是相反的。一切疏泄都跟肝气相关，肝气动才能疏泄。如果肝气过旺，肾气弱，那就会疏泄无度了，肾就不能固涩了，所以就用山萸肉来收涩肝气。

凡是往外走的，都叫疏泄。比如，大小便能够排出去，都是肝的疏泄功能在起作用。有人一郁闷就便秘；郁闷肝就郁了，肝郁则疏泄功能失常，所以人就便秘了。大便滑泄，则是因为肝疏泄的太过了，肝疏泄太过，大便就解得多，或解的次数多。在治泄、治痢疾的时候，要注意治肝，调节肝的疏泄。

出汗也跟肝的疏泄有关。汗为心之液，心和肝合作，产生出汗这种生理现象，必须肝疏泄的功能正常，汗才能很好的出来。如果肝疏泄不利，那么可能就不出汗了。如果肝疏泄太过，人可能会大汗淋漓。

汗为心之液，肾之液则包括尿液和精液。精液藏于肾中，要肝气动，也就是情欲动，才能疏泄出来。如果肝气过旺、肾气过弱，就疏泄无度了，肝气旺而肾气弱的人就容易早泄，其疏泄的功能得不到封藏制约。

肝和肾在这个时候是矛盾的，肾要封藏，要固住，不能疏泄出来，肝又要把它疏泄出来，那么这两脏开始较上劲了。当肾气旺的时候，肝想疏泄，肾不让它疏泄，那么就要很长时间才能疏泄；当肾气弱的时候，肝要疏泄，肾没办法，马上就疏泄出来了，所以当我们要补肾的时候，就要收敛肝气，用山萸肉的收涩作用。

山萸肉是收涩肝肾之气。其味酸，能泄肝，杀一杀肝的气焰；还能柔肝养阴，使肝的疏泄的作用柔软下来。加上其本身固有的养阴固肾功能，所以对于肝气是疏泄太过而肾气不固的遗精、大小便不禁、虚汗，都有收涩作用。

固涩精气，收敛心神

肝主疏泄，不仅是生理上的疏泄，也包括情绪上的疏泄。比如，你想说的话敢于说出来，想表达的东西能够有办法表达出来，也是肝气在疏泄，所以往往肝气旺的人话多，因为它需要疏泄。我们既要疏泄生理的物质，也需要疏泄自己的情感、思想。但话又说回来，话说的多了，也是要耗伤精气的，所以山萸肉不但可以固涩有形的东西，还可以用来固涩无形的东西，也就是固涩精气，收敛心神。

所以山萸肉还能安心神，对心气虚的心悸、精神不能集中等也有很好的作用。当然这要跟其他的药配伍。肾一虚，人容易精力不集中，所以补肾方中经常用山萸肉，就有助于交通心肾，安神定志，让人精力集中。

固脱

收涩的作用如此强大，所以山萸肉能够固脱。

什么叫固脱？正常的人是阴阳交抱的，阴中有阳，阳中有阴。当人要死的时候，阴阳就要离绝了。阳往上奔，阴往下走。阳往上奔表现为出汗，只有出去的气没有进去的气；阴往下走表现为洞泄亡阴，大便止不住了。

所以，经常在急救的时候用山萸肉来固脱，让阳不至于从上脱，阴不至于从下脱，阴阳依然能够交抱在一起。它不但能够固脱，还能平补阴阳，既补阴又补阳。所以在生死反掌的时候，经常要用到山萸肉这味药，力挽狂澜。在这个时候用山萸肉的量就比较大了。

张锡纯经常用山萸肉来进行急救。如果事情比较紧急，还可以加上大剂量的党参，这个方法经常用于穷人。穷人没钱用人参，什么参附汤、独参汤就没法用了，咱们就用山萸肉配党参，效果是一样的！此时山萸肉用量就非常大，往往用到二两、三两。二两相当于现在的60克。

利九窍

山萸肉还有利九窍的作用。九窍就是人体的孔窍，头上有七窍，下边有二阴，加起来就是九窍。这九窍都有不利的时候，有可能被东西堵住了，也有可能是气机不利，影响出入。这些情况都可以考虑用山萸肉，它有通窍的作用。

有人要问了，一个固涩的药，怎么还能通窍呢？大自然就是这样的，这又是事物的两面性。九窍不通是因为精气不通，因为人的精气是要自由出入往来于九窍的，精气不足，则无法在九窍间自在往来出入。所以，精气不足则九窍不利。用山萸肉固涩，补益精气，那么九窍自然通利了。通利和固摄看上去好像是矛盾的，实际上又是统一的，就好比佛和魔只在一念之间，固涩和通利也只有一步之遥。

六味地黄丸用山萸肉

六味地黄丸里面用山萸肉，它的用意其实是非常多的。地黄是能补肾的，但地黄的收涩性不足，不能帮助肾的封藏，所以要加一味山萸肉。山萸肉本身能够养肝肾之阴，同时又能收涩肝肾，它能把地黄补的阴收涩住。光收涩住还不行，后面又加了茯苓、泽泻来利水，通肾气，一边收涩一边通利，把精气收涩住，把邪气通利才出去。这是六味地黄汤用山萸肉的第一重作用。

第二重作用，补肾还得注意养肝，山萸肉味酸入肝，是肝肾同养的，它跟着养肾的地黄，大补肝肾之阴。肾水生肝木，肝阴足了，肾的消耗就小了。

第三重意思，山萸肉色红入心，地黄色黑入肾，地黄和山萸肉在一起用，也有交通心肾的意思。

山茱萸与吴茱萸

最后，顺便提醒大家，山茱萸和吴茱萸是两种截然不同的东西，吴茱萸是一味大热的药，温肝阳的；山茱萸则是一种小红果，养肝阴的。

为了区分起见，我们经常把山茱萸写成山萸肉，这样就能让人感觉它是一种养阴的药，而吴茱萸可以写吴萸，或者写泡吴萸，以示区分。

山萸肉一定要去核

此外，用山萸肉一定要把核去掉。现在从药店买的山萸肉中有时候会有核，一定要把它拣出来。山萸核是不能入药的，因为它有滑精的作用。山萸的皮和肉是固涩的，而核不但不能固涩，反能滑精。这种现象还有很多。比如麻黄是可以发汗的，而麻黄根恰恰相反，它是收汗的。还有我们即将讲到的枸杞，枸杞子是性温的，而地骨皮又是性寒的。相反的性质，往往存在于同一植物身上。

开山萸肉这个药的时候，也要用矛盾的眼光去看它，不要把它的作用定在某一端上，如果说山萸肉只是一个收敛的药，你就漏掉了很多内容。

药，有时候有些东西是很难讲的。讲了这一面就漏了那一面。比如你讲了山萸肉固涩的一面，就容易忘掉它还能利九窍。你讲了肝肾同源，就忘了肝肾之间还有矛盾。所以，我一直在强调思维的开放性和灵活性。我们要用开放和灵动的思维去看中药，也要用这种思维来听任何人讲的课。我们现在学中医，你如果仅仅局限于疾病本身，局限于病理生理，那么往往容易走入一些定论，一旦走入定论，你的思维就失去了鲜活性。而人体永远是鲜活的，疾病永远是变化的。用很死的思维面对这些变化的疾病会很麻烦。所以，我们一定要学会怎么思考。

枸杞

关于枸杞，以前我们在讲地骨皮的时候已经讲了一些。

枸杞子

枸杞是一种灌木，在宁夏长得很大，在一般地方只是两三尺高的一种小灌木。枸杞子是温肝肾的药，它可以生津助阳，温身暖血，可以填补真阴，同时还能退虚热，善于补益肝肾。枸杞子是以红润、粒大而紧、肉厚子少为最佳。有的枸杞子，籽特别多，肉特别薄，这就没那么好了。宁夏是枸杞的地道产地，其实，整个西北的枸杞子都非常不错。

张景岳的左归饮、右归饮、左归丸、右归丸里都用枸杞子，通过养肝达到温肾养肾的目的。肝肾都处在下焦，下焦容易积累寒气，下焦是藏精的，精得温则化，所以在养肝肾，滋补肝肾之阴时经常要用一些偏温的药，但也不能太温，太温会补出火，枸杞子甘温而不燥，用之最宜。

枸杞沐浴

枸杞全身都可以入药，枸杞叶也叫天精草，根皮叫地骨皮。枸杞叶嫩时可以食用，老了以后还可以用来洗澡。

古代的养生家很注重用枸杞来沐浴，《本草纲目》引用《洞天保生录》："正月一日，二月二日，三月三日，四月四日，以至十二月十二日，皆用枸杞叶煎汤洗澡，令人光泽，百病不生。"

后来明朝有位叫高濂的养生家，他的《遵生八笺》也非常推崇枸杞沐浴，他说用枸杞沐浴，但没有说用哪个部位，是用枸杞子、枸杞叶、还是地骨皮？很多书里讲的都不一样，这需要我们去判断。其实他的本意是枸杞子、枸杞的枝叶、枸杞根同用，因为沐浴是要洗全身的，用枸杞的全身来养人的全身，这是最为有效的。

枸杞叶是走表的，我们洗澡也是洗身体的最表层，所以枸杞的叶子是要用到的。枸杞子可以起到滋润肌肤的作用，可以通过皮肤的吸收来补肝益肾。地骨皮则是去虚热的，它往骨头里走，清全身的虚热，所以还要放入少量的地骨皮。这是古代很常见的养生泡澡方。

养生的天时地利人和

有人会问，为什么非得要正月一，二月二，三月三日这些日子呢？因为养生治病，要讲究天时、地利、人和。

人和是指一个方子方法到底有没有效，很大程度取决于你的心态。当你心态好的时候，这个方即使差一些，也能对你起很大的作用。当你心情不好的时候，再好的方法到你那也不行。

地利呢？北方到处都有枸杞，但一定要用宁夏产的地道药材，这就是地利。

最令我们难以置信的就是天时，哪一天用这个。之所以说每年的正月初一、二月初二、三月三来用，很大程度上是出于心理考虑。哪怕你没有严格遵循这个时间，但是在心里也必须要建立天时的这种观念。正月初二、二月初三、三月初四难道就不能用么？也可以用。过去每年只要求用十二次，这是最少的要求，因为枸杞产于西北，当时运输条件也不发达，对于中原人来说，枸杞历来就比较昂贵，吃枸杞的机会就不多，更何况用它来泡澡呢。所以古人很节制、很节约。当然，现在用这个东西，可以多多益善了。

Chapter 5 Medicines for Nourishing Heart Yin

Wheat

Wheat is sown in autumn, and it grows in winter, flourishes in spring, and gets harvested in summer. Wheat obtains the energy of the four seasons of a whole year, so it is taken as the top grain of the five cereals (wheat, rice, two different kinds of millets and beans). It is sweet-cool and non-toxic in nature, going into the heart channel of Hand-Shaoyin. When used as medical herb, wheat produced in the north to Huaihe River in China (called Huai Wheat) is the best of all. So, in prescriptions, when wheat is needed, it is always written as "Huai Wheat", that is to say, the wheat produced in the south of China is not suitable for medical use.

Huai Wheat and Ganmai Dazao Tang

Summer is subsumed to fire, corresponding to the heart; wheat is harvested in summer, going into the heart, and it not only nourishes the heart Yin, but also nourishes the stomach Qi, tranquilizes the mind, and eliminates heat to stop annoyance.

Zhang Zhongjing's **Ganmai Dazao Tang** (Liquorice Wheat Jujube Decoction) contains three herbs: wheat, Gancao and Dazao (jujube), mainly for treatment of women's visceral mania, stemming from the five internal organs' dysphoria rooted in the heart. The heart fire and heart Yin deficiency can cause a person to be irritable, so it needs to clear the heart fire and nourish heart Yin with this formula, in which wheat is the monarch herb. Gancao and Dazao go into the spleen meridians, and the spleen is the source for Qi and blood generation and transformation. Hence, only when the source of Qi and blood is sufficiently replenished, can it then provide better conditions for nourishing heart Yin with wheat. This formula is quite sweet in taste, which can help to relieve both the physical and emotional depression.

Wheat and Cooked Wheaten Food

Is it workable if one just eats steamed bun and noodle everyday now that-wheat can nourish heart Yin?

It is certainly unadvisable since the steamed bun or noodles are made from the peeled wheat, while the wheat to be used as herb must be the whole grain. Wheat rind is cold in property, the flour is only the powder of the wheat kernel, which is partially warmer. Many Chinese medicines are parched with the wheat bran in that it is to take advantage of the cold property of the wheat bran to weaken the warm property of the warm medicines in order to make the medicines become mild in property. The rice is just opposite to wheat in property. The rice bran is inclined to warmth, while the rice without bran is partially cool, that is, the rice we eat every day is a little bit cool in property.

The wheat flour is warm in property. The steamed bun or noodles can only appease our hunger, replenish nutrition, harmonize stomach Qi, reinforce our physical strength and build up muscles, but they do not have medicinal value. Of course, wheat as a medicine is not well suitable for daily food.

Blighted Wheat

In the process of washing wheat, the plump grains will sink in, and the non-plump grains, i. e. , the blighted wheat, will float up, but the blighted wheat has the efficacies of nourishing heart Yin, bringing down the deficiency heat and stopping the abnormal perspiration due to general debility.

In the antiperspirant formula, the blighted wheat is frequently used together with Huangqi (radix astragali), Longgu (ossa draconis) etc. The raw Huangqi can tonify Qi and strengthen the exterior, and Longgu is also an astringent medicine.

How can the blighted wheat stop sweating? Sweat is the fluid of heart, so, when the heart fire is vigorous and the heart fluid is disturbed by the heart fire, perspiration will be induced. When the blighted wheat is used to nourish the heart Yin sufficiently, it will repair the impairments caused by sweating. Meanwhile, the blighted wheat can also clear away the heart fire. When the heart heat retreats, there will be no fire to disturb the heart fluid, and therefore, perspiration will not be induced so easily.

The blighted wheat is actually shriveled wheat, but why are they shriveled? They are not fully endowed by the nature, that is to say, they are in a state of deficiency.

By the season of Grain Full (8th solar term), the wheat will need pulp filling in its growing period. Before the wheat is ripe, and if one opens and squeezes the wheat kernel, he or she could see some wheat pulp, which is actually the quintessence of wheat. When wheat is ripe, the pulp will become hardened. Only when the pulp is fully filled, can wheat become a healthy and complete grain. In case that it is not fully filled, it will be in a state of deficiency. But just because of its deficiency, it is able to treat the symptoms of deficiency.

In the case of heart Yin deficiency and fire, the blighted wheat will draw to the like of the human physical conditions. This again suggests that we should take advantage of the normal states of some medicines for some cases and the abnormal states for some other cases. When wheat is used as an herb, it does not mean that the more fully-grown the wheat is, the more valuable its medical value will be. Of course, in the formula of **Ganmai Dazao Tang**, the well-grown wheat can be used. The shriveled wheat cannot be ground into too much wheat flour, and the flour out of the shriveled wheat is in poor quality as well. So, few people would like to eat such flour, but it can be used as medicine. This is what Chinese people do and know how to make the best use of things.

Examples of Pathological Substances as Medicines

Here are some other similar examples, like silkworm, it can be used as medicine, but it does not mean the healthier the silkworm is, the better it will be as medicine. As a matter of fact, when silkworm is used as medicine, the best one is the silkworm that dies naturally, that is, Baijiangcan (silkworm larva), which is the best for medicine.

In addition, there are many other things that are used for their pathosis. For example, the bamboo damaged by moths will discharge a lot of sap staying on the joints of bamboo, which is called Tianzhuhuang (tabasheer) after it is dried up.

A bug smitten by the hyphae in soil will grow a grass called Dongchong Xia-cao (cordyceps sinensis) or other type of cordyceps like Jinchanhua (isaria cicadae miquel). Some other bugs survive if without being smitten by hyphae. So, only those bugs killed by hyphae can become cordyceps. So cordyceps, too, is the pathological condition of bugs. Therefore, the flora and fauna, both in their normal or abnormal states, can be used as medicine.

As the English saying goes, "call a spade a spade", what I want to say here is that "medicines are medicines; animals and plants are animals and plants", and there exist some differences between them. For example, atractylodes, there are two types, and the medical atractylodes is aromatic and dry, which can tonify the spleen; Again, there also exist two kinds of eclipta, and only the eclipta that can be used as medicine is called Hanliancao (eclipta alba). Besides, many similar plants have the same name, but some of them are the same plants or animals with different names for them in different states like the normal and pathological states, or existing in different seasons, for example, ox horn and bezoar refer to the different things from oxen. So, never simply take animals and plants as the Chinese medicines.

Baiziren (Platycladi Seed)

Baiziren is the seed of cypress. Let us get to know cypress tree first before analyzing the seed.

Cypress Subsumed to Shady (Yin) Wood

The Chinese character "柏" (bǎi, means cypress), the lateral radical in the left is "木" (mù, means wood) and the other side is "白" (bái, means white). The white color goes into the lungs, dominating astringency and subsumed to Yin.

A tree normally has dense leaves to the east and south sides, and sparser leaves to the west and north sides, excluding the trees along waters, where the leaves are thicker to the water side. The opposite is true of cypress, which has dense leaves to the west and north and sparser leaves to the east and south.

On the shady side of a mountain, cypress trees tend to grow very vigorously, while on the sunny side, cypress trees tend to grow a little weakly. For instance, on the hills in Changping county in Beijing, one can see more and dense cypress trees on the western and northern hillside, but on the southeastern hillside, the cypress trees become almost half sparser. Similarly, cypress trees in the north of China are growing more flourishingly than those in the south. In short, the cypress tree is subsumed to the shady (Yin) wood and it likes shade.

Cebaiye (Cacumen Biotae)

Cypress leaves can be used as medicine, called Cebaiye (cacumen biotae). In human body, Qi is subsumed to Yang, and blood is subsumed to Yin, and cypress is subsumed to Yin as well. As the saying goes "like draws to like", so cypress leaf goes into the blood system. Cypress tree is of wood, subsumed to the blood system, which means it goes into the liver meridians. Cypress corresponds to the season of autumn, and it is subsumed to metal, which means it can also go into the lungs and large intestine channels for purifying and descending effects. This is to deduce the properties of cypress leaf according to the **Wuxing Doctrine**.

The **Wuxing Doctrine** is a tool of Chinese traditional learning. Without such a tool, one may not go on further with thinking. The western modern philosophy puts stresses on casting aside the preconceived ideas or stereotypes and going back to the thing itself. However, thinking needs tools, without which one may become very clumsy.

Then, what is the efficacy of cypress leaves? The cypress leaves function to treat the symptoms of "Yin failure to converge Yang". That Yin does not converge Yang will manifest the symptoms of bleeding, sweating etc. In case that the lungs and the large intestine fail to properly play their purifying and descending functions, it may result in pathogenic fire in blood or mass formed by blood stasis. In such a case, the cypress leaves can be helpful. In addition, the cypress leaf is aromatic, which means it can remove dampness. Hence, cypress leaves can also eliminate dampness and heat in blood. Generally, leaves have permeable effects, and the cypress leaves can disperse dampness and heat outwards.

Baiziren Soothing Nerves and Moistening Intestines

Cypress trees also grow in the south of China, and bear seeds in autumn. The outermost shell of the cypress seed is like a flower. When peeling it open, one can see some seeds inside like rice grains. The outer part of the seed is a hard putamen. When it is cut open, in most cases, it is found empty inside. But the cypress tree in the north is quite different since it enjoys the favorable climatic and geographical conditions sufficiently. Once I visited the hills behind Changping town, I saw some visitors picking some Baiziren and peeling them open. I saw some oily kernels inside the seeds like rice grains. Having seen these oily kernels, I immediately understood that there are climatical differences of Yin and Yang and the four different seasons; and there are also geographical differences of the east, west, south and north. I did not pick any Baiziren during my visit to Changping, since I had formed a mindset that nothing is available inside the seeds from my visiting experience before in the south, and such a mindset has become a subconsciousness in my mind. In fact, the same plant growing in different places will definitely manifest some different characteristics. So, wherever one visits, he or she will surely have some gains if he or she can make careful observation with curiosity.

Baiziren can nourish heart, tranquilize the mind, and relax the bowel. All these efficacies are related to its natural properties. The kernel is the core of a plant. In TCM, many sorts of kernels ware being used, like Hetaoren (walnut kernel), Taoren (peach kernel), Xingren (apricot kernel), Baiziren (platycladi seed), and Suanzaoren (wild jujube seed). A small piece of cypress seed, buried in soil with sufficient conditions guaranteed, can grow into a big tree, which also has a very long-life span. This signifies that this seed contains great life vitality, and it also contains all information of the tree. Thus, it is clear that the seed has great potential.

The core/kernel means it can go into the heart, which tells us that all kinds of seeds or kernels more or less have the efficacy of going into the heart, so does Baiziren. But Baiziren is different from the other seeds or kernels in that it additionally has fragrance, so it can go into the heart more. Fragrance generally enjoys the efficacy of opening orifices, and the heart has its orifice, hence, Baiziren can open the heart orifice. Besides, Baiziren is very oily and it is able to moisten and nourish the heart. Therefore, it is used as a medicine for nourishing heart Yin, which means it can also tranquilize the mind. In addition, its oily and lubricant properties can help to relax the bowel. Those who suffer from insomnia due to disorderly defecations will find Baiziren more helpful.

But Baiziren should not be taken for too long time. Those who always use Baiziren because of insomnia or troubled defecations may, on the contrary, suffer from accumulation of dry stool due to the double properties of Baiziren. Baiziren is an aromatic medicine, and its fragrance can easily result in dryness. Although Baiziren is not too much fragrant, after a long-lasting use of it, fragrance will also play its role to result in dry stool, so, stop using Baiziren little now and little then even if it is able to relax the bowel in order to avoid the dry stool.

The balance of the body can be achieved so long as the liver-Qi is ascending and the lung-Qi is descending properly. However, in case that there is only ascending but no proper descending, the human body will fall into troubled conditions. The lung Qi takes descending function as its normal and smooth circulation, and the lung dislikes Qi's reversal upwards. In case that the lung Qi fails in its purifying and descending functions, the heart in between lung lobes will become uneasy. That's why tranquilization of heart and mind is closely related to the lungs. The heart is the monarch organ, and the lungs are the assistant organs, that is, metaphorically, one is the emperor, and the other is the prime minister. In order to relieve heat, the lungs must be appeased first. Baiziren can promote lungs for purifying and descending. At the same time, Baiziren can go into the large intestine to lubricate feces and help relax the bowel easily and smoothly so as to facilitate the lung fire to descend much easily. When the lung Qi descends, it will not disturb the heart, which will contribute to tranquilization of the heart and mind as well. This is the principle of nourishing heart and tranquilizing mind by Baiziren. One should not think that the process of nourishing heart and tranquilizing mind is a different thing from relaxing the bowel. In fact, these effects are the two in one. When **Shennong Bencao Jing** (**Shen Nong's Herbal Classic**) talks about a medicine, it often lists a lot of efficacies of the medicine. It does not mean to let us apply them mechanically, but help the readers find the relationship among these efficacies. Therefore, the readers ought to ponder why such two efficacies are put together, and what are the connections between them. Such connotations are not directly listed, but they are indeed implied in the book of *Shennong Bencao Jing*.

Suanzaoren (Wild Jujube Seed)

Suanzaoren, as an herb, is often used with Baiziren for nourishing the heart Yin.

Tranquilizing Mind by Suanzaoren From the Perspective of Channel Tropism

Wild jujube plant is a kind of date tree growing on the hills in north China. On the barren hills, the more stone the hills are covered with, no other plants available there, the more likely the hills will be able to grow wild jujube trees. Suanzaoren goes into the heart, liver, gallbladder, and spleen meridians. It is sweet and sour in tastes and mild in property (neither cold nor hot, neither warm nor cool).

Entering the liver, Suanzaoren can tranquilize the mind and astringe the liver Qi in order to help the liver to settle down the soul that it has stored up. Insomnia and dreaminess often arise from the failure of the liver to store up the soul. For such a case, Suanzaoren can help converge the soul into the liver.

Entering into the heart, Suanzaoren can astringe heart Yin, which is the highlighted role of Suanzaoren. Sweat is the fluid of heart, and sweating means the heart Yin is dispersing outwards. So, to astringe heart Yin can help to guard against too much sweating. Suanzaoren can be used for restraining sweating in sleep. As for shedding tears in sleep, Suanzaoren may also be added for treatment based on syndrome differentiation.

In case that gallbladder Qi deficiency arises or gallbladder meridian has deficiency heat, Suanzaoren may also be used for treatment.

The liver being uneasy, the mind not astringed or gallbladder meridian having deficiency heat, all of these can easily lead to insomnia, so Suanzaoren is an important medicine for treatment of insomnia.

Raw and Parched Suanzaoren

There are two types of Suanzaoren: the raw and the parched. Both of them can be used as medicine, but they have slightly different functions.

The parched Suanzaoren refers to the Suanzaoren that is just slightly fried, but not too much. The slightly parched Suanzaoren is very fragrant, so it can go into the heart and spleen, and astringe the fluid of body. That is to say, it is especially effective for treatment of insomnia due to the heart and gallbladder Qi deficiency.

But how to use the raw Suanzaoren? Generally speaking, the raw herb has a partially discharging function and it can disperse the deficiency heat in the gallbladder meridians. As discussed in the above sections, the coldness and coolness can help one refresh himself, while heat can make one feel dizzy and giddy. The gallbladder heat always makes the patient feel dizzy and sleepy, but he/she always fails to have sound sleep and will be susceptible to wake up. After waking up, he/she may feel drowsy again.

Insomnia has various manifestations. For some people, the more sleepless, the more sober they will feel, and even they feel terribly sober; for some other people, the insomnia will make them dizzy and sleepy, even always in a half-sleeping state, and so they always feel very tired after waking up. Those who suffer from insomnia due to serious endogenous heat or gallbladder heat will often feel dizzy and tired. They want to take a sleep, but they could not fall asleep. Under that circumstance, the raw Suanzaoren can help them fall asleep deeply. By the way, the raw Suanzaoren can also be good for treatment of the over-sleeping case. In short, Suanzaoren has effects of two-way regulation.

How can Suanzaoren nourish the heart and tranquilize mind? First, let us see the differences between the wild jujube and the common date. Generally, when buying dates from market, everyone would like to select the dates with thinner skin and thicker pulp and smaller stone. But for the wild jujube, it is just the opposite, and it has thicker skin, thin pulp and bigger stone inside. Both of them are of date. But why the common date is so largely different from the wild jujube? Is it the nature that endows them with the different energy? That is not so. Everything is equal in the nature. It can be said that the nature endows each of the jujube/date with equal energy, but only the common date gives the energy it receives from the nature to its pulp, so its pulp is so fat and sweet that it can nourish the spleen and nothing is left inside the core stone, while the wild jujube stores the received energy tightly in its stone so that the stone of the wild jujube is so fully developed while the pulp is left to become very thin. Hence, Suanzaoren can be used to nourish the heart.

A piece of date can tell us the phenomena of "fire generating earth" (based on the **Wuxing Doctrine**). Here, the fire refers to the stone of date, and the earth refers to the pulp. The pulp is fully developed in that the stone does not converge too much energy, and spares the energy for the pulp of the dates. While as for jujube, its fire does not generate the earth so that it could not have so thick pulp that it develops into a qualified Suanzaoren. For the common date, the fire has generated the earth to transform itself into sweet pulp, while the wild jujube stores the fire in its stone that can then go into the heart for nourishing heart Yin.

The wild jujube can store the energy endowed by the nature in its stone just because of its property of astringency.

Astringency here means to converge and control sweating, so all kinds of deficiency sweating can be astringed with Suanzaoren. It is especially effective for the sweating arising from heart-Qi deficiency. When one is in tension, he or she is often prone to sweating since tension actually indicates heart deficiency. Sweat is the fluid of heart, so heart deficiency will result in sweating. This is a normal physiological reaction. In case one is in the pathological state, he/she is also prone to a cold sweat, which is often resulted from heart Qi deficiency. In such a case, Suanzaoren can be used to converge the heart Qi and tranquilize the mind.

Guipi Tang

Suanzaoren are used in two extremely typical formulas. One is **Guipi Tang**, and the other is **Tianwang Buxin Dan**.

Guipi Tang contains the herbal ingredients: Renshen (ginseng), Huangqi (radix astragali), Baizhu (white atractylodes rhizome), honey-fried Gancao (liquorice), Muxiang (costustoot), Baifuling (white poria), Yuanzhi (polygala tenuifolia), Danggui (angelica sinensis), Longyanrou (longan aril), Chao

Zaoren (parched jujube kernel) .

The four herbs of Renshen, Baizhu, honey-fried Gancao, Bai Fuling together make **Sijunzi Tang**. Besides, Huangqi added here is to intensify the effect of tonifying the spleen and Qi. Muxiang added here is for refreshing and tonifying the spleen. Menawhile, the spleen dislikes dampness, so Fuling is used here for excreting dampness and tonifying the spleen, plus Yuanzhi for intercommunication between the heart and kidneys. By the way, never forget to replenish blood at the time of tonifying Qi since Qi and blood always go in parallel. Then, Danggui is added here for tonifying Qi and replenishing blood simultaneously, but which is more inclined to replenish blood. And then, add the sweet and warm Longyanrou to tonify the spleen and nourish the heart. And last, add Chao Zaoren to tranquilize mind by nourishing the heart. **Guipi Tang** is normally used to treat the impairment of spleen due to excessive worries. **Guipi Tang** is a formula for tonifying both the heart and spleen.

According to the ***Wuxing Doctrine***, the heart fire generates the spleen earth. The heart and spleen are like the mother-child relationship. In reality, by the time when the heart requires nourishing, it may not be enough to nourish the heart (the mother) only since the spleen (the son) fails to make a good show. The excessive worries may get the heart and spleen exhausted, resulting in pathogenic heat, drowsiness and insomnia. Excessive worries can cause insomnia, spontaneous perspiration or night sweat, or even some other symptoms due to the heart deficiency like insomnia, palpitation, spontaneous perspiration or night sweat; or the symptoms due to the spleen deficiency like poor appetite, even irregular menstruation, more leucorrhea. All these symptoms arising from excessive worries can be treated with **Guipi Pill**. The spleen and stomach are the sources for Qi and blood generation and transformation, so it may not be enough to tonify heart Yin only, and it is also necessary to replenish the source of the heart blood. Therefore, in **Guipi Tang**, more attention is given to tonifying the spleen.

Tianwang Buxin Dan

Tianwang Buxin Dan and **Tianwang Buxin Pill** are actually made with the same formula, in which Baiziren and the parched Suanzaoren are used together.

Tianwang Buxin Dan contains the herbal ingredients of Renshen (ginseng), Xuanshen (radix scrophulariae), Danshen (radix salviae miltiorrhizae), Fuling (poria cocos), Yuanzhi (polygala tenuifolia), Jiegeng (platycodon grandiflorum), Sheng Dihuang (radix rehmanniae recen), lipuored Danggui (angelica sinensis), Wuweizi (fructus schisandrae chinensis), Tianmendong (asparagus cochinchinensis), Maidong (radix ophiopogonis), Baiziren (platycladi seed), parched Suanzaoren (wild jujube kernel), coated with Zhusha (cinnabar).

Coated with Zhusha (Cinnabar)

Tianwang Buxin Dan is a small pill coated with impalpable powder of cinnabar, which makes the pill look reddish. That is why it is called "Dan" (which means reddish pill). Zhusha (cinnabar) must be used with caution now, but *Shennong Bencao Jing* says it can be used for a long time. In fact, when the ancients used the Chinese character "服" (fú) (this character in Chinese has a lot of different meanings like "taking orally", "coating", "wearing" etc.) here in the phrase of "服药" (fú yào, means taking medicine), it has the similar meaning to the character "服" (fú) in the phrase of "衣服" (yīfú, means clothing). That is to say, the character "服" (fú) in these two phrases shares the similar meaning "to wear". It does not mean to swallow cinnabar all the time, but means the behavior of using cinnabar including "to wear". For example, put a small bag of cinnabar of 1 to 3 *qian* under children's pillows, and it is not necessary to eat cinnabar. That will help to tranquilize the mind, and children will have sound sleep with less dreams at night.

Some pathogenic factors are tangible, like wind, coldness, heat, dampness, dryness and fire, which are all tangible and able to impair the tangible human body, while some others are intangible, like the evil spirit and monsters of all kinds in the nature, which are intangible and will be able to infringe upon the human mind. Cinnabar has a function of suppressing these invisible pathogenic factors.

Cinnabar is very heavy in texture, so 3-*qian* cinnabar is not much in size visually. Cinnabar can be taken for external use, but should not be used for oral administration except for the case of absolute necessity. **Tianwang Buxin Dan** coated with cinnabar is for oral administration use, for instance, **Tianwang Bux-in Dan** produced by Beijing Tongrentang Co. Ltd. still contains cinnabar with quite small dosage. So, when it is definitely needed, just to take very little of it orally will be helpful for tranquilizing the mind.

When cinnabar is used for coating pills, it must be ground into very fine powder, and that is why in prescriptions cinnabar is often written as "flying cinnabar", which means to fly cinnabar over water. Just think about it. If such a heavy-quality substance like cinnabar can suspend in water, it indicates that the cinnabar is extremely fine, even impalpable. So, such a method is used to produce the fine powder of cinnabar, i. e., keep on grinding the cinnabar until it can fly up. This is also a technology for processing herbal medicines.

Tips for Tianwang Buxin Dan

For tonifying the heart, the first thing to do is to tonify the spleen. For such a purpose, of course, Renshen has to be used. Danshen and Xuanshen are used together with Renshen. Xuanshen is used here for clearing heat and tonifying the kidneys; Danshen is used to promote blood circulation in order to remove blood stasis. Once the heart Yin is impaired and the heart blood is consumed and dissipated, the blood stasis will arise easily. In that case, Danshen shall have to be used. Accompanied with the impairment of heart Yin, the kidney fire will arise too, so Xuanshen is used here. By the way, Danshen goes into the heart, and Xuanshen goes into the kidneys, functioning to intercommunicate between kidneys and heart.

Fuling and Yuanzhi also function to intercommunicate between the heart and kidney. The heart lies in the upper, and Jiegeng used in this formula can carry the medical effects to go upwards. At the time of using Qi-dominating medicines, the medicines for nourishing Yin and generating blood, like Sheng Dihuang and Danggui, should also be used. In case that more heart Yin is consumed, it would be harder to astringe the mind. Hence, Wuweizi is used to help converge the vital life essence of the five internal organs, which is to converge the mind as well. In fact, Baiziren and the parched Suanzaoren also have the astringing function, however, they are not strong enough to perform the convergence, so Wuweizi has

to be used instead. Wuweizi is endowed with five different tastes, of which especially, the sour as the principal taste takes the converging effect. And then, add
Tianmendong and Maidong to nourish the lung Yin, by which the heart Yin is
nourished.

Modifications of Shengmai Yin

There is another formula hidden in the formula of **Tianwang Buxin Dan**, i.
e., Renshen (ginseng), Maidong (radix ophiopogonis), and Wuweizi (fructus
schisandrae chinensis), forming the well-known formula of **Shengmai Yin**,
which is also to nourish heart Yin. Therefore, it can be considered that **Tianwang Buxin Dan** is a formula expanded based on that of **Shengmai Yin**.

Renshen in this formula brings out Xuanshen and Danshen. And furthermore, Renshen, Fuling and Jiegeng are combined to imply the effects of **Shenling Baizhu San**. Renshen reminds us of Xuanshen, Danshen, Fuling and
Jiegeng. And then, Fuling reminds us of Yuanzhi subsequently. The whole
process of this formula composition is just like the process of friends introducing
one after another, and finally, a group of people work together to make a great a-
chievement. Maidong brings out Tianmendong, Sheng Dihuang and Danggui, all
of which are used for nourishing Yin. Wuweizi is used for the astringing purpose,
but for fear of its insufficient astringing strength, so it brings out two assistants,
i. e., Baiziren and parched Suanzaoren. Of course, in the ancient formula,
Tianwang Buxin Dan should be washed down with bamboo leaf decoction since
bamboo leaf goes into the heart meridians and helps clear the heart fire to go out
of the body with urine. This formula can be used for all the symptoms like disturbance of mind, distraction, palpitation, insomnia, fatigue, forgetfulness,
spermatorrhea in dream, heat in hands and feet, and ulceration in the mouth and
tongue, all of which arise from the excessive deficiency of heart Yin. By the way,
this formula is used under the condition that the patient has a thready rapid
pulse, which means Yin is impaired, accompanied with the pathogenic heat.

Converging Mind to Nourish the Heart Yin

The parched Suanzaoren and Baiziren can nourish heart Yin. Meanwhile, all the medicines for nourishing the heart Yin can converge the mind as well. In fact, the efficacy of Suanzaoren and Baiziren is not so powerful to nourish heart Yin directly, but only because of its slight oiliness. Their major efficacy lies in its convergence. That is to say, to converge mind is to nourish the heart Yin.

The heart is the monarch organ, so the slight oiliness of Suanzaoren and Baiziren means nothing for the monarch organ at all. The heart is like an emperor, and it receives a lot of worships. All the internal organs are serving it, so it does not need any special medicine to nourish it. But the monarch's profligacy is staggering, so the most important thing is to let it reduce its profligacy. How does the monarch heart squander its life essence? Too much energy consumption by a person will largely impair Yin and blood. So, when nourishing the heart, one has to pay much attention to the convergence of mind. Try not to let mind go beyond, or otherwise, it will cause some impairment, resulting in insomnia or palpitations. Generally, consumption of human body includes two major parts: one is the life essence of kidney, and the other is the mind. Both the heart and kidneys need converging. The life essence refers to the material level, while the mind refers to the spiritual level, or the consciousness level, both of which require converging.

第五章 养心阴药

小麦

小麦是秋天播种、冬天生长、春天茂盛、夏天收割，得一年四季之气，所以是五谷之长。它是甘凉无毒的，入心经。入药的小麦，以淮河以北产的为好，南方的就不行了，处方里通常写作"淮小麦"。

淮小麦与甘麦大枣汤

夏季属火，对应心，小麦夏天收割，是入心的，不仅养心阴，还能养胃气、益心神，消热止烦。

张仲景的甘麦大枣汤就是由这三个药组成的：小麦、甘草和大枣，主要是治疗妇人的脏躁症，脏躁症就是五脏烦躁不安，其根源在心。心有火，心阴亏虚，人就会烦躁，所以要清心火、养心阴，因此这个方子的君药就是小麦。甘草和大枣入脾经，心火生脾土，且脾为气血生化之源，补足了气血的源头，也为小麦养心阴提供了更好的条件。这个方子会很甜，甘以缓之，不仅会使身体，而且会使情绪得到舒缓。

小麦与面食

有人说，既然小麦还有养心阴的作用，那我天天吃馒头、面条不就行了吗？

这是不行的，因为馒头、面条是用小麦去皮后磨面做成的，而入药的小麦必须是整个麦粒。小麦皮是性寒的，面粉只是小麦的肉，是偏温一点。很多中药要用麦麸来炒，就是利用麦麸的寒凉之性，让温药不至于太温，药的性质就会变得平和一些。稻子跟小麦正好相反，它是糠偏温、米偏凉，所以我们吃的米是偏凉一点的。

面粉是性温的，光吃面粉就只能充饥，增加营养，和胃气，增气力，长肌肉，没有特别的药用价值。当然，如果是药，那就没法天天吃了。

浮小麦

淘洗小麦，粒子饱满的就会沉下去，不饱满的就会浮上来。把这些不饱满的小麦收集起来，就是浮小麦。它依然是养心阴的作用，且还能退虚热，止虚汗。

止汗的方中经常用到浮小麦，往往配生黄芪、龙骨等。生黄芪能益气固表，龙骨也是收涩的药。

浮小麦为什么能止汗呢？因为汗为心之液，现在心热旺盛，心液被心火扰动，所以就出汗了。浮小麦养足了心阴，就把出汗带来的损伤给修复了；它还能清心热，心热退了就再也没有火来扰动心液了，汗就不容易出。

浮小麦其实就是瘪的麦子，为什么这些小麦是瘪的呢？因为它得到的自然的赋予不够全，属于一种比较虚的状态。

到了小满的时候，麦子就需要灌浆，麦子没成熟时，把它剥开挤一下，里面就会有浆冒出来，这是麦子的精华，成熟后，里面就变硬了。浆必须灌满，才是一颗健康完整的麦子，如果没有灌满，它就处于虚的状态。但正因为它虚，才能以虚治虚。

当人体心阴虚而生火的时候，浮小麦能跟人体的状况同气相求。这又提示我们，有些药要用它的常态，有些药要用它的病态。瘪的小麦就是一种病态。小麦入药，并不是小麦越好药用价值越高。当然，你在甘麦大枣汤中可以用好小麦。瘪了的麦子，碾不出多少面粉，碾出的粉的质量也不好，所以人一般都不吃，恰好可以来做药，这就叫物尽其用。中国人最懂得物尽其用，因为中国人懂得珍惜。

病态入药举例

类似的例子还有很多。例如，蚕可以入药，但并非越健壮的蚕越好，入药的偏偏是那种自然病死的蚕，也就是白僵蚕，入药最好。

还有很多东西都是用它的病态。比如竹子被虫蛀了，流出了很多汁液，留在竹节中间，干了，就是天竺黄。

一只虫子在土里，被菌丝所侵袭，长出一棵草，这就是冬虫夏草，当然也可能是其他的虫草，如金蝉花等。有的虫子没有被菌丝侵袭，它存活下来了，只有被菌丝弄死的虫子才能成为虫草。所以虫草，也是虫子的病态。动植物的常态可以入药，病态也可以入药。

药是药，动植物是动植物，他们之间还是有区别的。比如苍术就有两种植物，入药都是香燥健脾的；旱莲草也有两种，入药都叫旱莲草，还有很多相近的植物，都是一种药名。有的则是同一种植物或动物，分常态和病态，或者分不同的时期、不同的部位，又有很多不同的名字，比如，牛角和牛黄，能一样么？所以咱们不能把中药跟动植物简单地等同起来。

柏子仁

柏子仁就是柏树的子，要弄懂柏子仁，我们先看柏树。

柏为阴木

柏字，一个木字旁，一个白。白入肺，主收敛，属阴。

一般的树，都是东、南面的树叶茂密，西、北边的树叶稀疏一些。当然这要排除在水边，在水边又不一样，在水边则是靠近水的那一面叶子稠密一些。柏树正好相反，它偏西、偏北的叶子比较稠密，偏东、偏南的比较稀少。

山的阴面，柏树长得往往非常旺盛，而阳面的柏树则长得稍微要次一点。我们去年秋天一起去北京昌平县的山上，就看到，山坡西面、北面柏树明显多一些，而东南面的柏树几乎要少一半。同理，北方的柏树长得比南方更茂盛，结子更多更饱满。总而言之，柏树它是阴木，它是喜欢阴的。

侧柏叶

柏叶也可以入药，叫侧柏叶。在人体，气为阳，血为阴，柏属阴，同气相求，所以柏叶入血分。柏树为木。为木而属血分，这意味着它入肝经。同时，因为柏树跟秋天相对应，跟西边相对应，那么它又是属金的，所以它又入肺、入大肠经，这意味着它能肃降。这就是在用五行的思维推演柏叶的性能。

五行，是中国传统学问的思维工具，抛开它，我们就没法思维了。思维要抛开成见，回到事物本身，这是西方现代哲学强调的，但思维又要有工具，没有工具，你就会变得非常笨拙。

那么，柏叶的作用是什么？柏叶主治阴不敛阳。阴不敛阳则有出血、汗症等。肺与大肠不能很好的肃降，也容易导致血中有火，导致血症。柏叶都可用到。另外，柏叶是芳香的，芳香就能化湿，所以柏叶还能化血中的湿热。叶子能透散，柏树叶能把湿热往外透散。

安神润便的柏子仁

南方也有柏树，秋天也结柏树子。柏树子最外边的壳有点像一朵花，把它剥开，里边的子就像米粒，外边还是一个硬壳，把这层硬壳再剥开，里边往往是空的，什么都没有。但北方的柏树得天时地利比较足，就不一样。我们去昌平县城后面的山上玩的时候，看到柏子我没有采，有朋友摘了些柏子，剥开里面是像米粒一样很油润的柏子。看了以后我马上明白了，天有阴阳四时差异，地也有东西南北区分。南方的柏树没有仁，北方的柏树有仁。我当时之所以不采，是因为之前在南方形成了这种思维定式，把这种思维定式带进了潜意识。其实一种东西在不同的地方，它还真的就不一样。我们每到一个地方，都要带着一种好奇心来观察，才会有收获。

柏子仁可以养心安神、润肠通便的，它为什么有这些功效呢？这又要联系到它的自然属性。仁是植物的核心所在。中药有很多用仁的，比如说核桃仁、桃仁、杏仁、柏子仁、酸枣仁。一颗小小的柏子仁，埋在土里，有了充足的条件，就能够长出一棵大树，柏树的寿命也是很长的。这意味着这颗仁里边蕴藏着生机，它蕴含的是整个树的全部信息，可见它的能量之大。

是核心就能入心，所以各种仁都或多或少的有入心的作用。柏子仁也不例外。柏子仁跟别的仁不同的是，它还有芳香，这样就更入心了。因为芳香能开窍，心有窍，它能够打开心窍。柏子仁是很油润的，能滋润，又养心，所以是一味养心阴的药。养心阴就意味着它能安神。其油润性又能润大便，对于因大便不好而睡不着的人，就更应该用柏子仁了。

但柏子仁也不能久服，如果因为睡觉不好、大便不好经常吃这个药，大便反而会变得燥结。为什么呢？这又是药的两面性。因为柏子仁是一个芳香的药，芳香就容易燥，柏子仁虽然不是太芳香，但用久了，芳香也会起作用的，因香而燥，大便也就燥了，所以柏子仁暂时用一下，它能够润大便，用得久了，反而又能使大便干燥，这是我们需要注意的。

肝气在升，肺气在降，这样才能够达成人体升降的平衡，如果只升不降，那么人就要出问题。肺苦气上逆，肺气以降为顺，肺气如果不肃降，处在肺叶之间的心就会不安宁，所以心不安宁跟肺有很大的关系。心为君主之官，肺为相辅之官，一个是皇帝，一个是宰相。要安心先得安肺，柏子仁能够促进肺的肃降，同时又能入大肠、润大便，让大便解得更快，更容易让肺火往下走，肺气下降就不会扰心，这样就有助于心的安宁，安心就是安神，所以它有养心安神的作用。我们不要以为养心安神与润肠通便是两回事，其实这些作用是一体的。《神农本草经》它讲一味药的时候，往往会把很多作用列出来，这并不是让你去套，而是让你发现这些作用之间的关系，我们要想它为什么这两个作用会在一起？它们之间会有哪些联系？这些联系，《神农本草经》并没有直接告诉你，这是书背后的东西。

酸枣仁

常与柏子仁一起用于养心阴的还有酸枣仁。

从归经看枣仁的安神作用

酸枣是北方山上的一种枣树，贫瘠的山上，越是石头多，不长别的就越容易长酸枣。酸枣仁入心、肝、胆、脾四经，味甘、酸，性平，它不寒不热、不温不凉。

入肝，它就能够安魂、收摄肝气，让肝所藏之魂安定下来。失眠多梦，往往因为肝不藏魂，酸枣仁能敛魂入肝。

入心，是酸枣仁的重头戏，它能够敛心阴。汗为心之液，出汗往往是心阴外泄，敛心阴就能收汗。睡觉时出汗，可以用点酸枣仁；睡觉时候流眼泪，也可以在辨证论治基础上加一点酸枣仁。

如果胆气虚或者胆经有虚热，也可以用酸枣仁来平息。

肝魂不安、心神不敛或者胆经虚热，都容易导致人失眠，所以酸枣仁是治疗失眠一味重要的药。

生枣仁与炒枣仁

枣仁有生熟之分，都可以入药，功效略有差异。

炒枣仁，也只是就是微微炒一下，不能炒得太过。微炒就很香了，香则入心脾，它能够收敛津液，对于心胆气虚的失眠是很有用的，所以治失眠要用炒枣仁。

生枣仁怎么用呢？一般生的东西就偏泄，它能够泄胆经的虚热。我们在前面讲过，寒能令人清，热能令人昏。有胆热的时候，人就昏昏沉沉的，贪睡，又睡不好，睡得浅容易醒，醒后还是昏昏沉沉的。失眠也分很多种情况，有的人是越失眠越清醒，头脑清醒得都可怕。还有一种失眠是昏昏沉沉的，像是睡着了又像是没有睡着，醒来又特别累，这是一种失眠。如果是火重，胆热的这种失眠，往往就是神昏倦怠，白天他想睡觉，但又睡不着，这时候用生枣仁，因为枣仁可以让人睡着，还可以治睡眠多，总之它有双向调节的作用。

酸枣仁为什么能够养心安神呢？首先我们要看一下酸枣与一般枣的区别。我们平时吃枣，买枣，都是挑选皮薄肉厚核小的。但是酸枣正好相反，它没有哪一条符合我们的要求，它皮厚肉少核大。同样是枣，为什么普通的枣和酸枣有这么大的区别呢？是大自然赋予它们的能量有多有少吗？不是这样的。大自然是很公平的，可以说它赋予每颗枣的能量是一样的，只是普通的大枣把自然界赋予它的能量放到了果肉上，所以果肉特别肥美，味甘养脾，它的核里面就没什么东西了。酸枣则把能量紧紧地藏在果核里面，所以果肉很薄很少，果核非常发达，能够养心。

在一粒枣上，我们就能够看出火生土，看出火土相生。火是果核，土是果肉。果肉发达，是因为果核没收敛多少能量，都给果肉了，这是普通的枣；酸枣呢，它的火就不生土了，它不长那么厚的果肉，一心地来发展自己，所以长成了那么好的一颗酸枣仁。普通的大枣，火已经生成土了，化作了甘美的果肉，酸枣则把这个火封藏在果核里，所以枣仁入心，供人们养心阴之用。

酸枣为什么能把天地赐予它的能量收藏在果核里面呢？这是因为它有收敛性。

收敛就能敛汗，各种虚汗可用酸枣仁来敛。它对心气虚导致的很多出汗，尤其有效。人在紧张的时候容易出汗，因为紧张实际就是心虚，汗为心之液，当心虚的时候就会出汗。人在紧张的时候出汗是正常的生理反应，当人进入病态以后，也容易这样出冷汗，这往往是因为心气虚，此时就要用酸枣仁来收敛心气心神。

归脾汤

用到酸枣仁有两个很典型的方剂：归脾汤和天王补心丹。

归脾汤：

人参、黄芪、白术、炙甘草、木香、白茯苓、远志、当归、龙眼肉、炒枣仁。

参、苓、术、草，就是四君子汤，外加一味黄芪，加大了健脾补气的力度，又加木香，醒脾健脾。脾苦湿，故用茯苓渗湿健脾，配上远志，又能交通心肾。我们在补气的同时千万不要忘了补血，气血是并行的，所以，后面紧接着加当归，当归既补气又补血，且偏于补血，此时气血都兼顾到了。后面再加龙眼肉，甘温，补脾养心。最后加炒枣仁，炒枣仁在这里就是起养心安神的作用。归脾汤一般治劳心过度、思虑伤脾，它是一个心脾两补的方子。

心火生脾土，心和脾是母子关系。要来养心，光养心是不够的，心神在这时候为什么需要养呢？是因为他的儿子不争气。思虑伤脾、劳心过度，把母子都累得够呛，所以导致身体发热困倦失眠。人要是操心过度，就会失眠而且自汗盗汗。还有很多一系列的心虚、脾虚的症状，如失眠、心悸、自汗、盗汗等，跟心虚有关。还有脾虚，吃得少，甚至是女子月经不调、白带多，这些都跟脾虚有关。凡是因为劳心过度，思虑伤脾，导致了很多症状，都可以用归脾丸。脾胃是气血生化之源，光补心阴还不行，还要把心血的源头给补足了。所以，在归脾汤里面它更注重的是补脾。

天王补心丹

天王补心丹和天王补心丸其实是一个方子。这里柏子仁和炒枣仁是一起用的。

天王补心丹：

人参、玄参、丹参、茯苓、远志、桔梗，生地，酒当归、五味子、天门冬、麦门冬、柏子仁、炒枣仁、朱砂为衣。

朱砂为衣

天王补心丹是把它做成小药丸，把朱砂飞成极细的粉末，薄薄地滚在小药丸的最表层，让药丸看起来是红的，所以叫丹。朱砂现在一定要慎用，但《神农本草经》里说它可以久服，是怎么回事呢？其实，古人讲服药，跟"衣服"的服近似，有佩戴的意思。并不是让你经常吃朱砂，而是说，一切使用朱砂的行为都是"服"，包括佩戴。比如，用一钱到三钱朱砂做一个朱砂包，放在小孩枕头下，不用吃下去，也能起到镇心安神的作用。小孩晚上的梦就会少，睡的就安稳，深睡眠的时间就会长。

邪气有的是有形的，有的则是无形的。风、寒、暑、湿、燥、火，这是有形的邪气，伤有形的肉体。自然界的一些精灵鬼怪，则侵害人的精神，这是无形的邪气。朱砂对这些无形的邪气就有镇摄作用。

朱砂是很重的，所以三钱朱砂也不多。朱砂不能内服，外用还是可以的，但如有必要，也可以内服。天王补心丹用朱砂就是内服的。像同仁堂产的天王补心丸，依然有朱砂，不要吃太多就是了。有必要的时候吃一点，它能够镇摄心神。

朱砂为衣，必须研得非常细，所以开方子写朱砂的话写成飞朱砂，就是把朱砂放到水里飞过。朱砂那么重的东西居然能够在水里面悬浮起来，说明这个朱砂已经非常非常细了。所以我们提炼朱砂的细末，常常用这个办法。没有飞起来的朱砂再继续研，继续飞。这也是药物炮制的一个工艺。

天王补心丹用药提示

因为补心先补脾，当然要用人参了，丹参和玄参是人参带出来的，它们都是参。玄参清热养肾，丹参活血化瘀。因为心阴一旦受损，心血耗散，就比较容易在体内产生瘀血，所以就要用到丹参。心阴受损，肾火也就会腾起来，所以要用到玄参。丹参入心，玄参入肾，也有交通心肾的意思。

茯苓、远志也是交通心肾的。桔梗则载药上行的。心是处在上面，用一味桔梗载药上行。用了这些味主气的药，接着再加养阴生血的生地、当归。因为心阴损耗得多，心神就不易收敛，所以用五味子来收敛五脏之精气，也是为了收敛人的神气。其实，柏子仁、炒枣仁也有收敛的作用，嫌它们收敛得不够，就加上五味子。五味子有五种味道，以酸味为主，酸就能收敛。加天冬、麦冬，它们是养肺阴的，通过养肺阴来养心阴。

生脉饮的扩充

天王补心丹中暗藏着另一个方子：人参、麦冬、五味子，这是大名鼎鼎的生麦饮，也是养心阴的。可以说，天王补心丹就是由生脉饮扩充而来的。

人参带出来玄参、丹参，而且，参苓桔梗，又有参苓白术散的意思。通过人参还带出来玄参、丹参、茯苓、桔梗，茯苓又带出来远志。这就像朋友介绍朋友来，然后一群人在一起，干成了某件事。麦冬把天冬、生地和当归也带来了，都是养阴的。五味子是收敛的，它怕自己收敛的不够，又带了两个部下，一个柏子仁，一个炒枣仁，这不全带齐了？当然在古法里面，天王补心丹要用竹叶汤来送下去，竹叶也是入心经的，能清心火从小便而出，用竹叶汤送下也是起这个作用。因为心阴过虚导致神志不安、心烦、心悸、失眠、疲惫或者健忘、梦中遗精、手脚热、口舌生疮，都可以用这个药。用这个药，脉必须是细数的，细数就意味着伤了阴而且生了热。

收摄心神方能补心阴

我们看到炒枣仁和柏子仁，它们是补心阴的，补心阴的药都能收敛心神。其实，枣仁和柏子仁直接补心阴的作用倒不是太大，只不过是有一点油润性而已，它们主要的作用在于收敛。收敛心神就是在补心阴。

心为君主之官，用得着你用那点儿枣仁、柏子仁的油润性来补吗？人家根本不稀罕。心就像皇帝一样，它受的供奉非常的多，五脏六腑都在供奉它，不稀罕你那点药，所以不需要专门用药去补它，那怎么办呢？但君主挥霍起来也是惊人的，只要让他少挥霍一点就行了。心君怎么挥霍？就是心神不收。如果一个人耗神过度，就会大量的伤阴、伤血。所以我们平时养心，就是要注意收敛心神，不要让心神外越，心神外越是很伤人的，会导致失眠、心悸。人的消耗主要有两个方面，一是肾精，一是心神，心和肾，都要收敛，精是物质层面的，神是精神层面，或者说意识层面的，都要注意收敛。

Chapter 6　Medicines for Nourishing the Spleen Yin

Shanyao (Chinese yam)

Obtaining Harmonious Qi from the Earth

Shanyao (Chinese yam), as an herb, is for nourishing the spleen Yin. In **Shennong Bencao Jing**, it is called "薯蓣" (shǔyù, means yam), and here "薯" (shǔ) is equivalent to "署"(shǔ, means "to arrange"). "蓣" (yù) here is equivalent to "预"(yù), which means "to get ready". It is read in some books that when farmers plant yam, they first poke a hole in the soil with a stick, and then put a piece of yam into it. The yam will grow to fill the pre-poked hole. In the pre-arranged space, yam can grow into the shape the farmer wants, so in such a way, yam is said to grow into a long-straight stick. I once saw in Hebei province of China some peculiar-looking yam, which may grow to stretch itself naturally without the pre-poked holes.

The top-quality yam is produced in Huaiqing, Henan Province of China. Huaiqing is a place where many good quality herbs are produced, like Huai Niuxi (achyranthes root), Huai Shudi (radix rehmanniae praeparata produced in Hua-iqing), Huai Shanyao (Chinese yam) etc. The yam produced in Huaiqing is mainly used as medical herb, which is actually little different from the yam sold in the vegetable market.

Yam going into the lungs, spleen and kidney meridians, it can nourish Yin, tonify Qi, astringe intestine to stop diarrhea, and secure the life essence, so it is a medicine for nourishing the spleen Yin. Yam grows in the earth, from where it obtains the harmonious Qi. The yam produced in Huaiqing, Henan province is regarded as the best yam since Huaiqing is located in the Central Plain, which is a very massive land with quite thick soil. Most of the people born in Henan have physically stocky build and very good physique. The yam produced in Henan has obtained the life essence of the soil, so it can nourish the spleen Yin.

Shanyao Disperses Pathogens

Yam is white in color, and it can go into the lungs, which means it is permeable and able to open hair pores to disperse the pathogens under the skin. Those who have the experience of peeling yam know that the yam mucus sticking to the back of hands will cause itches, which is just because it opens the pores and its permeability stirs up Qi and blood. In case that any other pathogenic factor exists in your hands, it may also be dispersed at the same time of itching.

There is a folk formula: first, break Chuanxiong into small pieces, then crush and mix the peeled yam and pieces of Chuanxiong together with some white sugar. The crushed mixture can be used to cure lumps in breasts. When applying it to the breasts, the patients will feel terribly itchy. After a few applications, the lumps will become smaller. Besides, some surgical pain, in case of lasting too long, might become hard and stiff, indicating that some pathogenic factors in between the skin and flesh are not dispersed, for which this folk formula may also be helpful.

This is what has been described in some books, and I think it makes some sense, but I have never tried such a formula before. Of course, as for treatment of the breast diseases or pain, there are more suitable and effective formulas for the specific symptoms, and also formulas for nursing and maintaining health.

Securing the Life Essence and Intensifying Yin

According to the *Wuxing Doctrine*, Yam is subsumed to the earth; the earth can generate metal; and the metal is then able to generate water. Therefore, yam can enter the kidneys. And in the meanwhile, it has a little astringent taste, signifying it can secure the life essence. In brief, yam is a medicine with two-way properties of dispersion and convergence.

Yam can secure the life essence, tonify the kidneys and intensify Yin. To intensify Yin is to make the astringing function of the kidneys further reinforced. Yin dominates astringency and quietness. The stronger Yin one has, the quieter he will become, and the more likely the life essence can be secured. What on the earth has stronger Yin? It is turtle. Turtle is quite inactive, and it is able to endure the loneliness, so it enjoys longevity.

Yam is an astringent produce, but never think that to eat yam can improve libido. This is not necessarily the case at all. The yam as a medical herb can secure the life essence and help abstain from sexual desire.

Do Not Take It for Granted That Shanyao Tonifies the Spleen

It is often claimed that yam can tonify the spleen. It cannot be so over-general since Baizhu and Cangzhu can also tonify the spleen. But they are different from yam. It is known that the spleen dislikes dampness. Cangzhu and Baizhu are aromatic and dry, which can tonify the spleen, remove dampness and nourish the spleen Yang, while yam is moistening, which, in fact, is to nourish the spleen Yin.

By the way, never think that yam can cure all kinds of the spleen deficiency just because it can tonify the spleen. Yam itself is sticky, and it only nourishes the spleen Yin when the endogenous dampness is heavy and the spleen is trapped by dampness; When the gastrointestinal dyspepsia arises and the coating on the tongue is thick and greasy, yam will not be suitable since the spleen itself is too weak to carry on T&T functions. Otherwise, the spleen will feel more difficult to transport and transform the sticky substance, and the dampness of yam may further trap the spleen and stomach Qi.

Moreover, some sorts of yam are also powdery after being steamed. As a matter of fact, all the lumpy root-type produces are powdery, which can cause Qi stagnation. For example, eating too much sweet potato or white potato at a meal will make one feel uncomfortable, which is mainly attributed to Qi stagnation. And the same is true for yam. Yam can tonify the spleen, signifying that yam is indeed helpful for treatment of the spleen Yin.

Examples of Uses of Shanyao

Yam can be used for those patients who have very small tongue in size with relatively dry coating on the tongue and have no phlegm. However, yam must not be used for those who have fat and big tongue marked with indents around, and thick and greasy tongue coating or slippery pulse.

Those who suffer from diabetes are particularly prone to hunger, so yam plus

Huangqi will be helpful for relieving the symptom. Diabetes is particularly easy to lead to hunger due to the spleen Yin deficiency, signifying that there is stomach heat. The endogenous heat can cause the trouble of indigestion, and therefore, the food is discharged before it is digested completely. That is why patients suffering from diabetes will be susceptible to hunger. Under such circumstances, yam will be quite good for tonifying the spleen Yin, plus Huangqi for tonifying the spleen Qi so that the spleen could become invigorated. In case that the patients have partially thin feces, Cangzhu can be added as an adjuvant medicine to resolve the dampness and tonify the spleen. This treatment may slightly alleviate the sticky property of yam.

Liuwei Dihuang Tang also contains yam. Just like tooth extraction and filling, when the dentist is going to fill a tooth in between two teeth, the teeth next to the middle one at both sides must be well secured. Dihuang tonifying the kidneys is like filling the middle tooth, and "the two teeth beside" here refer to the liver and spleen.

Shanyurou is used in the formula for astringing the liver, and yam for consolidating the spleen, and then Dihuang for tonifying the kidney Yin. In this way, the kidneys will be properly tonified and the healthy Qi can be then well converged, too.

Of course, this may not be an appropriate example, but these images can help us to remember what we are learning. Medical science is actually a very interesting learning. Those who are learning it should have curiosity and interest under all circumstances. Even in the face of a serious illness, they should also keep a very easy state of mind so that they may take everything light-heartedly rather than become panicky.

第六章　养脾阴之药

山药

得土气之冲和

山药是养脾阴的药，《神农本草经》中叫薯蓣，薯，通署，就是部署，蓣，通预，就是预备。有书上说，当地人种山药，先用木棍在土里戳一个洞，然后再放一块山药进去，山药就在这个洞里生长，正好把预先戳好的洞长满。预先部署好一个生长的空间，山药就能长成你想要的形状，所以山药都是直直的一根，据说山药就是这么长出来的。我在河北还见过长得奇形怪状的山药，可能当时没有扎木棍，让它随便长了。

山药是河南怀庆产的最好，怀庆产很多好药，比如怀牛膝、怀熟地、怀山药。怀庆府产的山药主要用来入药。而平时我们吃的山药是做菜用的，还是有一点区别的。

山药入肺、脾、肾三经，可以养阴益气、涩肠固精，是一味养脾阴的药。它长在土里，得土的冲和之气。为什么以河南怀庆府的山药最好呢？因为这里地处中原，中原是一个很厚重的地方，土气很重。你看河南人，长得都很敦实，体格特别好，不像我们太瘦。河南的山药得土气，所以能够养脾阴。

山药散邪

山药又是白色的，能入肺，入肺意味着它能透散，透散就能打开毛孔，就能把皮下一些不好的东西给散掉。有过削山药经验的朋友都知道，千万不要把山药的粘液粘到手背上，一粘到手背上就会痒，痒是因为它打开了毛孔，其透散之性动了你的气血。这时候如果你的手里还有什么毒，可能就趁着痒透散出去了。

有一个偏方，先把川芎打成细末，再把去皮的山药与川芎末一起捣碎，再加点白糖，就可以用来治疗乳房中的结块。当你把它涂上去以后就会痒，奇痒无比，你忍着，多涂几次，乳房结块就会变小。还有外科的一些疼痛，疼的太久了就很硬，一股邪气在皮肉之间散不去，也可以用这个偏方来涂。

这是书中讲的，我没有用过，不过觉得它还是有道理的。当然我们治疗各种乳腺疾病或疼痛症，还有更为对症的方法，有整体调理的方子，也非常有效。

固精强阴

山药属土，属土就能生金，金又能生水，所以它能入肾，同时又有一些涩味，涩意味着能固精。所以山药不但有透散的作用，还有固涩的作用。这又是一味药的双向作用。

山药能固精、补肾、强阴。强阴就是让肾的固涩的功能更进一步加强。阴主收敛，主静，阴越强，人就会越安静，精气就越能固。什么东西的阴最强呢？乌龟。乌龟不爱动，能耐得住寂寞，所以它很长寿。

山药是固涩之品，所以不要以为吃了它就会让性欲怎么膨胀，并没有这回事。真正用来入药的山药不是这样的，它能固精，使人容易节欲。

不能笼统认为山药健脾

人们都说，吃山药能健脾。其实不能说得这么笼统。白术、苍术不也健脾吗？但它们跟山药是两种不同的东西。脾苦湿，脾不喜欢湿，苍术、白术主要是香燥的，健脾而化湿，这是养脾阳的。山药滋润，其实是养脾阴的。

我们不能因为山药健脾，就认为只要是脾虚它都能包治。山药本身是黏黏糊糊的，它只是养脾阴，当体内多湿，脾被湿气困住了；当肠胃消化不良，舌苔比较厚比较腻的时候，用山药反而不行，因为脾本身就运化无力了，再运化这种黏黏糊糊的东西就更费力，山药的湿气又进去，会进一步把脾胃之气困住。

而且，有的山药还是有粉性的。你把它蒸熟，它就是粉粉的。一切块状根类的东西，都有粉性；凡是粉性的东西，都会滞气。比如红薯、土豆，吃多了都会不舒服，主要是因为滞气，山药也是这样。说山药能健脾，是因为它对脾阴虚确实有帮助作用。

山药的使用场合举例

如果病人舌头伸出来，很小，且舌苔也比较干，同时又没有痰，这个时候你就可以用山药；如果舌头胖大有齿痕，苔厚腻，此时千万不要用山药；如果脉滑，也不要用山药。

糖尿病人特别容易饿，如果用山药配黄芪，他就不会这么容易饿了。糖尿病之所以特别容易饿，是因为脾阴虚，脾阴虚就会有胃热，而邪热不能杀谷，所以吃的东西还没来得及很好地吸收消化，就被排掉了，所以会饿。此时山药养脾阴就是再好不过的了，再加上黄芪补益脾气，脾就振奋了。如果大便偏稀，还可以略微放一点苍术化湿健脾，这样就可以把山药黏黏糊糊的性质稍微地减轻一点，这是一个佐药。

六味地黄汤中用到山药，为什么呢？就像拔牙和补牙，补中间这颗牙的时候，边上的两颗牙你也要注意到，要把它固定好。地黄补肾，好比补中间的这颗牙，旁边那两颗牙一个是肝，一个是脾，用山萸肉把肝固涩住，再用山药把脾固住，固涩住了肝脾之气，再用地黄养肾阴，这样肾就能够得到很好的养护，正气就能得到很好的收敛。

用山萸肉把肝固涩住，再用山药把脾固住，固涩住了肝脾之气，再用地黄养肾阴，这样肾就能够得到很好的养护，正气就能得到很好的收敛。

当然这是一个不恰当的例子，我们可以这样去想，这些生动形象的东西有助于我们把知识记住，医学其实是一门很有趣的学问，我们无论在什么情况下都要带着一种好奇、快乐、有趣的心态去面对它。即使是面对一个大病，也要有一种很轻松的心态，这样就不至于慌了手脚。

Chapter 7　Medicines for Nourishing the Lung Yin

Yuzhu (Radix Polygonati Officinalis)

Yuzhu, also called "Wēi Ruí" in Chinese. It is often used as an ornamental plant in the south of China, and some people grow it in vases. Its leaves are like bamboo leaves, and the pairs of white flowers look like aeolian bells. Its root is used as medicine. The medicinal slices sold in the pharmacy are snow-white, which look quite moistening.

Yuzhu is sweet and slightly bitter in tastes and mild in property. It is neither cold nor hot, nor warm, nor cool, and it is mainly used for tonifying the spleen and moistening the lungs.

Clearing and Tonifying the Lung Yin

Yuzhu is characterized with white flowers, white roots, and moistening property that is to the lungs' preference, hence, it can moisten the lungs. Each of the five internal organs has its own preferences. The lung likes to be moistened; the kidney likes to be consolidated; the liver likes to be dispersed; the spleen likes to be properly tonified; and the heart likes to be nourished. So, each organ should be treated with different tactics, i. e. , to tonify the spleen, to moisten the lung, to consolidate the kidney, to soothe the liver and to nourish the heart. Yuzhu, white in color, can moisten the lungs. It is listed in the category of the medicines for nourishing the lung Yin.

The febrile diseases can impair Yin, especially the lung Yin. In that case, it is necessary to moisten the lung and clear the heat as well. Yuzhu is often used to nourish the lung Yin and treat the impairment of Yin due to febrile diseases.

Yuzhu has an advantage of nourishing the lung Yin but not converging the pathogens. It is a very salubrious plant, and it is not sticky as Shudi.

There are two kinds of body nourishing, i. e. , clear nourishing and turbid nourishing. The clear nourishing is just like refreshing with clear water, while the turbid nourishing is like applying fertilizer. Shudi, for example, belongs to the turbid nourishing. Although Shudi is nourishing, yet it is quite turbid, sweet in taste and sticky in property. The turtle shell is of turbid nourishing, too, or even more. And the decoction of Yuzhu is as clear water with slightly sweet taste. Besides, Lugen is also of the clear nourishing. In general, the lungs require clear nourishing, while the kidneys require turbid nourishing. Actually, at the time of Yin deficiency with pathogens, only the clear nourishing can be done. By the time when the pathogens are eliminated completely, the turbid nourishing can be started.

Application of Yuzhu to Rheumatism Treatment

According to the ancients, Yuzhu can be used for treatment of all kinds of pains including headache, osphyalgia (backache) and the symptoms of Yin deficiency accompanied with rheumatism. In addition to its efficacy of nourishing Yin deficiency, Yuzhu can also clear rheumatism.

Many pains or numbness superficially manifest the trouble of rheumatism, but in essence, such pains or numbness just arise from physical weakness or deficiency. In case of Yin deficiency, all the wind-cold damp pathogens will start their intrusion. At this moment, only dispelling the wind and dispersing the dampness may not be sufficient since the physical health conditions of the patients cannot hold the dispelling and dispersing. Now many patients instantly try to use the medicines of Wutou (aconite), Weilingxian (radix clematidis), Chuanwu (aconite root), Caowu (radix aconiti agrestis), Qianghuo (notopterygium root) and Duhuo (radix angelicae pubescentis) to search for the wind and clearing the dampness whenever they encounter rheumatism. In fact, one has to make an assessment about whether such medicines are appropriate or not. When the patient is in good health and at the very early stage of rheumatism, he can be treated in the way of searching for the pathogenic wind and clearing the dampness. But in case that the patient is too thin/weak or sick for a long time, he/she may not be able to endure such dry and severe medicines any more since he/she is not physically strong enough. Therefore, for those who mainly suffer from Yin-deficiency accompanied with various symptoms of arthralgia and rheumatism may have to

take Siwu Tang as the monarch medicine, which is to nourish blood before the treatment of arthralgia and rheumatism plus Yuzhu. This is the way of clear nourishing without impeding elimination of the pathogens. And then, on that basis, add some other medicines for searching for wind and eliminating dampness.

But Yuzhu is slow in nature, and it cannot be obviously effective for use only once or twice, which means it has to be used in a long term. Slowness in nature does not mean it is bad. The chronic diseases require treating with slow-featured medicines while the acute diseases require treating with quick-featured medicines.

Shashen (Radix Adenophorae)

Shashen is divided into the south Shashen and north Shashen. The former one is thick and big in size with fluffy texture and is partial to clearing heat, while the latter one is dense in texture and is partial to nourishing Yin. They are the different plants, but similar in nature.

Shashen is white in color, sometimes also called Baishen. According to the Chinese herbal medicine incompatibility principle, "Lilu (veratrum nigrum) is incompatible with Renshen (ginseng), Shashen (radix adenophorae), Danshen (radix salviae miltiorrhizae), Xuanshen (radix scrophulariae), Kushen (radix sophorae flavescentis), Xixin (asarum), Chishao (radix paeoniae rubra) and Baishao (radix paeoniae alba)". so Shashen cannot be used together with Lilu. By the way, Shashen is a clear medicine, and it is white in color, entering into the lungs. It is also slightly bitter with descending effect, corresponding to the fact that the lungs dominate purifying and descending. The fire is supposed to go downwards, and Shashen assists the lungs for purifying and descending. In fact, it is helping lungs to purge Qi downwards, that is, Shashen helps the lungs discharge the pathogenic fire. If the lungs Qi ascends in a counterflow, the pathogenic fire will reverse upwards, too. Shashen can be used for discharging the pathogenic fire and moistening the lungs. Shashen as a nourishing medicine gives the kidney exactly what it wants in many respects.

Moistening the Lungs to Relieve Cough

In the treatment of diseases related to the lungs, Shashen is often used for relieving a cough arising from Yin deficiency.

Cough may arise from many reasons, which are usually narrowed down to the unsmooth lung Qi or lung Qi reversing upwards. When the lung Qi is not smooth, it will reverse upwards, and consequently, the lung fire will also become stronger, resulting in cough. Shashen can be used to moisten the lungs to relieve cough.

Of course, it is not only Shashen that is used, but also Baibu (radix stemonae), which is also a common medicine for relieving cough. Regardless of the cold cough or hot cough, Baibu steamed or parched with honey can be effective for both of them. Kuandonghua (flos farfarae) and Qianhu (radix peucedani) may also be added, of which Kuandonghua is for warming the lungs, i. e., to warm up the healthy factors of the lungs, while Qianhu is for clearing the lungs, i. e., to clear the pathogenic factors. Hence, with the help of warming and clearing treatments, the cough will then come to a stop. Besides, Sangye (mulberry leaf) and Pipaye (loquat leaf) may also be used. Sangye is for ascending while Pipaye is for descending, which will then be able to straighten out the lungs Qi. What's more, Jiegeng (platycodon grandiflorum) and Xingren (apricot kernel) are effective, too. Jiegeng is for ascending while Xingren is for purifying and descending, which is also straightening out the lung Qi.

The pairs of herbs mentioned above are all for curing cough. It should be noted that the herbal pairs of Baibu and Shashen, Sangye and Pipaye, Qianhu and Kuandonghua, Jiegeng and Xingren are all frequently used.

In case that there is deficiency heat in lungs, one has to consider to use Sangbaipi (cortex mori) and the like. Of course, in the case of much phlegm, Shashen will not be suitable, since Shashen is for nourishing the lung Yin. Otherwise, the more the lung is nourished, the more phlegm there will be since the fluid to be replenished through nourishing will form phlegm again when it circulates inside. Shashen is generally used for treatment of cough arising from Yin deficiency of the lung.

Shashen for Treatment of the Intestinal Bleeding

Shashen can also be used for treatment of intestinal bleeding.

How come the intestine bleeding arises? The lung and the large intestine are mutually related for the exterior and interior. When the lung suffers from heat, the large intestine will also have heat consequently. The heat can impair Yin collaterals. And then, the blood heat will descend, causing the intestinal bleeding. Therefore, the lung should be moistened first in order to eliminate the heat from its source, after which the large intestinal bleeding will be relieved gradually. Of course, only Shashen may not be enough for treatment of this disease, and some special herbs like Diyu (sanguisorba officinalis) and Huaijiao (fructus sophorae) and the like are also needed.

Consideration of Both Nourishing and Moistening the Lungs

Shashen is for nourishing the lung Yin that is a very important nourishing treatment for the five internal organs. All the nourishing, whatever it is, must give consideration to the lung moistening as well since the lungs are subsumed to metal which generates water/fluid (according to **Wuixng Doctrine**). All the fluid in human body comes from the lungs. **Huangdi Neijing** says, "all food taken will go into the stomach", which means that after the food in the stomach is ground and digested, the spleen will dominate to ascend the clear in order to transport the food essence (the refined nutritious substances) to the lungs. The lungs are connected to all vessels. All the essential substances of food are transported to all the vital organs and each part of the whole body through close collaboration among the liver, heart, spleen, lungs and kidneys in parallel in order to carry on the metabolism.

The lungs are like the canopy over an imperial carriage. It is located at the highest point in the body among the five internal organs, corresponding to the sky in the divinatory symbols. When the lungs start to "rain", the human body will get moistened. Just as rain can moisten the whole nature. So, for nourishing Yin, one has to nourish the lung Yin so that sufficient water/fluid can be formed, which then guarantees the lung has sufficient Yin to "rain" water/fluid over the whole body. In fact, the lung not only generates the kidney fluid, but also generates fluid for the whole body. That is why it is necessary to nourish the lung Yin first before nourishing Yin of the five internal organs.

It is relatively dry in the north of China, so the medicines for nourishing Yin and moistening dryness like Shashen, Maidong and Lugen etc. are frequently and largely used, especially in the northwestern areas. In the past, the four famous doctors in Beijing like *Xiao Longyou*, *Kong Bohua* and so on had always used Shashen and Maidong in an extremely large dosage.

Therefore, for nourishing Yin of any organs, the first thing to do is to nourish the lung Yin, which is the knack of nourishing Yin. There is a saying in TCM: "It is easier to get a thousand formulas, but it is harder to get a knack. " A lot of TCM learners try to learn from the experienced herbalist doctors by copying formulas or prescriptions, which in fact, is a very silly way to learn TCM. They finally found their copy work useless since they could get thousands of formulas or prescriptions from books like *Compendium of Materia Medica* or *Prescriptions for Universal Relief*, but they are still unable to make diagnoses of diseases for patients.

The importance of formulas or prescriptions does not depend upon the number, but upon how to make the best use of them. If a doctor can make good use of formulas, a few effective formulas probably can help him survive. Otherwise, he may fail to survive even he has got a large number of formulas. And therefore, whenever one tries to learn from the experienced doctors, he or she should try the utmost to learn the knacks embedded in the formulas.

For example, **Liuwei Dihuang Tang,** after Maidong and Wuweizi added on the basis of its formula, can then go into the lungs to open the fluid source, and become more powerful for tonifying the kidneys. Similarly, the efficacy of **Siwu Tang** for nourishing blood may be doubled after Shashen and Maidong are added on the basis of its formula.

Substitution of Shashen for American Ginseng

Shashen is very cheap, but it has a very powerful efficacy, and sometimes it can even play the function of American ginseng. In many cases, Shashen is used to substitute for American ginseng since American ginseng, sweet and cold in properties, has the similar efficacy to Shashen for moistening lungs.

American ginseng and Renshen are put in the same category, and in many books American ginseng is listed in the same group as Shashen. Genseng is slightly warm in nature, especially the human planted Renshen, with the property of fire in it, so it is not that cool and moistening. Renshen used in all of Zhang Zhongjing's formulas is actually quite cool and moistening, which is said to be the ginseng produced in Shangdang, Shanxi province of China. And also, it is said the ginseng used by Zhang Zhongjing has been extinct, or it was equivalent to the American ginseng, or it was equivalent to Shashen. Anyway, there are many different opinions, but in fact, it depends upon the herbal quality and change of time.

In the case of the lung heat, unless Renshen or American ginseng is a must, Shashen can be used instead since it not only has the same efficacy as Renshen to nourish Qi and Yin and clear the lung heat as well, but also it is similar to American ginseng. The mere difference between Shashen and American ginseng is that the former one has less potency of nourishing Qi. For instance, in **Shengmai Yin**, Shashen can substitute for American ginseng.

Shengmai Yin is a commonly used in summer, and in the formula, Maidong can nourish the lung Yin, and Wuweizi can astringe the lung Qi. However, in case the lung heat arises, American ginseng would be better, but Dangshen can be a choice as well.

Shashen for Curing Pulmonary Tuberculosis

Shashen is also used frequently in the treatment of tuberculosis, and usually used together with Baibu. Western medicine also proves that Shashen has the function of killing mycobacterium tuberculosis that TCM would not describe in such a way.

Baibu is pesticidal herb, too. The domestic cats and dogs who suffer from parasites on the body can be bathed frequently with Baibu (30g) decoction, which can help to get grid of or guard against parasites. Similarly, children who suffer from lice in hair may also use Baibu decoction to wash. Those who have very particular demand, if any, can also add some Sangye (mulberry leaf) and

Juhua (chrysanthemum). By the way, Baibu is effective for all kinds of cough. Those who suffer from cough are susceptible to pneumonia because of bacterial infection. Baibu enjoys the pesticidal function, which means it can sterilize all kinds of bacteria.

In the past, a lot of consumptive diseases were regarded as tuberculosis, or called as pulmonary tuberculosis. Those patients who suffer from pulmonary tuberculosis often have a short and soft cough, which is even more terrible, signifying there is lung fire coming up to fume the lungs, so the patients will feel itchy at throat, then causing cough. Such cough can eventually make the patient lose his vital life essence and remain in low spirits. The cough with phlegm is much easier to treat, but on the contrary, the cough due to deficiency fire is much harder to treat since it is often related to the state of mind, the liver and kidneys. Therefore, the patients who suffer from pulmonary tuberculosis need to rest for recuperation at ease. As to treatment, use the clear nourishing medicines like Shashen (radix adenophorae), Tianmendong (asparagus cochinchinensis), Maidong (radix ophiopogonis), Baibu (radix stemonae), Wuweizi (fructus schisandrae chinensis) and Sangbaipi (cortex mori). Sangbaipi is for clearing deficiency heat in the lungs; Wuweizi is for converging the lung Qi; and Baibu is for relieving a cough and sterilizing the mycobacterium tuberculosis. Tianmendong, Maidong and Shashen are for moistening the lung.

As a matter of fact, medication is not the only solution to all problems. The patients need to be quiet for recuperation, have a pleasant state of mind, relax themselves, and keep away from anger and resentment. Or otherwise, it would be harder for them to recover since the liver is subsumed to wood, and wood generates fire, and fire restrains metal. Those who get angry will start coughing since wood-fire impairs the metal (i. e. , the liver-fire is attacking lungs). When the liver fire suddenly runs up, the irritated person will start coughing, which is called the irritated cough. Such a case would be a disaster for the patients who suffer from pulmonary tuberculosis.

Shashen for Curing Chronic Cough

Shashen is often used for treatment of long-lasting chronic cough arising from unknown reasons or mixed reasons. TCM doctors often use Chuan Beimu (Bulbus fritillariae cirrhosae), Pipaye (loquat leaves), Tianhua Fen (radices trichosan-this), Gancao (liquorice), Sangbaipi (cortex mori), Baibu (radix stemonae), Tianmendong (asparagus cochinchinensis), Kuandonghua (flos farfarae) and Shashen (radix adenophorae) for the treatment of chronic cough.

In principle, cough can impair the lung if it lasts long time. Meanwhile, the impairment mainly takes place to the lung Yin, for the lung likes moistening. Therefore, those who suffer from a long-lasting cough must nourish the lung Yin first with herbs of Shashen, Tianmendong and Maidong. In case that the cough lasts long, there surely exists deficiency fire in the lung, so Sangbaipi shall have to be used to clear it. The long-lasting cough may also cause some cold-heat com-plication, so, Kuandonghua is used here to warm the lung Yang; and Sangbaipi is used to purge lungs of the deficiency fire. At the same time, the long-lasting cough may also result in phlegm in the lung, which may be reduced with Beimu (fritillaria). Beimu is divided into Zhe Beimu (thunberg fritillary bulb) and Chuan Beimu (bulbus fritillariae cirrhosae). Chuan Beimucan moisten the lung and reduce phlegm, and Zhe Beimu is more powerful for resolving phlegm, so they can be used according to the specific symptoms. For example, for the physi-cally weak patients who suffer from a long-lasting cough and impairment of the lungs, Chuan Beimu is used to moisten the lung and reduce the phlegm; for the physically strong patients who suffer from a long-lasting cough and have more thick phlegm, Zhe Beimu is used to reinforce the phlegm resolving effect. The lung likes purifying and descending, and dislikes Qi reversal upwards, so Pipaye is used to descend the lung Qi. Tianhua Fen is also used for resolving the phlegm, and Baibu for relieving cough simultaneously.

Contraindications of Shashen

Never use Shashen for the patients who catch a cold, especially, at the early stage of a cold.

At the time of a cold, the exogenous pathogens attack the body surface. The exterior symptoms have to be eliminated in the first place rather than in a rush to tonify the lungs. Exogenous pathogens on the body surface will cause trouble to the lung Qi, resulting in phlegm formation and coughing. In that case, if Shashen is abused due to coughing, the lung Yin to be nourished will be fully transformed into phlegm to obstruct the flow of the lung Qi, causing chest distress, more phlegm and even pulmonary edema.

Also, in the case of thick and greasy tongue coating, Shashen should also be used with caution since the thick and greasy tongue coating indicates that there is serious phlegm and turbidity in the body, which may arise from improper function of the spleen and lung Qi. In that case, stop tonifying the lung. Otherwise, the more one tonifies the lung, the worse he or she will feel.

Also, if the patient feels distressed in chest, stop using Shashen immediately.

Shashen is a common medicine. People in the modern society often suffer from Yin deficiency, so Shashen is very frequently used because of the dry climatic conditions. But in fact, the southerners in China also use Shashen frequently since the southerners sweat a lot. And in the meantime, most of the southerners are physically thin, and are susceptible to Yin deficiency, hence, they need to tonify Yin of the five internal organs, for which the lung Yin needs tonifying first. That is why Shashen will have to be used.

第七章　养肺阴之药

玉竹

玉竹，又叫葳蕤。在南方经常作为观赏植物，有些人家会种在花盆里。它的叶子有些像竹叶，一对一对的小白花开得像风铃，很清俊的样子。入药取根部。在药店里看到的饮片是雪白的一片一片，有种很滋润的感觉。

玉竹性味甘、微苦，是平性的，它不寒不热、不温不凉，主要用作补脾和润肺。

清补肺阴

玉竹开的是白花，根也是白的，很润，肺喜欢润，所以它能润肺。五脏各有喜好，肺喜润；肾喜固；肝喜疏散；脾喜健运；心喜养。五脏各有其喜好，所以对待每一脏的政策都不一样，健脾、润肺、固肾、疏肝、养心。玉竹色白润肺，所以我们把它放在养肺阴的药里边。

我们知道，热病会伤阴，尤其是伤肺阴。此时应该怎么办？要润肺，还要清热。玉竹经常用来补肺阴，用来治疗热病伤阴。

用玉竹有一个好处，它在补肺阴的同时又不收敛邪气。玉竹是一种非常清爽的植物，不像熟地那样粘糊糊的。

人体的滋补有清浊之分，就是清补和浊补，清补就好比浇清水，浊补就好比施肥。比如熟地就是浊补的，虽然滋养，但是它很浊，味道很甜，粘糊糊的；龟板更浊。而我们单用玉竹熬出来的汤就跟水一样，略微有一点甜味，它很清；还有芦根也是清补的。一般来说补肺的药都是清补，补肾则要浊补。阴虚有邪的时候只能清补，待到无邪气方能浊补。

玉竹在风湿病中的应用

古人讲，凡是遇到头痛、腰痛，阴虚又有风湿的病症，就可以用玉竹。玉竹除了补虚，还能清风湿。

很多身体痹痛，表面上是风湿之邪在作怪，本质上是人体虚了，阴虚则风寒湿邪入侵，你能只祛风散湿吗？人体这时候是没有这个本钱祛风散湿的。现在很多人一遇到风湿，马上就用乌头、威灵仙、川乌、草乌、羌活、独活这些搜风散湿的药。但是我们要先看看这个病人是不是适合用这些药，如果病人身体很好，病又是初犯，你可以这样来给他搜风散湿。但是如果这个病人已经瘦得不成样子了，或是病了很久，再用这些燥烈的药就不行了，因为他已经没有这个本钱了。所以，如果遇到以阴虚为本，同时又有风湿等各种痹症的病人，方中往往就要用四物汤为君，治风先治血，加上玉竹，清养而不妨碍驱邪，在此基础上稍加搜风散湿之药。

但是玉竹的性质是非常的缓慢的，如果只用一次两次，根本一点感觉都没有，所以要久用。性缓就不好吗？也不是。性缓有性缓的用处，缓病就要用性缓的药，急病就要用性急的药。

沙参

沙参有南沙参和北沙参之分，南沙参粗大，质地蓬松，偏于清热；北沙参质地致密，偏于养阴。南北沙参是两种不同的植物，但性质相似，所以放在一起来论。

沙参是白色的有时候也叫白参，也属于五参的一种。"诸参辛芍叛藜芦"，所以它跟藜芦不能在一块用。沙参是一个很清的药，色白能入肺；又因为它微苦，苦就能降，正好跟肺主肃降相应了。火应该是往下走的，沙参助肺气肃降，其实就是在帮助肺泻火。肺气上逆，火就会上逆，沙参是肃降肺气的，所以就可以泻火。肺是喜欢滋润的，沙参正好也是一味比较滋润的药。沙参在各个方面都投合了肺的喜好，所以是养肺之品。

润肺止咳

治肺的时候会经常用到沙参，比如阴虚咳嗽。

人为什么会咳嗽？原因有很多，无论是什么原因，都会归结为肺气不顺或者肺气上逆。肺不润，肺气就会上逆，肺火也会大，人就会咳嗽。可以用沙参来润肺止咳。

当然不止用沙参一味药，还可以用百部，这也是止咳最常用的一味药，不管是寒咳、热咳，都可以用百部，可以用蒸的百部，还可以用蜜炙百部。还可以加款冬花和前胡，款冬是温肺的，前胡是清肺的，温肺是温了肺的正气，清肺是清了肺的邪气，一温一清，咳嗽就止住了。还可以加桑叶、枇杷叶，桑叶是升的，琵琶叶是降的，一升一降就能够理顺肺的气机；又可以用桔梗和杏仁，桔梗是升提的，杏仁是肃降的，一升一降也是在理顺肺气。

上面是治疗咳嗽的几对药，需要我们记住。百部配沙参，桑叶配枇杷叶，前胡配款冬花，桔梗配杏仁，这些都是经常用的。

如果肺里面有虚热，咱们还得考虑到桑白皮之类的。当然如果痰非常多，就不宜用沙参了，因为沙参是养肺阴的，补进去那么多水，又得到很好的流通，就成了痰饮，那就越补痰越多了，所以沙参一般用于肺阴虚的咳嗽。

治肠红下血

沙参还能治肠红下血。肠红是一个很委婉的说法，其实就是下血。

为什么会下血呢？因为肺跟大肠相表里，当肺有热的时候，大肠也会跟着有热，热伤阴络，血热下行就会导致肠红出血。我们先润肺，从源头上把热清掉，把肺润好，这样大肠下血也就会慢慢变少。当然治这个病也不止沙参一味药，治疗这类病还有一些特别的药，比如地榆、槐角之类。

滋补必兼顾润肺

沙参是养肺阴的，养肺阴在养五脏之阴当中是非常重要的。一切滋补都要兼顾到滋补肺，因为肺属金，金生水，人体的水液是由肺这里来的。《黄帝内经》讲"饮食入胃"，吃喝到了胃里，经过消磨，脾主升清，把食物的水谷之精微转输到肺，肺朝百脉，水精四布，五经并行，使津液最终由肺输布到五脏六腑四肢百骸，输布到人的全身。

肺为华盖，在五脏最高处，相当于天，对应的卦也是干卦。肺要下雨，人体才能得到滋润，就象天下雨整个自然界才能得到滋润一样，所以我们如果要想养阴，就得先养肺阴，要让天上有足够多的水，让肺阴足够把雨降下来，降到全身。肺金生肾水，其实它不仅是生肾水，它能生全身之水，所以补五脏之阴，就要先补肺阴。

北方比较干燥，像沙参、麦冬、芦根等这些养阴润燥的药就会经常用、大量地用。尤其是西北用得会更多。过去京城有萧龙友、孔伯华等四大名医，他们沙参、麦冬用得就特别多。

所以，一切养阴，不管养哪一脏之阴，首先要先养肺阴，这是养阴的一个要诀。中医经常是"千方易得，一诀难求"。很多人去跟老中医学习，其实都是在傻傻的抄方子。抄那么多方子，一点用都没有。任何一本书中都有很多方子，买一套《本草纲目》或者《普济方》几万个方子你都有了，但你可能依然不会看病。方子不在于多，而在于怎么去运用，你会运用，可能几个方子就能打天下，不会用，抄的再多也没有用。方子很容易得到，而方子里面的诀窍就很难得到了，所以千方易得，一诀难求，方子里面体现了诀，别人不告诉你，你永远不知道这个诀是什么。

方子不在于多，而在于怎么去运用，你会运用，可能几个方子就能打天下，不会用，抄的再多也没有用。方子很容易得到，而方子里面的诀窍就很难得到了，所以千方易得，一诀难求，方子里面体现了诀，别人不告诉你，你永远不知道这个诀是什么。

例如，在六味地黄汤的基础上加麦冬、五味子，就是入肺的，开启了水之上源，其补肾的作用就会更加强。我们还经常在四物汤的基础上加沙参、麦冬，也会使养血效果倍增。

沙参代替西洋参

沙参是很便宜的药，但是它的作用非常大，有时候甚至会有西洋参的作用，在很多场合替代西洋参。因为西洋参也是甘寒润肺的。

西洋参和人参是一类的，但是它在很多书里跟沙参列在一起。人参略微的带一点温性，尤其是现在人工种植的人参，都有一股火性在里面，不是那么凉润。张仲景方子里的人参都是很凉润的，有人说是山西上党的人参，有人说张仲景当年用的那种人参现在已经绝种了，还有人说那就相当于现在的西洋参，还有人说相当于现在的沙参，各家的说法不一样，这也取决于它们用药的质量，取决于它们的时代。

在有肺热的时候，只要不是非要用人参或西洋参不可，就可以不用，我们可以用沙参来代替。沙参有参的作用，能够养气阴，还能够清肺热，跟西洋参很相近，只不过补气的力度小一些而已。比如，我们在生脉饮里都可以用沙参来代替西洋参。

生脉饮是夏天常用的方剂，麦冬养肺阴，五味子收敛肺气，如果有肺热的话可以用沙参，如果没有肺热，则用西洋参比较好，用党参也可以。

用于肺痨

　　沙参还经常用在治疗结核病，一般跟百部相配伍。西医也发现沙参有杀灭结核杆菌的作用，当然我们中医不这么说。

　　百部也是一味杀虫的药，如果家里养的小猫小狗身上长了虫子，可以每次用三十克百部，熬一锅水给小动物洗洗澡，它身上的虫子就没有了，以后经常这样洗洗，也不容易生虫子。有的小孩子头上长虱子，也可以用百部熬水洗头，要是讲究，还可以在里面加点桑叶、菊花。为什么百部不管什么咳嗽都可以用呢？因为人老咳就容易咳出肺炎来，为什么会咳出肺炎来？因为有细菌感染了。百部能杀虫，这也意味着它能杀灭各种细菌。

　　过去有很多虚劳就属于肺结核，也叫肺痨，这种病人往往发出短促而轻声的咳嗽，这样咳反而很可怕。这意味着有一股游丝一样的肺火一直往上来熏你的肺，你的喉咙就会感到痒，所以就会这样咳。这种咳嗽最后能咳得人精气神都没有了。如果咳嗽有痰，反而好治。难治的是虚火咳嗽，因为它往往跟心情有关，跟肝肾有关。所以这种肺痨的病人需要安心静养，用药一般就是用这些清养的药，比如沙参、天冬、麦冬、百部、五味子、桑白皮。桑白皮也是用来清肺里的虚热，五味子是敛肺气的，百部能够止咳，还能杀灭结核杆菌。天冬、麦冬、沙参是来润肺的。

　　当然光用药是不行的，还得让病人安心静养，心情愉悦，身心轻松，不要发怒、不要窝火、不要憋气。不然的话肝属木，木生火，火克金，这样就不行。人有时候一生气一着急就咳嗽，这就是木火刑金，肝火腾地一下子就上来了，人就得咳嗽，我们通常说这种人是被气得咳嗽。这种情况，对于肺痨患者来说，简直是灾难。

用于慢性咳嗽

　　沙参还经常用于治疗慢性的咳嗽。这种咳嗽就是时间长，不明原因，可能什么原因都有的咳嗽。我们经常用川贝、枇杷叶、花粉、甘草、桑白皮、百部、天冬、款冬花、沙参这些药来治疗。

　　究其原理，咳嗽的时间一长就会伤肺，伤肺主要伤的是肺阴，肺喜欢润，所以咳得久了，我们首先要补肺阴，那么沙参、天冬、麦冬肯定是要用的。咳嗽久了，肺里面肯定会有虚火，所以用桑白皮去清肺其虚火。咳嗽久了，肺里面可能会寒热夹杂，所以用款冬花来温肺的阳气，用桑白皮来泻肺的虚火。同时，咳了那么久，肺里面肯定有痰，用贝母来化痰。贝母分浙贝母和川贝母，川贝母能润肺化痰，浙贝母化痰的力度大一些，可根据具体的情况来用。比如病人瘦瘦的，咳得又久，肺又受了伤，就用川贝来润肺化痰；如果病人身体比较强壮，虽然咳得也久，但依然很强悍，浓痰多，那可以用浙贝母，加大化痰的力度。肺是喜欢肃降的，肺苦气上逆，所以用枇杷叶来降肺气。花粉也是可以化痰的，同时加百部来止咳。

沙参的使用禁忌

沙参在感冒的时候要禁用，尤其是刚感冒，千万不要用沙参。

因为感冒的时候，外邪侵犯人的体表，有表症首先要解表，不要急于去补肺。外邪犯表会导致肺气不利，肺气不利就容易生痰、容易导致咳嗽。这时候如果你见到咳嗽就滥用沙参，补很多肺阴进去，会全部变成痰，痰浊大起，很快就把肺堵住了，出现胸闷、痰多，甚至肺积水等。

还有，舌苔厚腻的时候也要慎用沙参。舌苔厚腻，意味着体内痰浊比较重，痰浊重又是因为脾和肺的气机不顺畅。这样的情况下，就不要过于补肺了，因为越补越不行。

还有，如果感觉到胸闷，也不要吃沙参了。

沙参是一味常用药，在现代人普遍阴虚的情况下，沙参会用得很多。北方用的更多，因为气候干燥。其实南方也还是会经常用，因为南方人出汗多，而且南方人瘦，容易阴虚，需要补五脏之阴，补五脏之阴就要补肺阴，沙参肯定就要用到。

Chapter 8   Animal Medicines for Nourishing Yin

Honey

Quintessence of flowers, Mild, Sweet and Moistening

Honey is produced by bees. Honey bees include drones, queen bees, and worker bees. The drones are black in color and big in size. The drones are only responsible for copulating with the queen bees, after which they will die. Some drones may not die after mating, but they are just flying around idly, and finally they are often expelled by the worker bees. The worker bee is neither a drone nor a queen bee, but neutral without gender difference or sexual desire. Worker bees collect nectar from flowers to produce honey, indicating that honey is also neutral and mild in properties.

Bees are living in a large swarm in order, and even if they are disturbed for a while, they will restore their order very quickly as they used to be, indicating that they can keep harmonious. The honey brewed by such a creature can also make the vital organs of human body in order. So, honey can harmonize the five internal organs, appease the six hollow organs, and reconcile Qi, blood, Ying and Wei systems in the human body.

Honey is brewed from the quintessence of various flowers by worker bees. In spring, there is harmonious and vital Qi in between the sky and the earth, as it is written by *Fan Zhongyan*, an outstanding thinker and litterateur in *Song* dynasty in his work ***Notes of the Yueyang Tower***: "Spring warms the air, and the sun is clearly shining". Harmony is the precondition of vigorous growth. Without harmonious environment, there will be no growth/development. Spring is a harmonious season, in which the harmonious energy is clearly and sufficiently reflected in the plants whose quintessence is converged in flowers. And then, the quintessence of flowers is in the Huafen (pollen), from which the worker bees collect and store the spring harmonious and growing energy into honey.

In supermarkets, many different kinds of honey are available, like the so-called Huaihuami (flos sophorae honey), Juhuami (chrysanthemum honey),

Youcaihuami (rape flower honey) etc. As a matter of fact, these are just terms made by businesses, which finally overreach themselves. How is it possible that the worker bees only fly to certain flowers to collect Huafen (pollen) for brewing · particular honey. If it is really true, the honey brewed in such a way might not be that good. Only the honey with the quintessence of hundreds of flowers converged and brewed together can make the pure and essential substance that contains the vital life essence. Honey is the top-grade stuff that is highly praised by the ancients for maintaining good health.

Honey goes into the channels of the heart, spleen, lung, stomach, and the large intestine. It is aromatic in scent, signifying that it can open the orifices; and it is sweet in taste, signifying that it can also go into the spleen and the heart channel of Hand Shaoyin. Flowers dominate dispersion, suggesting that honey also has the dispersing function. Generally speaking, the sweet food usually stays in the spleen and stomach, for instance, the Chinese date may stay in the Middle Jiao and cause stagnation. But the honey is an exception that it enjoys both activating and dispersing effects though it is sweet. After getting into the spleen, it can easily promote transportation of the vital life essence to lungs.

Functions of Honey

The raw honey, also called whitish honey, is white in color, going into the lungs and causing mild laxation. Many people like to eat honey for treatment of constipation. Honey does have certain effect in this aspect. It can harmonize Ying and Wei systems, moisten the vital organs of human body and clear heat. Compared with the raw honey, the refined and processed honey is more powerful in its potency for tonifying the spleen and stomach, but will lose its efficacy for clearing heat since it has changed to be warm in property after being processed. For medical use, Choice of either the raw honey or the processed honey depends on the specific cases and symptoms.

Honey can relieve pain. Pain often arises from acuteness or urgency, that is, some parts of the body are not quite relaxed. Acuteness or urgency will result in obstruction, causing pains, which can be alleviated with sweet taste, that is, relax the functions of the body so as to relieve the pains.

Honey can also eliminate toxins. Many Chinese medicines are processed with honey, such as, Baibu (radix stemonae), it is processed with honey. Fuzi (radix aconiti carmichaeli), in case of being misused, can cause botulism, which could be detoxicated with honey. Honey is similar to Gancao (liquorice) in many respects, and it can reconcile hundreds of medicines. Therefore, honey is frequently used to make patented medicine pills, i. e., honeyed pills, in which honey not only acts as a binder, but also plays a reconciling role to form the pills of integrated harmony. The ancients called the pill ("丸", Wan in Pinyin) as "roundness" ("圆", Yuan in Pinyin). It is round in shape, and harmonious integration in medicinal efficacy.

Honey can moisten stool. *Zhang Zhongjing* in the section of Yangming Diseases of his book **Shanghan Lun** recorded a formula called **Mijian Dao** (Honey Decoction Guideline), which is to put honey in a copper ware and refine on the fire to a certain level of heat, and rub the refined honey into a honey strip while it is hot. Then cool it to a warm state and plug it into anus for treatment of constipation arising from Yin deficiency and large intestine dryness.

Contraindications of Honey

Those who suffer from the spleen and stomach deficiency or the kidney Qi deficiency should not eat honey since they always have loose bowels, suffering from diarrhea or semifluid feces many times a day due to the spleen and stomach deficiency, failure of astringency and the kidney Qi deficiency slipping. By the way, the kidney deficiency can result in down-slipping of stool, leucorrhea and seminal fluid, which is called the kidney Qi deficiency slipping. Those who suffer from these symptoms should stop eating honey.

Those ladies who suffer from more leucorrhea should not eat honey, either. Some ladies who suffer from more leucorrhea, serious impairment of Yin and dry stool should not eat honey either, or otherwise, the more honey they eat for treating their dry stool, the more leucorrhea they may suffer from, and the drier the stool will become, which makes a vicious circle. In addition, those who suffer from more phlegm should be cautious about eating honey, too.

Guiban (Turtleshell)

Natural Thinking and Institutional Thinking

Once I saw a faucet in the community was running to water the lawn in a raining day while the worker was standing beside. I asked: "It is raining. Why do you still keep on watering here?" The worker looked up at me, and said it was a rule. And then, he went on his watering work.

Different people follow the different ways to think. Some people follow the nature, which is called natural thinking, while some other people follow the rules, which is called institutional thinking. These are two different ways of thinking. Those who keep closer to the nature will have more natural thinking; Those who keep closer to the rules will have more institutional thinking. Those excellent doctors, regardless of Chinese medical doctors or western medical doctors, are particularly following the natural thinking, that is, to follow the principles and the way of nature to give treatment flexibly according to specific symptoms rather than to follow the stereotyped rules and regulations.

The quack doctors follow the institutional thinking more, and they always do what the books say. TCM should follow the natural thinking completely. If one throws away the law of nature and just sticks to some classic formulas, he or she would be the same as the above-mentioned watering man who switches from natural thinking to the institutional thinking.

Therefore, those who come from farmland have more frequent contact with the nature and have primitive and living experience usually will follow the natural law with natural thinking way to handle problems; on the contrary, those who were born in families of the public officers will have chances to face the interpersonal relationship, some rules and regulations and power tactics, so they will strongly follow the institutional thinking more, and handle affairs according to regulations.

But some people may challenge me, "What do you think about the saying ' The poor family brings up a prime minister, and the thatched cottage can also shelter a senior officer'". In fact, this involves their experiences in their childhood, but also their natural thinking since the natural thinking is alive, flexible, and even wild with great vitality. Those who follow the natural thinking can undertake the great events and achieve great success as well.

TCM puts much stress on the natural thinking, experiences Yin and Yang, and observe all things on earth based upon the natural thinking way. Here are some animal medicines like Guiban (turtleshell) and E-jiao (donkey-hide gelatin). They are flesh and blood stuff. As medicines, they can be used for tonifying Yin. However, how to use and when to use such tonics should be weighed on the basis of the natural thinking.

Renmai (Renmai Channel) And Dumai (Governor Meridian)

A lot of medicines have been discussed for tonifying Yin, like Sheng Dihuang, Shudi, Tianmendong, Maidong and the like, all of which are herbal medicines. When the human body suffers from the loss of life essence and blood to certain extent, the herbal medicines will be insufficient to bring the required tonifying effects, as such, the flesh and blood stuff will have to be used inevitably. The turtle can be used to tonify the primordial Yin, corresponding to the deer in the fire-associated formulas. The turtle as medicine goes to Renmai (Renmai channel), and the deer as medicine goes to Dumai (governor meridian). The former one is to tonify Yin, while the latter one is to tonify Yang.

There is a debate about getting through Renmai and Dumai. Is there a way to get through these two meridians? Renmai dominates Yin, and Dumai dominates Yang. In human body, Yin and Yang exist harmoniously, and they are interconnecting and communicating with each other. Generally, Renmai and Dumai are open, but only to a different extent of opening for different people. Renmai goes along the front of the body, and Dumai mainly goes along the back of the body. The two meridians of Renmai and Dumai have an intersection at the gingival junction, just above the two large incisors, where the outside is the philtrum, and the inside is Yinjiao acupoint. Renmai and Dumai just intersect at the gingival point.

Whenever one suffers from heatstroke coma or malaise, just try a nip or massage at the philtrum immediately, which is equivalent to massage Yinjiao acupoint. This massage action, in fact, is to get through Renmai and Dumai meridians. Those who suffer from coma will have Yin and Yang obstructed. What they need most immediately in such an emergency is to have the two meridians of Renmai and Dumai get through, for which massage at the philtrum will be very effective. **Guilu Erxian Jiao** is one of the commonly used patented medicine containing the herbal ingredients of Guijiao (tortoise plastron gelatin), Lujiao (deerhorn gelatin), Renshen (ginseng), and Gouqizi (fructus lycii). Guijiao and Lujiao here are for tonifying Renmai and Dumai respectively, which also implies to get through the two meridians of Renmai and Dumai. In brief, regardless of the meridian therapy or the medical treatment, they both mean to get through Renmai and Dumai meridians.

As for the ordinary people, Renmai and Dumai meridians can only get through to a certain degree but not further, while for a *kungfu* man, he may get through Renmai and Dumai more effectively, and the degree of Yin and Yang intersection in his body is different from the ordinary people, which is to a higher level, so the principle of "practicing for proving" must be followed. Some people often ask about how to get through Renmai and Dumai, and even ask for proving it. But, in fact, proving it to oneself would be much better than letting others prove it. How to prove it to yourself? One must practice *Kungfu* until he gets through Renmai and Dumai by himself. Then, the result will prove itself naturally.

The word "Ren" in the term of "Renmai" actually implies an "important mission". What mission does it have? When human being stands upright, there is only one vertebra supporting at the waist where flesh stays to form the belly. Can we imagine that a lumbar vertebra is able to support the body? In fact, the bone is merely a visible support, and there is another invisible backbone to support the body, i. e., Renmai. It supports the human body in the front so that one can hold his head high. There is another channel called Chongmai, which is corresponding to Renmai. And literally speaking, Chongmai has an uprush potential and it circulates in parallel to that of Renmai in a long section. Such an uprush energy and vitality are also the support for the human body.

In the front of the body are Renmai and Chongmai, and at the back are Dumai and Bladder meridian. The bladder meridian and Dumai at the back are largely in parallel. Dumai dominates Yang of the body, and the bladder meridian is also one of the most vigorous meridians of Yang. When a person is vigorous in

Yang, Dumai will be very tight, which will not easily lead to hunchback. The senior-aged people are susceptible to hunchback because of both Yin and Yang deficiency. When Yang is in deficiency, Dumai will become loose, which means Dumai cannot hold the back; at the same time Renmai is also deficient, which means it becomes weaker to hold the weight, and Chongmai then fails to rush up. As such, the body will naturally lean forwards. Therefore, on the one hand, the front side shrinks and lean forwards, and on the other hand, the back side becomes loose and fails to hold, and the trunk of the aged people start to bend down and become hunchbacked. Hence, Renmai and Dumai do exist and impose great influence on human body configuration.

Tortoise and Its Plastron

Tortoise is quite familiar to everyone, and it is slow in action and low in body temperature. It may take no food continuously for a few months, but enjoys longevity. Generally, the tortoise was born in a dark and wet place. It likes hiding more, signifying that it can tonify the kidney and enjoys the astringing and storing properties. Longevity suggests that it has very tenacious vitality. Low body temperature suggests it is able to nourish Yin. There are many kinds of tortoises including mountain tortoise, sea tortoise and river tortoise, among which the river tortoise is the best. For medical use, the river tortoise plastron will be the best, but now most of the tortoise plastron in pharmacies are from the sea tortoise shell. The shell of one sea tortoise shell can be over a dozen *jin* in weight, while the best shell of a river tortoise could be possibly sized as an adult hand palm, weighing only a few dozen grams or around a hundred grams. Attention is required to that the sea tortoise shell cannot be taken for medical use.

The tortoise plastron is sweet-salty in taste and cold in property, going to the liver, spleen and kidney meridians, and it can tonify the primordial Yin (kidney Yin). I have once seen a very big mountain turtle, whose carapace was broken in some way with some very thick white liquid coming out of the crack. This actually is the primordial Yin in the tortoise shell. The tortoise shell is very heavy in its texture, so it has the efficacy of suppressing Yin and subduing Yang. Those who suffer from Yin deficiency will lead to Yang floating above, so the suppressing medicines can help restrain the floating Yang. The tortoise plastron as a medicine has the function of tonifying the primordial Yin on the one hand and suppressing the floating Yang on the other hand. It is often used for treatment of the primordial Yin deficiency, hyperactivity of liver-Yang or Yang floating outside.

In general, in case that only Yin deficiency arises without the primordial Yang floating outside or hyperactivity of liver- Yang, Shudi will work. Otherwise, it may also suppress and subdue Yang simultaneously while Yin is tonified. Yin may not grow if it fails to obtain its Yang. In that case, the tortoise plastron will not be quite suitable. Moreover, the tortoise is an intelligential creature, and it should not be indiscriminately slaughtered and abused, but should be used with restraints.

Dabuyin Jian

There is a well-known formula called **Dabuyin Jian** (Decoction for Greatly Tonifying Yin) for treating Yin deficiency accompanied by Yang floating outside. **Dabuyin Jian** contains the herbs of Guiban (tortoise plastron), Shudi (radix rehmanniae praeparata), Huangbai (phellodendron amurense), Zhimu (rhizoma anemarrhenae), and Zhujisui (pig spinal cord), which can also be made into pills, called **Dabuyin Pill**. This is a heavy dosage for tonifying Yin and replenishing fluid. **Liuwei Dihuang Pill** is not so powerful as **Dabuyin Pill** in respect of tonifying Yin and replenishing fluid. Of course, as for Yin deficiency with accompanying heat, **Dabuyin Jian** is wonderfully effective.

Guiban tonifies the primordial Yin and subdues the floating Yang; Shudi goes into the kidneys to tonify the primordial Yin; Huangbai and Zhimu can clear the floating heat. The floating heat often arises in the Lower Jiao from Yin deficiency so Huangbai and Zhimu are used here for clearing it. Zhujisui itself can tonify Yin, and also plays the role of enhancing the other medical efficacies to guide the effects of Zhujisui into the human spinal marrow where the bone marrow is converged. This formula can be made into either decoction or pills.

Talking about **Dabuyin Pill**, I have to remind that Guiban may be crushed into powder if it is used in decoction since the fine powder may help to be extracted with more life essence while it is decocted; or Guiban may also be broken into small pieces, but it has to be decocted for a longer time. For making pills, it must be ground into fine powder, or otherwise, it will stick in the intestines to form abdominal mass and cause indigestion. The medicines like tortoise plastron, human fingernails, carbonized hair and the like all should be ground into very fine powder in case of making pills.

Crisp Tortoise Plastron

The raw tortoise plastron is inclined to tonifying Yin, but it can also remove stasis. For intensifying its force of removing stasis, the tortoise plastron requires processing. Break the tortoise plastron into smaller pieces, and stir to parch it with sand until it is burning hot, then sift off the sand quickly and spray vinegar over it, after which the tortoise plastron will immediately blow out lots of small bubbles, and become crispy in texture. This is the so-called crisp tortoise plastron.

The crisp tortoise plastron can remove stasis and nourish Yin, but simply its effect of nourishing Yin is relatively weaker. The crisp turtle shell and the processed crisp tortoise plastron are often used together, which can play a very effective function of resolving hard lump. This recipe is often used for treatment of various abdominal masses and lumps. In the book of *Shibing Lun (Treatise on Seasonal Diseases)*, there is a **Shuangjia Souxie Fa** (double-shell formula for searching pathogens) that contains crisp turtle shell and crisp tortoise shell. In case that it is not powerful enough, add pangolin scales to form a tri-shell formula for searching pathogens, which can be used for resolving various hard lumps in the body. The tri-shell formula is much stronger and even can be used for treatment of the liver cirrhosis and the like. Hardening is equivalent to lump or abdominal mass formation. In a word, on the basis of soothing and nourishing the liver and promoting blood circulation to remove blood stasis, the two-shell formula or the tri-shell formula can be used to soften hardness to dissipate stagnation.

E-jiao (Donkey-hide Gelatin)

There are many legends about E-jiao (donkey-hide gelatin), which specially refers to the donkey-hide gelatin made in Dong'e, Shandong province of China.

Preparation of E-jiao

According to the ancient method, it would be very complicated and particular for making E-jiao: choose the hide of an especially black donkey that grows up by eating the grass on the Shi'er hills and drinking the water of Langxi river in Shandong province of China. The adult donkey shall be slaughtered on the day of winter solstice. Take the donkey hide and scrape off the hair from the hide, and then soak the hide in the water from Langxi river for seven days. After that, cut the prepared hide into small pieces and put in a porcelain pot with the water from Dong'e well (the water must be gradually added), and then start to boil it over the mulberry wood fire for three days and nights into gelatin. In this process, the dregs must be strained off, and also some herbs or ingredient excipients are added to extract gelatin. One may have the experience that while boiling the pig's foot and stewing it slowly over slow fire, he or she would find the soup would gradually become sticky, and then boil into gelatin. The donkey hide can also be slowly boiled into gelatin, too, i. e., E-jiao (or Dong'e E-jiao, or Dong'e Donkey Hide gelatin).

The top-quality E-jiao is dark deep green in color and faint scent in smell. But this medicine is so famous that many people step into production of it so there are lots of jerry-built products, and it becomes harder to get the genuine E-jiao being prepared according to the above-mentioned traditional method. A recent report said that now most of E-jiao was made with the hides of mules, horses, cows, pigs and so on as raw materials. This is not the creation of the modern people, but it was there in the ancient time. Suppose the raw materials are not genuine and pure, the final product of E-jiao will smell very unpleasant.

Black Donkey Hide

Why should E-jiao be made with the black donkey hide? The donkey, in the **Wuxing Doctrine**, is subsumed to fire, but the black color is subsumed to water, so the black donkey is an image that can coordinate water and fire. The hide is subsumed to the lung which in turn dominates the hide and hair. The hide is permeable because of the hair pore in it. E-jiao is used for nourishing blood and Yin and tonifying the kidneys. E-jiao is made by boiling the black donkey hide, suggesting the inter-promoting relation between metal and water/fluid since the hide is subsumed to metal and the kidney is subsumed to water/fluid.

In addition to nourishing Yin, E-jiao can also dispel wind, moisten dryness and reduce phlegm. By the way, donkey meat is very good for nourishing Yin, but it should not be eaten too much, especially the elderly people. Otherwise, it would be similar to eating more chicken, easily stirring up pathogenic wind. The donkey hide also attracts wind, and it can enter the liver meridians to replenish blood. Just as the weather in spring, it not only rains but blows wind as well. In the gentle breeze and fine drizzle, all plants will grow flourishingly and prosperously. The gentle breeze means growth, corresponding to the spring and vitality, so does Yin nourishing. In the antanemic medicines (blood nourishing medicines), some medicines related to wind need to be added. For instance, E-jiao contains "wind", and at the same time, it enjoys the moistening function as well, that is to say, E-jiao contains both "wind" and "rain".

Similarly, **Siwu Tang** contains "wind" and "rain", too. The herbs of Danggui and Dihuang in it are for nourishing Yin, i. e., "the rain", while Chuanxiong in it is a moistening agent in "the wind". "The wind" is aromatic and moving freely.

With both "wind" and "rain" available, its nourishing potency will be intensified. In case that it only rains without wind, the rain will become stagnant; or in case that it only blows wind without rain, it will blow drier and drier. Only wind and rain combined together can bring up vitality. When the function of nourishing Yin is more powerful than that of stirring up the wind, it can drive away the wind. To nourish Yin can drive away the wind, and to nourish blood can drive away the wind, too. As it is known, the principle goes like "treatment of the pathogenic wind is to start with the blood treatment, after which the pathogenic wind will extinguish itself naturally". So, when Yin is sufficiently nourished, the pathogenic wind will finally die away naturally.

Therefore, a black donkey hide is endowed with multiple meanings of coordinating water and fire, inter-promoting metal and water, gentle breeze and fine drizzle etc., and it has obvious effects for nourishing Yin and moistening dryness.

Water to Be Used for Making E-jiao

The medicines for nourishing Yin are usually greasy and can induce phlegm. However, E-jiao can reduce phlegm. Why is it so?

It has been mentioned that E-jiao is made with the black donkey that drinks the water of Langxi river. Langxi River originates from Hongfan Spring, which is subsumed to Yang. The water to be used for boiling E-jiao is from E-jing Well, and the well water is subsumed to Yin.

E-jing well is an ancient well located in Dong'e county of Shandong province of China. The water from this well is crystal clear with heavy texture. It is "interlinked" with the underground water of *Jishui* river origin, while Jishui water is linked to heart. In *Huangdi Neijing· Líng Shū*, there is an article named "*Jīng Shuǐ*" (Meridians and Waters), it records the ground waters and rivers, which are interlinked with the vital organs of human body and the twelve meridians, among which *Jishui* river goes to Shaoyin Channel, i. e., to the heart.

But how is the E-jing water interlinked with *Jishui* river? The big rivers on the ground often have some invisible parts underground as we often see some swirls in the large rivers. Of course, some water is flowing in a swirling current, and some swirls exist just because of holes in the riverbed, connecting to the underground river. In fact, there are rivers on the ground and underground. The rivers on the ground are equivalent to the channel of Yang, while the underground rivers are equivalent to the channel of Yin. The ground rivers can be seen on the map, but the underground rivers cannot be seen. Well, the underground rivers are more worthy of studying, and they are actually interconnected to the ground rivers.

E-jing is just a well. The expert drillers of wells all know that a well should be made in the water vein, where the underground water passes. E-jing well may be right at the point where the underground river is interconnected with Jishui water system, so the water from E-jing well is quite special. The water in E-jing well is subsumed to Yin while the water from the Langxi river is subsumed to Yang, which refers to the intersection of Yin and Yang. The water from E-jing well goes to the heart, and the black donkey hide goes to the kidneys, which refers to the intersection of the heart and kidneys. Therefore, in the process of tonifying Yin, pay attention to the intersection and concordance of Yin and Yang.

The water in E-jing well is clear with heavy texture, which tends to descend in property. After drinking, the drinker will feel it quickly going downwards to resolve phlegm and wash away the waste inside the body downwards without stagnation. Therefore, E-jiao can not only replenish blood but also disperse blood stasis.

E-jiao Siwu Tang

E-jiao is a common medicine for treatment of blood trouble, which is associated with a very famous formula called **E-jiao Siwu Tang**, containing the ingredients of **Siwu Tang** plus E-jiao.

Siwu Tang is nothing more but a formula containing four herbs. If one wants to further intensify its potency for replenishing blood, he or she has to add the refined life essence of the flesh and blood, that is, E-jiao (donkey-hide gelatin), not only for nourishing blood, but also slightly dispersing blood stasis and clearing the floating heat since E-jiao goes to the lungs and kidneys while **Siwu Tang** mainly goes to the liver and kidneys. However, **E-jiao Siwu Tang** not only goes to the liver, lungs and kidneys, but also takes into account of Qi and blood, so it is more powerful for nourishing blood.

E-jiao Siwu Tang is also frequently used for miscarriage prevention. After all, E-jiao is made from the black donkey hide. The hide can even wrap up the whole donkey, so it is imaginable its efficacy for securing the fetus. This is just deduced from the perspective of imagination. In fact, the efficacy of **E-jiao Siwu Tang** for miscarriage prevention is to be achieved through sufficiently nourishing blood, after which the fetus will be secured naturally. From all angles, we can be convinced with the truth of miscarriage prevention with **E-jiao Siwu Tang**. Therefore, when talking about the efficacy of an herb, one must try to explain it from different perspectives in different ways, sometimes in a right reasoning way, sometimes in a false reasoning way, sometimes in the medical way, sometimes in a pharmacological way, and sometimes in an imaginal thinking way. The imaginal thinking way may look preposterous, but it can give us some inspiration or enlightenment, or even not, at least it is a tool, and will be helpful for understanding the efficacies of medicines.

Contraindications of E-jiao

E-jiao should be used only when it is really needed.

When it is needed to nourish blood or to give treatment of blood deficiency and fever arising from tuberculosis, or to prevent miscarriage, E-jiao, or **E-jiao Siwu Tang** can be used; or when the primordial Yin deficiency arises, E-jiao can be then used together with tortoise plastron gelatin and deer-horn gelatin. But it is not advisable to take E-jiao for daily tonic use.

E-jiao, in any case, is a medicine, and it is not advisable for the healthy people to take it. As mentioned above that it is very particular about the production of E-jiao. There seems to have some mysteries under cover, so many people take it as a tonic food; or some people may just imagine it is good for nourishing or tonifying uses. And therefore, they abuse E-jiao over and again, which then results in price boom with sudden huge profits, and this again stimulates some businessmen to take risk in profiteering from making counterfeit and shoddy products.

第八章　养阴类动物药

蜂蜜

百花之精，平和甘润

蜂蜜是蜜蜂所产。我们知道，蜜蜂有雄蜂、雌蜂，还有工蜂。雄蜂是黑色的，个头也不小，蜂王则是雌蜂。雄蜂只负责跟蜂王交配，交配完了死了。有的不死就游手好闲到处乱飞，往往就被工蜂驱逐出去。工蜂既不是雄蜂，也不是雌蜂，它是中性的，没有雌雄之分，没有情欲。蜂蜜是工蜂采花酿出来的，这意味着蜂蜜也是中性、平性、平和的。

蜜蜂群居而不乱，即便被外界干扰一下，乱了一会儿，它们会马上调整，又恢复以前那样的井然有序了，而且它恢复得特别快。这意味着它能和。这样一种动物，酿出的蜂蜜也让人体的五脏六腑井然有序。所以蜂蜜能和五脏、安六腑，调和人的气血营卫。

蜂蜜是采百花之精酿造而成的。春天，天地之间是一种和谐的生发之气，范仲淹的《岳阳楼记》讲"春和景明"。和谐，是生发的前提，不和谐是不能发展的，春天是和谐的季节。和谐之气在植物上体现得尤其充分和明显，而植物的精华又在花上，花的精华又在花粉。蜜蜂采花粉来酿蜜，可以说是把春天的冲和之气、生发之气收藏起来了。

我们在超市里经常可以看到什么槐花蜜、菊花蜜、油菜花蜜，其实，这只是商家做出来的概念，这些概念又弄巧成拙。哪有蜜蜂只采一种花的？如果真的只采一种花，酿的蜜反而没那么好，蜜蜂要采百花之精，将其和合在一起，酿成蜂蜜，才是天地间最纯的、最精华的东西，体现了春天的生发之气与和谐之气。所以蜂蜜是养生之上品，所以古人非常推崇它。

蜂蜜入心、脾、肺、胃、大肠经。它芳香开窍，开窍就入心经；芳香味甘则入脾；花主散，蜂蜜作为花的精华，它也能散。一般甘味的东西会守在脾胃，比如说大枣，就会守中，产生壅滞，唯独蜂蜜甘甜活泼，能发散，入脾后很容易游逸精气，上输入肺。

蜂蜜的作用

生蜂蜜又叫白蜜，色白入肺，还能润下，很多人喜欢吃蜂蜜来治疗便秘，确实有一定的作用。它能和营卫，润脏腑，还能清热。把蜜进行提炼，进行炮制就成了熟蜜，也叫炼蜜。熟蜜补脾胃的作用更强了，清热的作用就没有了，因为它经过炮制，性质变温了。入药用生蜂蜜还是用熟蜂蜜，要根据具体情况而定。

蜂蜜还能止痛。因为痛往往是因为急，也就是体内某些部位不够缓和，急则不通，不通则痛。那么，甘以缓之，让人体各方面的机能缓下来，缓下来就不急了，不急就不痛了，这就叫缓急止痛。

蜂蜜还能解百药之毒，所以我们很多药都用蜂蜜来炮制。前面我们讲的百部，就是用蜂蜜来制的。附子等中药误用，会引起中毒，可以用蜂蜜来解。蜂蜜和甘草有很多相似的地方，它能调和百药，所以我们制作药丸的时候也经常用蜜丸，就是用蜂蜜来调和的。蜂蜜在其中不仅起粘合剂的作用，还起一个调和的作用，让这些药在一起和合成一个圆融的整体，所以，古人把丸叫"圆"，形状上它是圆的，药性上它是圆融的。

蜂蜜能够润大便，张仲景在《伤寒论》的阳明病篇有一个方子就是叫蜜煎导，把蜂蜜放在一个铜器里边，放到火上炼，炼到一定的火候，趁热搓成长条，放温后塞到肛门里，治阴虚大肠干燥的那种便秘，效果还是挺好的。

蜂蜜的使用禁忌

脾胃不实、肾气虚滑的就不要吃蜂蜜了。这种人表现为老是拉肚子，大便比较稀、比较溏，一天上好多次厕所，这是因为脾胃不实，不能统摄，还因为肾气虚滑。肾气虚了，不但大便容易滑，白带、精液都容易往下滑，这叫肾气虚滑，这样的人就不要吃蜂蜜了。

女子白带多的也不要吃蜂蜜，有的女子白带多，伤阴伤得也比较重，大便还干，大便一干她又吃蜂蜜，越吃蜂蜜白带越多，白带越多，大便越干，恶性循环。此外，如果痰多，吃蜂蜜也是要慎重的。

龟板

自然思维与制度思维

前几天，正下着雨的时候，我在小区看到给草坪浇水的水龙头依然在喷水，而且管草地的工人也在。我问：天上都下雨了，你怎么还在这里浇水呀？工人茫然地抬头看了我一眼，说这是规定，然后继续浇水。

人和人的思维是不一样的，有的人遵循的是自然，这叫自然思维；有的人遵循的是制度，这叫制度思维。这是两种不同的思维。跟自然接触得比较多的人，自然思维会多一些；跟制度接触得比较多的人，制度思维就会多一些。优秀的医生，不管是中医还是西医，讲究的是自然思维，就是遵循自然之理、自然之道，灵活变通，很少有条条框框。庸医更多的是遵循制度思维，书上怎么规定的，就按书上的来做。中医应该是完全遵循自然思维的，你要是把自然之理丢掉，去守一些方子，就从自然思维跳到制度思维上来了。

庸医更多的是遵循制度思维，书上怎么规定的，就按书上的来做。中医应该是完全遵循自然思维的，你要是把自然之理丢掉，去守一些方子，就从自然思维跳到制度思维上来了。

所以，一个从农村走出来的人，跟自然接触得比较频繁，有着很原始、很鲜活的经验，那么他的自然思维就要多一些，他处理问题的方式会遵循自然；一个累世公卿的，祖祖辈辈在机关里做事的，他接触的是一些人际关系、一些制度、权术，那么他的制度思维比较强一些，必须按规定办事。

但又有人讲"寒门生宰相，白屋出公卿"，这是什么意思呢？这跟他小时候的历练有关，也跟他的自然思维有关，自然思维是一种鲜活、灵动，甚至很狂野的思维，是很有生命力的，能够做大事，成大事。

中医要讲自然思维，从自然思维中去体会阴阳，体察万物。我们这里讲的龟板、阿胶是动物药，是血肉有情之品，可以补阴。但这个补阴之品什么时候当用，什么时候不当用，我们要根据自然思维去把握。

任督二脉

补阴的药前面我们讲了很多，生地、熟地、天冬、麦冬之类，但这些都是草木，当人体的精血亏到一定程度的时候，草木是补不了的，那就得用到血肉有情之品。乌龟是大补真阴的，跟火部方药的鹿相对应。龟是通任脉的，鹿是通督脉的。一个补阴，一个补阳。

近期有关于打通任督二脉的争论。到底是否存在打通任督二脉呢？任脉主阴，督脉主阳，人是阴阳调和的，他需要阴阳交抱，阴阳之气要互相沟通。所以在每一个人的身上，任脉和督脉都是通的，只是通的程度不一样。任脉在身体的前面，督脉主要在身体的后面，它们有一个相交之处就是在龈交，也就是在两个大门牙的上方。外边是人中，里边就是龈交穴，任脉和督脉在牙龈这个地方相交。

人要是中暑昏迷或者不舒服，赶紧揉一揉人中，也就相当于揉了龈交这个穴。这个小小的动作，其实就是在沟通阴阳，也就是在打通任督二脉。人一昏迷，阴阳就更加不通了，要把它通过来怎么办？赶紧打通任督二脉。这时候揉人中就有打通任督二脉的作用。龟鹿二仙胶是我们很常用的一个方剂。它的组成是龟胶、鹿胶、人参、枸杞子。其中龟板是补任脉的，鹿角是补督脉的，也有打通任督二脉的意思。所以不管是经络疗法还是药物疗法，都含有打通任督二脉的成份。

在普通人这里，任督二脉只能打通到这个程度，在练家子那里，他能把任督二脉打得更通，他体内阴阳交汇的程度跟普通人不一样，这是一种更高的境界，我们要遵循一定的路子，先修后证。有人总是说，任督二脉怎么通？你证明给我看。让别人证明给你看，不如自己证明给自己看。中国的学问都是自己证明给自己看的。如何证明给自己看？你先得练这个功夫，练到能打通任督二脉，你就证实了，不修你就证实不了。

任脉的"任"其实有"重任"的意思，它负担着什么样的重任呢？我们直直地站在这里，腰部只有脊椎骨在撑着，肚子这一圈全是肉，一根腰椎骨把我们撑起来吗？其实，骨头只是一个有形支撑，还有另外一个无形的支柱在支撑我们的，这就是任脉，它从前边把我们支撑起来，这样，人才能够昂首挺胸地站着。跟任脉相对应的还有冲脉，我们光从字面上来理解，冲脉就有一股往上冲之势。冲脉的循行跟任脉在很长一段是平行的，它这股上冲之气也是人体的支撑。

前边有任脉和冲脉，后边则有督脉和膀胱经。膀胱经和督脉在背部很大的程度上是平行的。督脉主一身的阳气，膀胱经也是阳气最旺盛的一条经脉。当人阳气旺的时候，督脉就会很紧，督脉一紧人就不容易驼背。人到老的时候就容易驼背，那是因为阴阳两虚，阳虚了督脉就松了，督脉一松，背上就拉不住；同时任脉也虚了，任脉一虚，它负重的能力就减弱了，冲脉它也冲不起来了，这样一来，身体自然的就会往前面倾。前面在缩、在倾，后面又松了拉不住，人的腰自然就弯了，背就驼了。所以任脉和督脉是存在的，而且对人的体形都有非常大的影响。

乌龟与龟板

我们可能都见过乌龟，它行动迟缓，体温很低，可以好几个月不吃东西，还长寿，一般它生在阴湿之处，比较喜欢躲藏。比较喜欢躲藏，意味着它能入肾，有封藏之性。长寿意味着它的生命力非常的顽强。体温低，也意味着它是入阴的。乌龟有很多种，有山龟、海龟、河龟，其中以河龟最佳。入药的龟板，以河龟板最好，但现在药店很多都是海龟的龟板。一个海龟的龟板能有十几斤，河龟的龟板巴掌大的最好，只有几十克或者一百来克。但海龟板是不入药的。

龟板甘咸寒，入肝、脾、肾三经，是大补真阴的。我曾经看到过一个很大的山龟，背上的甲壳不知道怎么被磕破了一点，伤口就有一些很浓很浓的白浆流出来，这就是龟板里面的真阴。龟板是甲壳类的，质地很重，有镇阴潜阳的作用。当人阴虚的时候，阳气就会往上浮越，于是用重镇的药把往上浮越的阳气给镇压下去。龟板一则补真阴，二则镇浮越之阳，所以经常用在真阴大虚、有肝阳上亢或有浮阳外越的时候。

一般的情况下，如果只是阴虚，并无真阳外越、肝阳上亢，用熟地就行了，如果潜镇的话，补阴是给补了，但同时又潜镇了阳气，把真阳都给潜镇住了，阴不得其阳也不能生长，所以这时候用龟板反而不好。更何况龟是一种有灵性的动物，用的时候一定要有节制，不能滥用，滥杀无辜是不好的。

大补阴煎

治真阴大虚而浮阳外越，有一个很有名的方剂叫大补阴煎。大补阴煎的组成是龟板、熟地、黄柏、知母、猪脊髓这五味药，也可以做成丸药，叫大补阴丸。这是一个补阴壮水的重剂。六味地黄丸补阴壮水的力度不如大补阴煎大，对于这种阴虚有热用大补阴煎是极好的。

龟板补真阴、潜浮阳；熟地入肾，大补真阴；黄柏、知母清浮游之热，因为阴虚，所以生热，这种热往往在下焦，所以用黄柏、知母来清；猪脊髓本身可以补阴，又起到药引子的作用，以猪的脊髓入人的脊髓，而脊髓也是骨髓的集中之地，引药力入脊髓，使之迅速发挥作用。这个方，无论是做成汤剂，还是做成丸剂都可以。

讲到大补阴丸的时候，我们要提醒一下，龟板在入汤剂的时候，可以把它打成粉，打成粉它出汁就多，也可以打成小块，要久煎。如果要入丸剂，要注意把它研成极细的粉末，不然它就会粘在肠子里出不来，就容易生出症瘕、积滞。鳖甲、人指甲、血余之类的药都是这样的，要碾成极细的粉末，才能入丸药。

酥龟板

生龟板偏于补阴，但也能散结，如果要增强其散结的力度，就要对龟板进行炮制。把龟板打成小片，拌沙炒得滚烫，然后迅速筛去沙子，喷上醋。龟板在醋里一呛，马上就要鼓出很多泡来，质地也变得酥脆，这就成了酥龟板。

酥龟板偏于散结，兼养阴，只是养阴的作用比较弱。它经常跟酥鳖甲一块用，酥鳖甲也是经过了炮制的鳖甲。二者一起用，软坚散结的功能非常好，经常用于治疗各种症瘕，也就是体内的各种结块。《时病论》中有一个双甲搜邪法，就用酥龟甲、酥鳖甲。如果嫌不够你还可以加穿山甲，那就是三甲搜邪法，体内的很多结块都可以用这个来化。加了穿山甲，力度会更大，甚至可以用于肝硬化之类的病的治疗。因为硬化就相当于这地方结块了，也相当于症瘕。在疏肝养肝、活血化瘀的基础上，用二甲或三甲来软坚散结。

阿胶

关于阿胶的传说非常多。阿胶，就是山东东阿这个地方产的胶。

阿胶的制法

阿胶要是按照严格的古法制作的话，是非常复杂也非常讲究的。要取用一种黑驴的皮，这种黑驴必须是吃狮耳山的草、饮狼溪河水的黑驴。养大了的驴要在冬至这一天把它杀了，取它的皮，刮掉毛，在郎溪水里浸泡七天。然后切成小块，放在瓷锅里面渐渐加入阿井的水，用桑木火煮三天三夜，就煮成胶了。在这个过程中，可能还要滤掉渣滓，还要加进去一些药或者收胶的辅料。我们煮猪蹄，小火慢炖，汤会黏黏的，要是一直熬的话也会熬出胶来。驴皮慢熬也会熬出胶。驴皮熬成的胶就是阿胶。

好的阿胶是深墨绿色的，气味清香。但是因为这个药太有名了，大家就都去做，偷工减料的就多。所以，真正按照上面讲法做的阿胶就少了，鱼目混珠，假的居多，真的就比较难得了。最近有一个报导，说现在阿胶都是用什么骡子皮、马皮、牛皮、猪皮，甚至旧皮鞋、废皮箱的皮为原料做的。这并不是现在才有，古代就有了。用的皮要是不地道的话气味是非常的难闻。

黑驴皮

为什么制作阿胶要用黑驴皮呢？驴在五行中属火，黑色属水，黑驴有水火既济之象。皮是属肺的，肺主皮毛，而且皮上面有毛孔很通透。阿胶是用来养血、滋阴、补肾的，用皮熬成，有金水相生之义。因为皮毛属金，而肾属水。

除了养血滋阴，阿胶还可以驱风、润燥、化痰。驴肉很能养阴，但不能多吃，尤其老年人不能多吃，吃多了就跟鸡肉似的容易动风。驴皮也跟风同气相求的，能入肝经而补血。这就好比春天，光下雨还不行，还得起风。在和风细雨中，植物会才能长得飞快。和风意味着生长，对应春天，对应生发之气。补阴也是这样的，往往在补血的药中都要加入风药。阿胶就有风在里边，同时又滋润，可以说是有风有雨。

我们看四物汤，其中也是有风有雨的。当归、地黄养阴，这就是下雨了。为什么要用川芎呢？川芎是风中润剂，芳香走窜，这就是风。

有风有雨，它滋补的作用就强。如果光下雨不起风，那么雨就呆滞了；如果光起风不下雨，就会越吹越干。有风有雨，才能有生机。当滋阴的作用比动风的作用更大时，就能驱风，养阴可以驱风，养血也可以驱风。"治风先治血，血行风自灭"，养阴养得多的时候，风自然就没有了。

所以，一个黑驴皮，有水火既济、金水相生、和风细雨等多重含义，其养阴、润燥的作用是显而易见的。

制作阿胶所用之水

养阴的药都容易滋腻、生痰，但阿胶却有化痰的作用，这是为什么呢？

前面我们讲了，制作阿胶所用的黑驴，要喝狼溪水。狼溪河发源于洪泛泉，它是阳性的。熬制阿胶用的阿井水则是阴性的。阿井是山东东阿县的一口古井。这口井的水很清，质地很重，它跟济水相通，而济水是通心的。《黄帝内经·灵枢》中有一篇就叫作《经水》，就是讲大地上的河流，跟人体的五脏六腑、十二经脉是相通的，其中济水能通少阴，是通心的。

阿井是山东东阿县的一口古井。这口井的水很清，质地很重，它跟济水相通，而济水是通心的。《黄帝内经·灵枢》中有一篇就叫作《经水》，就是讲大地上的河流，跟人体的五脏六腑、十二经脉是相通的，其中济水能通少阴，是通心的。

阿井的水为什么和济水相通呢？地上的大河往往还有看不见的地下部分。我们经常会在比较大的河里看到漩涡。当然有些水是打着漩涡流的，还有些漩涡是因为河底有洞，通地下的暗河。地上有河流，地下也有河流。地上的河流相当于人体的阳脉，地下的河流相当于阴脉。我们看地图能够看到地上的河流，却看不到地下的河流。地下的河流更值得研究，而且地下的河流往往与地上的河流是相通的。

阿井是一口井。会打井的人都会说，井要在水脉上打，水脉也就是地下水经过的地方。阿井可能正好就打在与地下河与济水相通的那个地方了，所以井水很特别。阿井水属阴，狼溪水属阳，这是阴阳相交。阿井水通心，驴皮又通肾，这又是心肾相交。所以，补阴时要注意阴阳相交、阴阳和合。

阿井水清，而质地很重，性下趋，喝下后，会迅速往下走，这就可以化瘀，涤荡体内的污垢，迅速往下走，不停留在人体内形成疾病，这叫瘀化下行不作痨。所以，阿胶不但能补血，还能化瘀。

阿胶四物汤

阿胶是血证的常用药，有个很有名的方剂叫阿胶四物汤，就是在四物汤的基础上加一味阿胶。

四物汤只不过是四味草木之药，如果要进一步加大补血的力度，就要加一味血肉有情之品，也就是阿胶，不仅能够补血，还稍微有些化瘀的作用，同时能清浮游之热。因为阿胶同时通肺、通肾，而四物汤主要是通肝、肾的，阿胶四物汤走肝、肺、肾，兼顾了气血，所以养血的力度会更大。

阿胶四物汤在安胎的时候会经常用。毕竟阿胶是驴皮熬的，驴皮连一头驴都能裹住，所以对胎就有一定的固摄的作用。这是从形象思维的角度看的。其实，阿胶四物汤安胎是通过养血，血养足了，胎自然就安了。从各个角度都能讲得通阿胶安胎的道理，所以，有时候我们得正着讲，有时候可以歪着讲；有时候可以从医理、药理的角度去考虑，有时候可以用一些形象思维。形象思维说出来的可能是一些荒诞不经的东西，但是它能给我们一些启发，即使不能给我们启发，它也是一种工具，至少对我们记忆药的作用有所帮助。

阿胶使用禁忌

阿胶，也是当用则用，不当用的时候就不要用了。

需要补血，有血虚、痨热，或需要安胎的时候，可以用阿胶，或者阿胶四物汤。真阴大虚的时候，可以用阿胶配上龟胶、鹿角胶使用。但用来作为一种日常补品，我认为大可不必。

阿胶是一味药，没事好端端的就不要乱吃药了。正是因为阿胶这味药在制作的时候有太多讲究，它就有了一层神秘的色彩，很多人就拿它做补品，没事也吃。很多人出于自己的欲望，总认为补一补好，于是滥用阿胶，结果把它的价格抬上去了，高价就会产生暴利，有暴利就会让很多人铤而走险。作假的人多了，大家都吃不到真的了。

Volume 6
Atractylodis of Genera - Earth-associated Formulas and Medicines

Chapter 1 Introduction of Earth-associated Formulas and Medicines

The Middle Part and Four Dimensions

Out of the five-category formulas and medicines represented by the five elements (wood, metal, water, fire and earth) in the **Wuxing Doctrines**, four have been discussed so far with only the element of Earth remaining. It may seem that four fifths of the content have been covered. In fact, that is not the case. Metaphorically, if "the *Tao* of formulas and medicines" were taken as the human body from the perspective of content, what have been discussed and analyzed in the previous volumes could be equivalent to the part of the four limbs merely. The earth-associated formulas may be taken as the trunk of the whole body: this category is the most complicated, but also the most important part in the whole book. The other four elements are corresponding to the four directions (east, west, south and north) and four seasons (spring, summer, autumn and winter) respectively, while the earth corresponds to the middle part and the growing summer. As it is known, the actions of the four seasons go like: sprouting in spring, growth in summer, harvesting in autumn and storage in winter. Amongst these four actions, there actually exists one more action, i. e., the transformation. The growing summer takes place between Xia Zhi (the Summer Solstice), which falls on June 21st or 22nd in the solar calendar, and appears to have the longest day of the year in the Northern hemisphere, and Li Qiu (autumn beginning), which falls on September 22nd or 23rd in the solar calendar, marking the arrival of the autumn, and the day and night are of equal length in the Northern hemisphere.

This is the time when transformation and transportation occur significantly. The actions of the four seasons are related to the action of the earth property. A Chinese idiom says, "the earth (promotes) sprouting and earth (promotes) growth". In fact, earth not only promotes sprouting and growth, but also dominates harvesting and storage. These attributes are related to the earth properties in the same way as the four limbs are connected to the vital organs of the human body.

The meridian-collateral diagram shows that the twelve main channels run throughout the body and connect the internal organs to the limbs. Learning about the channels will provide a better understanding of the internal organs and trunk. The above four volumes build up the knowledge regarding the most complicated properties. Each of the other properties has its own dynamic movement, whereas the earth is a stabilizer to the four actions. The earth is responsible for collection, transformation and dispersion. Taking the central government as an example, the central government collects data/information throughout the country, interprets and analyzes, then spreads the final decision to the whole country. Which of the organs can play the similar functions in the body? It is the spleen and stomach that are located in the "central area". This volume will analyze the earth-associated herbs and focus on the earth-spleen and its corresponding T&T functions.

Transportation and Transformation (T&T)

The conception of T&T is crucial in TCM. Transportation is a dynamic process that occurs within the body. In this process, the extraneous materials entering into the body are transformed into the nutrients that the body needs.

Before analyzing the formulas and medicines in the earth category, it is necessary to develop a deep understanding of the conception of T&T, after which it will be easier to understand this volume about the earth-associated formulas and the principles of TCM in general. T&T is essential in the body and is also necessary for using the herbs in the other categories. Tonifying Yang without proper T&T would lead to endogenous heat, whereas tonifying Yin without proper T&T would lead to phlegm accumulation. What is the point of taking herbal medicines like Guiban (tortoise plastron) and Dihuang (rehmannia) if the body cannot digest and absorb it? The worst part of malfunctioning of T&T is that, although the body can excrete a portion of the undigested medicine, the remaining portion staying inside the body may cause harm. Therefore, the T&T function of the spleen is crucial to the body, as it transforms foreign materials into substances that the body can use and then transports and distributes to the whole body.

Characteristics of the Earth

The properties of the earth can be analyzed from the prospective of Chinese culture. China is named as Zhong Guo (the Central State). It is neither because Chinese people think that the universe rotates around this country, nor that Chinese people are arrogant but because this place possesses the properties of "the Central Land".

What is the "the Central Land" characterized?

"The Central Land" is subsumed to the earth according to **Wuxing Doctrine**. Thus, it has the property of the earth. But what is the property of the earth? It has the capacity to accept wastes. All wastes and unusable substances are dumped to or buried in the earth.

The waste buried in the earth disappears after a certain period of time. Where does the waste go? It is transformed by the earth into part of soil.

Chinese people possess the similar qualities. They accept different concepts, religions and cultures with humility. In the Han dynasty, the people accepted Buddhism when it was first introduced into China. They also accepted Christianity when it came to China. Chinese people not only accept concepts, but also integrate the foreign ideas into Chinese culture. These are the characteristics/qualities that Chinese people share with the Earth.

Some people claim that Chinese traditional culture is the integration of Confucianism, Buddhism and Taoism. However, it is difficult to differentiate the three in Chinese culture. Chinese culture is by nature the product of trans-culturalism and has the capacity to integrate many ideologies. Each person may ask himself or herself whether the body is made of the rice, vegetables or pork that he/she eats over the years. Of course, not.

Transportation and Transformation (T &T) Is a Process of Pain and Filth

T&T is a painful and filthy process and even disgusting. One cannot see the process of T&T taking place inside his or her body. Yet, if the food were vomited in these processes, it aways makes people feel sick. The result of T&T is comfortable, and as ascending the clear and descending the turbid are carried out, the nutrients of fluid and grain will be transported or distributed to the whole body. Again, after Xiazhi (the summer solstice), the growing summer dominates the T&T when it is humit and hot. Generally, by this season, the diseases spread under the influence of unpleasant odor due to fermentation, which always makes people feel rotten. However, this process generates the life essence for the great harvest in autumn and storage in winter.

It is comfortable to stay in an air-conditioned room during the growing summer. Yet by doing so, the connection of the body to nature is disturbed, affecting the normal T&T function. Therefore, during summer, one should be cautioned not to contradict the nature. Appropriate exposure to the heat of summer is beneficial to the body. Human reaction to the nature is either accommodated or unaccommodated. The unaccommodated condition will trigger the body's T&T functions, assisting the body to switch from the unaccommodated state to the accommodated state. A similar process occurs with food ingestion, even when ingesting the top-quality food, the body still regards it as a foreign material, and therefore, the body will reject it to some degree. Since the food ingested is rejected and required by the body simultaneously, how does the body deal with it then? It is the T&T function of the spleen and stomach that the body maintains the necessary nutrients and eliminates the unnecessary turbid substances through excretion.

The transformation of food into the nutrients is more obvious for children. Children often react to foods that they are exposed to for the first time, like stomachache or even diarrhea, after which they usually won't have reaction to that food again later on. Why is it so? It is because the rejection reaction by the stomach to the food that it has not previously been exposed to. For example, for a friend's visit, one will definitely show his welcome and invite the friend to have a cup of tea. However, if it is a stranger who comes to visit, one may have a sense of heightened alertness. He may chat for a while and, if the stranger turns out to be trustworthy, he might invite the stranger into the house. This is also a T&T process of interpersonal relationship. Therefore, T&T takes place in the nature, society and the human body at any given point in time. If T&T is properly a-chieved, the unfortunate thing can be turned into fortunate thing, and the fortunate thing might become better. However, if T&T is done improperly, the reverse case will happen. In Chinese, there are a lot of idioms and sayings related to the importance of transformation like: "transform a critical issue into a minor one, transform a minor issue into none", "transform the bad into the good", "transform the ill luck into blessings" and "transform hostility into friendship". These sayings imply the T&T conception. Hence, T&T is a crucial process for health.

There are two regular patterns when it comes to children's dietary habits. First, when a child is experiencing diarrhoea, don't panic, but try to recall whether he/she has ingested any food that he/she has never been exposed to. If that is the case, there is no need to panic. It is most likely the process of trans-formation taking place. This process is painful and might cause vomiting or diar-rhoea. The child often recovers after vomiting or diarrhea. Second, children's di-et should not be excessively varied. If they occasionally ingest new food and ex-perience some reaction, transformation function is improved by exposure to that food, and the body's capacity will be gradually improved as well to accept differ-ent foods. However, if a child is constantly being exposed to new foodstuffs and the body is unceasingly reacting to varied foods within a short period, the spleen and stomach may be harmed, which consequently impairs T&T function of the spleen and stomach. Therefore, children's diet should remain simple, and their caregiver should assess the timing of the introduction of new foods into the diet.

In summary, proper T&T functions are crucial to a person's wellbeing. The process of transforming the bad things into good things and transforming the anti-gen into body requirement is painful, but the result is favorable. This also applies to human life: people stay proactive and ambitious through continuous T&T. It is sometimes necessary to bear hardship since it enforces body to carry on T&T. Those who have lived their lives in favorable circumstances may find difficulties to get out of hardship sometimes. This is due to their lack of ability to transform themselves. Many people may experience such encouraging words by the other people when in trouble, "look at a matter from the angle of the good point". In other words, that is to encourage those in trouble to facilitate transformation in case of encountering difficulties, although the situation might be unfavorable and hard to bear. In case of failure of proper transformation, they may take the matter to heart, and they may either give up or become manic. Furthermore, there are a lot of people who display closed mindedness. What causes this bigoted behavior? It is a result of a mental disorder/barrier. Otherwise, no one would have such behavior against others. Some people have no difficulty accepting new concepts or people or ideas. This is due to their ability to transform the new concepts or people or ideas. Those who lack such ability often have mental barriers and/or depression. This is like a person who doesn't do physical exercises may easily suffer phlegm accumulation and stasis, for which the treatment is to transform himself and do more exercises. This process of transformation and physical exercise is usually painful.

Understanding of Transformation and Transportation in TCM

T&T is a wide-scoped conception, which is involved with T&T in the human body and that regarding herbal reactions. T&T is the function of the earth, to which the spleen corresponds. Therefore, tonifying the spleen is the best way to promote T&T function. In terms of tonifying the spleen, Baizhu (white atractylodes rhizome) is an important herb. Hence, Baizhu will be taken as a representative for the formulas and medicines in the earth-associated formulas and medicines.

Baizhu and Cangzhu (rhizoma atractylodis) are both named as Zhu in **Shennong Bencao Jing**. However, they are different herbs, in which Baizhu will be analyzed first, followed by Cangzhu, and then the other herbs that are for tonifying the spleen. The spleen governs T&T function, mainly for the Middle Jiao T&T function. However, T&T in fact occurs in the Upper, Middle and Lower Jiao, and these are often termed as "pneumatolysis", for which lots of herbs will be discussed in the following sections.

There are various transformations in TCM, such as, reducing phlegm, removing blood stasis, resolving dampness and retention, which are, in fact, either e-liminating foreign substances, or turning them into substances that human body needs. Phlegm comes from the body, but it is not involved in body physiology. Thus, Phlegm becomes a foreign substance. In a normal situation, the body will try to eliminate it. For example, in case of phlegm in the throat, the body will react to cough it out since phlegm is a foreign substance that the body wants to e-liminate. Another example is about the blood stasis. When the blood is "dead" and becomes immovable, blood stasis will occur. Blood is an essential substance in the body, but since transportation function is impaired, the flow of blood is al-so impaired, resulting in blood stasis, which is no longer what the body needs. Thus, it must be eliminated. Phlegm and blood stasis, to a great extent, are re-sulted from impaired T&T function.

With proper T&T function, the body can transform the foreign substance (e. g., foodstuff) into essential substance (e. g., Qi and blood). However, if the T&T function is impaired, the essential substances start to become foreign sub-stances. Qi and blood are essential substance in the body, but with impediment of T&T function, Qi fails to circulate properly, resulting in phlegm; and blood fails to flow properly, leading to stasis; and fluid fails to flow properly, producing dampness. If one is going picnic on a sunny day, he/she may not feel wet even if he/she lies on the grass (though there is humidity in the soil and grass). Such moistness is needed by the nature. However, in case of the stagnant water, it will become wet. The same phenomenon is also true to the human body.

The foreign substances like phlegm, blood stasis, dampness, and retention are attributed to the impairment of the normal T&T function. Therefore, it is im-portant to take care of the Middle Jiao, i. e., the spleen and stomach when one is trying to resolve/transform these foreign substances. He or she should not use herbs only to resolve phlegm/stasis, he or she should also attach great importance to T&T function of the Middle Jiao in order to strengthen the spleen in respect of its T&T function.

The so-called obstruction of Qi and blood circulation discussed in the previ-ous volumes refers that Qi and blood fail to circulate and flow properly to maintain normal physiological functions. For example, when TCM says that the disharmony between the heart and the kidney may cause insomnia, it does not mean that the heart and the kidney have stopped communicating completely but means that the heart and the kidney have not fully coordinated. Again, TCM says insomnia would also be caused by the liver failing to store "Hun" (the spirit or soul). That means the liver is not governing "Hun" as effectively as it should do in a healthy state, indicating the different level of severities. The mildest situation is when the patient experiences sleep disturbance and more dreams. In the more severe cases, there arises sleep talking in dreams. In the most extreme cases, somniloquy may occur when one is awake. In that case, it will be diagnosed as mental disease, which occurs due to failure of self-control.

Vague Description and Understanding of Transformation and Transportation

As a matter of fact, nothing is absolute, and the same is true in TCM. The vagueness in languages requires some extra interpretation for helping to understand the content. Especially in the process of learning TCM, a lot of the concepts require a great deal of interpretation. For example, in a book of medical case reports about the syndromes of meteorism or paralytic stroke, there is one formula recorded for treatment, but it is impossible to record every detail of the treatment. Writing a book about TCM formulas is just like taking notes in mathematic class, and only the most important parts are recorded. Therefore, while reading the book, one should try to interpret the case and the formula together, and think beyond what is written. Regarding the TCM formula recording books, its interpretation varies from reader to reader. A lot of TCM concepts require a proper interpretation by the readers themselves.

Furthermore, understanding is also a sort of transformation. Conversation with the others often requires transformation of the information that one receives. He or she might find some words offensive, or he or she might disagree with certain opinions, but through proper transformation, he or she might find some points helpful. Refusal to transform or direct rejection of different opinions of the others would be like inducing vomiting straight after eating something without transformation and digestion, or talking about a book without fully understanding its content. Therefore, it is important to transform and understand what has been learnt.

Baizhu and Cangzhu, especially Cangzhu, tonifies the spleen in order to strengthen the T&T function in the body. Besides, the herbs for resolving blood stasis, reducing phlegm, and opening the orifices on the one hand help clear the obstruction for T&T function, and on the other hand, help promote the T&T function.

第六卷 术之属－土部方药

第一章 土部方药概论

中部与四维

五行已经讲完了四个，只剩下土部一个了。大家可能会觉得现在已经讲完五分之四，只剩下五分之一了，其实不然。如果说方药之道像一个人体，那么前面已经讲完的四个部分如同四肢，还没有讲的部分类似躯干。讲完四边的四肢，现在讲中间的躯干，中间是最复杂的。四周对应东西南北，对应春夏秋冬；中间对应中土，在季节上它对应长夏。我们知道春生、夏长、秋收、冬藏，在生、长、收、藏的中间还存在一个"化"。所以在春、夏、秋、冬中间，从夏至到立秋以后这段时间属于长夏季节，长夏季节它就要"化"。中，就意味着运化。春生、夏长、秋收、冬藏其实都跟土有关，有个成语叫"土生土长"，其实是"土生土长"、"土收土藏"，都跟土有关。就好比四肢都跟五脏六腑有关一样。

我们看经络图，十二经脉都跟手足有关，五脏六腑都有经脉，要么延伸到手上，要么延伸到脚上，我们把四肢上的所有经脉讲完，那么对五脏六腑也就更了解了。先把十二经脉讲完，然后再讲五脏和躯干，这样就好讲了，所以我们前面讲的四部方药等于讲了东西南北四维，有了四维再讲中央，就好讲了。虽说好讲，但实际上也难讲，因为四维比较简单，是四个方向、四个维度，而中央意味着集中、运化、扩散到四周。人体的中央，或者说自然的中央，我们可以把它对应到社会组织上的中央，即中央政府。中央政府意味着要把东西南北四周的地方上的信息集中起来，进行运化，然后制定政策，以各种形式发散到地方上去。这种社会组织的中央，跟人体有某些相似之处。哪里是人体的中央呀？脾胃。脾主中土。所以讲土部方药，也就是属于"中"的这些方药的时候，首先要讲到人体的中央——脾土；其次要讲到一个特别重要的概念，就是运化。

运化

运化这个概念在中医里非常重要。"运"就是运行，身体本身就在运，在这个过程中，外来的东西被化掉了。任何东西进入体内都要经历运化的过程，自身的"运"，把外物"化"成我们需要的东西，这就叫运化。

讲土部方药，首先仔细品味一下运化的含义。体会清楚了运化的含义，认识土部方药就会比较简单，对中医医理的理解也会比别人高一筹。不管是养阴的水部方药，还是养阳的火部方药，无论哪类方药，都需要运化。如果补阳不能运化就会上火，补阴不能运化就会生痰。龟版和地黄，吃下去不消化有什么用呢？不要认为不消化就能原样排出来。可能一部份排出来了，另一部份积聚在体内形成了一些不好的东西，不为利反为害，不为福反为祸，这就比较麻烦了，所以需要运化。把外物运化成自己的，这是脾土的功能。脾土属于中央，这也是中央的功能。中央要把外在的东西运化成自己的东西，再输布到四旁。

土的特征

土到底有哪些性质？这可以从我们中国的文化来讲。中国为什么叫中国？是不是中国人一向总以为自己在宇宙的正中心呢？是我们中国妄自尊大？其实没有这种意思。中国人是很谦卑的，传统文化尤其谦卑，怎么能说我们妄自尊大呢？中国之所以叫中国，是因为这片地域有"中"的特征。

"中"有什么特征呢？

"中"在五行属土，它就有土德，有土的特征。那么土有什么特征呢？我们不需要的水、不需要的垃圾都是往地上扔，往地上扔意味着这些东西其他地方不能接受它。一张废纸不能总夹到书里边吧？书里边不能接纳它，桌子上不能放它，只能扔到地上，扔到土里，土能接纳它。土是能接纳万物的，任何废弃不用的东西，最后都是被扔到土里。

扔到土里的东西，过些时间就没了。它怎么就没了呢？它被运化掉了。所以土是最能接纳、最能运化的。很多垃圾埋在土里，天长日久它们也成了土了。你去年埋在土里边的西瓜皮今年还能找到吗？肯定找不到。哪去了？它被土运化掉了。

中国人也是这样，不管外界来了什么思想，什么宗教，什么文化，我们都能接收，而且都能很谦卑的、很谦逊的接收。汉朝的时候佛教传到中国，我们接收；后来基督教，我们也接收，不排斥；叫我们留辫子我们就留辫子，叫我们剪辫子我们就剪辫子。流行穿中山装了或者穿西装了，我们马上也跟着改，不像有的国家直到现在还穿着他们的衣服。中国人非常能够接纳，这就是土德。中国人对新鲜的事物总是保持着惊喜，保持着欣赏的态度，保持着接纳的态度，然后又运化成自己的。佛教在印度都没有那么发达，后来到了中国，有了禅宗，这是佛教跟中国的传统文化交融的一个结果，也就是中国文化把印度佛教的东西经过运化的结果。宋明理学也是如此，你说它是儒学还是道学？还是佛学？这些它都有。

中国传统文化，有人说就是儒、释、道三教合一。这种观点对吗？我觉得这是不对的。为什么呢？因为儒、释、道这三家是无法厘清界限而分彼此的。中国文化就是中国文化，你不能说这个是儒，那个是释，那个是道，不是。中国文化它是一个有机的整体，在这里边，它把什么思想都运化开来。比如我们的身体，一个人他长了几十年，主要吃的就是米饭、蔬菜和肉类，你不能说我们的身体是由饭、菜、肉组成的。

运化是一个痛苦和肮脏的过程

运化，是一个非常痛苦、非常肮脏的过程，甚至可以说是一个非常恶心的过程。为什么这样说呢？比如吃下去的东西，在肠胃里边运化，这个运化过程我们看不见；但如果这时候正在肠胃中运化东西被吐了出来，这东西是很令人恶心的。食物在肠胃里边运化，其结果是好的，是升清降浊，将水谷精微输布到全身，令人很舒服；但过程却是很肮脏、恶心的。再比如，夏至过后的长夏季节主运化，气候湿热，闷浊的空气中到处弥漫着臭味，还有疾病的蔓延，这时候让人很难受；但正是这样一个过程，春生夏长的东西，通过运化，得以变成了秋收冬藏的精华。

那么，长夏季节，我们在屋子里边吹空调，好不好？你舒服了，但你就减弱了运化那个痛苦的过程，这会影响身体的运化。所以夏天该热的时候，咱们一定要热一下，千万不要过于贪凉。人在大自然里边，有适应的时候，也有不适应的时候。这种"不适应"能够促进人体的运化，帮助人体从"不适应"状态调整到"适应"状态。我们吃饭也是的，哪怕你吃最好的东西，对于身体来说都是一个异物，当然这个异物起码它是能吃的，既然能吃，说明它跟我们的身体有同气相求的那一部分，但哪怕再同气相求，它对于我们的身体来说依然是个异物，人体对它依然有排斥的一面。有排斥的一面，也有需要的一面。饮食既需要又排斥，那怎么解决这个矛盾呢？那就需要我们的脾胃来运化，就是取其精华，去其糟粕，把需要的吸收过来，把不需要的化做大小便排走。

这个过程在小孩子身上表现得更明显。小孩吃一点他从来没有吃过的东西，往往要么肚子疼，要么拉肚子，但以后再吃这个东西就不再拉肚子了，为什么？因为他忽然吃之前从来没有吃过的东西时，肠胃会有排斥反应。好比一个熟人到家里来了，一进来就赶紧让他喝茶；一个生人到到家里来，我们就会有所排斥，一般会先聊几句，试探试探，然后可能感觉挺好，一起喝起茶来了，这也是一个人际关系运化的过程。所以说自然、社会、人体无时无刻都是在运化。如果运化得好，坏事也能运化成好事，好事能运化成更好的事；运化得不好，好事也能运化成坏事，坏事能运化成更坏的事。有一句话叫"大事化小、小事化了""化腐朽为神奇""逢凶化吉""化金戈为玉帛"，都蕴含"运化"之道，有这个能耐就能很好地化，没这个能耐那就坏了。

小孩子吃东西有两点规律：第一，小孩子拉肚子时，不要紧张，要先想一想他有没有吃从来没有吃过的东西。如果是吃了从来没有吃过的东西，那你就不要慌张，他很有可能是正在运化呢，要记住运化的过程是痛苦的，可能让人呕吐，也可能让人拉肚子，拉完就没事了，不用过于紧张。还有一点，小孩的饮食不要过于复杂。如果是偶然吃了一下没有吃过的东西，拉了一次肚子，运化了一次，在这个运化的过程中，人体也进步了一点。如果饮食过杂，天天变着法地给他吃没吃过的东西，生怕亏了他似的，今天这个，明天那个，然后他老是坏肚子，这样就会伤了脾胃，最终导致运化不利，这样反而不好。所以小孩子的饮食可以稍微单一一些，每吃一种新东西的时候，要瞅准时机，不要一味的给他新东西去吃，吃的不要太杂。

所以人一定需要非常好的运化能力。把坏事运化成好事，把异己的东西运化成对自己有好处的东西，过程虽然痛苦，但结果是好的。人生也是这样，只有在不断的运化中才能积极进取，所以说人要吃点苦，因为吃苦就是在运化，那是迫使人行动起来去运化，一直在顺境中度过的人，他运化能力就差，遇到不如意的事情他就运化不掉。我们经常说"你要想开啊……"，就是说，这件事情对于你来说虽然是不好的事情，但你必须要把它给运化掉，必须有运化能力，若运化不掉，那就容易想不开了，想不开要么疯了，要么怎么样怎么样去了，这就是运化能力差。还有人有很多的偏见，什么是偏见呢？所有的偏见都是思想障碍。没有思想障碍，人是没有偏见的。有的人很通达，四通八达，说明他运化能力好，不管什么东西在他那里都能行得通，没有障碍；如果他运化能力不好，就会思想障碍多，或意志消沉。就好比人运动的少，就容易生痰生瘀，那还得去化，还得去动，还得去经历这个痛苦的运化的过程。

中医理解的运化

运化是一个大的概念，在后面讲到人体的运化、药物的运化作用时，先要有这个大的观念为基础。运化是土的功能，对应于人体就是脾的功能，想要运化得好首先就要健脾，健脾有一味重要的药，就是白术，所以土部方药就以白术为代表。

白术、苍术，《神农本草经》笼统的都叫作术。其实白术和苍术还是有区别的，所以我们先讲白术，再讲苍术，以此继续扩展，引出一批健脾的药。因为脾主运化，这主要是中焦的运化。上焦、中焦、下焦都存在运化的过程，这个运化在很多地方又叫气化，上焦有气化，中焦有气化，下焦也有气化，随后我们还要讲很多气化的药。

化在中医里有很多种，比如化痰、化瘀、化湿、化积等，其实是在把异己的东西消灭掉，或者说把它变成对自己有用的东西。痰是人体生出来的，生出来以后它不参与正常生理活动，成了异己的东西，正常情况下人体会将其排出。比如喉咙里有一口痰，肯定是想把它咳出来吐掉，这就说明它是一个异己的东西，我们要把它排出来。还有化瘀血，血死了，行不动了，就成了瘀血，血本来是我们自己需要的，因为运化不动而成了瘀血，就不再是人体需要的了，就要把他排出去。所以人体之所以会有痰和瘀，很大程度上都是因为运化的能力不行了。

运化的能力好，你会把异己的东西（食物）变成自己的东西（气血）；运化的能力不好，你会把本该属于自己的东西也给丢了，使其变成异己的东西。气、血都是我们需要的东西，但由于运化不好，气行不通生了痰，血行不成了瘀，水行不通就成了湿。水也应该行得通的，我们到自然界里面去看，比如说，大晴天的，我们到一块草坪上去能感觉到湿的吗？感觉不到。躺在草地上也不会弄湿身子，但草坪里面是有水的，自然界就需要这种状态的水，它有湿度，但不是潮湿。如果是一潭死水行不通了，就成了湿，人也是这样的。

痰、瘀、湿、积等异物，都是因为我们的运化能力不行而导致。因此往往在化痰、化瘀、化湿、消积的过程中，都要注意中焦脾胃，要健脾以增强自身运化能力，不能只用化痰、化瘀的药，而不注重中焦的运化功能。

当然前面讲的气行不通，血行不通，是指气运行得不到位，血行不通就是血运行得不到位。比如心肾不交导致失眠，只是心肾交得不到位。还有，中医所说的肝不藏魂，也是说肝藏魂藏得不到位，即使是不到位也有轻重之分。最轻微的肝不藏魂就是睡觉睡的不踏实、不安稳、多梦；严重一点，他老说梦话；再严重，他醒着也说梦话。什么人醒着也说梦话呢？疯子。他自己控制不住自己。

模糊表述与理解运化

中医没有一个绝对精确的表述。不光是中医，其他地方的表述也是不够精确。学中医的时候，很多东西需要配合着理解，看很多医案，比如说某个鼓胀或中风，也就写一个方子。这一个方子怎么能把人家那么大的病治好呢？分明不是的。每个病都是有一个治疗过程的。一开始先要把这个病控制住，然后怎么治这个病，怎么病变药变，病好后还有一个善后的过程。所以，治病是有一个过程的，但是一般的医书不可能把整个过程全写写下来。写医案的人就像我们做数学笔记，把最关键的记下来，至于具体的演算过程就不记了。如果不配合着去理解，你觉得那么大的病就这样一诊，就这一个方子就够用了，从这个角度理解那它就是错的。所以说，书不存在对错，只有读书人存在对错。

还有，我们听到一句话，也需要去运化，理解也是一种运化的过程。听到任何问题、任何话你都要去运化它。有些话可能你听得有些逆耳，不太同意，但是你只要运化一下，吸收里边对你有用的东西，或者有些东西激发了你的一些想法。如果你拒绝运化，马上就排斥，就好比吃下去的东西不消化，然后又呕了出来；又如你看一本书，没有把内容消化好，就匆匆忙忙地讲出来。所以我们学一个东西，看一个东西，都需要运化，这样就比较完善了。

白术、苍术，尤其是白术，它通过健脾增强人体的运化能力。再讲一些化瘀的、化痰的、消瘀的、开窍之类的药。这类的药一方面在给人体的运化开辟道路，扫除障碍；另一方面也能促进人体的运化。

Chapter 2 Baizhu (White Atractylodes Rhizome)

Medical Properties of Baizhu

Rectangular Stem Enters the Middle Jiao

Baizhu is a perennial herb and its root can be used as medicine. The root of Baizhu is lumpish and the stem is in a rectangular shape.

Rectangular stem as medicine can enter the spleen. Generally, for any plants, if the roots take rectangular shape, when used as medicine, they could surely go to the Middle Jiao, going to the spleen to aid T&T function.

In addition to Baizhu, Huoxiang (ageratum) also has a rectangular stem. There are two types of Huoxiang, i. e., the common Huoxiang and Guang Huoxiang. Guang Huoxiang refers to ageratum (produced in Guang Dong and Guang Xi provinces of China), whose efficacy is of the best. The stem of Guang Huoxiang is rectangular, too. Thus, it can enter the Middle Jiao and can transform and clear damp-heat.

Skills about Collecting Herbs

On mountains, one can see various herbs that he might have never seen before. What should he do then? He can learn the properties of each herb through observation and tasting, and then find its therapeutic efficacy. That is a quite special skill for collecting herbs. In ancient times, doctors collected the right herbs for the right time and the local conditions from mountains for their patients.

Experience and observation can help the herbal collectors to understand the properties of herbs, for instance, both Baizhu and Huoxiang have rectangular stems, but Baizhu is less aromatic than Huoxiang in scent. Huoxiang goes to the body surface and enters the Middle Jiao because of its strong aromatic property and rectangular stem. Thus, Huoxiang is an effective herb to resolve dampness. Baizhu, on the other hand, is less aromatic with less flavor and strong taste, plus its rectangular stem, so Baizhu enters the body's interior.

Similarly, for treatment of diseases, doctors may seldom encounter the same case with the exact symptoms as recorded in *Shanghan Lun*. Hence, doctors must observe the case carefully and treat diseases based on syndrome differentiation, rather than copy the formulas in **Shanghan Lun**. The same is true to collecting herbs.

Now treatment of diseases is still done based on syndrome differentiation, but how about collecting herbs? Now fewer people have the right skills to collect herbs based on syndrome differentiation. Most of the TCM doctors are limited by the herbs recorded. However, diseases are constantly changing with various forms, so one should not be limited to the herbs in **Shennong Bencao Jing** (**Shen Nong's Herbal Classic**), but observe and experience the herbal properties and collect right herbs for the right time and the local conditions.

While collecting herbs, one should know that the sweet herbs can enter the spleen; the yellow-colored herbs are subsumed to the spleen (the earth); and the herbs with rectangular stem, like Baizhu, suggests that it can enter the spleen. With such understanding of comparative state (pharmacological method state) in mind, one can collect herbs wherever he or she is around the world, even if in a place where he or she has no idea about the herbs available, he or she still can identify its therapeutic efficacies of each herb based on its growing environment, along with its properties, color, appearance, smell and taste.

This is how the well-known TCM doctors have been practicing since the ancient time. The written dosage in the book is for reference only. They can use other herbs to substitute herbs unavailable at the time of writing prescriptions with the dosage adjusted according to the quality of the herbs.

Tonifying the Spleen and Resolving Dampness

Baizhu is collected in winter and it can enter the spleen and stomach channels to "tonify the earth-spleen and resolve dampness". To tonify the earth-spleen means to strengthen the spleen for its T&T functions. According to the **Wuxing Doctrine**, the earth restricts fluid. Thus, the earth-spleen can transport and transform fluid-dampness.

The soil/earth absorbs rain and becomes moist, but not to the point that this moistness becomes dampness. Small rain moistens plants but does not turn the soil into mud. That is the optimal moisture for the plants to grow, and also the optimal moisture that the earth-spleen needs. Heavy and continuous rain will turn the soil into mud. Many plants require moist soil, but cannot survive in the mud. Therefore, the spleen dislikes dampness. The spleen needs moisture but not dampness, as each and every thing has its own threshold.

Earth can restrict fluid, and the earth-spleen can transform and transport fluid-dampness. However, in case there is too much fluid, the function of this restriction cycle will fail. So, the spleen dislikes dampness.

Baizhu is bitter, sweet, warm, and pungent in tastes and properties. Bitter taste makes it have the function of drying dampness. So, the bitterness in the taste of Baizhu acts to dry the dampness that the spleen rejects. Sweet taste enters the spleen to satisfy the spleen because the spleen prefers sweetness. Baizhu is warm in property and the "spleen is a moistened soil, and it will start to carry on its T&T functions in the warm condition". So, it can be seen that the properties enjoyed by Baizhu: bitterness, sweetness and warmth work together to meet with what the spleen prefers.

Baizhu is aromatic in scent, so it can refresh the spleen as it provides the spleen with what it prefers, while the other herbs do not. For example, Huoxiang has a rectangular stem, but it is not sweet. Comparing with Baizhu, Huoxiang has less potency for tonifying the spleen. As a medicine, the whole Huoxiang plant is used, especially the parts above the ground. But for Baizhu, only the root is used as medicine. This creates another difference between the two herbs. Both Huoxiang and Baizhu have rectangular stems, but they can be differentiated from the parts that are used as medicines, the shape, the scents, and tastes.

Processing of Baizhu

Fresh Baizhu root has whitish juice when it is cut apart. The root is soft after being dried up either in the sun or in a cool place. Baizhu bought from markets is often very dry, but it will become soft again after certain time.

Raw Baizhu is often used when the spleen Yin is in deficiency with endogenous fire. However, it is difficult to get raw Baizhu but usually only fried Baizhu available in the pharmacy. In such a case, some other herbs available may be used instead for treating the endogenous fire.

Raw Baizhu has a thick viscosity. It can slow down the circulation of Qi and result in Qi obstruction. In order to prevent Qi obstruction and stagnation, raw Baizhu can be used in combination with Fuling and Chenpi. Chenpi harmonizes the stomach and regulates Qi, and Fuling can alleviate fluid retention whilst purging the spleen Qi. What if Chenpi and Fuling are not appropriate to use for the patient? One can slice the raw Baizhu and soak it in rice-rinsed water/fluid (water used to rinse rice before the rice is cooked). Once the white pulp is fully diffused out, dry it in a cool place. This processing method is usually used in the southern areas of China. I have never seen this method performed in the north of China. Baizhu has severe dryness property that may be intensified after it is parched. Therefore, the parched Baizhu is not appropriate for patients with endogenous fire. The rinsed Baizhu no longer has the capacity to cause Qi stagnation and becomes more moistening. Such a moistening property enhances the capacity of Baizhu to nourish the spleen Yin. In the north of China, the parched Baizhu is commonly used. However, such Baizhu is parched with earth since earth is neutral and enters the Middle Jiao.

Two-way Regulation of Tonifying the Spleen

Baizhu has the double functions of both inducing and reducing sweat. It reduces sweat in case that the patient is suffering from abnormal sweating; and it induces sweat in case that the patient is not sweating normally. Therefore, Baizhu has two-way regulating functions.

All herbs that have two-way regulating functions can enter the Middle Jiao, enjoying T&T capacities. For example, **Xiaochaihu Tang** has a lot of two-way regulating functions. It enters the Shaoyang meridian and goes to gallbladder meridian. Anyway, each herb in the formula should be analyzed: Chaihu (radix bupleuri) enters the liver and gallbladder; Huangqin (scutellaria baicalensis) is often said to enter the Upper Jiao and the lung. However, as Huangqin is yellow in color, it also enters the Middle Jiao and the spleen; Renshen (ginseng) enters the Middle Jiao doubtlessly, so does Banxia. Overall, in this formula, most of the ingredient herbs enter the Middle Jiao and have a two-way regulating function.

The two-way regulating function of Baizhu on sweating is achieved by tonifying the spleen. Once the spleen is functioning properly, the human body will recover to the normal sweating condition.

Contraindications of Baizhu

Baizhu is used with a quite large dosage in some formulas, which in fact is inappropriate. Although Baizhu is seemingly neutral, there are some contraindications in many cases.

Patients with the kidney deficiency should take Baizhu with caution since the spleen-earth restricts the kidney-fluid. When the spleen-earth is over consolidated, it can even more restrict the kidney-fluid, resulting in further kidney deficiency. For instance, Baizhu is not used in **Liuwei Dihuang Tang**. There are some exceptions, however, depending on the specific cases, for instance, Baizhu may be combined with Shengdi or Shudi.

Furthermore, Baizhu can obstruct the circulation of Qi. As mentioned before, this can be avoided by rinsing Baizhu in rice-rinsed water, or using it together with Fuling or Chenpi, or frying it. However, this property of Baizhu is not entirely inhibited, it is merely relatively reduced. Since Baizhu has the property of obstructing Qi circulation, it should not be used when there occurs exogenous pathogenic influence. Once the circulation of Qi is obstructed, the pathogenic factor is also trapped within the body and will be difficult to be dispersed out of the body.

Other troubles, such as ulcers and skin diseases, are in fact the clinical symptoms of Qi obstruction. The patient will suffer from pain in case the pathogenic factors stay on the body surface and is not properly dispersed. In that case, Huangqi is recommended. The efficacies of Huangqi include tonifying the spleen and Qi, promoting healing of ulcers, stopping sweating and consolidating the exterior. However, Huangqi does not block Qi. Therefore, Huangqi can be substituted for Baizhu to tonify the spleen and Qi when necessary, for example, in the case of skin diseases.

Baizhu is dry in property, and will remain slightly dry even after being rinsed. It surely benefits the patient who suffers from severe dampness. However, it is not suitable for those patients who are not suffering from dampness and whose tongue is slim and dry since such patients are in the condition of spleen Yin deficiency. In that case, Baizhu, if used, will worsen the spleen Yin deficiency.

In addition, Baizhu should be used with caution for patients who suffer from insomnia. For instance, when insomnia is due to liver Qi stagnation, resulting in irritation, which then worsens the liver Qi stagnation. Once the causes of such insomnia are diagnosed, doctors usually prescribe **Xiaoyao San** plus some herbs that can nourish the heart Yin. However, sometimes that treatment worsens the insomnia. Why is that so? Chaihu is ascending, due to which Qi is dispersed with the ascending effect. Furthermore, Baizhu is dry in property. When the kidney fluid loses its moistness, fire will stir up. The dryness of Baizhu aggravates the fire, resulting in worsening of insomnia. So, this should be taken into consideration in case the insomnia is not improved effectively in treatment.

Formulas Related to Baizhu

Zhizhu Pill

Baizhu can tonify the spleen, and its general efficacy is for ascending purpose. Therefore, it can be more effective for treatment of spleen Qi sinking, for which there is a famous formula called **Buzhong Yiqi Tang**. All ptosis taking place in any parts or organs in human body are generally attributed to the failure of the spleen Qi to ascend. The main efficacy of **Buzhong Yiqi Tang** is to upbear the spleen Qi, so many ingredient herbs used in **Buzhong Yiqi Tang** are for the purpose of ascending of Qi. However, only promotion of the spleen Qi to ascent is not enough, and there should be a counteractive action to balance the ascending effect as well. The stomach dominates descending. Transformation in the Middle Jiao is done through the interaction of the ascending of the spleen Qi and the descending of the stomach Qi. The famous formula of **Zhizhu Wan** includes Baizhu and Zhike (fructus aurantii), in which Baizhu is for ascending purpose while Zhike is for descending purpose, satisfying the spleen and the stomach respectively. Therefore, this formula is used to regulate the ascending of the spleen Qi and descending of the stomach Qi. In fact, there are different versions for this formula of **Zhizhu Wan**. The formula is named after the above two main ingredient herbs. As for some other ingredient herbs, it varies according to the specific cases.

Use of a fixed formula with fixed herbs is like narrowing ones thinking to a frame. I prefer to analyze formulas with fewer ingredient herbs. Especially, the typical formulas with two ingredient herbs are particularly worth spending time in analyzing them in details. Normally, TCM holds the idea that formulas with three ingredient herbs represent the sky, earth and human respectively; formulas with four ingredient herbs represent the four seasons and a complete life cycle (sprouting, growing, harvesting and storing) or the monarch- minister- assistant-envoy respectively; formulas with five ingredient herbs represent a complete five properties cycle (sprouting, growing, transforming, harvesting and storing respectively); formulas with six ingredient herbs represent a complete Six Yáo (which, in the *Book of Changes*, refers to the symbols "- -"); formulas with seven ingredient herbs represent a complete cycle of seven days of a week; and formulas with eight ingredient herbs incorporate the eight Guà (refers to a divinatory symbol). The more ingredient herbs a formula has, the less worthy it may become for analyses. One should value formulas with fewer ingredient herbs since he or she can form big formulas based upon them. Obviously one can prescribe a large formula in clinical practice either because of the practitioner's experience or unnecessary addition to the formula. While in study, the TCM learners should begin with the smaller formulas.

We will therefore start with **Zhizhu Tang** for discussion of Baizhu. **Zhizhu Tang** is often modified according to specific cases. For instance, Fuzi (radix aconiti carmichaeli), Rougui (cassia bark), Ganjiang (rhizoma zingiberis) can be added when the coldness symptom is severe; or Huanglian (coptis chinensis) can be added in the formula when the heat symptom is severe since Huanglian enters the Middle Jiao. Other herbs, such as Maidong (radix ophiopogonis), Lugen (rhizoma phragmitis) and so on can also be added to this formula according to the specific symptoms. In case the descending of the stomach Qi is severely impaired, Zhishi (fructus aurantii immaturus) should be used; in case stomach Qi descending is not so severely impaired, Zhike (fructus aurantii) may be used instead; in case dampness symptom is severe, Cangzhu (rhizoma atractylodis) should be used. However, if dampness symptom is not severe, Baizhu may be used. A simple formula, **Zhizhu Tang** suggests that two different Zhu (atractylodes) can be used in combination, telling us that the spleen dominates the ascending and the stomach dominates the descending, for which herbs should be chosen accordingly.

Overall, Baizhu is inclined to a tonifying efficacy. It targets the deficiency of the spleen and stomach. Baizhu should not be used in case there is an excessive syndrome (a physically strong patient is running a high fever or suffering from such disorders as blood stasis or constipation) . The so-called deficiency refers to that of the healthy Qi, for which Baizhu can be employed for tonifying use. However, if pathogenic Qi is too vigorous or there arises excessive pathogen, Baizhu should be used with caution, or especially, stop using Baizhu when the patient is suffering from vomiting, diarrhoea and/or abdominal distension due to the excessive pathogenic factor(s) . Otherwise, Baizhu would worsen the syndromes.

Sijunzi Tang

Sijunzi Tang amplifies the function of Baizhu.

Sijunzi Tang contains the ingredient herbs of Renshen (ginseng), Baizhu (white atractylodes rhizome), Fuling (poria cocos), and Gancao(liquorice) .

Sijunzi Tang is a major formula for tonifying Qi. Many formulas are made based on modification of this formula. Renshen and Baizhu tonify the spleen. Fuling and Gancao enter the Middle Jiao. Therefore, this formula supports the point of view "to tonify the spleen means to tonify the Qi'. Although this view is perhaps slightly imprecise, it is helpful for understanding.

Regarding **Sijunzi Tang**, Renshen is said to be the monarch herb. In fact, the monarch-minister-assistant-envoy in TCM are not fixed. I prefer to take Baizhu as the monarch herb in this formula. Baizhu can tonify Qi, too, but only it is not so strong as Renshen. Renshen reinforces the efficacy of Baizhu of tonifying Qi. Baizhu also transforms dampness, although its capacity to resolve dampness is not so strong as its Qi tonifying function. Therefore, Fuling is used to intensify the effect of Baizhu on transforming dampness. Baizhu tonifies the spleen, yet it is not as strong as Gancao in this regard. Therefore, Gancao, too, strengthens the spleen-tonifying effect of Baizhu. **Sijunzi Tang** can be taken as a formula that tonifies the spleen (the source of Qi and blood generation and transformation). Hence, once the spleen is healthy, there will not arise the problem Qi deficiency.

Sijunzi Tang with Chenpi and Banxia added can reduce phlegm and break blood stasis. **Erchen Tang** is composed of Chenpi and Banxia, and it is the primary formula used to reduce phlegm. Phlegm forms when the spleen is in deficiency. In this case, it is necessary to reduce the phlegm in order to clear the channel for Qi, which in turn improves Qi and blood generation and transformation. Chenpi regulates Qi circulation and harmonizes the stomach. Banxia calms down the adverse-rising energy and harmonizes the stomach, especially for the treatment of Qi adverse-rising of the stomach.

Qi deficiency is often accompanied by Qi stagnation. In fact, Qi deficiency means the insufficiency of Qi, and Qi stagnation means Qi is blocked by phlegm. **Sijunzi Tang** should be used to tonify Qi in case that Qi deficiency arises. Chenpi and Banxia should be used to resolve the phlegm due to Qi deficiency. What should be done in case that there arises the false deficiency of Qi, which is the blockage of Qi due to phlegm retention? Use Muxiang (costustoot) rather than some other aromatic herbs to regulate Qi since Muxiang enters all the Tri-jiao (the Upper, Middle and Lower Jiao). Muxiang can be used to regulate Qi regardless of the location of Qi stagnation in any of the three Jiao. In addition, Sharen (fructus amomi) should be used as it can dredge the primordial Qi of the spleen and the kidney, purges the stagnation and disperses Qi. These herbs, combined with **Sijunzi Tang**, make a new formula called **Xiangsha Liujunzi Tang**, which tonifies the spleen, reduces phlegm, disperses Qi and resolves blood stasis.

Lizhong Tang

There exists only one herbal ingredient difference between **Lizhong Tang** (Decoction for Regulating the Middle Jiao) and **Sijunzi Tang**. **Sijunzi Tang** contains Renshen (ginseng), Baizhu (white atractylodes rhizome), Fuling (poria cocos) and Gancao (liquorice), while Lizhong Tang contains Renshen (ginseng), Baizhu (white atractylodes rhizome), Ganjiang (rhizoma zingiberis) and Gancao (liquorice). In these formulas, Renshen, Baizhu and Gancao are essential. Fuling should be used in case there is severe dampness. Ganjiang should be used when the syndrome involves coldness.

"The spleen is taken as the moist earth, so it begins to carry on its transformation function when in warmth". Ganjiang warms the Middle Jiao. Transformation will proceed well once the Middle Jiao is warm. Fuzi can be added when Ganjiang is not sufficient to warm the Middle Jiao. Fuzi has a powerful warming function and enters all parts of the body. It warms the spleen when it is matched with herbs that enter the spleen. Fuzi also enters the kidney, especially when its dosage is large or if it is decocted for a long period of time. For example, the dosage of Fuzi in **Fuzi Lizhong Tang** is usually relatively large. Or if it is decocted for long time, it will enter the kidney, then promoting the spleen through the kidney.

In addition to Renshen, Baizhu and Gancao, Fuling is used in case there is dampness; or Ganjiang is used in case there is coldness; or both Fuzi and Ganjiang are used in case the coldness is severe. From here, the logic behind the classic formulas can be understood. Anyhow, one should try the best to understand the principles adopted in the classic formulas rather than rigidly confine oneself to the classic formulas only. Once the learners have mastered the principles and rules in TCM, they may also be able to make classic prescriptions by themselves.

Wuling San

Wuling San contains the ingredient herbs of Fuling (poria cocos), Zhuling (grifola), Zexie (rhizoma alismatis), Gui (cassia), Baizhu (white atractylodes rhizome).

Wuling San is a formula for removing dampness through diuresis. Why is Baizhu used in this formula?

Fuling, Zhuling and Zexie are all used for relieving fluid retention. Fuling removes the dampness retention in the spleen, while Zhuling and Zexie remove the dampness retention in the kidney. Gui can be either Guizhi (cassia twig) or

Rougui (cassia bark). Use Guizhi in case the cold pathogen has obstructed the body surface since the obstruction can impair Qi transformation in the Foot Taiyang channel. Or if there is no exogenous pathogenic influences, Rougui is used to give a treatment of deficiency due to coldness in the Lower Jiao and the improper Qi transformation in the kidney channel. Baizhu promotes Qi transformation of the spleen, then helping to remove fluid retention. The proper Qi transformation can help remove fluid and then let it flow out easily through the bladder. Such Qi transformation is not that of the bladder itself but of the overall body. This means any impairment of Qi transformation in any part of the body can potentially affect fluid metabolism. Therefore, Baizhu is used to tonify the spleen in order to promote the overall Qi transformation. Rougui or Guizhi is used to promote the Qi transformation in the kidneys and bladder. Once the kidneys Qi and spleen Qi are moving properly, the dampness will be eliminated more easily.

As mentioned above, the kidney deficiency refers to the deficiency of the healthy Qi. When there is vigorous pathogenic Qi, Baizhu would be an appropriate choice, as the proverb says that earth can be used to bridle water flood whenever it comes. Baizhu not only can promote Qi transformation but also help remove the fluid retention. Guizhi and Baizhu in **Wuling San** play the function of promoting Qi transformation.

This also suggests two techniques for prescribing herbs. First, once the disease is correctly diagnosed, the herbs to be selected should not go against the diagnosed diseases. Second, it is important to strengthen Qi transformation. As it is well-known that Fuling, Zhuling and Zexie are effective for relieving fluid retention. However, in many cases, they are not so effective, indicating that Qi transformation is very critical. **Wuling San** modified by adding Baizhu or Cangzhu and Guizhi or Rougui can promote Qi transformation of the spleen and kidney to an extent of twofold results with half the effort in the respect of relieving fluid retention. Some herbs directly target the disease symptom itself, accompanied by some other herbs for Qi transformation. Both aspects should be addressed in order to achieve the maximum therapeutic effect.

第二章　白术

白术药性解

方茎走中焦

白术是一种多年生的草本植物，根部入药。白术的根是成块状的，茎是方的。

方茎能通脾。只要植物的茎是方的，那么它肯定能走中焦，能够通脾，助运化。

方茎的还有藿香。藿香分为普通藿香与广藿香。广藿香就是广东、广西产的藿香，作用最好。广藿香的茎就是方的，能够走中焦，清化湿热。

采药的功夫

如果我们去采药，山上草木各种各样的，可能很多是你不认识的。那怎么办？即使你不认识这个东西，也要体察物性，去观察、去品尝，然后确定这个东西到底该如何用。这是采药的比较高的境界。古时医生都会亲自给病人采药治病，会因时制宜、因地制宜。

我们还可以继续体察，同样是方茎的，白术的香味要弱一些，藿香的香味强烈一些。香味强烈就会走表，方茎入中焦，既走脾胃又走表，那化湿的作用就很好。白术芳香弱一些，气比较轻、味比较重，再加上它的根入药，所以它是往里走的。

看病也是这样。很少有一个病是规规矩矩、老老实实，就跟《伤寒论》写的一模一样的在那里等着你去治，等着你去用《伤寒论》里边的大青龙汤、小青龙汤。没有这么规矩的病。你还是需要观察这个病，辨证论治。采药也是这样的，所以采药看病都需要功夫。

现在看病依然在讲辨证论治。而采药呢？懂这个的人就越来越少了。中药成了一个僵死的学问，局限于具体多少味药。病是千变万化的，药也是千变万化的，并不只是《神农本草经》上列的那些药，它那些药也是一些例子。我们能采得到就采，采不到我们再体察物性，然后因时制宜、因地制宜地来用药，能采到什么药就用什么药。

我们采药的时候，遇到甘甜的，就知道它能入脾；遇到黄色，也知道它属于脾土；如果看到它的茎是方的，像白术那样，也提示它入脾。其余以此类推。有了这种取象比类的思维，我们即使到了南美热带雨林里，你也能采到治病的药。即使所有的植物你都不认识，也能根据那个地方的天地、环境，再根据这些植物的性质、颜色、形状、气味，仔细的辨别，就会知道它到底治什么病，到底在什么时候可以用。

自古大医用药，都是这样用的，但他在写书的时候，写到白术多少、地黄多少、生姜多少，都是代表方剂、参考剂量，在具体的方子里，没有这个药，可以用那个来代替；这个药品质好，可以少用点，那个药品质差，可以多用些，这种灵活变通的能力，现在很少有人能做到了。

补土除湿

白术是冬季采，入脾经和胃经，它的作用可以用"补土除湿"来概括。补土就是补脾，脾土是主运化的，土克水，脾土能够运化水湿。

下雨了，土吸收了雨水，就变成了湿土，但又不是太湿。如果雨不大，下到庄稼地里刚刚把土润湿，土没有变成泥，而是一种很松、很软、很滋润的土，很适合作物的生长。这是脾土最佳的状态。如果雨下得过多了，土就更加潮湿，变成了泥巴，这样就不好了。很多植物适合在潮湿的土壤里边生长，在泥里它反而不能生长，这就叫脾恶湿。脾需要湿但又不需要太湿，任何事情都要有一个限度。

土克水，脾土能够运化水湿，但是如果水太多了它就克不动了，所以脾又恶湿。

白术的性味是苦、甘、温，气是辛香的。苦能燥湿，脾恶湿，正好用苦味来燥湿。甘味是入脾的，脾喜欢甘甜的味道。白术是温性的，"脾为湿土，得温则运"，脾喜欢温的，正好白术的苦、甘、温的性质都是脾喜欢的。

白术的气是芳香的，芳香可以醒脾。白术之所以能健脾，是因为它对脾可以说是投其所好，送其所要。脾喜欢什么，它就给脾什么。其他的药则不同，如藿香虽然也是方茎，但它没有甘甜的味道，补脾的能力要稍微弱一些。不补，它与白术的性质有天壤之别了。又因为藿香是全草入药，主要用地上的部分，包括茎、叶，白术是根入药，全草入药与根入药，又不一样。虽然都是方茎的，它们又可以从入药的部位、形状、气味上来进行区分。

白术的炮制

新挖出来的生白术，把它切开，里边有白色的浆汁，直接晾干或者晒干，它还容易软。买到的生白术一般都会很干燥，但放一段时间，一回潮它就软了。

一般脾阴不足而且有火，经常要用生白术。药店里边现在可能都抓不到生白术，只能抓到炒白术，实在抓不到生白术，你就不用。有火怎么办呢？可以再配别的药。药是死的，人是活的。

生白术有粘滞性，容易滞气。用了生白术，又怕它闭气，可以配上茯苓、陈皮。陈皮是和胃理气的，茯苓能够利水，也是宣通脾气的。有火，又怕它滞气，又不想用陈皮和茯苓，那怎么办呢？你可以把生白术放在淘米水里漂。白术先切成片，然后泡在淘米水里，把里边的白浆全部漂出来，再把它晾干。这叫漂白术，南方有，北方没有见过。因为白术本身就有一定的燥烈之性，一炒就更燥烈了，体内有火的人会受不了，所以就用漂白术。漂白术不滞气，还有滋润性，能养脾阴。北方一般都是用炒白术，就是用土炒的白术，土性平和，而且是入中焦的。

健脾的双向调节作用

白术还有发汗的作用，其实它不仅能发汗，它还能收汗。当汗太多的时候，它能把汗收回去一些；当不出汗的时候，白术又能发汗，它有双向调节的作用。

凡是对人体机能具有双向调节作用的药，往往都是入中焦的，都是有运化能力的。比如，小柴胡汤对人体也有很多双向调节作用的。它走少阳，走胆。我们不要把一个方子孤立起来看，我们看小柴胡汤的药物组成，柴胡是入肝入胆；黄芩呢？你能说它就是走上焦入肺的吗？不一定，黄芩的黄就是入脾的，也会走中焦；人参肯定走中焦不用说了；半夏也走中焦。所以小柴胡汤它为什么能够主半表半里，为什么有那么多的双向调节的作用呢？因为其中走中焦的药还是非常多。当然这话不严谨，但对我们会有很多启发。

白术对汗有双向调节作用，依然是靠健脾，脾一健运，汗自然就恢复正常了。

白术使用禁忌

白术在很多处方里用量较大，这是误区，白术这味药似乎很平和，但它也有很多禁忌，很多情况下是不能乱用的。

肾虚之人，慎用白术。因为土克水。把土培养得太强大了，就更加克水，肾就越来越虚。六味地黄汤一般就不用白术，当然这也不是太绝对的。白术配生地或熟地，这也是一种配伍，也是可以用的，这是要根据具体情况来看的。

还有，白术有个特点就是闭气。前面虽然说过，用淘米水去泡，就不闭气了；或者加上茯苓、陈皮就不闭气了；炒了，就不闭气了。其实闭不闭气，不是非此即彼，这些方法，只不过是让白术闭气的力度小了一点。既然闭气，所以感冒有表邪就不要用白术这类的药。气机闭住了，邪气就不容易透散。

还有一些溃疡、皮肤病之类的，其实就是气闭。邪气在体表，没有很好透散，就会痛，这时候不如用黄芪。黄芪的作用，不但能够补脾益气，还能托疮生肌、收汗固表，黄芪不闭气，白术闭气，遇到这种皮肤病非得健脾益气时，用黄芪代替白术。

白术性质是燥的，即使是漂白术，还是偏燥。湿气重，用了当然好；如果湿气不重，舌头伸出来小小的、干干的，用它就不好了。病人本身就脾阴虚，用白术脾阴就更虚了。

还有失眠的人要慎用白术，比如肝郁失眠，失眠就烦，烦就更加肝郁，肝郁气滞，辨证都准确了，普通的大夫会用逍遥散加些养心阴的药，这是常规的思路，有时候越喝这个越睡不着觉，为什么呢？柴胡是升散的，神气随着这个药升散掉了；白术是燥性的，"水流湿，火就燥"，一燥，火就越来越大，越是让人睡不着觉。遇到失眠，如果治疗起来没有疗效，可以从这些方面去考虑。

白术相关方剂

枳术丸

白术能健脾，从整体上讲它的作用是往上升的，所以当脾气下陷的时候，用白术会比较好。治疗脾气下陷，有一个很有名的方子，叫补中益气汤，身体各部位的一切下垂，都是因为脾不能升。补中益气汤主要是升提脾气，所以其中很多药都是往上升的。但脾也不能一味地往上升，有升就得有降。上升，把水谷之精微往上带到肺里，再由肺来播撒到全身，但不能光升不降，什么在降呢？胃主降。在一升一降中，脾和胃完成了中焦运化这个艰巨的任务。体现在药上，有一个很有名的方子叫枳术汤，一味枳壳，一味白术。术是往上升的，枳是往下降的，正好适应了脾升胃降的这种格局，所以这个方子是用来调节脾胃的升降的。枳术汤也有多种版本，因这两味药，就叫枳术汤，至于后面应该加什么药，可根据具体情况而加，就不把它们固定在一个方子里了。

把很多的药固定到一个方子里，就等于把自己的思维固定到一个框架里面了，所以我们讲方子的时候，喜欢讲药味比较少的。两味药组一个方子，值得大讲特讲，因为它有典型性。三味药组一个方子这是天地人；四味药组一个方子是一年四季，生长收藏、君臣佐使；五味药组一个方子，那是生长化收藏，走完了五行；六味药的方子走的是六爻；七味药的方子走完了七日的一个来复；八味药的方子则合八卦；再更多的药的方子，可以就说不用那么太值得重视了。我们要重视小方子，再根据这些小方子，来组成大方子。船小好掉头。当然，在临床上你能开出一个大方子，这可能是你的功夫，也可能是你在堆砌；在学习当中，咱们还是从小方子入手。

所以我们在讲白术的时候，首先讲枳术汤。当然，枳术汤也是可以变化的，如果寒象重，可以加附子、肉桂、干姜之类；如果热象重，可以加黄连，因为黄连也是走中焦的，还可以加麦冬、芦根之类；如果是胃气不降很严重，枳可以是枳实，如果没那么严重，枳可以是枳壳；如果湿象特别重，术可以是苍术，如果湿像没那么重，术又可以是白术。一个枳术汤，就提示这两个术可以一块用，提示脾主升胃主降，用药根据具体的情况来选择。

从整体来讲，白术是偏补的药，它能治脾胃的虚，如果是实症的话，就不能用它了。虚就是正气虚，白术能补正气虚。如果邪气太旺、邪气实，那么用白术就要注意了，因为实邪引起的呕吐、拉肚子、腹胀，就千万不要用白术。此时它是有实邪，白术一补，邪气就更加厉害。病不但不好，反而更加严重。

四君子汤
四君子汤这个方子，是把白术的作用放大了。

四君子汤：

人参、白术、茯苓、甘草。

它是补气的主方，很多方子都是由它演变而成的。人参补脾、白术补脾，茯苓、甘草都是走中焦的。所以，应了那句话："补气就是补脾。"这句话有点不严谨，但我这么一说你那么一听，帮助理解，理解了就可以把它忘了，过了河可以拆桥。这桥虽然修得不漂亮，但它能帮我们过河，这才是最重要的。

四君子汤里，有人说人参是补气的，是君药，其实，君臣佐使是没有固定的。我更倾向于把白术做君药：白术也补气，只是补气的力度没有人参那么强。加人参，把白术补气的作用放大；白术也可以化湿，但化湿的力度还不够大，加茯苓利湿，把白术化湿的力度放大；白术还可以补脾，但补脾的力度没有甘草强，再加甘草把白术补脾的力量放大。我们可以把四君子汤理解为健脾的方。脾为气血生化之源，脾健运好了，就不愁气虚啦。

四君子汤再加上陈皮、半夏，就具有消导、化痰的意思。陈皮、半夏就是二陈汤，是化痰的主方。脾虚就生痰，生痰就要化痰，把痰化掉，道路扫清，气血生化的能力也就更强了；陈皮理气和胃，半夏降逆和胃的，如果胃气逆，就更适用。

气虚还往往伴随着气郁。气虚就是气少了，气郁就是气被痰堵住了。气虚就用四君子补气；气一虚它又生了痰，再用陈皮、半夏化痰。因为有痰，气被堵住了，导致了气虚的假象，那怎么办呢？先要把气理过来，再加木香。为什么要用木香而不用别的芳香药呢？因为木香不但走中焦而且通三焦，三焦哪一焦的气有阻滞，都可以用木香来通。砂仁能通脾肾之元气，开郁宣气。这就成了香砂六君子汤，健脾化痰，行气解郁。

理中汤

理中汤跟四君子汤只差一味药，四君子汤是参、术、苓、草，理中汤是参、术、姜、草。参、术、草是必用的，如果湿重，就加茯苓；如果有寒象，就加干姜。

"脾为湿土，得温则运。"干姜是温中焦的，中焦温了，运化自然就好了。如果觉得加干姜还不够温，那就再加点附子。附子大热，通行全身，跟着走脾的药就主要温脾。附子还能入肾，尤其是量大的时候，它马上就往肾里走，或者熬药的时间长的话，也会往肾里走。像附子理中汤中附子的量一般稍微大点，或者熬的时间长点，它就会往肾里边走，形成肾火生脾土的局面。

在人参、白术、甘草的基础上，有湿就加茯苓，有寒就加干姜，寒重就加附子，附子、干姜一块用。所以，经方是很有道理的。但我们不要局限于经方，更重要的是要从经方里面去找它的规律，找它的道理。规律和道理找到了，然后我们的每一个方子也都可以说是经方。我们应该追求这样的境界。

五苓散

茯苓、猪苓、泽泻、桂、白术。

五苓散是一个利湿的方子，我们以后讲化湿的时候还要讲。今天我们主要讲五苓散中为什么要用白术。

茯苓、猪苓、泽泻，这三味药都是利水的，茯苓利脾里的水，猪苓、泽泻利肾的水。桂，当寒邪闭表，阻碍足太阳膀胱经气化的时候，就用桂枝；当没有外邪、下焦虚寒、肾经气化不利的时候，就用肉桂。白术则是促进脾的气化的。要利水，一定要促进气化，这样会事半功倍。且利出的水会从膀胱走，"气化则能出焉"。有气化，膀胱里面的水才能出来。这个气化并不是膀胱本身的气化，既然叫气化，那么全身都存在气化。这就意味着只要有一个地方气化不行，它就能影响全身，影响水液的排泄。所以用术健脾，促进全身的气化。用肉桂或桂枝促进肾和膀胱的气化。肾气、脾气通了，水湿也就容易利出来了。

肾虚是肾的正气虚，现在有水了，是邪气盛，当然用白术，水来土掩嘛，也有土克水的意思。白术不仅促进气化，更让水利出去。这是五苓散中用桂、术的意思，都是在气化上做文章。

这也提示了用药过程中的两个技巧。第一个，即使完全辨证对了，在药物的选择上，我们还是要注意，要丝丝入扣，不能选择与病有违背的药；还有一个，就是要促进气化。要利水，单纯利水，单用茯苓、猪苓、泽泻就够了。但是为什么很多情况下，用茯苓、猪苓、泽泻效果不好呢？气化很关键。五苓散加了术和桂，促进脾和肾的气化，利水就事半功倍。所以，有的药是直接治病的，有的药是促进人体气化的。两方面都要兼顾到，用药疗效才能得到很大提高。

Chapter 3   Cangzhu (Rhizoma Atractylodis)

Analyses of Medicinal Properties of Cangzhu

Similarities and Differences between Cangzhu and Baizhu

Cangzhu looks like Baizhu, yet they are quite different herbs.

Cangzhu is bitter, pungent, and sweet in tastes, and warm in property. It enters the meridians of the lung, spleen, stomach, large intestine, and small intestine. Cangzhu is aromatic in scent, and it can dry dampness and tonify the spleen. Cangzhu can also induce sweat. Cangzhu has the capacity to exorcise evil spirit because of its strong aromatic scent; and it can reduce phlegm because of its effect of tonifying the spleen. Cangzhu is much more aromatic than Baizhu (Baizhu is only slightly aromatic). The aromatic property is helpful for refreshing and tonifying the spleen. Overall, Baizhu is relatively mild while Cangzhu is much stronger and always has a quick effect in treatment. Baizhu has much more powerful effect for tonifying use than Cangzhu. In clinical practice, Cangzhu has no tonifying effect. In case of spleen deficiency accompanied with heavy dampness, Cangzhu and Baizhu can be used together.

"Tonifying the spleen to dry dampness" means that it has a stronger efficacy on tonifying the spleen than drying the dampness. It could also mean that Baizhu tonifies the spleen in order to dry the dampness. Cangzhu has a stronger potency for drying dampness comparing with that for tonifying the spleen. It also dries the dampness in order to tonify the spleen. Both Cangzhu and Baizhu can induce sweat, but Baizhu is weaker in this regard.

Cangzhu Dries Dampness

Cangzhu is an herb that can dry dampness. All the therapeutic effects of Cangzhu are involved with dampness. It can induce sweat. So, can it be used to induce sweat in a cold/flu? That is not necessarily the case. Cangzhu is used to induce sweat only when Qi circulation is obstructed or the pores are trapped due to dampness. According to **Shanghan Lun**, in case of external attacks, patients often suffer from adiaphoresis due to obstruction of the body surface by the cold pathogens. However, all pathogenic factors like wind, coldness, heat, dampness, dryness, and fire can block the sweating pores with only different degrees of severity. Both coldness and dampness are Yin pathogens that can block the pores. Hence, when the pores are blocked by cold pathogen, Mahuang (ephedra) and Suye (perilla leaf) can be used to induce sweat; and when the pores are blocked by damp pathogen, Cangzhu should be used to induce sweat.

Such description is seldom seen in books, so the learners need to understand the implied information behind the words. For example, in **Shanghan Lun**, it only discusses the pores being blocked by cold pathogens. But the TCM learners should think about what other pathogens can block the pores and inhibit perspiration. Dampness is one of such pathogens. Therefore, Cangzhu is used to induce sweat when the pores are blocked by dampness. Meanwhile, dampness can also cause flowing sweat, which may take place in case that damp-heat stays at the body surface, disturbing the harmony of the Ying (nourishment Qi) and Wei (defense Qi). In that case, Cangzhu is used since Cangzhu has a two-way regulating function of inducing sweat. Cangzhu accomplishes this target by both tonifying the spleen and drying dampness.

In clinical practice, one might find a prescription that he writes for a patient is effective, and then he might wonder which of the herbs in that prescription is responsible for such an effect. Such thinking is quite wrong. The effect of a prescription is not merely achieved through specific herbs, but the composition of all the herbal ingredients. Another case is that a patient has been taking herbal medicine for a certain time, but one day he might say to the doctor that the formula he just took is incredibly effective, and would ask the doctor to stick to the same formula. This thinking is also wrong.

Processing of Cangzhu

Cangzhu is a perennial herb. The top-grade Cangzhu is produced in Maoshan in Jiangsu province of China since Cangzhu grows there enjoys a sweet taste. As mentioned previously, Cangzhu is bitter, pungent, and sweet in tastes, which is stated based on the properties of Maoshan Cangzhu. Cangzhu produced in the

other places is much bitterer and pungent in tastes with less sweetness. Generally, bitterness and pungency are of much stronger tastes. It is better for an herb to
have the properties of both strength and mildness, which are the properties of
Cangzhu produced in Maoshan. Maoshan Cangzhu is small in size, thin but solid, oily and lubricating with hair on the surface. Therefore, it is also called Mao
(hairy) Cangzhu.

When Mao Cangzhu is sliced open, many red spots will be exposed on the
cross section, called Zhusha Dian (spot of oil cavity), indicating this herb can
enter the heart. It has been mentioned above that Cangzhu has some effects on
sweating. As it is known in TCM, sweat is the fluid of the heart, suggesting Cangzhu can enter the heart meridian. The heart governs fire; fire and earth promote
mutually. Cangzhu produced in Hubei province of China is second best in quality, but it is larger in size and has a more pungent taste with less sweetness. So,
this type of Cangzhu has less therapeutic effect as an oral medicine compared to
Mao Cangzhu. However, this does not necessarily mean that one should disregard
it completely. It can still be used in other ways, for example, to be used for per-
fume satchel. Even the Cangzhu produced in the north of China can also be used
in such a way.

As to the selection of herbs, it is better to choose the veritable medicines,
that is, the herbs with the most powerful effects. In case of unavailability of the
veritable medicines for the time being, the ordinary herbs may also be used. In
that case, the herbs should be processed for compatibility, of which the aim is to
suit the herbs to the therapeutic requirement. It is worthwhile to study the processing of Cangzhu. In the previous section, the rinsing method for Baizhu has
been mentioned, that is, using the rice-rinsing water. The same method may also
be used for Cangzhu, and it is better to process it with the rinsing water of glutinous rice. After rinsing, scrape off the skin layer and slice the rinsed Cangzhu.
And then, parch it with sesame seeds or sesame oil until the herb turns yellow or
brown. This processing method is rarely used these days, but it was a common
practice in ancient times. Cangzhu is very dry and strong, and sesame seeds are
moistening. The processed Cangzhu with sesame seeds (i. e. , using the corrigent
for treatment) can make Cangzhu become mild. Similarly, the rinsing water of

the glutinous rice is used for the same purpose. In such a way, one can take the advantage of the property of driness of Cangzhu, and on the other hand, he or she also controls its dryness within the acceptable range in order to suit the human body. In fact, processing of herbs is a challenging technique that must be handled carefully.

There is another processing method for Cangzhu, which is performed after White Dew (15th solar term) (name of season in lunar calendar, around September 7 or 8). Cangzhu is fully soaked in the rinsing water of glutinous rice and dried up on the rooftop day and night for one month, and let it absorb the moisture at night. After having been processed in such a way, it is named Shen Zhu (holy rhizoma atractylodis), which would have a stronger therapeutic effect. There is a famous formula named **Shenzhu San**, containing so-processed Cangzhu. **Shenzhu San** is **Pingwei San** plus Huoxiang (ageratum) and Sharen (fructus amomi). After White Dew, the nutrients of Cangzhu starts to condense in the roots. Hence, Cangzhu harvested after White Dew has more nutrients in its roots, making it more effective. After White Dew, Autumn Qi is dominant and there will be more dew. Dew is cooling and moistening. Cangzhu absorbs the nutrients of the rice and becomes mild once it is soaked in rice-rinsing water. It then absorbs Yang Qi of the sun during its exposure to the sun and the moisture of the dew at the night. It becomes less dry and more moistening. The roofs of houses in the past were constructed with tiles, which at least have two layers. One layer of the tiles is facing upward while the other layer is facing downwards. Meanwhile, tiles have good permeability and can screen the light of the sun. Cangzhu placed on the tile can absorb the human Qi in the house, too. By the way, try to avoid excessive exposure to rain. The herbs should be covered when it rains.

Pingwei San

Many formulas are involved with Cangzhu like **Pingwei San** (Stomach Harmonizing Powder) and **Sanmiao San**.

Analyses of Pingwei San Formula
Pingwei San contains the ingredient herbs of Cangzhu (rhizoma atractylo-

dis), Houpo (mangnolia officinalis), Chenpi (pericarpium citri reticulatae) and Gancao(liquorice)

Pingwei San is a commonly used formula, of which the monarch herb is Cangzhu. Just like **Siwu Tang** and Danggui (angelica sinensis), where **Siwu Tang** reinforces the function of Danggui. **Pingwei San** reinforces the function of Cangzhu. Cangzhu is aromatic and severely dry in property, and it can play both descending and ascending functions. Cangzhu also harmonizes the stomach and dries dampness. Houpo is added to enhance the drying and descending effects of Cangzhu. Houpo is also an aromatic herb that can transform dampness. Cangzhu is aromatic, drying, and slightly sweet. What if Cangzhu were not sweet? One can then add Gancao, which by nature is sweet. As **Pingwei San** acts to harmonize the stomach, Chenpi is used in the formula to regulate Qi and harmonizes the stomach. Therefore, using Houpo, Chenpi and Gancao with Cangzhu together can strengthen the function of Cangzhu. In clinical practice, **Pingwei San** is often used for the symptom of dampness. In case that there is necessity to break severe stagnation of Qi, Qingpi (the green tangerine peel) can be used instead of Chenpi. Cangzhu is substituted with Baizhu if and when there is spleen and stomach Yin deficiency accompanied by a slim tongue body and a dry tongue coating.

The spleen and stomach are subsumed to the earth. *Huangdi Neijing* (*the Internal Canon of Huangdi*) states that the heaving earth is called ' Dun Fu. "Fu" means mound. A city named "Fu Yang" in Anhui province of China tells us that on the south of the mound ("Yang" here refers "in the south"). "Bei Jian" is the term used for a concaved area of ground, or a sinking in the ground. On the mound, it is easier to be dry. Fluid always accumulates in the sinking/low places, where it is usually damp. Neither the mound nor the sinking is good. Therefore, it is necessary to even out and harmonize the surface in order to achieve a balanced state, that is, neither overly dry, nor overly fluid-filled and damp. This also applies to the spleen and stomach. It should not be well-distributed in terms of moistness. Whenever there is imbalance, it must be harmonized and regulated.

A large dosage of Lugen (rhizoma phragmitis), Yuzhu (radix polygonati officinalis), and Shanyao (Chinese yam) can be used to nourish spleen Yin when dryness occurs due to "Dun Fu"-mound influences. And if there arises dampness in the spleen and stomach due to the presence of the "Bei Jian"-sinking influences, then use herbs that can transform dampness to fill the "sinking". Once the "sinking" is filled up, the spleen will not accumulate dampness anymore even when it "rains". However, fluid may accumulate again in case that the dampness is removed without filling the "sinking". The function of **Pingwei San** is to fill/even out the "sinking" where it is prone to accumulate fluid. Now, it may be easier to understand the use of **Pingwei San**. It dries dampness and harmonizes the spleen and stomach in order to optimize their functions.

Xiangsha Pingwei San

There are many modifications of **Pingwei San**. For example, a famous formula named **Xiangsha Pingwei San** is an herbal powder with Xiang and Sha added on the basis of the formula of **Pingwei San**. Regarding the two additional herbs of **Xiang** and **Sha**, there is argument about what herbs they really refer to. Some people think they are **Muxiang (costustoot)** and **Sharen (fructus amomi)**, while some others think that they are **Xiangfu (rhizoma cyperi)** and **Sharen**. In fact, it depends upon the specific case. Sharen dries dampness, and it is inappropriate for those patients who are suffering from thirst and dry mouth since Sharen is aromatic and dry in nature, and too much Sharen can worsen the syndromes of thirst and dry mouth. Muxiang enters the Tri-jiao while Sharen enters the spleen and kidney and enters the Lower Jiao, too. Therefore, use Muxiang and Sharen in addition to **Pingwei San** when it is necessary for herbs to enter the Tri-jiao, the spleen and kidney; otherwise, use Xiangfu and Sharen in addition to **Pingwei San** when it is necessary for herbs to enter the liver, spleen, and kidney.

Some people claim that "**Xiangsha Pingwei San** can be prescribed for anyone". For example, when a patient comes up with a syndrome that cannot be diagnosed, but he insists on some medicines, for such a case, **Xiangsha Pingwei San** may be the proper formula to prescribe. This formula is mild and harmonizing, and it is effective for many cases with various symptoms. Xiang and Sha regulate Qi and **Pingwei San** harmonizes the Middle Jiao, the spleen and stomach. The transformation of the Middle Jiao can be strengthened once the spleen and stomach are harmonized. Thus, the patient will feel relieved and comfortable. In addition, the herbs that regulate Qi, such as Muxiang and Sharen or Xiangfu and Sharen can soothe Qi once the transforming function is restored, and the patient will surely feel better. As such, **Xiangsha Pingwei San** has gained popularity.

Modifications of Pingwei San

Pingwei San can be used whenever there is an impairment of the Middle Jiao, the spleen and stomach. There are many modified versions of **Pingwei San**. The book named *"Yixue Chuanxin Lu"* (*Records of Medical Treatment and Herbs*) thoroughly analyzes various modified versions of **Pingwei San**. For example, **Pingwei San** is modified by adding Gehua (flos puerariae), Gegen (radix puerariae) and Zhijuzi (semen hoveniae) in case the patient regularly consumes alcohol; or by adding Shanzha (fructus crataegi) in case the patient eats a lot of meat; or by adding Caoguo (amomum tsao-ko), Qingpi (the green tangerine peel), Ganjiang (rhizoma zingiberis) in case the patient extremely loves eating a lot of fruit.

Excessive fruit is harmful to the health for some people. Fruits are not always good for all people since fruits are in general cold and damp in property. In case of cold dampness in the spleen and stomach, fruits may worsen the conditions. Therefore, the more fruits the patients have, the paler they may look, and the poorer appetite they may suffer. Fruits can provide moisture to healthy people. However, in case a person suffers from dampness, especially cold dampness in the spleen and stomach, fruit does not provide moisture to the body. Cold dampness in the Middle Jiao prevents body fluid T&T, resulting in failure of Qi and blood to be transported and distributed to the face. Hence, it will not provide moisture, either.

If the patient has severe dampness and the spleen is in a state of extremely Yin deficiency, Baizhu can be substituted for Cangzhu in **Pingwei San**, and again add Lugen (rhizoma phragmitis), Maogen (couchgrass root) and even Danggui (angelica sinensis) and the like to tonify the spleen and stomach Yin. By the way, in the case of coldness in the spleen and stomach, **Pingwei San** may be used together with **Liangjiang San** that refers to the two ingredients of Ganjiang (rhizoma zingiberis) and Gaoliangjiang (galangal).

Formulas are generally modified in clinical practices based on specific cases and syndromes.

Shenzhu San

Shenzhu San is the modified **Pingwei San** with addition of Huoxiang and Sharen. Huoxiang is used since Chenpi, Cangzhu and Houpo in **Pingwei San** all enter the Middle Jiao and the interior parts of human body, while Huoxiang not only enters the Middle Jiao, but also clears dampness and heat. However, Huoxiang functions at superficial level. With addition of Huoxiang, the formula can benefit both the body's exterior and interior. Thus, its function of transforming dampness is intensified.

After Xiazhi (the Summer Solstice, the 10th solar term) around the 20th-22nd June in the lunar calendar, summer heat pathogens become active. Summer heat is the combination of dampness and heat. It forms when the damp and heat entangle with one another. The entanglement of the damp and heat is in fact the entanglement of Qi between the sky and earth. When heat in the sky descends and the damp on the ground ascends, they will be entangled in between where human live. Similarly, the damp and heat Qi also exist inside the human body. When the exogenous dampness and heat trap the body surface, the endogenous damp and heat will impair the spleen and stomach. In such a case, use of Huoxiang and Sharen based on the formula of **Pingwei San** can strengthen the spleen, harmonize the stomach, clear heat, and dry dampness. Therefore, for **Shenzhu San** and **Xiangsha Pingwei San**, what one needs to do is to keep in mind when to use it and what for it to be used.

In fact, while **Shenzhu San** is used to smoothen Qi circulation, Huoxiang can be used all year round, especially, when the patient is suffering from failure of sweating, poor digestion, and poor appetite due to the interior and exterior disharmony. **Shenzhu San** is named so since the monarch herb in this formula is **Shenzhu**, i.e., the processed Cangzhu dried on the roof of house after Bai Lu

(White Dew, the 15th solar term, around Sept. 8), and it is mild in property.

Other Formulas Related to Cangzhu or Its Compatibility

Ermiao San

Ermiao San (literally means "Two Wonder Powder") is another well-known formula related to Cangzhu. As its name suggests, **Ermiao San** is a medical powder composed of two wonderful herbs.

"San" here means powder, into which the herbs are crushed. "San" also implies its property of dispersing outwards. Dampness and heat in the spleen and stomach needs dispersing. The formulas for dispersing purposes are all called ' San', for example, **Pingwei San**, **Shenzhu San** and **Huoxiang Zhengqi San**.

Ermiao San was formulated by Zhu Danxi, a medical expert in Yuan dynasty. He was adept at nourishing Yin and tonifying the spleen. Most of his prescriptions are inclined to Yin nourishing. Of course, most of his patients needed Yin nourishing at that time, so he had more experience in the field of Yin nourishing. Zhang Zihe, a medical expert in Jin dynasty, was adept at purging, i. e., to help the patients to induce sweating and vomiting, and have loose bowel. As a matter of fact, most of his patients needed such treatment, and Zhang Zihe himself was also more experienced in this field.

Ermiao San contains only Cangzhu and Huangbai (phellodendron amurense). Cangzhu resolves dampness. Huangbai is bitter and cold, entering the Lower Jiao to clear pathogenic heat.

Sanmiao San

Later on, another modified formula named **Sanmiao San** (literally means "Three Wonder Powder") was developed based upon **Ermiao San** by adding one more herb Niuxi (radix achyranthis bidentatae), either Chuan Niuxi (radix cyathulae) or Huai Niuxi (achyranthes root). However, attention is called that Chuan Niuxi should be used in the cases of blood stasis or the damp-heat inclined to the blood system with more conspicuous symptom of pulse slip at the left side since Chuan Niuxi goes to the blood system; otherwise, Huai Niuxi should be used instead in the case of damp-heat staying in the Qi system. For instance, those who suffer from high blood pressure with a symptom of blushing face should use Huai Niuxi since Huai Niuxi goes to the Qi system and has a descending function so that it can suppress the liver Qi and reduce the blood pressure. **Ermiao San** is a wonderful formula, and it becomes even much better after Niuxi is added to make into the formula of **Sanmiao San** since Niuxi (either Chuan Niuxi or Huai Niuxi) has the property of going downwards and can direct the other herbs to go downwards rapidly.

By the way, from the perspective of medical function, Jiegeng (platycodon grandiflorum) takes the opposite direction comparing with Niuxi. Jiegeng can lift the other herbs upwards rapidly, up to the throat only. Therefore, Jiegeng is not used for diseases related to the head, but it can be used for diseases related to heart, lung, chest, and throat. Niuxi can descend all the way to the feet. Suppose that it is required to lift the medical effects to the head, Shengma (rhizoma cimicifugae) may be used instead. Besides, Sangye (mulberry leaf), Juhua (chrysanthemum) and Manjingzi (fructus viticis) all guide medicines to the head.

Niuxi in **Sanmiao San** plays a function of guiding medicine to lead Cangzhu and Huangbai downwards plus the intrinsic properties of Cangzhu and Huangbai of clearing damp-heat in the Lower Jiao. The effects will be intensified then. This formula can be used in both the powder and decoction forms with the same effect.

Cangzhu Used with Xuanshen (Radix Scrophulariae)

Cangzhu and Xuanshen are often used in a pair by the Medical expert Zhu Chenyu for the treatment of diabetes.

Many pairs of herbs are used for the treatment of diabetes. There is a book called *Shi Jinmo Duiyao* (*Shi Jinmo on Herbal Pairs*, written by Shi Jinmo who is one of the four famous TCM experts in the modern times in China). The most brilliant and valuable facet is that he simplified a lot of formulas into pairs of herbs, which helps TCM doctors to acquire a deeper understanding of formulas.

Cangzhu is dry and severe in property, while Xuanshen is moistening. Diabetes is mostly characterized with a condition of dryness since the sugar escapes through urination. The patients suffering from diabetes often have a very good appetite since such a disease always arises from the pathogenic dryness, then bringing about the consequences of failures of the spleen, kidney and stomach to distribute fluid and food nutrients properly throughout the body. The nutrients of fluid and food run off through urination. Thus, the body cannot be properly nourished and moistened, but the urine becomes sweet. Similarly, some areas along a river are barren and not even a blade of grass grows, for instance, some area along the Yellow River, which causes water and soil erosion, making the river become yellow. Sugar is sweet, while sweet is subsumed to the earth. Metaphorically speaking, the Yellow River is a model for diabetes.

What should we do to control the soil erosion? The best way is to moisten the areas by inducing rain. Rain promotes the growth of grasses and plants that will reinforce the riverbed and control the water loss and soil erosion. Similarly, for treatment of diabetes, the patients also need body conditioning with some moistening herbs like Sheng Dihuang (radix rehmanniae recen), Shanyao (Chinese yam) and so on to nourish the Yin of the lungs, spleen and kidneys. However, these moistening herbs, if used in large amount, may affect the T&T functions, which then results in thin sloppy stool. In that case, Cangzhu can be used as a corrigent herb to restrain the moistening herbs. As a matter of fact, in the herbal pair of Cangzhu and Xuanshen, Cangzhu only plays the function of corrigent herb, while Xuanshen plays the functions of generating body fluid to quench thirst and mobilizing the body fluid circulation in order to nourish the kidneys, but Xuanshen can cause thin sloppy stool. That's why Cangzhu is used for counteracting purpose. Besides, Cangzhu may also counteract the other moistening herbs in the formula and astringe the life essence of the spleen. When a patient is suffering from diabetes, the life essence of the spleen may run out. Therefore, in the process of treating diabetes, the fluid and nutrients not only have to be replenished, but also astringed at the same time, which is also part of the function of Cangzhu. After that, the patient may not suffer from thin sloppy stool any more, signifying that the damp-heat in the spleen and the stomach is cleared away and that the T&T function is enhanced as well.

第三章　苍术

苍术药性解

苍术与白术的异同

苍术和白术有一点相近，但其实是差异很大的两味药。

苍术味苦、辛而甘，它是温性的，入肺、脾、胃、大肠、小肠这五经。苍术有芳香的气味，能够燥湿健脾，能发汗。又因为它非常芳香雄烈，所以还能辟邪。苍术能化痰，是因为它能健脾。要论起芳香雄烈来，苍术的作用比白术要大得多，虽然白术也芳香，但它没有苍术那么芳香。芳香就能醒脾、健脾。总体说来，白术是一味比较缓、比较柔的药，苍术的性子就比较刚烈，而且发挥起作用来也比较急、比较快。要论补益性，白术要远远优于苍术，苍术基本上没有补的作用了。在临床上，如果脾虚同时湿气又比较盛的话，经常苍术和白术一起用。

有人总结说："白术是健脾燥湿，苍术是燥湿健脾。"

"健脾燥湿"，意思是说它健脾的力量大，燥湿的力量稍微小一点；还有一种含义，就是白术是通过健脾来燥湿的。苍术燥湿的力量强，健脾的力量倒在其次；还有一种含义，就是苍术是通过燥湿来健脾的。苍术、白术都有发汗的作用，只不过白术发汗的作用比较弱。

苍术燥湿

苍术是一味燥湿的药，它发挥的任何作用都跟湿有关。它能发汗，那么治感冒能用它来发汗吗？未必。只有湿困无汗，当身体的气机、毛孔被湿困住了，才可以用苍术来发汗。以前学《伤寒论》，学外感病的时候，经常会看到人体不出汗，是因为肌表被寒所遏，其实风、寒、暑、湿、燥、火都能扼住毛孔，只是程度有深浅而已。寒是一种阴邪，能遏住毛孔，湿也是一种阴邪，也能遏住毛孔。所以当毛孔被寒邪遏住的时候，可以用麻黄、苏叶；被湿邪遏住的时候，就得用苍术来发汗了。

这些一般书上讲的不是太多，我们要看文字的背后。比如《伤寒论》，它表面上只讲了汗毛孔被寒邪所遏住，看到这个就要想到，除了寒邪，还有哪些邪气能够遏住人的汗毛孔，让人不出汗呢？湿邪是其中之一，所以当湿困无汗时就要用苍术来发汗。湿邪还能让人汗出不止，当湿热在人的肌表，扰乱了人的营卫，会让人出非常多的汗，这时候依然要用苍术，所以苍术有双向调节的作用，有汗能止汗，无汗能发汗。它是健脾和燥湿两种功能共同发挥作用的效果。

以前有人刚学医的时候，给人开了一个方子，方子有效了，他很高兴，但他马上冒出一个疑问，说不知道是哪一味药的效果。其实这种思维就是错的。开了一个方子并不一定是某几味药的效果，而是它们共同作用的结果。不要再想从这个方子里找出到底是哪几味药在发挥作用了。还有这种情况，某病人一直吃药，某一次他对你说：大夫啊，这次药效果特别好，你就按这次开吧。这种观念也是错误的。这次的效果好，是因为有前面很多次的铺垫，这一次开始发挥作用了，效果好了，并不只是说这一次的方子开的好，以前的方子就不好了。所以我们开方子的时候要注意到这个，不能因为病人说某一次方子吃的效果好，你就按那次的方子走，这是唯方唯药的侥幸心理。

苍术的炮制方法

再回到苍术。苍术是一种多年生的野生草本植物，江苏南京附近茅山产的最好。茅山的苍术有甘味，前面讲了，苍术是味苦辛而甘，这就是按照茅山苍术的性味来说的。普通苍术苦、辛比较明显，甘味少。苦、辛都是比较刚烈的气味。但药要能刚中有柔、刚柔并济，茅山苍术就有这个特点。茅山苍术并不大，很小很瘦，很坚硬，有一定的油润性，表面有很多毛，所以又叫毛苍术，即叫茅苍术，这两种写法都对，它们是同一种药。

把茅山苍术切开，会发现里边有很多小红点，叫朱砂点，这意味着它能入心。前面我们说了苍术对汗有作用，汗为心之液，也说得通。归经之说不可拘泥。心是主火的，火土相生。比茅山苍术稍微再差一点的是湖北这一带的，它的块头较大，辛烈的气味更加的强，甘味就少。这种苍术用来做内服药的时候，就远远不如茅苍术了；但我们不能因为它不如茅苍术就弃而不用，它也有它的用途。例如我们可以用它来做熏香，做香囊，这样就用湖北的苍术，甚至北方的苍术都可以。

在选择药材的时候，最好要选择地道药材，当不能选择地道药材的时候，普通的药材也可以用，我们还可以在炮制或配伍上下功夫，总之要让药符合我们的作用要求。苍术的炮制也非常的讲究，前边我们讲漂白术是用淘米水来浸泡，苍术也可以用淘米水来浸泡，最好用糯米的淘米水来浸泡，浸泡好了以后再把它的皮刮掉，切成片，然后跟芝麻一起炒，或者加芝麻油来炒，炒得通黄，当然这种炮制的方法现在比较少见，过去是这么要求的。为什么要与芝麻一起炒？因为苍术是很燥烈的，芝麻是油润的，芝麻油也是油润性的，用芝麻来炮制苍术，够让苍术的燥烈之性小一些，这相当于反佐。为什么用淘糯米的水来浸泡呢？因为淘米水也是很滋润的，也是企图把苍术的燥烈之性减小，一方面要用它的燥烈之性，另一方面又要控制它的燥烈之性，控制到人能够适用的范围，这是中药炮制方面需要拿捏的一个技术。

还有一种炮制苍术的方法，是在白露节（一般在西历 9 月 7 日、8 日）后，依然将苍术用淘米水来浸泡，泡透以后把它晾到房顶上，日晒夜露一个月，这种苍术更好，叫神术。有一个很有名的方子叫神术散，用的就是这种苍术。神术散就是在平胃散的基础上加藿香、砂仁。苍术到白露节后，精气就往根部收了，所以白露节后采的苍术，根部精华就比较多，药力就比较足，白露节后能得秋气，露水多，露水是凉润的，辛香燥烈的苍术用淘米水浸泡，得到了米的精华，就稍微润了一些。再日晒夜露，白天得到太阳的阳气，晚上得到露水的滋润，那么它的滋润性就更好一些，燥烈之性就小一些。为什么要把它晾到房子上边呢？过去的房子是那种瓦房，瓦至少得有两层，有朝上的那一层瓦，还有朝下的那一层瓦，瓦是很通透的，能遮光避雨，还能透气，苍术放在瓦房上边晾晒，能得屋子里的人气。有人问：如果下雨怎么办？下雨就得把它盖起来，不能让它淋着雨，老淋雨不行。一般秋天的雨水也比较少，这时候正是秋高气爽。

平胃散

与苍术有关的方子很多，我们主要讲两个，一个是平胃散，一个是三妙散。

平胃散方名含义
平胃散：
苍术、厚朴、陈皮、甘草。

平胃散是一个很常用的方子，它的君药为苍术。它为什么能成为我们重点介绍的方子呢？就像以前我们讲四物汤和当归一样，四物汤以当归为君药，它把当归的作用放大了。平胃散是把苍术的作用放大了。我们知道苍术是芳香燥烈的，可升可降，它能够平胃，能够燥湿，为了加大它燥湿的功能，为了加大它往下降的作用，所以加了厚朴，厚朴也是一味芳香化湿的药。前面讲了，苍术辛香燥烈，它需要略微带一点甘甜。如果苍术实在没有甘甜怎么办呢？我们加点甘草，那它不就辛香燥烈中有了甘甜吗？平胃散要和胃，所以加了陈皮，陈皮是理气和胃的。因此在苍术的基础上加上厚朴、陈皮、甘草，其作用就被放大了。在临床中，只要遇到了湿气，我们就经常会用到平胃散。当然，在必需破气的时候，陈皮可以换成青皮。在脾胃阴虚的时候，舌头小小的，舌苔上没有什么津液和水分，这时候就不能用苍术，可以把苍术换成白术。

　　平胃散为什么叫平胃散呢？我们知道，脾胃是属土的，土是有高有低的。《黄帝内经》讲，当土凸起来的时候叫"敦阜"，"阜"是小土堆的意思，安徽有"阜阳"，本意就是小土堆的南面，山东还有个"曲阜"；当土陷下去的时候叫"卑监"。当土凸起来的时候容易干；当土陷下去了，四周都很高，只有这块土地就容易积水，就会比较湿。太高了、太低了都不好，所以我们要把它弄平整，这样才能干湿得当。脾胃也是这样，不能让它这一块湿，那一块干，或者说不能太干或者太湿，要让它干湿很均匀，高低就要调节一下，平一平。

　　如果遇到"敦阜"，出现了燥，怎么办呢？就要大量用芦根、玉竹、山药之类的来润养脾阴。那如果是"卑监"，脾胃湿气太多，就要来化湿，把陷下去的地方填平。填平后这一块就永远不会湿了。如果不把这里填平，只把湿气燥了，等到下次下雨时，这里依然会很湿。平胃散的意思就是把它这个卑监容易受潮的地方填平。借用这个比喻，就可以知道平胃散的方意之所在了，它不仅燥湿而且还要让脾胃达到平的状态。

香砂平胃散

　　平胃散的加减也非常多。例如有一个很著名的方剂叫香砂平胃散，就是在平胃散的基础上加上香、砂，那么香、砂是哪两味药呢？不确定。有人认为是加木香和砂仁，有人认为是加香附和砂仁，到底是哪两个呢？要看情况而用。砂仁也是燥湿的，当你口干的时候就不要用砂仁了，因为砂仁芳香，香就能燥，砂仁如果用多了，会让你更口干的；木香是通三焦之气的，砂仁是通脾肾之气的，还能够直达下焦。所以如果需要通三焦脾肾之气，可以木香砂仁加上平胃散。如果要通肝脾肾之气，那就用香附砂仁再加平胃散。

有人讲"香砂平胃散，一天开到晚"，为什么可以这么说呢？比如，你作为一个医生，来了个病人，不知道他是什么病，但你也不能就愣着，好歹得给人家一个方子，开个什么方子呢？香砂平胃散。这并不是教我们不会看病开方子就给人家开平胃散，而是说香砂平胃散这个方很平和，且对很多病都有效果。香砂是理气的，平胃散是平中焦、平脾胃的，只要脾胃一平，中土在中焦运化的力度就强了，人就要舒服很多，再加上木香砂仁或者香附砂仁这几味理气的药，中焦运化的好了，然后再把气一理，人自然就舒服了，所以香砂平胃散有很强的普遍性。

平胃散加减

凡是中焦伤了，脾胃伤了，都可以用平胃散。平胃散的加减法非常多。有一本书叫《医学传心录》，这本书里面讲香砂平胃散的加减法，讲得比较详尽。比如病人平时喝酒比较多，可以在平胃散里面加上葛花、葛根、枳椇子；病人平时吃肉多可以加上山楂。如果平时特别爱吃水果，要在里面加上草果、青皮、干姜之类的。

水果吃多了也不好，不是所有人都能随便吃的。水果本身是寒湿的，当脾胃有寒湿比较重的时候，越吃水果，脸色越黄，食欲越不振作；水果对于健康人来说，能补水，但对于脾胃有湿、尤其是有寒湿的人来说，越吃水果越补不了水，寒湿困在中焦，脾不能运化津液，气血不能输布到脸上，它就不能补水。这是题外话。

如果病人湿重，脾阴又非常虚，你可以把平胃散的苍术换成白术，再加上芦根、茅根甚至当归之类的，来养他的脾胃之阴；当病人脾胃有寒的时候，平胃散可以合上两姜散。两姜散就是干姜、高良姜。

方子的加减都是需要在临床中根据具体的情况来定的。

神术散

神术散就是在平胃散的基础上加上藿香、砂仁。为上么要加藿香？因为平胃散里的陈皮、苍术、厚朴这些药都是走中焦，是往里走的。藿香也是走中焦的，是去湿热的药，但它能走表，加了藿香就表里通透了，化湿的作用就更好了。

夏至到了，暑邪就会比较盛。暑是由湿热二气组成的，湿和热交织在一起就成了暑邪。湿热交织其实就是天地之气交织，天上热气往下来，地上湿气往上走。湿气和热气就交织在中间，在中间的是人，人就在湿热之气的交汇之处。天地之间是湿热之气，同样人体里面也是湿热之气。外面的湿热之气困住人的体表，里面的湿热之气伤人的脾胃。把藿香、砂仁和平胃散配在一起，既健脾又平胃、又清热、又燥湿，这些作用全有了。所以，关于神术散、香砂平胃散，我们没必要记它有什么作用，只记它在什么时候能用就行。

要宣畅三焦之气用神术散，一年四季都可以用藿香。尤其是病人表里不通的时候，汗出不来，消化又不好，食欲也不好，可以用神术散。为什么叫神术散呢？因为它的君药是神术，就是白露以后放在房顶上晾的苍术。它的性质非常的平和。

苍术相关其他方剂或配伍

二妙散

跟苍术有关的还有一个名方叫二妙散，顾名思义，就是两个很好的药在一起构成的散。

散就是散剂，就是把药打成粉，要么来吞，要么用水煎煮。散，取它往外散的意思。脾胃的湿热需要散，所以，我们用的药都是叫散，比如平胃散、神术散、藿香正气散。

二妙散是朱丹溪的方子。朱丹溪擅长养阴，也擅长攻下、健脾，他是一位思想很圆融的大师。只不过他的病人需要养阴的比较多，在他处方用药的时候就偏于养阴，所以后来以至于有人说他是养阴派的。当然，因为他的病人需要养阴的多，所以在他养阴方面就有一些心得。张子和是攻下派的，攻下派喜欢汗、吐、下，就是让人出汗，呕吐，拉肚子。

二妙散仅有两味药，苍术和黄柏。苍术除湿，黄柏苦寒，走下焦而清热。

三妙散

后来又出现一个方子叫三妙散。就是二妙散的基础上加一味牛膝，可以用川牛膝，也可以用怀牛膝。如果有瘀血可以用川牛膝；没有的话，可以用怀牛膝。因为川牛膝是入血分的，怀牛膝是入气氛的。或者如果说湿热偏于血分，左脉滑象更明显，就用川牛膝。如果湿热在气分，比如有的人血压比较高，脸红红的，就用怀牛膝，因为怀牛膝还有往下潜镇的作用，镇肝气，能够降血压。二妙散的作用已经很妙了，三妙散加入一味牛膝就更妙了。川牛膝也好，怀牛膝也好，都有往下走的作用，它能够引导各种药迅速地往下走。

顺便说一下，跟牛膝作用相反的有一个药是桔梗，桔梗能够把各种药迅速的往上升提，升提到咽喉。所以头上病一般不用桔梗，心、肺、胸、咽喉的病可以用桔梗。它升提到嗓子眼，就再不往上走了。牛膝能一直降到脚。有人会问，你如果要一直升到头顶怎么办？那就用升麻了。什么桑叶、菊花、蔓荆子都是走头的，这些都是引经药的作用。

牛膝在这里就是引经药，它把苍术、黄柏往下引。苍术、黄柏本身就能除下焦的湿热，加上引经药，它的作用就会更好。叫三妙散，就是说可以做成散剂用。我们也经常会在汤剂里用，直接把这三个药开在汤剂里，作用也是一样的。

苍术配玄参

苍术配玄参，是祝谌予老先生在治疗糖尿病时经常用的一组药对。

治糖尿病有很多对药。有一本书叫《施今墨对药》，其高明之处在于把很多药方简化成对药，也就是一对一对的药，使人对这个方子有更深一层的认识。

苍术是一味燥烈的药，玄参是一味滋润的药。而糖尿病是以燥为主，糖尿病的人都干巴巴的，糖都到哪里去了？都去尿里面了。这种病人饭量还特别大。这是一个由于燥邪引起的病，脾肾胃不能很好地输布人体的水谷精微，水谷之精微流失了，人得不到很好的滋养，尿还很甜腻。黄河流域的很多地方，寸草不生，水土就很容易流失，水土流失，黄河的水都黄了，土都到水里去了。不恰当地讲，黄河就是一个糖尿病的模型。

怎么来治糖尿病？怎么来治水土流失呢？就要来滋润这个地方，让这个地方总下雨。下雨，就会长草木。长草木，河床就能固定住，就能减少水土的流失。这样来治理它，治理黄河，治理人体，只要有耐心，慢慢这样来治理，是可以的。治疗糖尿病时候用的药，往往都比较的滋润，像生地啊、山药啊，养肺阴、养脾阴、养肾阴的药，都会用，但是用多了这些滋润的药，人体的运化能力不行，这些药马上又成了那种很稀的大便，又排出去了，那怎么办呢？可以用苍术，来反佐这些滋润的药。其实苍术配玄参，苍术只是一个反佐。玄参是养肾的，是能生津液止渴，它是调动人体水液循环的一味药；但玄参能让大便变稀，就加一味苍术，来反佐。它不但反佐玄参，而且反佐方子里边其他的所有的滋润的药，所以苍术在这里边，它有一个敛脾经的作用，能收敛脾的精气。当人得糖尿病的时候，他脾的精气，已经耗散得比较多了。所以一方面要来补他的水分、补精气，另一方面，要让这些补进去的精气能够收敛起来。所以，要用到苍术。用了苍术以后，大便就渐渐不稀了。这意味着脾胃的湿热被清掉了，也意味着人体的运化能力增强了。

Chapter 4　Chenpi (Pericarpium Citri Reticulatae) and Other Qi Regulating Medicines

About Regulation of Qi

In the earth-associated category of formulas and medicines for tonifying the spleen and T&T, there are many herbs that can promote the T&T functions in the body. Cangzhu and Baizhu are the most typical herbs among them, since Cangzhu tonifies the spleen to dry dampness, while Baizhu dries dampness to tonify the spleen. Therefore, Cangzhu and Baizhu are taken as important examples to illustrate the importance of tonifying the spleen in order to have smooth T&T functions.

The Critical Elements of Transformation and Transportation: Qi, Blood, Spleen and Stomach

The T&T functions rely on the spleen, but how the spleen carries out these functions relies on the Qi and blood circulation in the whole body. Qi is invisible, but it is the driving force of all the physiological movement in the body. Blood is visible, flowing with Qi circulation, and Qi is attached to blood. Therefore, Qi and blood are subsumed to a Yin-Yang pair, as they are interconnected and inseparable. The circulation of Qi and blood promotes the T&T functions in the body. So, Qi and blood must be regulated into smooth circulation in order to guarantee proper T&T. Otherwise, T&T functions may be impaired, which will then induce phlegm or result in blood stasis in case of failure of proper Qi or blood T&T. Phlegm and blood stasis will further impede circulation of Qi and blood. Therefore, regulation of Qi and blood is an important approach to promote the T&T functions.

The formulas and medicines for promoting T&T functions will be involved with the natural herbs or animal medicines that go into the Qi system or blood system or both. However, these medicines will have some effects of regulating Qi and blood to some extent.

However, the regulation of Qi and blood depends upon the internal organs of the body. Therefore, in order to clearly understand the regulating process of Qi and blood, the relationship between the internal organs and Qi and blood must be analyzed.

Functioning of the Qi-regulating Medicines

When talking about Qi, one should keep in mind the importance of harmony. The Chinese idiom says "harmony brings wealth", so in the interpersonal communication, peace and harmony is very important. Similarly, for Qi system, harmony is also very critical in order to keep smooth circulation of Qi. The harmonized Qi circulation in the body is like a gentle wind that can activate the vitality of human body. Therefore, Qi must also flow smoothly. There are two criteria for the Qi in the human body: one is to keep it in a harmonious state, and the other one is to maintain its smooth circulation. Qi stagnation may induce phlegm. Hence, Qi should be regulated in order to reduce phlegm.

The internal organs of the body must be taken into consideration while Qi regulating herbs are being analyzed since each organ (of the liver, lung, spleen, heart, and kidney) has its own Qi. Regulation of Qi refers to that of all organs, but the priority among the priorities of regulation is the stomach Qi regulation. As the saying in TCM goes, "live when the stomach Qi is in order, or die when the stomach Qi is in disorder". Besides, the stomach is the "sea" of all the internal organs, since the stomach receives the fluid and grains, and all the internal organs are closely related to the stomach. Meanwhile, the stomach is an organ that is rich in Qi and blood. Hence, Qi and blood in the body can circulate in order only when the stomach Qi runs smoothly, or otherwise, most of the Qi and blood will be impaired at the points where stomach Qi does not run smoothly, then directly affecting the overall circulation of Qi and blood in the body. The regulation of stomach Qi should be taken as the key focus. Based on this concept, let us begin with the medicines that regulate the stomach Qi, from where we may go further to analyze the formulas and medicines related to regulating Qi of the other internal organs of the body.

Among the medicines that regulate the stomach Qi, Chenpi is the most typical one. As a matter of fact, Chenpi is orange peel or tangerine peel. When orange peel is used as medicine, the longer on shelf, the better it will be. It is often stored on shelf for quite long enough until it becomes dark in color. That is why it is called Chenpi (literally means old peel).

Category of Citrus Genus

From the perspective of TCM, many plants are precious since almost all the parts on the whole plant can be used as medicines, such as mulberry tree, lycium, cassia tree and bamboo. Each and every part of these plants can be used as herb. The same is true to the citrus plant/orange tree.

About the Citrus Medicines

According to the place of origin, Chenpi produced in Xinhui, Guangdong province of China comes the best in medical effect, followed by the Chenpi produced in Fujian province with little weaker medical effect. However, the orange peel produced in Zhejiang province is not qualified to the normal standard of TCM for medical use, but it may be used as a substitution for emergency use. Anyway, if Xinhui Chenpi is not available for the time being, the other Chenpi may be used instead, but it depends on the other herbs used in the formula.

Based on the maturity and time of storage, there are various types of tangerine peel, including Qingpi (pericarpium citri reticulatae viride, or the green tangerine peel), Chenpi and Jupi (orange peel). Chenpi may also be processed into salted Chenpi and Shenbei Chenpi. As a matter of fact, different parts of an orange tree can be used as medicines for different purposes, like Juhong (exocarpium citri rubrum) and Jubai (tangerine endocarpium), Juluo (tangerine pith), Juhe (tangerine seed) and Juye (tangerine leaf), which are respectively named according to the parts of the fruit that are collected. Besides, there is another type of Juhong called Huazhou Juhong (exocarpium citri rubrum) produced in Huazhou, Guangdong province of China, different from the regular Juhong. Another type of fruit called Zhi (trifoliate orange) looks like orange, as it is known that the tangerine fruits produced from the tangerine tree growing to the south of Huaihe river in China is called tangerine orange, but the that produced from the tangerine tree growing to the north of Huaihe river is called Zhi (trifoliate orange), including Zhishi (fructus aurantii immaturus) and Zhike (fructus aurantia) when used as medicines. In addition, the category of citrus genus also covers kumquat, ponkan, grapefruit, citron and oranges. From this brief introduction, one may have a rough idea and an overall understanding of the herbs in the category of citrus genus.

In general, all the herbs mentioned above are used for harmonizing the stomach, regulating Qi and reducing phlegm. However, they are different to some extent in terms of their clinical application. So, sometimes all the herbs related to the orange tree may be used together or substituted for one another, but sometimes they have to be used specifically and separately based on the syndrome differentiation, like Juhong and Jubai.

Qingpi (Green Tangerine Peel)

Orange trees blossom and bear many oranges, however, it does not mean that every fruit can fully grow into a mature orange, since some of them may fall from the tree before they are mature. However, such unripe oranges have very provocative, pungent and fragrant taste with strong bitterness. The peel of these small and unripe oranges is called Qingpi. The peel of the ripe orange is called Jupi (orange peel), which is milder than Qingpi in property.

According to TCM theory, green color indicates the herb goes to the liver, so Qingpi enters the liver meridian. Furthermore, the unripe orange is still in its rising and dispersing stage, which also indicates that it can enter the liver. Therefore, Qingpi is often used as a guiding herb to direct the medical effects to the foot Jueyin meridian.

Comparing with Chenpi, or the peel of the ripe orange, Qingpi is much stronger and more vigorous(like an energetic young man) for regulating Qi than Chenpi (like an old man). Qingpi is widely used in clinical practice to get rid of the stale and bring forth the fresh. And also, Qingpi is often used in combination with Chenpi. Chenpi regulates Qi while Qingpi breaks the Qi stagnation. To put it directly, Qingpi has much stronger effect for regulating Qi.

Jupi (Orange Peel) and Chenpi

Jupi will become Chenpi after it is left in a dry and cool place for around three to five years, or even longer. Chenpi is much milder in properties than Jupi, but Jupi is milder than Qingpi.

However, a lot of Chenpi are not from Jupi stored on shelf for 3 or 5 years, but are made by some special processing methods. Such processed Chenpi are even better in effect.

For example, the salted Chenpi is the Chenpi processed with salt. Chenpi goes to the stomach and functions to regulate Qi. However, after it is processed with salt, the salted Chenpi can go to the kidneys. Besides, the spleen is the source of phlegm, the lungs store the phlegm, and the kidneys are the root of the phlegm. When the kidney Qi is impaired, the spleen is prone to producing phlegm and the lungs are subsequently prone to accumulating phlegm. Therefore, salt orhalite is used to process Chenpi for regulating Qi and resolving phlegm, while clearing the root of the phlegm and smoothing the kidney Qi. Furthermore, the halite-processed Chenpi can soothe Qi, promote the secretion of body fluid and dispel the effects of alcohol, so it can be used as a snack as well.

Shenbei Chenpi is the processed Chenpi with addition of Renshen (ginseng) and Chuanbei (bulbus fritillariae cirrhosae). As it is already known, Chenpi regulates Qi, and however, in this process, Qi will be consumed. Therefore, Renshen is added to tonify Qi or nourish the vitality in order to avoid any impairment of Qi in the process of regulating the Qi and resolving the phlegm. Sometimes, Chenpi may not be strong enough for resolving the phlegm. So, Chuanbei is added, which can resolve the phlegm and moisten the lungs without causing impairment of the lungs. Shenbei Chenpi is not frequently used right now, but the TCM learners should keep in mind its functions of tonifying effects without causing stagnation and resolving phlegm without causing impairment.

Juhong (Exocarpium Citri Rubrum) and Jubai (Tangerine Endocarpium)

Fresh orange peel can be separated into two layers. The outer part is red, called Juhong (exocarpium citri rubrum) and the inner part is white, called Jubai (tangerine endocarpium). Usually, the orange peel is used as a whole, but sometimes, they are used separately in some particular cases.

Juhong is the most exterior layer of an orange. The lung dominates and corresponds to the skin and hairs, and the pores on the surface of the orange are quite similar to the pores on the human skin. Therefore, Juhong can enter the lungs to regulate the lung Qi. Furthermore, Juhong has a strong aromatic scent that can easily disperse. Hence, Juhong has a stronger dissipating potency than regular Jupi.

In contrast, Jubai is the interior layer of the orange peel, and it is partially sweet with slight aromatic scent in nature. It enters the spleen and stomach to regulate Qi. Jubai is not so sweet that it does not has so strong dissipating potency, but it has a stronger effect for tonifying Qi.

Another type of Juhong called Huazhou Juhong, also known as Hua Juhong, as mentioned in the above section. It is produced in Huazhou in Guang Dong province of China. Such type of Juhong, to be exact, is the whole orange rather than the exterior layer of the orange peel for the regular Juhong. This type of Juhong is also one of the citrus genius, but it has a thicker peel and less pulp, warm and dry in properties. It has similar functions to Chenpi, but with a more powerful drying property and more effective for regulating the Qi and resolving phlegm and dampness. However, the supply of Hua Juhong is quite limited because of its limited production. By the way, the most valuable Hua Juhong is produced in Lanyuan, so it is called Lan Juhong. Due to rarity, Hua Juhong or Lan Juhong sometimes is substituted by shaddock peel, which also has certain effect of regulating Qi.

Juluo (Tangerine Pith)

Juluo is a white stringy substance on the interior of the orange peel, which can help to get through collaterals in human body. However, Juluo is very valuable because of its limited supply.

There are channels and collaterals in the human body. Collaterals are the extremely fine vessels. The chronic diseases always stay in the collaterals since pathogens always travel with Qi to circulate to every point throughout the body.

When phlegm arises in the body, it will travel with Qi to enter the collaterals of body, resulting in numbness. Generally, once the pathogens enter the collaterals, it will be difficult to eliminate them. At the early stage when the pathogens start to attack the human body, they often stay in the major channel, i. e. , the foot Taiyang bladder channel, from where they are much easier to be cleared. However, once they scatter into the collaterals, some herbs for collaterals will have to be used to guide the medical effects of the other herbs to the collaterals in the human body to search for and eliminate the pathogens. For such cases, Juluo will be the best choice.

Juluo usually starts from the Qi system to resolve phlegm and dredge the collaterals. It is often used with Sigualuo (loofah sponge), the dried pulp of loofah, which can dredge the collaterals, too, but it tends to target the blood system. Therefore, when the pathogens invade the collaterals, Juluo and Sigualuo are often used together as herbal ingredients, in addition to their own effect of resolving phlegm, to direct the medical effects of the other herbs into the collaterals where the pathogens stay.

Juhe (Tangerine Seed)

Juhe is the seed of orange, which, slightly greenish/bluish, can enter the liver channel. It is often used to treat hernia. Hernia is related to the liver channel and the testes. Juhe and lychee seed are often used as paired herbs, specifically for treating the diseases related the testes, not only because they look like the testis, but also Juhe especially has the functions of entering the liver channel to regulate Qi.

Hernia occurs along the pathway that the liver channel traverses, so it can be treated by soothing the liver. In the case that the Qi of the Middle Jiao is sinking, the way of tonifying Middle Jiao and Qi should be adopted; in the case of the liver stagnation, Xiaoyao San may be used. Generally, hernia is accompanied by liver coldness, so, on the one hand, Xiaohuixiang (fennel), or even Wuzhuyu (fructus evodiae), Guang tangerine seed and lychee seed are added/used to regulate Qi, and on the other hand, as guiding ingredient herb to direct all the other herbs to the desired channels where they should go.

Both the testes of the males and the breasts of the females are at the nodes of the liver channel, where the diseases usually can be treated with Guang tangerine seed and lychee seed. These two herbs can also be used to treat diseases involving the breast tissue.

Juye (Tangerine Leaf)

Juye also enjoys some aromatic scent, suggesting that it can regulate Qi as a medicine. Juye is light in weight and it does not fall even in winter. Generally, herbal leaves often have dispersing functions, and green color signifies they can enter the liver. Juye, as a medicine, is a very effective herb for the treatment of diseases related to the breast, especially for the treatment of lobular hyperplasia of breasts. It can regulate the liver Qi and remove stasis.

Another magical effect of tangerine leaf is to remove fishy smell, which is also a kind of toxin. That is why people feel sick when they are exposed to fishy smell. Humans have an instinct to differentiate toxic substances from edible, non-toxic substances through the olfactory and taste receptors. In general, the pleasant smell is good for the body, for instance, the delicious dishes, and the scent of flowers. The unpleasant smell will be judged by the human organs as foul odor and make humans feel sick. Seafood or fish is beneficial to the body, but the fishy smell is stink, which can make some people feel uncomfortable. Tangerine leaf can help to eliminate the fishy smell. Similarly, perilla leaf and fresh ginger have the same functions to remove the fishy smell.

Jurang (Tangerine Pulp)

Generally, Jurang is not used as a herb, but the sweet orange can be moistening, so it can moisten the spleen and harmonize the stomach, especially the sweeter orange, since it not only regulates Qi, but also moistens the spleen and lungs. Try to avoid the sour orange since the sour tangerine pulp may cause Qi stagnation, which then is prone to inducing phlegm.

Let us observe the people around us. We may find that those who are relatively fatter or are suffering from a lot of phlegm usually dislike the sour food or fruits. However, those who are thin or skinny and are not suffering from phlegm may like the sour food. Children typically have no phlegm, so they may like to eat the sour orange, but the elderly, on the contrary, seldom like the sour taste because of phlegm accumulation, and the sour orange may worsen the condition.

Zhi (Trifoliate Orange)

There is another plant called Zhi (trifoliate orange), for which *Yanzi's Spring and Autumn Annals* (a book about the statements and actions of Yan Ying, the prime minister of the vassal state Qi in Spring and Autumn period of the ancient China) states that the tangerine tree growing to the south of Huaihe River in China is called orange tree, but when the tangerine tree is planted to the north of Huaihe River, it will become Zhi, a kind of bitter orange. In fact, Zhi is a plant that is quite like the tangerine tree. However, after it is planted in the northern areas to the north of Huaihe River, it evolves into a different plant due to the different terrain and climate changes. Zhi, as an herb, includes Zhishi (fructus aurantii immaturus), or just the peel, known as Zhike (fructus aurantii).

Each year, Zhi tree blossoms and bears many small fruits, but it does not mean that every small fruit can fully grow into a mature one, since some of them may fall from the tree before they are mature. The fallen fruits are then cut into slices, dried up and made into herb called Zhishi. The other fruits keep on growing into yellowish and mature fruits, the peel of which is called Zhike. In China, Zhi trees are often planted in Shaanxi province of China, and as herb, Zhishi or Zheke produced in Shangzhou of Shaanxi province is the best in quality. The thorns on Zhi trees are bitter, pungent, and cold in properties.

Zhike (Fructus Aurantii) and Zhishi (Immature Bitter Orange)

Zhike enters the lung and stomach channels to play a dispersing function. Fundamentally, Zheke has a stronger effect of regulating Qi.

According to the TCM theory, the Qi of the liver ascends from the left side and the Qi of the lung descends from the right side inside the body. Zhike is often used to assist the descending of lung Qi in case this function is impaired. As the rhymed formula in TCM says, "left Yujin (radix curcumae) and right Zhike

(fructus aurantii) ", referring that diseases and disorder along the left side of body often arise from the failure of the liver Qi to ascend normally, so Yujin may be used to soothe the liver stagnation in order to promote the ascending of liver Qi along the left side; Diseases along the right side of the body often arise from the failure of the lung Qi to descend normally, so Zhike may be used to promote the descending of the lung Qi along the right side. Both stomach and lung Qi have a physiological tendency to descend, for which Zhike in its property just complies with. Therefore, Zhike as a medicine can help to remove stasis along the lung and stomach channels, purge the lung of pathogenic fire, and clear obstruction of Qi in the chest.

Unlike Zhike, Zhishi is the immature bitter orange, having a stronger property than Zhike. Zhishi can relieve the stagnant Qi and eliminate the phlegm. Therefore, Zhishi can drive the sthenia pathogenic factors and go downwards rapidly. Besides, Zhishi can also open and unblock orifices.

Zhishi and Zhike can be substituted for one another for certain cases based on the relative importance or urgency. For example, Zhishi is used in the formula of **Wendan Tang**, but Zhike may be substituded for Zhishi as well in this formula in case the patient does not have sthenia pathogens. Another example is that Zhike may be substituted for Zhishi in the formula of **Dachengqi Tang** in case a milder descending effect is required.

Xiao Jinju (Small Kumquat) and its Proper Uses

Xiao Jinju is a much sweeter fruit, which can be eaten including the peel and its pulp except the seeds.

In the past, when Jupi and Chenpi were necessary, the Chenpi produced in Xinhui of Guangdong province was used in order to avoid any accidental impairment of healthy Qi in the process of Qi regulation. Or take the kumquat pie as a snack (by pressing kumquat into a pie, then mixed with some sugar and dried up as a special snack). Such a snack can function to reduce phlegm.

Both the old Chenpi (stored on shelf for many years) and the kumquat pie are very mild in properties, making the patient feel more comfortable. However, if Qingpi or Zhike is directly used to relieve the stagnant Qi, patients may feel uncomfortable. In brief, herbs should be used properly based on the syndrome differentiation. The use of stronger herbs does not always mean better effect.

In addition, there are some other citrus fruits whose properties may be understood by observing, tasting, and using in practice.

Divertive Uses of Chenpi Chenpi

All in all, both Chenpi and Jupi are pungent, bitter, and warm in properties. Pungent taste means it can run transversely and eliminate stagnation; bitter taste means it can go straight and drive Qi to descend downwards. Therefore, Chenpi can move freely in the body. When used with Baizhu, Chenpi or Jupi can tonify the spleen and stomach; when used with Gancao, Chenpi or Jupi can tonify the lung. It is not so effective when it is used separately.

Someone does suggest to eat orange with the tangerine pith since the pith has the function of dredging collaterals, but I do not approve it since the pith separately can purge the lungs and cause seepage of the spleen. Hence, I, on the contrary, suggest to eat the tangerine pulp only, especially the sweet orange rather than the sour orange. Besides, orange peel should not be eaten, either, except that the peel is processed with salt or sugar, or used together with some other herbs.

The effects of Chenpi depend upon the herbs that it is used with. It can play a tonifying function if it is used with the restorative herb(s); it may play purging function if it is used with the laxative herb(s); or it may play ascending or descending functions when it is used with the other ascending or descending herbs respectively. In brief, Chenpi does not have a specific property but follows the herbs that it is matched with. It becomes effective when used with effective herbs, or becomes ineffective when used with the ineffective herbs.

TCM doctors in the past seldom wrote Chenpi as the first herb in a prescription (which is an established practice in TCM, but is ignored sometimes in modern times) since the first herb in a formula usually represents that it is the monarch medicine, for which Chenpi cannot play such a function. Chenpi can only function as ministerial, assistant or envoy medicines in a formula because of its unstable property. A monarch medicine must have a specific property, and it always sets up certain concept in the prescription. If Chenpi were put at the first position in a prescription as a monarch medicine, it would cause confusion on choosing the ministerial, assistant and envoy medicines/herbs.

Tangerine peel can be cooked into a special dish with oil and salt plus some other seasoning and side ingredients. The same is true to the shaddock peel with the superficial layer scraped off.

Compatibility of Chenpi and Its Related Formulas

The critical point for understanding the compatibility of a herb is to know its properties/nature well. As for Chenpi, its fundamental nature and function can be summarized as "harmonizing stomach and regulating Qi".

Compatibility of Chenpi for Harmonizing Stomach and Preventing Vomiting

Chenpi used with ginger can prevent vomiting due to the cold attack since Chenpi can harmonize the stomach, and fresh ginger with skin can warm the stomach. Besides, fresh ginger has the function of reducing phlegm and enjoys the descending effect. By the way, if the vomiting arises from the heat attack, Chenpi should be used with Zhuru (bamboo shavings) instead.

Vomiting is often accompanied by phlegm, as well as food with saliva if there are food residues in the stomach. Some people vomit due to car sickness, but such type of vomiting varies from person to person. Some may feel phlegm in between the nasal cavity and throat, which would cause them to feel sick to vomit some food residues with a lot of phlegm. There are also some other causes, such as bumpiness, strange smell, psychological tension, or physical weakness that impair the T&T functions of Qi and then weaken the function of the spleen to up-lift the clear. Under these conditions, the food nutrients in the spleen and stomach is transformed into phlegm. Hence, Chenpi, fresh ginger and Banxia (pinellia ternata) are often used to prevent this type of cold vomiting.

For arresting the heat vomiting, Banxia may also be used together when Chenpi and Zhuru is used since Banxia can function to reduce phlegm though it is partially warm.

Compatibility of Chenpi for Calming Adverse-rising Qi and Stopping Hiccough

Chenpi and Zhuru can also be used to calm adverse-rising Qi and stop hiccough, especially the hiccough due to heat.

Heat hiccough usually is the hiccup singultation arising from the heat in the stomach, which may be stopped by drinking a glass of cold water. In case there exists coldness in the stomach, cold hiccough will occur, which will be stopped with a glass of hot water. Cold or hot water can help to regulate the temperature in the stomach.

Hiccup singultation stems from the disharmony of the stomach Qi, so Chenpi should be the first herb to use for its Qi regulating function. The doctor should make sure of cold hiccup or heat hiccup. Use Zhuru in the case of a heat hiccup; or use Dingxiang (clove) (an aromatic herb that can harmonize the stomach and stop hiccup) in the case of a cold hiccup. Furthermore, kaki calyx is an effective herb that is specialized for stopping both cold and heat hiccup.

For tackling the hiccup, there are many other ways, such as a sudden shock may also work in case one has uncontrollable hiccup since, at the sudden shock, he or she may suffer disturbance or dispersion of Qi in his body, after which he or she can calm down very quickly, and then, he or she will have a smooth Qi circulation. This process can help him or her to stop hiccup.

Erchen Tang and Reduction of the Phlegm Due to Heat

Erchen Tang contains Chenpi (pericarpium citri reticulatae), Banxia (pinellia ternata), Fuling (poria cocos) and Gancao (liquorice).

In the formula of **Ercheng Tang**, Chenpi and Banxia mainly function to reduce phlegm. The longer they are stored on shelf, the better they will become since the longer they are stored, the milder they will become, and the less impairment they may cause to the human body. Furthermore, if the phlegm is induced due to heat, Chenpi may be used together with Zhimu (rhizoma anemarrhenae), Beimu (fritillaria) and Gualoupi (trichosanthes peel) for reducing the phlegm. Among these three herbs, Zhimu clears heat, and both Beimu and Gualoupi are partially cold. Besides, Banxia can also be used though it is warm since warm transformation is necessary in the process of reducing phlegm, or otherwise, Yang may be damaged, which will slow down the effect of reducing phlegm and impairs the Yang Qi if only cold herbs are used.

Constipation and Harmonizing the Stomach

Stomach disharmony can cause vomiting, hiccup singultation, belch and e-ven constipation. Bowel motions are related to the large intestine and the stomach as well since the intestine and stomach are interconnected. Food moving from the stomach to the small intestine and then to the large intestine, is a descending process. The spleen governs the rising of the clear while the stomach governs the descending of the turbid. The separation of the clear from the turbid is carried out through the processing and descending of food from the stomach to the small intestine and on. In this process, the clear, that is, the food nutrients, keeps on rising due to the functions of the spleen. The turbid descends due to the functions of the stomach, as such the wastes are finally discharged out of the body.

In case the stomach is in disorder and the descending function of the stom-ach Qi is impaired, the large intestine Qi will fail in its descending function, too. As it is mentioned that the liver Qi ascends along the left side of the body and the lung Qi descends along the right side, the spleen and stomach in the Middle Jiao are the pivotal organs that are the power source to drive the clear to ascend and the turbid to descend. In fact, all the ascending and descending functions in the body are interrelated. The improper ascending of the liver Qi will surely result in an improper ascending of the spleen Qi. Similarly, the improper descending of the stomach Qi will surely impair the descending of the lung Qi, which then af-fects the descending of the large intestine Qi. A slight move in one organ may af-fect the whole body. Hence, the stomach disharmony can lead to constipation, for which the treatment should start with harmonizing the stomach.

As for constipation trouble, many methods can be adopted for promoting bowel movements. When stool builds up in the large intestine due to heat or damp-heat stagnation, Dahuang (rheum officinale) and Mangxiao (mirabilite) can be used to purge the bowels; when the feces are constipated in the large in-testine and becomes dry and hard, Mangxiao, as a salty herb, could be a good choice to soften the hard feces (regardless of the dry or sticky types), and drive feces out of the body.

Dahuang always keeps on moving downwards once it is taken. Dahuang is bitter and aromatic, which goes downwards in the stomach, the small intestine and large intestine. Thus, it will purge stagnation and function to dredge the bowels.

When Dahuang and Mangxiao are used separately, they have their own functions respectively. Dahuang relaxes the bowels with a little mild effect, but it can purge the excess heat in the blood system or purge the excess heat in the stomach and spleen. Mangxiao is mild, too, and has little impairment to the human body if it is used separately, and it only functions to soften the hard feces. However, Dahuang and Mangxiao, if used together, will have an extremely strong effect.

There are two other situations where constipation is related to Qi and blood:

One is called Qi constipation, which is related to the lungs since the lungs govern the overall Qi of the body. When the Qi in the body is not sufficient, the body may lose dynamic force to push stool downwards. Qi constipation can be treated with Chenpi to harmonize the stomach on the one hand, and Xingren (apricot kernel) to open the lungs on the other hand in order to strengthen the descending function of lung Qi. As such, with the stomach being harmonized and the lubricating property of the apricot kernel, it will be easier to relax the bowels.

Another one is called blood constipation, resulting from blood stagnation, for which Chenpi and Taoren (peach kernel) should be used. Chenpi, as is known, is for harmonizing the stomach. Taoren, as a type of seed, is rich in oil, and it has a moistening and descending function. Furthermore, Taoren can break stagnation in the blood and disperse blood stasis. Once blood stasis is removed, new blood will be regenerated and the normal blood circulation is restored, and then, the fluid in the large intestine will be replenished as well. Hence, in combination with the descending function of stomach Qi, it will be easier to relax the bowels, too.

Treatment of the stomach for harmonizing the Nine Orifices

All the above-mentioned vomiting, hiccup and constipation are involved with the orifices on the body, but they are all related to the stomach.

A TCM saying goes, "all the nine orifices are governed by the stomach", which means the diseases involved with the nine orifices are all related to the stomach. The so-called "nine orifices" refer to the seven orifices on the head: two ears, two eyes, two nostrils and the mouth, plus the two lower orifices: the genitals and anus. There are many diseases associated with the nine orifices, for which the treatment varies depending upon the different syndromes. However, one needs to keep in mind that "all nine orifices are governed by the stomach" in the process of treatment. Therefore, he/she needs to bear in mind the harmonization of the stomach. Chenpi or the similar herbs, when used appropriately, can greatly strengthen the effect of treatment. That is what TCM always says "the disharmony of the nine orifices should be tackled by giving treatment to the stomach", especially when the treatment has shown no good effect over a given period, to harmonize the stomach may break a new path.

From the above analysis, it can be seen the functions of Chenpi and its wide applicability of harmonizing the stomach. Even chronic rhinitis may also require harmonizing the stomach, since rhinorrhea is related to the stomach, too.

Medication Based on Syndrome Differentiation

In the above section, many medications have been discussed, like kaki calyx and Chenpi for preventing vomiting (both cold and heat vomiting), fresh ginger for cold vomiting, and Zhuru for heat vomiting. Clinically, all these medications are made based on the syndrome differentiation. TCM often mentions one term "medication based on syndrome differentiation", including two aspects: one is syndrome differentiation, and the other is medication, for which the first importance is to differentiate the various syndromes of cold-heat, Yin-Yang, exterior-interior and deficiency-excess. Some TCM doctors can make perfect syndrome differentiation, but they may not be good at making medication. As a matter of fact, medication is a very accurate and unique process, in which there are many ways and perspectives regarding selection of herbs, but at least one point should be kept in mind that the hot medicines should be used mainly for the cold syndromes, and the cold and cool medicines should be used mainly for the heat syndromes.

For instance, vomiting may show many different syndromes and stem from different reasons like the spleen deficiency, stomach heat, phlegm, blood stasis, disharmony of the liver and stomach, or any other reasons. Therefore, all these syndromes should be treated with different herbs accordingly. However, some herbs are specific for some specific diseases, for example, kaki calyx is used to stop hiccup that does not require the process of syndrome differentiation. Whenever hiccup occurs, kaki calyx will do. So, TCM doctors should take both the situations of "specific herbs for specific disease" and "specific herbs for specific syndromes" into consideration.

Once I followed my TCM teacher to see a patient who is a professor at a famous university and around 60 years old. He looked strong, speaking with a voice like a great bell, but he was suffering from high blood pressure, with quite red face and hot temper. My teacher used the formula of **Zhengan Xifeng Tang** but removed the herb Chuanlianzi (szechwan chinaberry fruit) since Chuanlianzi is an herb for purging the liver Qi, which was inappropriate for that professor's specific case. Therefore, my teacher's modification of **Zhengan Xifeng Tang** was for the purpose of imposing some suppression of the liver Qi but not too much, which was proved very effective for that case. That is what I mean that treatment must be done based on the syndrome differentiation of different patients ' cases.

Another case I heard about from a veteran doctor of TCM was that he had an old patient with chronic appendicitis, for which, in fact, there is a special and effective curing method. The first TCM doctor for the patient mainly used the bitter-cold medicines to eliminate dampness and heat for promoting blood circulation to remove blood stasis, which killed the pain. However, the patient started to have loose bowels, so, he came to the veteran doctor who diagnosed that the patient had yellowish and greasy coating on the tongue, an obvious symptom of dampness and heat in the Middle Jiao. So, the veteran doctor gave him the formula of **Lianpo Yin** for clearing the dampness and heat in the Middle Jiao, too, but was found ineffective. And then, the veteran doctor asked some details about the patient's life and got to know that the patient had diarrhea, showing some cold symptom instead of heat symptom since the patient still had stomachache now and then and liked to apply hot compress and pressure on the abdomen, which appeared to be the cold symptom, but the coating on the tongue showed serious damp and heat symptoms. Upon further inquiry, the veteran doctor got to know that the patient worked in an ice plant to do ice cream before he retired. Up to then, the veteran doctor traced back to the root of the patient's trouble: the combination of excessive exposure to coldness in his working time before and Yang deficiency in his old age now, as well as too much bitter-cold medicines he had used, which worsened his condition of Yang deficiency. According to TCM theory, the patient who suffers from Yang deficiency will show the symptom of coldness, while the patient who suffers from Yin deficiency will show the symptom of heat. Hence, the patient was treated with the method (for treating the cold diseases) of tonifying the spleen and warming the Middle Jiao, which easily solved the problem of loose bowels.

Tongxie Yaofang

Tongxie Yaofang is a formula involved with Chenpi. This formula was recorded in a book written by Zhu Danxi, medical scientist in Yuan dynasty. It contains four herbs: parched Baizhu (white atractylodes rhizome), parched Baishao (radix paeoniae alba), Fangfeng (radix sileris) and Chenpi (pericarpium citri reticulatae). This formula is famous because of its well- considered composition, good effects and wide application. Wood restricting the earth tells us that the liver and the spleen are prone to disharmony. Harmony among all the internal organs is the goal, but it is a very difficult goal to accomplish. The five elements in the *Wuxing Doctrine* have mutual restriction, thus, conflicts are often involved. But such conflicts can be mediated to some extent.

Parched Baizhu tonifies the spleen. Baishao purges the liver fire and nourishes the liver Yin. The liver is subsumed to Yin in physique but subsumed to Yang in function. The liver Yin deficiency may result in the excessive liver Yang. Baishao is sour in taste, and it can be used to purge the liver of pathogenic fire in its functions and nourish the liver in its physique. Baishao helps the liver to stay harmonized so that the liver will not attack the spleen. Fangfeng is pungent and dispersing in properties, so it can disperse and harmonize the liver Qi. Chenpi can harmonize the stomach Qi.

Tongxie Yaofang is, in fact, using Baizhu and Baishao to soothe the liver and spleen respectively, while Chenpi and Fangfeng in this formula function to mediate the other herbs.

This formula was initially used to treatthe diarrhoea with pain. Pain is often associated with the liver, especially the discontinuous pain, which is often associated with Qi disharmony due to the liver disorder. Diarrhoea, on the other hand, is related to the spleen. Therefore, the diarrhoea with pain in fact refers to disharmony between the liver and spleen. But now, this formula is also used for some other purposes through certain modification.

Houpo (Mangnolia Officinalis)

Houpo is the bark of magnolia tree. It is pungent, bitter, and warm in nature with aromatic scent, entering the spleen, stomach and large intestine channels with descending effect. As it is known, the stomach dominates descending functions, with which Houpo complies exactly. Therefore, Houpo is often used to assist the descending function of the stomach in case it is impaired. Especially, those who improperly take Renshen (ginseng) and Huangqi (radix astragali) may have the descending function of the stomach impaired, resulting in indigestion and gaseous distention, for which Houpo can be used for treatment.

Houpo Relieves Gaseous Distention

In the modern times, many people eat their head off every day, resulting in dyspepsia. Houpo can be added based on other herbs that resolve food indigestion to descend the food rapidly, for example, Shanzha for treatment of the meat indigestion, Caoguo (amomum tsao-ko) for treatment of vegetable and fruit indigestion, parched Daoya (fructus oryzae germinatus) for treatment of rice indigestion, roasted Maiya (malt) for treatment of wheat food indigestion. Furthermore, Jupi (orange peel) is added for harmonizing the stomach; Zhike (fructus aurantii) and Houpo are added for descending the stomach Qi. Meanwhile, in order to prevent an excessively descending consequence, Sharen (fructus amomi), an aromatic herb, may be added to refresh the spleen.

Houpo goes downwards, harmonizing the stomach and relieving the stomach distension. There are two types of stomach distension: excess distension and weak distension. However, in the modern times, most of the cases are of the excess distension which refers to Qi stagnation in the stomach and results in poor appetite. For such a case, Houpo will be a good choice. In TCM, there is a saying, "Eat Houpo meals and wear Rougui clothes", which means Houpo can make one has appetite, and Rougui can make one feel warm when he/she feels cold in the case of Yang deficiency. Rougui is a warm herb that can warm the kidney, which in turn, warms the whole body.

Use Houpo with Caution for Deficiency Distension

Those who are suffering from the weak distension must be cautious about the use of Houpo. Many people, especially the elderly, always suffer from the stomach distension, which usually stems from overeating, less physical exercises and failure of the spleen T&T due to deficiency. A small dose of Houpo can make them feel very comfortable, but Houpo cannot be used in a long run, and especially the elderly should stop using it where it should stop, since long and continuous use of Houpo may impair Qi.

The same is true to Laifuzi (radish seed). Some elderly people have heard that Houpo and Laifuzi are beneficial to the body, so they start to drink them as tea. They may feel good for the first try. However, long and continuous use will then result in distension again since the initial distension can be excess distension for which Houpo and Laifuzi can be effective. Long and continuous use of them may turn the excess distension into deficiency distension for which Houpo and Laifuzi will not be effective any more.

Meaning of "Harmonizing the Stomach"

In the previous section about **Pingwei San** (literally means "powder for harmonizing the stomach"), mound and sinking concerning the earth has been discussed as one can see that the rugged ground appears everywhere on the earth. According to the **Wuxing Doctrine** (the **Five-element Doctrine**), the earth at the high place represents the stomach earth that likes a little "rain" for coolness since "the stomach is dry earth and coolness can make it calm down". The spleen is like the sinking earth that is always moist, and it likes dryness and warmth instead of coolness. Therefore, TCM thinks "the spleen is damp earth that starts its T&T functions when it is warm". In that case, there is a conflict between the spleen and the stomach. In order to settle such a conflict, it is necessary "to level the earth", that is, to relieve the conflict between the stomach and the spleen so that these two organs can stay harmonious.

Pingwei San contains the herbal ingredients of Cangzhu (rhizoma atractylodis), Houpo (mangnolia officinalis), Chenpi (pericarpium citri reticulatae) and Gancao (liquorice). The function of this formula is "to level the earth", though its main function is to eliminate the dampness. Houpo is pungent, bitter, and warm in properties. Its warm and pungent properties can help disperse dampness, and its bitter property can help Qi go downwards. These effects of Houpo can precisely eliminate the stomach distension due to the damp pathogens or the failure of spleen T&T. **Pingwei San** might have been named as **Pingpi San** since all the herbs in the formula function to dry the spleen dampness, which is like leveling the mound to fill up the sinking and moist place so that the dry soil can absorb some dampness from the sinking place. As such, the spleen-earth will no longer be that damp again. This is the real intention of **Pingwei San**.

Muxiang (Costustoot)

In the previous sections of this volume, we have discussed a few earth-associated medicines/herbs that share a common feature: they are all aromatic. Baizhu is aromatic, and Cangzhu is more aromatic. The category of citrus genus includes Chenpi, Juhong, Zhishi, Youzi Pi (shaddock peel) are all aromatic though there exist some differences in their aromatic intensity. Houpo is also aromatic. All the aromatic herbs can refresh the spleen, which governs T&T. Thus, the herbs that assist T&T functions are often aromatic. Furthermore, the aromatic property can resolve the turbid and open the orifices. The differences among the properties of aromatic herbs determine that they are used for different purposes though they all have the effect to assist T&T function.

In addition to the above-mentioned aromatic herbs, there are many other aromatic herbs, too, such as Muxiang and Sharen.

Production Place of Muxiang

Muxiang is a type of vine that attaches onto the other trees. It blossoms in late spring and early summer. However, the medicinal part of Muxiang is the root rather than the vine itself. It is ready for use once the root is sliced and dried.

Muxiang produced in Guangdong and Guangxi of China is called Guang Muxiang, and that produced in Yunnan Province is called Yun Muxiang. Both are fine in quality. Second to that is the Muxiang produced in Sichuan province, which is called Chuan Muxiang.

Muxiang is also produced in many other places in the north of China, like Anguo city in Hebei province, Bozhou in Anhui province and Zhangshu in Jiangxi province.

Muxiang Enters the Tri-jiao Channel

Muxiang, as an herb for the Qi system in the Tri-jiao, is pungent and warm in properties. It always reminds us of it entering the Tri-jiao channel, the liver channel, and the spleen channel, as Houpo always reminds us of its functions of descending Qi and entering the large intestine; Chenpi always reminds us of its function of harmonizing the stomach; Qingpi always reminds us of its function of relieving the stagnant liver Qi; and Xiangfu always reminds us of its special functions of regulating the liver Qi. All of these tell us that each herb can remind us of something about its major and special functions.

The most important and special function of Muxiang is that it enters the Tri-jiao, promoting the circulation of Qi, descending Qi, and regulating the ascending and descending functions of the Tri-jiao. As a matter of fact, the primary functions of Muxiang are to purge the lung of pathogens (in the Upper Jiao), harmonize the spleen and stomach Qi (in the Middle Jiao), and soothe the liver Qi (in the Lower Jiao), which means Muxiang can regulate and promote the circulation of Qi in all the Upper Jiao, Middle Jiao, and Lower Jiao. Furthermore, Muxiang enters the lung, spleen, stomach, and liver channels, signifying that it regulates the Tri-jiao through these organs.

The Three Levels of Learning

There are three levels of learning, the first of which is the foundation. Some people may think that reading many books can be regarded as laying a strong foundation. However, it depends on what learning is referred to. For instance, the learning about TCM is based upon experience that not only refers to the medical experience but also refers to that in all respects of life. After all the experience and medical knowledge were merged into one's learning, he or she would lay a strong foundation about TCM. That is why there is an assumption that the old TCM doctors are more experienced in clinical practice.

The second level of learning is about temperament and personality, especially for TCM learning, which refers that a TCM doctor should have his own unique understanding about TCM.

The third level of learning is acquired from reading books. Those are the three levels of knowledge. Only when all these three levels of learning are integrated into one, can such a learning be applied in the real clinical practice and give effective treatment of diseases.

Identification and Contraindications of Muxiang

Muxiang is strongly fragrant and dry with a pure Yang property and a little fishy smell. Some people like the scent of Muxiang, but some others dislike it.

Muxiang, as an herb, is prepared by cutting it into slices. The top quality Muxiang looks grayish yellow with off-white pores in it, just like the dried bone. For some Muxiang, there seem some lipid-like substances in the pores because of oil exudation. Muxiang is sticky when it is chewed in the mouth.

All aromatic herbs have a drying property. One might find that his or her hands are slightly dry when he or she frequently touch the aromatic herbs since the aromatic herbs can consume the body fluid and worsen the Yin deficiency. Therefore, those who suffer from the Yin deficiency should take great caution of using Muxiang.

Muxiang is seldom used alone, but often used with herbs that nourish Yin.

For instance, those patients who suffer from Yin deficiency would need Muxiang and Sharen when they use Yin nourishing herbs in order to avoid failure of T&T of the Yin nourishing herbs. In such a case, Muxiang added is to open the Tri-jiao channels in order to assist T&T functions.

Xianglian Pill and Its Use for Treatment of Dysentery

Muxiang enters the Tri-jiao to regulate the circulation of Qi. The Qi stngnation and pneumatolysis obstruction in the Tri-jiao will result in a most typical symptom of dysentery, which is not like loose stool of diarrhoea but more like jelly substance. This, in most cases, is due to damp-heat trapped in the spleen and gastrointestinal system, causing Qi stagnation that affects the intestinal organs to carry on their normal T&T functions. **Xianglian Pill** is often used for those patients who suffer from dysentery.

There are many modifications of the formula of **Xianglian Pill**, but its key herbs are Muxiang and Huanglian (coptis chinensis). Huanglian is used to clear the damp-heat in the Middle Jiao, while Muxiang is used to regulate Qi circulation in the Tri-jiao (including the Upper, Middle and Lower Jiao). Once Qi has been regulated to circulate smoothly and the damp-heat is cleared, dysentery will surely be cured. This is the medical principle and functions of **Xianglian Pill**. In clinical practice, some other herbs are also used in addition to Muxiang and Huanglian. For instance, when **Xianglian Pill** is used to cure dysentery, especially the heat dysentery, it is often used together with **Baitouweng Tang**. By the way, **Baitouweng Tang** is also a classic formula used to treat dysentery.

Generally, in the formula of **Xianglian Pill**, the baked Muxiang is used instead of the raw Muxiang. The baked Muxiang is usually processed by parching the raw Muxiang wrapped with flour dough in a pot until the dough is completely dry (since the aromatic scent of Muxiang is very easy to disperse if it is not wrapped completely in a dough), after which the dried dough is removed. The baked Muxiang is milder than the raw Muxiang since it also absorbs the scent of flour in the process.

Furthermore, dysentery is involved with dysfunction of the lienogastric T&T. Therefore, for curing the dysentery, the baked Muxiang is better than raw Muxiang. For curing dysentery, damp-heat needs to be cleared and the Qi stagnation needs to be regulated gradually but not hastily since treatment of any diseases takes time, and any rush in using herbs may not bring good effects.

Some dysentery can cause pain, for which Baishao needs to be added since Baoshao, sour in taste, can play a converging function of holding the primordial Yin. Furthermore, dysentery is often involved with the liver. Baishao not only stops the pain, but also nourishes the liver and Yin, and it soothes the liver Qi circulation. Hence, Huanglian, Muxiang and Baishao are often used to treat dysentery.

Muxiang with Zhizi for Treating Stranguria and Regulating the Tri-jiao

Muxiang is often used for treating stranguria, too. There are five types of stranguria: Qi, blood, stone, grease, and exhaustion. The main manifestations of stranguria are urinary obstruction, odynuria, turbid urine, hematuria etc. As to hematuria, it must make sure whether pain occurs or not in the process of urination. If without pain accompanied with urination, that would be real hematuria that should be treated accordingly in the way of tackling blood trouble; however, if pain is accompanied in penis with urination, that can be diagnosed as stranguria, which is related to the damp-heat trapped in the Lower Jiao and an inappropriate pneumatolysis of the bladder. Therefore, regulating the Tri-jiao Qi circulation must be taken into consideration while treatment is given to stranguria.

In fact, many TCM formulas are available to target stranguria, such as **Daji Yinzi, Xiaoji Yinzi** and **Bazheng San**. However, these formulas are the basic formulas that should be modified for the specific cases. Herbs such as Muxiang and Zhizi are often used to treat stranguria.

Like the pair herbs mentioned above in the formula of **Xianglian pill**, Muxiang and Zhizi, as a pair of herbs, can regulate the Qi circulation and clear the floating heat in the Tri-jiao. Zhizi, cold and bitter in property, can clear heat and, to some extent, dry dampness.

Muxiang should not be decocted for too long time, and even some books state that Muxiang should not be exposed to heat and it does not need to be decocted. It is usually pulverized into powder and dissolved in the boiled decoction for use. In prescriptions, it is often clearly noted that Muxiang should be put in five minutes before the decoction is ready. If Muxiang is decocted too long over fire, its aromatic scent may escape. However, for treatment of dysentery, it is another different case in which Muxiang must be baked as mentioned above.

Muxiang with Xuanhusuo for Treating Pains due to Qi Impairment

Muxiang used with Xuanhusuo (corydalis turtschaninovii bess) can treat various pain due to Qi impairment. Xuanhusuo can regulate the liver Qi, and it is good for killing pains. However, if only Xuanhusuo is used, sometimes it may not relieve pain. Besides, it is not so effective for Qi regulation, and it needs to be intensified in order to reinforce its potency for Qi regulation. Hence, Muxiang is added to regulate Qi circulation in the Tri-jiao, and help relieve pains due to Qi impairment to some extent.

But it does not mean Xuanhusuo can be used to treat all pains due to Qi impairment. In fact, there are many herbs that can be used for regulating Qi circulation. Some pains may be addressed by some other herbs instead of Xuanhusuo, depending on the part where the pain occurs.

For instance, in case the pain is involved with the stomach, Chenpi and Muxiang will work. Of course, Xuanhusuo may also be added; in case the pain is involved with the lung Qi stagnation, Baidoukou (amomum cardamomum) may be used additionally since it can enter both the lung and spleen to clear the damp-heat; in case the lung Qi fails to circulate and disperse smoothly, Suye (perilla leaf) can be added since Suye, pungent and warm in property, goes to the exterior with dispersing effects and can assist the dispersing function of the lungs. Many diseases are related to Qi obstruction, which at the very early stage causes pains. However, long-lasting obstruction will finally induce phlegm. Hence, Muxiang is often used with some other herbs that reduce phlegm to reinforce the effect on reducing phlegm.

Zhuichong Pill

The formula of **Zhuichong pill** comes from the book of *"Zhengzhi Zhunsheng"* (*Standards of Diagnosis and Treatment*) written by Wang Kentang in the Ming Dynasty. It contains Muxiang (costustoot), Qianniu (semen pharbitidis), Leiwan (omphalia) and Binglang (areca-nut), used for tackling various parasites in the body.

Both Leiwan and Binglang can kill parasites. Besides, Binglang can also remove stagnation and descend Qi.

Each person has parasites in his or her body and can live in peace with parasites, and even some of these parasites are necessary for human body in order to maintain a healthy condition. However, when the body is suffering from any pathogens, the parasites may suddenly multiply and cause troubles. Generally, in case the damp-heat, blood stasis or phlegm occur in the body, causing a turbid condition in the body, the parasites would multiply, for which Binglang can be used to kill the parasites on the one hand, and relieve the stagnant Qi, disperse blood stasis, and promote digestion on the other hand so that it can eliminate all the pathogenic influences from the body.

Qianniu can relieve water retention. With Muxiang added to keep smooth Qi circulation, Qianniu and Binglang can rapidly drive pathogens out of the body through urination and bowel movements.

Sharen (Fructus Amomi)

Properties and Production Place of Sharen

Sharen, as an aromatic herb, enters the liver, kidney, spleen, and stomach channels to refresh the spleen and stimulate the appetite. It is pungent and warm in properties, and it is mainly used to remove the cold pathogens in the spleen and stomach. Sharen is mainly produced in Guangdong, Guangxi, Fujian, Yunnan, Hainan provinces of China. Some areas in the Southeast Asia and India also produce Sharen. However, from the perspective of clinical effects, Sharen produced in China is proved to be more effective clinically.

Sharen is an herbaceous plant, different from most of the other plants that grow upwards and blossom to bear fruit at the top. However, as for Sharen, a separate stem grows from the root, and the stem does not bear leaves but flowers and fruits only. The stem is short, looking like Sharen is growing on the ground. As it is growing along with the root, it tends more to enter the Lower Jiao.

Sharen has a shell, inside which are granules that stick together to form a ball, so it must be cracked open when it is used. By the way, attention is called here that Sharen should not be decocted for over 5 minutes, or it may be used directly by adding it to the boiled decoction after it is crushed.

Sharen Enters the Kidney and Astringes Qi

Sharen enters the kidney and descends Qi. As is known, the lung governs Qi circulation of the whole body, and the kidney astringes and stores Qi, for which Sharen can help the kidney in this function. Meanwhile, Sharen also directs the effects of the other herbs to the kidneys. Therefore, Sharen is also called Suo Sharen that implies that it has the property to converge and store the effects in the kidneys.

Aromatic Property of Sharenfor Drying and Resolving Greasiness

Generally, Sharen is used with a dosage of maximum 6 to 8 grams since it is an herb for regulating Qi circulation. Qi is intangible, and a small dosage will do. The larger dosage of Sharen may make the patients feel thirsty since the aromatic property of Sharen can dry dampness and consume Qi, and then consume the body fluid. In addition, Sharen goes downwards, and it can guide the body fluid to go downwards.

Sharen is often used as spice for stewing meat since its aromatic, and dry properties can help resolve greasiness, allowing fat in the meat to retain its aroma but not oily or greasy, especially in the process of stewing pork feet. The aroma of Sharen can also transform the turbidity and eliminate the stinking smell in the meat. Sharen can tonify the spleen and stimulate the appetite, but it should be used in an appropriate dosage, neither too much that may cause the meat to become tough nor too little that will not achieve the expected effect.

In the past, Sharen was often used to process Shudi (radix rehmanniae praeparata), for which Sharen was crushed and soaked or decocted in water, and then, such prepared water was poured over Dihuang (rehmannia). After that, the watered Dihuang was then steamed and dried nine times. As a matter of fact, the standard processing method of Shudi is by using Chenpi and Sharen since Sharen can resolve grease. Sharen can also help the spleen and stomach to transform and transport Shudi, and it can help the kidney to absorb and store the effects of Shudi, too.

Critical Medicine for Prevention of Miscarriage

All the pregnant women must take great caution of using the aromatic herbs including Muxiang. The aromatic herbs, such as Shexiang (musk) and Bingpian (borneol), are strictly prohibited, and the pregnant women should not even smell them since the aromatic scent has a spurting power, which might impair the fetus, or even cause miscarriage.

If the pregnant women suffer from the spleen and stomach disharmony or disorder of Qi circulation, Sharen can be used instead since it is mild and it can soothe the Middle Jiao and regulate Qi circulation. Furthermore, Sharen can tonify the spleen, upbearing the clear to prevent miscarriage. Besides, Sharen can also help the kidney to properly play its storing function, which, in turn, help the fetus become more secure.

Therefore, Baizhu and Sharen are often used to harmonize and settle the foetus. They are used in many formulas for preventing miscarriage. Normally, Kesha (referring to Sharen with the outer shell) is used in formulas.

Sharen should not be overused. Although it does not impair or consume qi, and can harmonize the spleen and stomach, improper use of it may bring the opposite to what one wishes. Hence, one must be flexible in the use of Sharen.

Pregnant women can use Sharen, but the lying-in women cannot since the aromatic and dry herbs consume blood, which is not good for the lying-in women who are in a condition of blood deficiency after delivery. Furthermore, what the women under such conditions need is to use some medicines to eliminate the lochia as possible rather than the herbs like Sharen for tonifying and storing purposes.

Sharen Used with Muxiang and Chenpi

Sharen, Baizhu and Chenpi used together can harmonize the stomach and tonify Qi, among which Baizhu tonifies the spleen and Qi, Chenpi regulates Qi circulation and Sharen can regulate the Qi of the spleen, kidney, and stomach.

As mentioned in the previous section, Muxiang and Sharen are used as corrigent herbs in the formulas for nourishing Yin, like **Liuwei Dihuang Pill** as a formula for nourishing the kidney Yin. Sometimes, **Liuwei Dihuang Pill** is not sufficient on its own, so, some doctors may additionally put in some Guibanjiao (tortoise plastron gel), Lujiao Jiao (deer-horn gel), E-jiao (donkey-hide gelatin) and even raw turtle shell, but such additional herbs are all greasy and stodgy, and can spoil the patients' appetite. In that case, Muxiang and Sharen are added to relieve the greasiness, and regulate the spleen and stomach in order to stimulate the digestive absorption. Furthermore, Muxiang regulates the Tri-jiao to promote the smooth transformation and transportation of the medical effects in the body; Sharen assists the kidney to play its storing function, allowing the effects of Yin nourishing herbs to be stored in the kidneys.

Sharen Used for Treatment of Cholera

Sharen can be used for treatment of cholera because of its functions of reconciling Qi circulation of the spleen and stomach, and its ascending and descending functions.

Let us see the two Chinese characters "霍乱"(Huo Luan, means cholera) , "霍"(Huo) means "suddenly", and "乱"(Luan) means "disorder". so "霍乱" (Huo Luan) literally means "a sudden disorder in the spleen and stomach". Essentially, the spleen controls the ascending of the clear and the stomach controls the descending of the turbid. In case that the spleen and the stomach are in a sudden disorder, the spleen will fail to upbear the clear, causing loose bowels; and the stomach will fail to descend the turbid, resulting in vomiting. Vomiting and diarrhea are the main symptoms of cholera.

In the summer, the way of eliminating dampness with aromatics can be followed to refresh the spleen and stimulate the appetite, for example, the formula of **Huoxiang Zhengqi San** and some other formulas may be used with some modifications by adding Huanglian (coptis chinensis) (for clearing the heat and descending the turbid) and Houpo (mangnolia officinalis) (for promoting the stomach Qi to go downwards and refresh the spleen) to remove the damp-heat in the Middle Jiao.

Sharen may be used, too, for Sharen, if used together with Huoxiang, Chenpi and Mugua (pawpaw), can treat cholera-induced muscle cramp. The patients who suffer from cholera will often experience muscle cramp in the calf. Mugua enters the liver to relax tension and direct Qi to go downwards. Huoxiang can go to both the interior and exterior of the human body to relieve the exterior syndrome, harmonize the Middle Jiao, and promote the Qi circulation between the interior and the exterior. Jupi (orange peel) regulates the stomach Qi. Sharen regulates the spleen, stomach, and kidney Qi. Therefore, all these medicines used together will play a very effective function in the treatment of cholera.

Besides, another type of cholera called dry cholera is also attributable to the sudden disturbance of the spleen and stomach Qi. The clear Qi fails to ascend but starts to descend; the turbid fails to descend but starts to ascend, and the turbid stuff cannot be vomited out. In that case, a severe cramp occurs in the stomach. This type of cholera is more severe and horrible than the ordinary cholera with vomiting and diarrhea. Just because of Qi stagnation, the pathogens stir up in the Middle Jiao, causing severe pains. A dry cholera has another name called twisted intestinal fever, for which the proper treatment must be given to drive the pathogens out of the body.

The first thing to do is by emesis promotion with braised salt water. Let the patient drink highly concentrated salt water and induce vomiting, after which the bowel movement will follow. Sharen is needed to add in the salt water to regulate Qi circulation and harmonize the stomach, which can bring about a much better effect.

第四章　陈皮与各种理气药

理气概说

在土部健运方药中，促进人体运化的药有很多，苍术和白术只是两个有代表性的药物，因为苍术和白术一个是健脾燥湿，一个是燥湿健脾，都跟脾有关，是用它们来说明运化以健脾为首要。因为脾主运化，要运化首先要健脾。

运化的关键在脾胃、气血

运化取决于脾，那么脾是怎么运化的呢？它要依赖全身气血的周流。因此讲到运化就非得讲到气血，气行于周身，血也是行于周身，气是人体一切活动的推动力。气是无形的，血是有形的，血随气走，气依附在血上，所以气和血也是一对阴阳，是交抱在一起、不可分割。气血的周流促进了人体的运化，要想运化正常，就要理气、理血。相反，如果气血不顺畅的话，那么运化也就不得力了。这就叫"失于运化"。气失于运化就容易生痰，血失于运化就容易成为瘀血。痰和瘀血堵在那里，又会进一步地影响气血的循行，所以理气和理血是促进人体运化的重要途径。

我们讲运化的方药，就要讲理气和理血这两大类药。这两大类的药非常多，因为人体以气血为本，而大自然中的这些东西，不管是动物也好，植物也好，它无非都是走气或者走血，有的同时走气、走血，走气走血也就或多或少的有一些理气、理血的作用，因此这两类的药我们会讲得多一些。

理气理血又取决于五脏六腑，所以我们从五脏六腑讲，讲到气血，从气血又讲到五脏六腑了，这样一来一回，我们对五脏六腑、对气血理解得可能会更加的透彻。

理气药如何起作用

我们先讲理气的药。气是以和为贵、以通为贵，和气生财，不论在哪里都要和气。人际交往要和和气气，身体的气也要和。身体的气一和就相当于和风，和风能够吹生万物。气还得通，所以气以通为贵，气堵了就不好了。衡量人体的气有两个准则：一个是和，一个是通。气堵了就成了痰。所以要理气化痰。

怎么讲理气的药？要结合五脏六腑。肝有肝气，肺主一身之气，脾有脾气，心有心气，肾有肾气，五脏六腑都有它的气。理气最重要的是理哪里的气？其实理哪里的气都重要，但我们认为理胃气是重中之重。得胃气则生，失胃气则死。有胃气则生，无胃气则死，这是一层意思。还有一层意思，胃为五脏六腑之大海。胃是受纳水谷的，五脏六腑跟胃都有关系。同时胃为多气多血之腑，胃气顺的话，那么气血也会顺；胃气不顺，那么人体的很大一部份气和血在这里不顺了，直接就要影响到整个人体的气血顺与不顺。所以理气以理胃气为主。所以说我们先讲理胃气的药，然后再延伸到理五脏六腑之气的其他的方药。

理胃气的药最有代表性的是哪一个？抓主要的就是陈皮。陈皮就是橘子皮。因为橘子皮放的年头越久越好，放陈得发黑了都可以，所以叫陈皮。

橘类

很多植物全身都是宝，整棵树上很多东西都可以入药。例如桑树、枸杞、桂，还有竹子，都是全身都能入药的。橘树也是如此。

橘类药概观

根据产地，广东新会产的陈皮最好；福建的力量就弱一些，但也可以用；浙江产的橘子皮就不堪入药了。不堪入药并不是说不能作为中药，而是说作为药物它是不达标的，你要是实在没办法也可以用。如果实在没有新会陈皮，随便一种橘子皮也可以凑合，看你怎么搭配。现在药方里很多陈皮就是普通的橘子皮。

根据成熟和储藏的时间，有青皮、陈皮、橘皮；根据炮制也可以分为盐陈皮、参贝陈皮；根据所取的部位，一棵橘树有这些药：橘红、橘白、橘络、橘核、橘叶。还有一种橘红叫化州橘红，跟我们普通讲的橘红又不一样。跟橘子相似的植物还有枳，橘生淮北称为枳。枳又有枳实和枳壳。另外，小金桔、芦柑、柚子、香橼、橙子，都属橘类。把这些东西从头到尾仔细地理一遍，能让我们对橘类的药物有个大体上的了解。

总体上讲，这些药都是和胃、调气、化痰的，但又因为它们确有不同，所以在作用上又会略有区别。中医也是这样，不严谨的时候，咱们可以把所有与橘子相似的药放在一起，想办法互相替代；严谨的时候，一片橘皮还得分成两层，分成橘白和橘红。

青皮

橘子开的花不大，但是很多。花谢后，结出特别小的橘子，一颗一颗的。但并不是每一颗都能长成大橘子的，在长的过程中，它会一批一批的掉。没有成熟的小橘子在地上，把它捡起来，发现橘子皮已经有很刺激的辛香气味了，但它还很苦，不能吃。这种掉下来的、特别小的橘子，把它青色皮剥下来，就是青皮；等到橘子红了，可以吃的时候，剥下来的皮，说严谨一点就叫橘皮，橘皮的性质比青皮要平和一些。

青入肝，青皮入肝经。又因为这种橘子还没有成熟，正处在一种升发的阶段，它还正在长，它本身依然有生发之气，生发之气也入肝，所以青皮就经常是足厥阴经的引经之药。

跟陈皮相比，或者跟成熟了的橘皮相比，青皮性子比较烈，没那么平和，它理气的力度比较强、比较烈、比较生猛。这就好比年轻人和老年人，年轻人往往脾气比较大。青皮在临床上也是经常使用的，它有推陈致新的作用，而且它经常与陈皮一起用。陈皮主要是理气的，青皮是破气的，什么叫破气啊？气停滞了，它能够给你冲击开，这叫破气，或者说理气的力度更大。

橘皮和陈皮

橘皮，在阴凉干燥的地方保存三五年甚至更长时间就成陈皮了，陈皮的性质就会更加平和。橘皮比青皮平和，陈皮比橘皮更加平和。

有很多陈皮，并不是把橘皮放在那里就可以变成陈皮，它还有很多炮制的方法，能够把它炮制得比放了三五年的陈皮更加管用。

比如盐陈皮，就是用盐炮制的陈皮。陈皮是理气的，走胃，用盐炮制过它就会走肾。陈皮本身就会理气化痰，痰是从哪里来的？脾为生痰之源，肺为贮痰之器，而肾则为生痰之本。当肾气不利的时候，脾就容易生痰，肺就容易贮痰，所以我们可以用盐或者青盐来制陈皮，可以理气治痰，同时可以治痰之本，能够利肾气。还有，青盐陈皮能够顺气生津，还能醒酒，它既是一种小食品，也是一种药。

还有参贝陈皮，是在炮制陈皮的时候加了人参和川贝。陈皮是理气的，理气时就会耗气，加人参就是用来补点气，这样在理气化痰的时候就不会伤气了；陈皮化痰的力度可能还不够，所以加一味川贝，川贝能化痰又不伤肺还能润肺。所以参贝陈皮是一个补而不滞、消而不伐的药。参贝陈皮现在用的不多了，作为一个知识，我们还是要了解一下。

橘红和橘白

把新鲜橘子的皮剥下来，可以看到它分两层。上面一层是红的，里面一层是白的。通常是把整个皮入药的，但是如果讲究的话可以分开，红的叫橘红，白的就是橘白。

橘红在橘子的最表层，肺主皮毛，橘子的最表层也会入肺。肺往往对应于最表层，而且橘子上面也有很多气孔，与人体的毛孔类似，所以橘红是入肺的，能理肺气。橘子有很香的气味，这种香气主要就集中在橘红这里，它太香了也有不足，一香就散，耗散的力度就比较大，所以橘红的力度比普通的橘皮要大一些。

橘白就正好相反，橘白是里面的，味偏甘，入脾胃，它甘多而辛少。它微弱的香气，依然能够理脾胃之气；香气不那么重，所以它耗散的就小，补的作用就大。

还有一种橘红是化州橘红，也叫化橘红，是广东化州产的，整个橘子叫橘红，它不是从橘子上面剔下来的那层红。这种橘红也是橘类，只是它的肉比较厚，瓤比较少。这是一种很温、比较燥的东西，跟陈皮的作用有相似之处，只是它的性质更燥一些。一燥，它理气的作用就强一些，但依然平和，化痰湿的作用很好。但是毕竟化州地方不大，化橘红产量很少，化州橘红又以赖园的最好，叫赖橘红，就更难找了。市面上有许多假的橘红，是用柚子皮冒充的，不过柚子皮也是理气的，也有一定的作用。

橘络

把橘子剥开后，里面有一层络，也就是白色的丝，抽出来，就是橘络。一个橘子抽不了多少橘络的，所以橘络这个药还是很贵的。橘络能够通人体的络。

人体有经脉，有络脉，络脉是很细的脉。久病入络，而痰随气走，无处不到。当人体有痰的时候，痰也会随着气走，进入人体的络脉。痰一旦进入了络脉，往往就会导致发麻，病到了络脉就比较难治，邪气在人体里，刚开始的时候，走最大的那条路，即足太阳膀胱经。这个时候最好打，也是最难打的，打得不好的话，他会从大动脉很快分散开去，进入人体络脉的时候，就要用一些入络的药，带着别的药到络脉里面，去把这些邪气搜出来。这就会用到橘络。

橘络是从气分化痰通络的，经常与丝瓜络一起用。丝瓜老了以后，里面就全是网络状的东西，把里面的子抖掉，再把外面的皮剥掉，剩下的就是丝瓜络。丝瓜络也能通络，它偏于通血分，所以橘络、丝瓜络经常一起用，当病入络脉的时候，它们可以作为药引子，把各种药引到络脉，它们也有直接化痰的作用。

橘核

橘核，就是橘子里面的核，有点微微发青，它是入肝经的，经常用来治疗疝气。疝气是跟肝经有关，且跟睾丸有关。橘核和荔枝核也是经常用的一对药，专门入睾丸。凡是睾丸有病就用它们来治。当然，并不仅仅是因为它们形状相似，更因为它们有理气的作用。尤其是橘核有理气的作用，同时它又入肝经，它就能够理肝气。

疝气的发病部位是肝经循行之处，可以通过疏肝来治；如果有中气下陷的，用补中益气；如果是肝郁的，可以用逍遥散。一般疝气间带着有肝寒，可以加小茴香甚至吴萸，里面加广橘核、荔枝核，既用来理气又是取它在形象上有相似之处，还可以用来做药引子，把这些药带到它该去的地方。男子的睾丸、女子的乳房是肝经的结节之处。广橘核和荔枝核能治肝经结节处的病，治乳房上的一些病，也可以用这两味药。这个就是相通的，我们可以从一个地方联想到另一个地方，这种联想能启发我们，再在临床中反复得到验证，就是和中医的医理相符的。

男子的睾丸、女子的乳房是肝经的结节之处。广橘核和荔枝核能治肝经结节处的病，治乳房上的一些病，也可以用这两味药。

橘叶

橘树的叶也是药，叫橘叶，也是很香的，香就能理气。橘叶很轻，到了冬天它也是不掉的。是叶子就能发散，青就能入肝。橘叶也是治疗乳房一切疾病的一味好药，它能理肝气而散结。尤其是乳房小叶增生，用它就比较好。

橘叶还有另外的一个妙用，可以用它来解鱼腥之毒。人为什么闻着腥味就非常的难受呢？因为腥味本身就是一种毒。人的嗅觉、味觉有一种本能的判断能力。一般来说，闻着舒服的对人体就有益，比如做菜只要闻着香，对人体就好；花香对人体也比较好，它闻着就比较舒服。对人体不好的东西闻着就不舒服，闻着不舒服的气味就会被理解为是一种臭味。鱼有对人体有有益的一部分，也有有害的一部分，它有一种鱼腥味，会让人感觉很难受，要把鱼腥味去掉，就可以用橘树的叶来解鱼腥之毒，放进去橘叶以后，鱼就不腥了。不腥，意味着这个毒解掉了。当然苏叶、生姜也可以来解鱼腥之毒。

橘瓤

还有橘瓤，就是一瓣一瓣的橘子，一般是不入药。当橘子很甜的时候，甘则润，就能润脾，还能和胃。吃橘子一定要吃甜的，甜的既能理气，又能滋润脾和肺；不要吃酸的，吃酸的就容易生痰。因为橘瓤跟橘皮的性质完全相反。橘皮是理气的，橘瓤则滞气。味酸且滞气，就容易生痰。

我们可以来观察身边的人。如果某人比较胖，或者痰比较多，你看他喜不喜欢吃很酸的东西，一般都不喜欢吃。那些没痰的人，瘦瘦的，吃点酸的倒没事。小孩子没有痰，橘子酸一点他也可以吃，老年人看都看不得这些酸的东西，因为他有痰，酸橘子能生痰。

枳

还有枳。《晏子春秋》里面讲，橘生淮南则为橘，橘生淮北则为枳。其实它是一种类似橘树的植物，只是它生长的环境变了，就长成了另外一种东西。枳，用在药里又有枳实和枳壳。

枳开小花，开花的时候结得满树都是。但是，不是每一个小小的枳都能长大、成熟，其间要不断地掉下来很多。掉下去的也不要浪费了，把它捡起来切成片，晒干，这个叫枳实。其他的枳继续长，长大就黄了，剥下皮来，就是枳壳。枳一般长在陕西，陕西商州产的最好。枳上面有刺，是苦、辛、寒的。

枳壳和枳实

枳壳入肺、胃两经。因为它已经成熟了，成熟了就发散开来，所以它能入肺，同时入胃经。从根本上讲，它也有理气的作用，且作用比较强。

肝从左升，肺从右降。当肺气不能很好地下降的时候，经常用枳壳来降肺。中医有一个诀叫"左郁金，右枳壳"。左边有病，是因为肝气不能很好地上升，用郁金，以解肝郁，让肝气从左往上升。如果右边有病，往往是肺气不能很好地下降，用一些枳壳促进肺胃之气往下降。因此，枳壳是一个往下降的药。肺气是往下降的，胃气也是往下降的，枳壳正好顺应了肺胃二经，或者说顺应了肺胃这两个脏腑的性质，所以它在肺胃二经上散结逐瘀、泻肺气、除胸痞。

枳实就不一样了，因为它还没有成熟，性子就比枳壳烈一些。它能破气行痰，能很快地降气，或者说把一些实邪往下降。它还有开窍，有通窍的作用。

枳壳和枳实有时也是可以通用的。我们没必要完全拘泥于书里讲的它归哪一经、到底有什么作用。根据轻重缓急，例如温胆汤用了枳实，如果病人实邪不重的话，我们不妨把枳实换成枳壳。又如大承气汤用的是枳实，如果怕它下降得太厉害，我们也不妨把枳实换成枳壳。

小金橘与用药的轻重刚柔

还有小金橘，这是可以一个一个连皮带肉一块儿嚼的，然后把里面的籽吐掉。小金桔也有化痰的作用，只是它的味道更加甘甜。

在过去用到陈皮这一类的药的时候，用橘皮、陈皮，如果怕伤正气，那就用真正的广陈皮，也就是广东新会产的陈皮。如果还不放心，还怕它理气理出毛病来，可以用金桔饼。金桔饼就是把小金桔压成饼，再拌上糖让它干燥，也是作为一种零食吃的，有化痰的作用。

用很多年的老陈皮，甚至用金桔饼，这种柔和的方式，会让病人比较舒服。如果你直接用青皮、枳壳去破气，病人就不舒服了。总之，药与病要匹配，什么样的人用什么样的药，而不是力度越大就越好。

此外，还有橙子、芦柑、柚子，这些东西都属于橘类。我们可以格物致知，去观察它、品尝它、体会它的性质。

陈皮无主见

总而言之，陈皮或橘皮，它的性质是辛、苦、温。辛，它能横行，能散结；苦，能直行，能往下降气，它能在人体内纵横驰骋。它的性质很活泼，配白术，就会补脾胃；配甘草，就会补肺；单用它一味反而不好。

有人说吃橘子不要把橘络剥掉，橘络可以通络，而且它对脾胃特别好。我不以为然，橘络入药可以，在吃橘子时单吃它，未必好，因为它反而泻肺渗脾。所以吃橘子时，就只吃橘子瓤。且橘子瓤必须是很甜的才好吃，不要吃酸的，吃酸的就会生痰。橘皮也不能吃。后来有用盐腌的，或者用糖腌的桔皮，这就可以吃了，它被炮制过，或者经过配伍，才能用。

陈皮跟着补药就补，跟着泻药就泻，跟着升药就升，跟着降药就降。它没有一定的性质，它跟着配伍的药走。它跟了得力的药就有得力的作用，不跟得力的药就没有得力的作用。

过去医家也有很多家法，在写方子的时候不要把陈皮写在第一位，因为写在第一位的往往是君药，陈皮不能做君药的，只能作臣药、佐药或使药。因为陈皮没有主见。一般君药要有主见，君药是定位的。如果把陈皮作君药定位，别人不知道你想干什么，那么后面的臣药，佐药和使药都不好配了，所以这是一个家法，或者说这是一种不成文的规矩，只是现在这样的规矩都慢慢地被大家忘记了。

橘子皮可以当一道菜，在做的时候要用油、用盐，就是说不会把橘子皮专门单独地去吃，还要放别的佐料和配菜，也是需要配伍。柚子皮也可以做菜吃，把柚子皮上面的一层表皮削掉，柚子皮有一层很厚的白瓤，可以切成丁，炒着吃。单吃的时候会感觉索然寡味，但是跟别菜配在一起，再加上一些调料，柚子的白瓤能吸收很多味道，味道会很美。

陈皮相关配伍和方剂

要理解一味药的配伍，首先要记住它的根本性质。陈皮的根本性质只有四个字：和胃理气。

陈皮和胃止呕的配伍

比如，陈皮配生姜，可以止呕。为什么呢？陈皮能和胃，生姜连皮用，能温胃。当胃气不顺的时候，用陈皮来理气，同时用生姜来温胃。生姜有化痰的作用，也有往下降的作用。我们说陈皮、生姜能止呕，并不是说所有的呕都止，它只能用于止寒呕。如果是热呕，可以用陈皮配竹茹。

呕往往伴随着有痰，如果胃里有食物的话，肯定还要呕食物，在呕食物的同时仍会有一些痰涎。有些人坐车的时候，晕车，会想吐。晕车的吐有很多种，其中有一种就是总感觉鼻腔和嗓子接头的地方有点痰，这种痰让他恶心，他呕的时候不仅呕食物，还会呕出很多痰，这就是痰呕。生姜是化痰的，陈皮和胃，它也能化痰。在坐车的时候，一是因为在车里颠簸动荡；二是因为闻了不习惯的气味；三是因为心理比较紧张，坐车坐得少；四是因为身体比较虚。所以气就运行得不通了，脾升清的功能就减弱了。脾不升清，那么这些水谷的精微，在脾胃里就化成痰了，不能很好地往全身输送，胃里就积攒了很多痰，所以通常用陈皮、生姜加半夏来止寒呕。

止热呕时，用陈皮、竹茹，也可以加半夏。半夏虽然偏温，但是它主要的作用还是在化痰上。

陈皮降逆止呃的配伍

陈皮、竹茹不但可以止热呕，还可以止呃逆，当然主要是治热呃的。

热呃是因为胃里有热导致的呃逆，胃里有寒也有可能导致呃逆，这就是寒呃了。有人说喝一杯水，呃逆就可以好了。如果是热呃，喝一杯凉水就好了；如果是寒呃，喝一杯热水就好了。为什么呢？因为水喝下去，首先是到胃里，水的温度也能调节胃里的温度。

呃逆起源于胃气不和，就要用陈皮来理气。接着要看它的寒热。如果是热就要用竹茹，如果是寒就要用丁香。丁香是一味芳香的药，也能和胃止呃。还有一个止呃逆的专用的药就是柿蒂，整个蒂都可以用，柿蒂是涩的，它也有很好的止呃的作用。柿蒂是止呃的专用药，不管寒呃热呃都可以用。

治呃逆方法还有很多。呃逆就是胃气不顺嘛，胃气不顺的原因可能是浑身的气不舒，可能是肝气不舒。遇到有人呃逆，你在旁边吓他一下，就可能止住。为什么呢？因为惊则气乱，或者说惊则气散。人体的气是不能乱的，他受惊的那一刹那，气就乱了，但马上他又会定下神来，神一定，乱了的气马上就理顺了。在这一乱一顺的过程中，气就顺了，气一顺，他就不再呃逆了。

二陈汤与热痰的化法

陈皮、半夏再加上茯苓、甘草，就是我们经常讲的一个方剂：二陈汤。

它为什么叫二陈汤呢？因为陈皮、半夏都是越久越好，因为越久越平和，对人体的损伤就越小。陈皮、半夏主要是用来化痰的。如果是热痰，陈皮可以同知母、贝母、瓜蒌皮这些药一起用，知母是清热的，贝母和瓜蒌皮也是偏寒性的。半夏也未尝不可用，虽然它是温药，但也不是太温，何况痰要温化才行，不能一味地用凉药，那样反而把阳气都扼杀掉了，化痰效果就会慢一些。

便秘与和胃

胃不和，不但会呕吐、呃逆、打嗝，还可能导致便秘。解大便本来是与大肠有关，但跟胃也是有关系的。因为大肠与胃是相通的，食物从胃到小肠再到大肠，是一个往下降的过程。脾主升清，胃主降浊，食物吃到胃里边，包括在小肠里边，都还存在一个泌清别浊的过程，泌出来的清，也就是水谷精微、营养物质，依然会往上升，这是脾的作用，糟粕往下走都是胃的作用，我们消化产生的这些糟粕，才能顺利地排出体外。

如果胃气不和，胃气不降，大肠之气也就跟着不降。中焦脾胃是一个枢纽，肝从左升，肺从右降，它的动力来源都在脾胃，都跟脾升清、胃降浊紧密联系。人体的升降是一体的，肝升得不好，脾升得必然不好，胃降得不好，肺降也必然受到影响，大肠的下降也会受到牵连。可谓牵一发而动全身。如果胃不和，就有可能导致便秘，大便降不下来。降不下来怎么办呢？也要从和胃开始。

通便的方法有很多，如果大便结在大肠里边了，不管是因为热结，还是因为湿热粘腻结在里边了，都可以用大黄、芒硝把它攻下去。如果是因为干结，结在大肠里边了，可以用芒硝来软坚散结。芒硝是一味咸药，咸能软坚，芒硝的作用就是让大便变软，不管是干结的还是黏糊糊的大便，它都能给慢慢的软化，软了就好往下排。

大黄一喝下去，它就一直往下走。因为它是苦的，苦就往下走，它又是芳香的，芳香就能走蹿，这味药到胃里边是往下降的，到小肠里边也是往下降的，到大肠里边它同样往下降，它这么一倒腾，有结的就不再结了，所以它也能通。

— 903 —

大黄和芒硝一起用的时候，它们的力度是非常大的，单用其中一种，力度会比较小。如果只用大黄，它能通便，但通便的力度比较小。小有小的好处，它能泻血分的实热，或者说泻脾胃的实热。如果只用芒硝的话，它泻下的力度也比较小，它只是把大便变软，其他的由人体自身来完成，这样，基本上就对人体没有什么伤害。

还有两种情况，跟气血有关：

气不通，人体没有足够的气把大便往下推，这叫气秘。为什么没有足够的气呢？这跟肺有关，肺主一身之气嘛，肺气不足造成了气秘。我们一面用陈皮来和胃，另一面加一味杏仁来开肺，肺肃降的功能强了。胃一和，往下降的功能就加强了，大便自然就下去了。况且杏仁是一种仁，有油性，能滋润肠道，让大便也容易往下降。

还有血秘，就是因为血不通导致的便秘。此时用陈皮和桃仁相配来治疗。陈皮依然是和胃的，桃仁是仁，里面有油，能滋润，而且桃仁是果仁，它能往下降，同时桃仁还能破血、化瘀。瘀血化掉了，新血就生出来了，血液循环就好了，大肠的水液就充足了，加上胃气往下降，大便就容易下来。

九窍不和，其治在胃

前面我们讲了呕吐、打嗝、便秘，这些都是人体孔窍的问题，它们都跟胃有关。

中医有一句话叫"九窍皆属于胃"，是说人体暴露在外面的九个孔窍的病都和胃有关。所谓九窍，是指头上的七窍：两耳、两眼、两个鼻孔，还有嘴巴，还有下面的两窍，也就是前后二阴。九窍疾病，是很多的，其治疗的方式当然是多种多样的，但在治疗的过程中，我们要记住"九窍皆属于胃"，要有一个和胃的思想，在适当的时候用一些陈皮之类的药，效果会大大地增强。这就叫"九窍不和，其治在胃"，尤其是在久治不愈的情况下，考虑和胃，会别开生面。

从这里也可以看出陈皮这味药的作用，也可以看出和胃这个方法有广泛的适用性。甚至慢性鼻炎也要和胃，因为流鼻涕也和胃有关。

辨证用药

前面我们讲的这些病，比如讲柿蒂止呕的时候，寒呕、热呕都可以用，陈皮也是寒呕、热呕都可以用。竹茹和生姜就不一样了，生姜只能用于寒呕，竹茹只能用于热呕，所以临床的功夫首先在于辨证。我们经常讲辨证用药，它包括两个层面，一个是辨证，一个是用药。辨证，首先是要区分寒热、阴阳、表里、虚实。有人辨证很对，但他不会用药。用药要精到。选药的途径、角度非常多，但至少，是寒症你就要用热药为主；是热症你就要用寒凉的药为主。

比如病人呕吐，同样是呕吐，他的症可能不一样，有的是因为脾虚，有的是因为胃热，有的是因为痰，有的是因为瘀血，有的是因为肝胃不和，有的是因为其他的原因，这就要用一些药来针对这些症候。还有的药是针对这个病，用一个柿蒂来止呃逆，这就不是通过辨证来用的，而是通过辨病来用的，只要是呃逆，柿蒂你就可以给用上，它就有效果，柿蒂就是针对这种病的药。有针对病的药，有针对症的药，这两个要结合来用。

过去我在师父那里看到一个病人，是北大的教授，年纪有六十来岁，还没有退休，个子很高大，声如洪钟。本来是身体很好的一个人，现在血压高，脸也非常的红，脾气也非常的大。用什么方子？镇肝息风汤，但他把里面的川楝子去掉了。因为川楝子是泻肝气的药，所以，就不要用川楝子来破他的气了，其他的药都可以用。可以去镇压他，但是，不要镇得太狠。这是根据这个人的具体情况用的，要分人用的。镇肝息风汤用到这个分上就用得比较精到了。

我又想起了另外一件事情，是听北京的一位老中医讲的。他当时遇到一个病人是慢性阑尾炎，因为病人年龄比较大，不敢做手术，找中医治疗了。本来中医治疗阑尾炎还是有一套方法的，而且很快。前面的医生主要用苦寒的药，清利湿热，活血化瘀。痛是好了，但后来病人老是拉肚子。于是病人换了医生到这位老中医这里来了。病人舌苔又黄又腻，这肯定是中焦有湿热。开了莲朴饮，也是清中焦湿热的方，吃了还是不管用。然后，这位老中医仔细询问。得知病人虽然拉肚子，但是拉出的东西并不是热辣辣的，还有很多寒象。有时候肚子还会痛，喜欢用热的东西敷在肚子上，而且喜欢按，这又像是一个寒症。但是从舌苔上看，又是一个湿热，很严重的湿热。那怎么办呢？再仔细询问才知道，这位病人在退休前是一家制冰厂的工人，是专门做棒冰、雪糕的，接触的寒凉太多了；而且病人现在年纪也比较大了。年纪大同样也会阳虚。还有，之前用了很多苦寒的药，这又进一步导致了阳虚。阳虚则寒，阴虚则热。所以他后来把这个病

— 905 —

当成一个寒病来治，采用健脾温中的方法，很快就把这个腹泻治好了。这就是追本求源。

痛泻要方

我们再讲一个与陈皮相关的方剂，痛泻要方，此方最早出现在朱丹溪的著作中。一共四味药：炒白术、炒白芍、防风、陈皮。这个方子之所以有名是因为它的配伍非常精到，效果非常好，适用面也非常广。木克土，肝脾一向不和。和谐是一种追求，人体的五脏六腑一定要和谐，但这种状态很难达到，五脏生克，它们各自之间都是存在矛盾的。但这个矛盾可以适当调解一下。

炒白术是补脾、健脾的；白芍泻肝火，能养肝阴。肝是体阴而用阳。它本质上是属阴的，但在功能上是属阳的。肝主升，升为阳。当肝阴虚的时候，肝阳就会上亢。白芍味酸，可以泻肝之用，养肝之体。它让肝自己把自己养好了，不要过于逞能，否则脾土就被克得很难受。防风，是一味辛散的药，能够辛散肝气、和肝气；陈皮能够和胃气。

这个方子其实是用白术、白芍把肝脾先好好地抚慰一下。白术是补偿给脾的，白芍是补偿给肝的，然后再互相劝一下。防风和陈皮是劝和的。

这个方子最初是用来治疗痛泻的。一切的痛往往跟肝有关系，尤其是阵痛。一阵痛一阵不痛是气痛，气不和往往跟肝气不和有关。腹泻则跟脾有关。所以痛泄破译开来就是肝脾不和。后来，痛泻要方不仅仅用来调和肝脾，它还有其他的作用。

厚朴

厚朴是厚朴树的树皮，味辛、苦，性温。厚朴有芳香的气味。它入脾、胃、大肠三经，性质是往下降的。脾主升，胃主降。厚朴主降，正好顺应了胃的性质。当胃下降力度不够的时候，经常用厚朴来推动胃往下走。胃下降的力度不够，就会导致胀满、不消化。有的人本来不该吃人参黄芪这类补药，这样补气的药吃多了也会导致壅滞，胀满，也可以用厚朴来消胀。

厚朴消胀

现代人饱食终日，每天吃得很多，有食积，可以在消导化食的基础上加一些厚朴，把这些东西迅速降下去。比如伤食腹胀，吃肉多了不消化，用山楂；吃多了蔬菜、水果就用草果；吃多了米饭就用炒稻芽；吃多了馒头、包子就用炒麦芽。另外可以加上橘皮来和胃，加枳壳、厚朴以降胃气。为防止降得过于厉害，还可以加一些砂仁。砂仁也是芳香的，芳香能醒脾。砂仁是先升后降，可以防止降得过于厉害。

厚朴是一个往下走的药，能平胃、消胀。胀分虚实，有实胀、有虚胀。实胀，是气真的壅滞在那里了，现代人一般实胀居多。一胀就吃不下饭，所以用厚朴是能够让人吃饭的药。胀消了，人就觉得还能吃些。所以中医有一句话叫"吃厚朴的饭，穿肉桂的衣"，什么意思呢？不想吃饭的时候，就考虑用厚朴；当特别怕冷、老要穿衣服的时候是阳虚，可以用点肉桂，你就可以少穿衣服了，因为肉桂是一个温药，它可以温肾，温肾就可以温人的全身。吃了厚朴，你就很能多吃饭；吃了肉桂，你就能少穿衣。咱们要这样去理解，而不能死板地去理解。

虚胀慎用厚朴

虚胀就要慎用厚朴。现在有很多人，尤其很多老年人，觉得比较胀，这往往都是因为不运动，吃得又比较多，脾虚不能运化。吃一点厚朴，也会感觉很舒服，但要适可而止，因为厚朴是不能久用的，老人尤其不能久用，久用会伤气。

不光厚朴是这样的，还有莱菔子，就是三子养亲汤里的萝卜子。有的老人在电视里面听说厚朴好，听说莱菔子好，就从药店里买来自己泡水喝，刚喝下去的时候感觉真舒服，就买来很多。吃一次舒服并不意味着吃一百次还舒服，可能吃到第十次你就吃过头了，结果吃坏了，肚子又胀啦，于是就多吃一些，结果是越吃越胀。这怎么回事呢？殊不知，以前那个胀是实胀，实胀用厚朴、莱菔子之类的就能消掉，消掉以后本来就不应该再吃这个。老年人脾胃之气本来就比较虚，存一点胃气已经很不容易了，又吃了这么多克伐消导、破坏脾胃之气的药，再胀起来就是虚胀了。虚胀有虚胀的治法，就不能再继续用厚朴、莱菔子之类的了。

"平胃"的含义

我们讲苍术的时候讲到平胃散，讲到土。土有高高隆起的土，也有低低陷下去的土，当土高低不平的时候，高处的土相当于胃土，"胃为燥土，

— 907 —

得凉则安"，它喜欢下点雨，喜欢凉凉的，这样的话它那上面就容易长东西。脾为湿土，就好比是那陷下去的土，里边总是潮乎乎的，甚至有一些积水，所以它就喜欢干、喜欢温、喜欢暖一点，它不喜欢太凉的，太凉了那一潭水就结冰了，所以，"脾为湿土，得温则运"。那脾和胃就是有矛盾的了，怎么样才能缓解这个矛盾呢？我们就要把土稍微平一平，让高出去的胃土不会高得太多，让陷下去的脾土不会陷下去太多，它们的矛盾不就缓和了嘛！

平胃散，是由苍术、陈皮、厚朴、甘草这四味药组成。它的意思是让土能够平一些，虽然它主要的作用是在燥湿。厚朴是辛、苦、温的，往下降。辛温则散湿，苦则下降。厚朴的辛温苦降就正好能够消除胀满，消除因湿邪，或因脾不能运化导致的胀满。平胃散其实是平脾散，这些药都比较燥，都是燥脾湿的，这就好比把胃高出去的燥土削一些下来，填到陷下去的湿土里边。这样它会把低洼里的一些湿给吸过来，然后脾土就没那么湿了。这就是平胃散的本意。

木香

前面讲了几个土部的药，细心的朋友可能会发现，这些药都有一个共同的特征：就是比较香。白术是芳香的，苍术更香。橘类，包括陈皮、橘红、枳实、柚子皮等等，虽然气味有差别，但它们无一例外，都是比较香。厚朴也是香的。芳香就能醒脾，脾主运化，所以运化的药往往都有芳香之气；同时，芳香还能化浊、开窍。这些香气之间虽然有差别，但是共同的地方就是能够促进运化。因为它们有差别，所以在用法上也有不同。

后面我们还会讲很多芳香的药。先讲两味：木香、砂仁。

木香产地

木香是一种藤，附着在其他的树上，到春末夏初的时候会开花，但它入药的部位不是藤而是根，切成斜片，晾干以后就可以用。

广东、广西产的木香，叫广木香，云南产的木香叫云木香，都是佳品。四川产的木香叫川木香，就没那么好了。

北方很多地方也产木香，如河北的安国、安徽的亳州、江西的樟树。

木香归三焦经

木香辛、温，归三焦经、肝经、脾经，是三焦的气分药。看到木香，首先就想到它是入三焦的，这是它与其他药不一样的地方。如果看到厚朴，就要知道它有一个特殊的作用就是降气，入大肠的，因为大肠是主降的。看到陈皮，第一印象就是和胃。看到青皮呢？就是它能破肝气。所以每一味药都会给我们一个第一印象，第一印象就是它区别于其他的药的地方，后面要讲的还有香附，它也是一味理肝气的药，它还有很多其他的作用，但它最主要、特殊的作用就是理肝气。

木香最主要、最特殊作用就是入三焦经。说木香是入三焦经的气分药，能够行气、降气、调三焦之气的升降。其实考究起来，首先木香能泻肺气，能和脾胃之气，还能疏肝气。泻肺气是走上焦的，肺属上焦；和脾胃之气，脾胃是属中焦的；它又能疏肝气，肝肾是属下焦的。这就意味着它上、中、下三焦之气都能理。同时，木香入肺经、脾胃之经和肝经，这也是通过分别入三焦的几个脏腑来实现它通调三焦之气的作用。

学问的三个层面

一个人的学问，要分三个层面：首先是根底。有人觉得，读了很多书，就叫学问有根底。这要看是什么学问，像中医这样的学问，它的根底是生活，生活的经验。，这种经验并不单是医疗的经验，还有其他生活的经验。结合自己的生活、结合自己的阅历，再结合医理，结合这些学问，医道自然也就成熟了，为什么老中医更好？因为他有很多生活的经验，他的学问有根底。

学问还要有性情、性格，尤其是像中医这样的学问。什么叫性格呢？就是要让这些东西讲出来就像是你讲的，有你个人的特色在里面，有你个人的思考在里面，有你个人的表述方式在里面。

第三是书本中获得的学问。只有将经验、性情和书本知识相结合，才能够学以致用。

木香的鉴别及使用禁忌

木香有纯阳之性，很香、很燥，稍微有一点腥气。有人很喜欢木香的气味，也有人很讨厌。

木香是根部入药，切成片。好的木香，皮是灰黄色的，里边有灰白色的小孔，就像枯了的骨头一样。放在嘴里咬一咬，能够黏牙。有的木香，小孔里有油脂状的东西，这是走了油。

凡是芳香的药，就会有燥性。如果你的手经常碰一些芳香的药，事后你会觉得手有点发干。因为你接触到了香燥的东西，会消耗津液，使阴虚的人更阴虚，所以阴虚的人用木香就要注意。

但单纯用一味木香的时候很少，木香往往是与很多滋阴一起用，例如阴虚的人，用了滋腻的药补阴，为了防止滋腻药不能运化，所以往往加木香，还加砂仁，在后边我们还要讲到。加木香的作用就是为了通三焦之气，来帮助运化。

香连丸与痢疾

木香通三焦而调气，能促进三焦气化，调气滞。那么，三焦气滞，气化不利，会导致一些什么情况呢？最典型的是痢疾，痢疾拉下来的是一些浓冻状的东西，不像普通的稀便，这往往是因为湿热盘踞在脾胃大小肠这一带，脾胃大小肠气滞了，水谷清浊不分，影响大小肠本身，以至于身体有用的东西都会转化成不好的东西往下排，一次排一点，但又不能完全排净，所以人得痢疾，经常会用到一个药：香连丸。

香连丸有很多种配方，它最主要的两味药就是木香和黄连。黄连是用来清中焦的湿热，木香则用来调气，调理上中下三焦之气。气调顺了，湿热清掉了，痢疾就会好得快。这就是香连丸这个方子的原理。当然痢疾并不是说只用这两味药就能管用，我们还可以加其他的药来辅助这两味药。香连丸在治疗痢疾尤其是热痢的时候，经常会跟白头翁汤一起用。白头翁汤也是治疗痢疾的经方。

香连丸里边用的木香，用的是煨木香，就是把木香用湿面团裹住，放在锅里炒，因为木香的香气跑得很快，所以要用面团把它全部裹住，这时候它的香气就不会全部发泄出来。等到把面团炒干以后，再把面团去掉，用里边的木香。木香经过这么一煨，油就少了，气也比较缓和了。而且面团属于五谷，用面团裹住煨一遍，能使木香得谷气，所以煨木香与生木香相比，它比较和缓。

还有一重意思，痢疾跟脾胃的运化机能失调有关，所以在用药时要兼顾脾胃，所以，治痢疾的时候，用这煨木香会比较好。痢疾的湿热需要缓缓地清，它的气滞也需要缓缓地调，不能太急，不是说药用得越急见效就越快。

有的痢疾会痛，那就加白芍。白芍味酸，酸就能收，能够收住真阴。而且痢疾往往跟肝有关，加白芍并不仅仅是因为白芍能止痛，它还能够柔肝养阴，能缓肝之急。黄连、木香、白芍，是在治痢疾时经常用的。

木香配栀子用于淋证理三焦

还有淋证，也经常要用到木香。淋证有五，气、血、石、膏、劳，主要表现为小便不通、尿痛、尿浊、尿血等。而尿血又要分别，要问他尿血的时候痛不痛，如果不痛，就是真正的尿血，需要按血证来治；如果伴随着阴茎疼痛，就是一个淋证，这也跟湿热困在下焦、膀胱气化不利有关。所以，治淋证一定要兼顾调理三焦之气。

治淋证有很多方子，比如大蓟饮子、小蓟饮子，还有八正散之类的，但这些方剂都只是基础的方剂，还要根据具体的情况来加减。所以木香、栀子这些药在治疗淋证的时候要经常用到。

木香调理三焦之气，栀子清三焦浮游之热。前面我们讲了香连丸，现在又讲了木香和栀子这对药，其实这两对药的结构是一样的，一个调气，一个清热。栀子是苦寒之药，能清热，也有一些燥湿的作用。

木香在用于理气的时候，是不能久煎的，甚至有的书上说它根本不能见火，不需要熬，一般是把它打成粉，然后在药剂里泡一泡，就能喝了。一般开方子的时候，木香要写上后下五分钟，在熬药的最后五分钟把它扔下去就行，它只能熬五分钟，就有作用了，如果久煎，香气就全跑掉了。当然治疗痢疾的时候，就要把它煨熟，就又要另当别论。

木香配玄胡索治一切气痛

木香配玄胡索能治疗一切气痛。玄胡索是调理肝气的，最善于止痛。但如果只用玄胡索来止痛的话，有时候止得住，有时候止不住。虽说它能调理肝气，但作用还有待提高，加一味木香，它的调气力度就更大了。木香调三焦之气，对于气痛是有一定作用的。

玄胡索治气痛，也有的气痛还是治不了，毕竟理气的药还有很多，因为气不顺，有时候你没有必要用玄胡索，可以根据痛的部位来合理的用药。

例如与胃有关，用陈皮就行了，木香、陈皮，同时还可以用一味玄胡索；如果与肺气不利有关，可以再加白豆蔻，白入肺，豆蔻入中焦，白豆蔻入肺脾两脏，能清化肺脾里面的湿热；如果肺气不能宣散，可以加苏叶，苏叶是往外宣散肺气的，它是一种辛温的叶子，能走表，能散，与理气的药一起用，就像一个屋子里面现在闷得比较厉害，一边要开窗子，一边又要在屋子里面加强通风。很多病都是跟气不通有关，气不通马上就堵在那里了，刚堵上的时候往往会让人痛，堵久了，最后形成了痰。所以，气滞就成了痰。木香通常又与其他化痰的药一起用，它可以加大化痰的力度。

追虫丸

追虫丸出自《证治准绳》，一共四味药：木香、牵牛、雷丸、槟榔，能够治疗体内的一切寄生虫。

雷丸就是杀虫的；槟榔能杀虫，还能破积、降气。

每个人体内都有寄生虫，只是人体和这些寄生虫相安无事，人体甚至需要一些寄生虫来维护体内生态；但当人体出问题的时候，这些虫会突然繁殖得非常多，这就比较麻烦。一般来讲，在湿热或者有积滞的情况下，或者有瘀血，有痰的情况下，体内比较污浊，这些虫就会失去正常的生长规律，繁殖得过多。所以用槟榔，一则杀虫，二则破气化瘀消食，它能把体内一切不好的东西全部扫荡出去。

牵牛是利水的，也是驱邪比较迅速的。再加一味木香，保证气机通畅，这样牵牛和槟榔就能够让人体的邪气从大小便迅速地排出去。

砂仁

砂仁的性状及产地

砂仁是入肝、肾、脾、胃四经的，也是一味芳香的药，醒脾开胃。它性辛温，能破寒气，主要破脾胃中的寒气。砂仁这味药，产于我国广东、广西、福建、云南、海南，东南亚、印度也有出产，但是，从现在用药的总体情况来看，还是国产的砂仁比较好，市场上国产的砂仁价格也更贵。仔细闻起来，国产砂仁的气味要温馨一些。

砂仁是一种草本植物，它结的果跟别的植物不一样。别的草就是往上长，在上面开花结果。砂仁则是从它自己脚下的根上单独长出一个茎，这个茎不长叶子，直接开花结果。而且这个茎非常矮，结的砂仁看上去就好像是结在地上一样，是附在根上另长出来的，那么它入下焦要多一些。

砂仁外面有一层壳，里面有很多小粒，在一起攒成一团。我们要把它砸碎用，熬的时间不能太长，只能熬个五分钟，甚至把它打碎了放到熬好的药里面泡就可以了。

入肾纳气

砂仁能够入肾，又能降气。我们知道肺主一身之气，而肾主纳气。肾要把人体的气往底下收，砂仁帮助肾纳气，也能够把其他药的药性往肾里面引。所以又叫缩砂仁。这是取它能够封藏的意思。

香燥解腻

我们平时用砂仁，顶多用到 6 克、8 克。因为它是一味调气的药，而气是无形的，轻轻地拨动它就可以了。砂仁用多了，会让人口渴。为什么？因为芳香燥湿耗气，消耗津液，而且它往下走，还能把津液往下引。

砂仁经常用在炖肉料中，它的香燥之性能够解油腻，使肉类肥而不腻，尤其是炖猪蹄，那是必用的；它芳香化浊，能够去掉肉类的腥臭；它健脾开胃，能让人胃口大开。但是，用量必须恰到好处，用的太少，杯水车薪不起作用，用得太多，肉就柴了，可见这个药的威力。

在过去制熟地的时候，经常会用砂仁。把砂仁捣碎，泡水，或熬水，浇到地黄上，再把地黄经过九蒸九晒。用砂仁、陈皮来制熟地，是熟地的标准制法，因为砂仁能够解滋腻，还能帮助脾胃运化熟地，还能帮助熟地往肾里边吸收、封藏。

保胎要药

孕妇必须慎用芳香的药，就连木香都要慎用。像什么麝香、冰片根本碰都不能碰，甚至闻都不能闻。因为芳香走窜得太厉害，易伤胎元，甚至引起流产。

那如果孕妇出现脾胃不和、气机不利，该怎么办呢？砂仁可以用，因为砂仁很平和，能够宽中、调气；同时，砂仁健脾，脾主升清，有升提的作用，能防止坠胎；砂仁还能帮助肾的封藏，肾封藏得好，胎也就更加坚固。

所以，白术、砂仁，经常作为保胎要药，出现在各种孕妇用的方剂中。孕妇用砂仁，一般用壳砂，也就是带着外壳的是砂仁。

　　当然，砂仁也不能用得太多，它虽然不耗气，能够和脾胃，但如果使用不当，也会适得其反，这要靠我们灵活地把握。

　　孕妇可以用砂仁，但是新产妇不要用，为什么呢？香燥耗血，而新产妇本身就处于血虚的状态，再多用香燥的药对她是非常不利的；而且新产妇需要尽可能地排除恶露之类，也不宜用封固之品。

砂仁配木香、陈皮

　　砂仁与白术和陈皮在一起能够和胃益气。白术是健脾益气的，陈皮理气，如果加一味砂仁，理脾肾之气，又理胃气，效果会更进一层。

　　前面我们讲了，木香和砂仁经常一起用于滋阴的药里，作为反佐。比如六味地黄汤是一个补肾阴的药，有时候光用六味地黄汤还嫌不够，有人就加入龟版胶、鹿角胶、阿胶，甚至加生龟版，这都是一些不易消化的、滋腻的药，吃多了，病人就容易不爱吃饭。那么，再加木香和砂仁，一则解腻，二则调理脾胃，促进人体消化吸收机能。而且，木香是调理三焦之气，能使药力运行顺畅；砂仁能促进肾的封藏，把这些养阴药很好地封藏在肾里。

砂仁与霍乱

　　砂仁能同时调和脾胃之气，能升能降，所以就能够用来治疗霍乱。

　　从"霍乱"这两个字的本身来看：霍，意思是"猛然"，霍乱，就是指脾胃猛然一下子就乱了。本来，脾主升清，胃主降浊，升降有序。现在猛然乱了，脾不能往上升清气，清气在下，人就会拉肚子；胃不能降浊，浊气在上，人就会呕吐，所以霍乱的症状就是上吐下泻。

　　怎么办呢？夏天可以用芳香化浊的方法来醒脾开胃，例如可以用藿香正气散，及其他的一些药，里面可以加一些黄连、厚朴，化解一下中焦的湿热，黄连能清热、降浊，厚朴也是促进胃往下降的，同时它的芳香能够醒脾。

　　当然砂仁也是可以用的。它跟藿香、陈皮、木瓜一起用可以治疗霍乱转筋。因为得了霍乱的时候，人经常会出现小腿肚子抽筋，加入木瓜走肝，用来缓急，同时能够引气下行；藿香既走表又走里，解表和中，通表里之气；橘皮是理胃气的；砂仁是理脾、胃、肾之气的。所以他们一起在针对霍乱，效果很好。

　　还有一种霍乱叫干霍乱，它也是脾胃之气陡然一下子乱了。清气不升反降，但该泻而泻不出来；浊气不降反升，该吐却吐不出来。这样，肚子里就绞痛。这比普通上吐下泻的霍乱要可怕得多。气闭住了，所以出不来。邪气一直在中焦搅和，让人痛得不得了，这种病又有个别名叫绞肠痧。怎么治呢？要让这些邪气有个出路，先让该吐的吐出来，该泻的泻出去，然后才好办。

　　首先催吐，用烧盐汤。就是烧得很浓的盐水，让病人喝下去，喝下去后就会呕吐，吐了以后，上通则下达，下面也能泻出来了。如果在盐汤里面加点砂仁，理气和胃，效果会更好。

Chapter 5　Medicines for Relieving Stagnation and Stasis

In addition to the aromatic herbs discussed above, let us see another two aromatic herbs: Xiangfu (rhizoma cyperi) and Chuanxiong (ligusticum wallichii). Both herbs are inclined to relieving stagnation and stasis, but Xiangfu is mainly used for relieving Qi stagnation and Chuanxiong is for relieving blood stasis.

Xiangfu (Rhizoma Cyperi)

Xiangfu is a perennial herbaceous plant that is quite common along waterside or in the fields. On its root, there usually grows one or two strip-type hairy rotundus called cyperus rotundus. Generally speaking, the long and gracile cyperus rotundus is relatively desirable, especially cyperus rotundus produced in Jinhua city, Zhejiang province of China has the best therapeutic effects. By the way, the hair should be removed prior to use.

Properties of Xiangfu

Xiangfu is pungent and warm with slight sweet taste. Xiangfu enters the liver, lung and Tri-jiao channels, that is, running in the whole body.

The lung dominates Qi circulation of the whole body. Soothing the liver and regulating the Qi of the liver and lung is the key to relieving stagnation and stasis. The Tri-jiao is the channel for regulating the fluid and fire in the body. Herbs that enter the Tri-jiao can promote the Qi circulation and relieve stagnation.

Xiangfu as a medicine is used for the Qi system and it can run in all the twelve meridians and the eight extra-channels, which means Xiangfu can travel in the Qi system of the whole body. All herbs that enter the Tri-jiao suggest that they have a wide range of effects and can act to regulate the whole body.

Besides, Xiangfu entering the liver channel implies that it also enters the blood system to regulate Qi in the blood. When used with herbs for the blood system, it can direct the medical effects of these herbs to Qi system to generate blood. That is why Xiangfu used with Danggui can nourish blood, and Xiangfu used with Danshen (radix salvia miltiorrhiza) can disperse blood stasis.

What is Stagnation/Stasis

Huangdi Neijing states that universe and earth have their own stagnation, all the four directions (east, west, south and north) and Wuxing (the five elements of wood, metal, water, fire, and earth) have their own stagnation respectively. The internal organs of the body also have their own stagnation and stasis respectively. In conclusion, there always appear Qi stagnation and blood stasis in the human body. Normally, Qi and blood circulate smoothly throughout the body. Once the circulation is impaired, stagnation and stasis will then occur. However, stagnation does not mean that Qi or blood comes to a complete halt. In fact, slight sluggishness, if any, can be called stagnation or stasis.

Tackling Qi circulation in any case is the principal way of treatment of both Qi stagnation and blood stasis.

Qi and blood are inseparable. Qi is the commander of blood, and blood is the mother of Qi, which means Qi, acting like a commander, leads blood to circulate in the whole body; but on the other hand, blood, acting like the mother of Qi, carries Qi to circulate. Therefore, Qi and blood are inseparable. Qi is subsumed to Yang and blood is subsumed to Yin. They often hold together. Where there is Qi, there will be blood, and vice versa. If there is only blood without Qi, blood stasis will soon occur, which will then intensify Qi stagnation. If there is Qi without blood, or if there is more Qi and less blood, that would be unimaginable.

Qi stagnation and blood stasis, if there is, must be treated through regulating Qi or dispersing stasis, for which Xiangfu is characterized with such functions. Whatever the stagnation belongs to, its ultimate source is in the liver. Therefore, to soothe the liver is the principal solution to relieving stagnation or stasis. The liver has a great influence on emotion, and Qi is also closely related with emotion. *Huangdi Neijing* states that "anger causes Qi to go up; joy makes Qi slow down; shock makes Qi dispersed; and fear causes Qi to go down". These tell us that emotions can regulate Qi directly. For example, one of the treatments for hiccup mentioned in **Huangdi Neijing** is to scare a person suffering from hiccup in a sudden. I personally tried this method once. One day, I was walking with a friend when he started hiccupping. In the street, there were no herbs available. Thus, when we walked into an isolated alley, I pretended to be scared out of my wits and grabbed him at the hand to run. In that situation, he was frightened and started to run with me in scare. After a short distance, we stopped. He asked me what was going on, and he looked much more frightened than I supposedly did. I replied, "Nothing. I was just trying to scare you to stop your hiccup". This method did work on him. Sudden shock can disturb one's Qi. When he calms down again, Qi in his body will become smooth, too. Such a sudden disturbance of Qi helps stop the hiccup. That also proves the physiological effects caused by emotions.

Yueju Pill

The liver is susceptible to stagnation, so the principal approach to relieving stagnation is to soothe the liver. Meanwhile, once the liver is stagnated, there will be an increasing pressure on the spleen. Therefore, the spleen must be tonified in the process of relieving stagnation. **Yueju Pill** is an effective formula for relieving stagnation/stasis.

Yueju Pill contains five herbs: Xiangfu (rhizoma cyperi), Cangzhu (rhizoma atractylodis), Chuanxiong (ligusticum wallichii), Shenqu (medicated leaven) and Zhizi (fructus gardeniae).

Five types of stagnation/stasis are noted in TCM: Qi stagnation, blood stasis, damp stagnation, food stagnation and fire stagnation. Qi stagnation refers to obstruction of Qi, which is the root of all stagnation. Blood stasis refers to the obstruction of blood. Qi and blood stagnation may also arise from severe dampness, which is called damp stagnation. Food stagnation refers to that stemming from over-eating, causing indigestion and impairment of the clear ascending and the turbid descending functions of the spleen and stomach. Fire stagnation refers to the Qi and blood stagnation due to the endogenous heat that restrains Qi circulation in the body.

The five herbs contained in **Yueju Pill** directly target at these five types of stagnation specifically. Xiangfu relieves Qi stagnation; Cangzhu dries the damp to relieve damp stagnation; Chuanxiong eliminates blood stasis; Shenqu promotes digestion and resolves food stagnation; and Zhizi clears fire, the floating heat in the Tri-jiao, relieving fire stagnation.

The degree of stagnation severity decides the dosage of each herb in this formula. For instance, in case that food stagnation does not occur, Shenqu may be removed from the formula; in case there arises cold symptom, parched Zhizi can be substituted for Zhizi, or even Zhizi can be taken out of the formula. In brief, this formula can be modified based on the real syndromes. However, **Yueju Pill** cannot be used for too long time since the five ingredient herbs are all partially dry but not moistening and can consume the vital Qi. In clinical practice, this formula is often modified based on the syndrome differentiation.

Xiaoyao San

The formula of **Xiaoyao San** is quite effective for relieving stagnation/stasis, and especially, it can be used in a long run.

Xiaoyao San contains the ingredient herbs: Chaihu (radix bupleuri), Baizhu (white atractylodes rhizome), Baishao (radix paeoniae alba), Danggui (angelica sinensis), Fuling (poria cocos), Gancao(liquorice) and Bohe (mint).

Chaihu can soothe the liver. Soothing the liver and relieving stagnation together is a frequent topic for treatment in TCM, but in fact, they are different processes. In order to relieve the liver stagnation, the tactics for relieving stagnation is use the herbs that can soothe the liver.

According to the **Wuxing Doctrine**, wood restricts earth, so the spleen (earth) will be affected if one starts to soothe the liver (wood). That is why Baizhu is used in this formula. The book **Jingui Yaolue (Synopsis of Golden Chamber)** states that "when diseases of the liver are confirmed, one needs to know that the liver can affect the spleen, and thus the spleen should be nourished first". Both Fuling and Gancao enter the Middle Jiao. Fuling used with Baizhu can promote the pneumatolysis function of the Middle Jiao. Gancao, sweet in taste, can nourish the spleen and coordinate the action of the other herbs in this formula.

Chaihu is pungent and dispersing in properties, which are to the liking of the liver. However, anything beyond its limits will become harmful. Ye Tianshi (well-known medical expert in Qing dynasty) said that Chaihu "robs the liver of Yin". That problem can be solved by parching Chaihu with vinegar or even with the blood of turtle; and it may also be solved by using Baishao as a corrigent herb in this formula. Baishao, sour in taste, can enter the liver; and it is cold and moistening, so it can purge the liver fire and nourish the liver Yin. Baishao plus Danggui is a paired medicine used for nourishing and regenerating blood. In the process of soothing the liver, Danggui and Baishao should be added since some liver Qi stagnation arises from Yin deficiency, for which Danggui and Baishao are essential herbs.

Bohe relieves the exterior syndromes, and it can reconcile the interior and exterior. Besides, it also assists Chaihu to disperse and relieve stagnation.

Comparing with **Yueju Pill**, **Xiaoyao San** is much milder, and it can relieve stagnation by way of regulating the five internal organs. In brief, **Xiaoyao San** not only can relieve the stagnation through soothing the liver, it can also tonify the spleen and nourish the liver Yin. Hence, **Xiaoyao San** has much broader applications than **Yueju Pill**.

The formula of **Xiaoyao San** may be modified by adding Zhizi in case of fire stagnation or fire due to stagnation, and Danpi (cortex moutan radices) in case of severe heat symptom, which then will be made into a modified formula called **Danzhi Xiaoyao San**, or **Jiawei Xiaoyao San** produced in Beijing Tongrentang of China.

In case of dampness arising, Cangzhu and Baizhu can be added to **Xiaoyao San**; in case of Qi stagnation, or severe liver stagnation, Xiangfu may also be put in additionally; in case of severe blood deficiency, Danggui and Baishao may not be sufficient for treatment, then Chuanxiong and Sheng Dihuang can be added. After all those modifications, we may have a formula called **Siwu Tang** (containing Danggui, Bai Shao, Chuanxiong and Sheng Dihuang).

The formula of **Xiaoyao Pill** has numerous modifications and it is frequently used in clinical practice. In the modern society, a lot of people are suffering from various stagnation/stasis that requires relieving in order to keep smoother circulation of Qi and blood and avoid further development of stagnation/stasis into various diseases. In many cases, **Xiaoyao Pill** is used to lay a strong foundation for curing diseases with other medicines since only after the Qi stagnation or blood stasis is relieved, the liver and spleen are reconciled and harmonized. And especially, when the liver is soothed properly, the diseases involved will be cured easily. Or otherwise, the phlegm or stagnation may not be resolved/ dispersed if the prior treatment foundation is not laid with **Xiaoyao Pill**.

Why Females are Prone to Stagnation/Depression

Women are prone to suffering from stagnation/depression, including both psychological depression and physiological stagnation/stasis comparing with the males. Generally, the psychological depression and physiological stagnation/stasis are closely inter-related. When a lady experiences emotional depression, she would suffer from the Qi stagnation and blood stasis simultaneously; when she suffers from the liver stagnation, she would feel depressed emotionally too, and vice versa. Xiangfu is frequently used in gynecology to relieve stagnation. That is why many books claim that Xiangfu is a panacea in gynaecology.

In TCM history, there have been many theories on the matter of women being prone to suffering from stagnation/ depression. One of the most popular theories claims that the stagnation is involved with much blood loss at menstruation every month, as such the liver is always in a state of Yin deficiency, resulting in hyperactivity of the liver Yang, and hence, the liver stagnation occurs easily.

Women easily become agitated or experience mood swings before or during menstruation since breast distending pain may occur when Qi and blood are unstable, or when there is a large amount of blood loss, or when there is severe liver stagnation. Therefore, the female liver stagnation/depression is closely related to the menstrual cycle, and it needs relieving physiologically and emotionally, for which understanding and sympathy from the males are very important.

Otherwise, breast hyperplasia, breast cancer, mastitis and some other gynaecological disorders may develop gradually in case that the liver stagnation/ depression finds no vent to relieve. As such, soothing the liver is very important for modern women and **Jiawei Xiaoyao Pill** can be taken as a necessary medicine at home.

Processing of Xiangfu

Xiangfu is particular for medical use since it needs very special processing and compatibility with other herbs in order to achieve the maximum herbal effects. Xiangfu enters all parts of the body, suggesting that it has no distinct target, and its effect will be scattered, hence, great attention should be paid to the its processing.

The raw Xiangfu can play its functions upwards in the body, and regulate the Qi circulation of the lungs and chest. Raw Xiangfu can be used when chest distress occurs, or when stagnation/stasis requires relieving at the body surface. The parched Xiangfu goes downwards, entering the liver and kidney and moving down to the waist and feet; the parched Xiangfu charcoal has Qi-regulating and hemostyptic effects; the parched child-urine-soaked Xiangfu can tonify deficiency; Xiangfu fried with salt fluid can enter the blood system and moisten dryness; Xiangfu fried with halite (a special salt with greenish color, going to the liver and kidneys) can tonify the kidney Qi; Xiangfu soaked and parched with liquor goes upwards and especially tends to enter the meridians and collaterals; Xiangfu soaked and parched with vinegar tends to enter the liver meridian to relieve the liver stasis and remove the Qi stagnation since sour taste can go to the liver. For instance, those patients who suffer from liver cirrhosis or those women who suffer from lumps or nodules in breasts should use the vinegar Xiangfu since breasts are subsumed to the liver meridian, and the mammitis or the lobular hyperplasia in breasts attribute to stagnation that has to be removed with the effects of Xiangfu. Furthermore, the hypochondriac pains, occurring below the costal region where the liver channel travels, also attribute to the liver Qi stagnation, for which vinegar Xiangfu is often used in the formula for treatment based on the syndrome differentiation.

Xiangfu can also be parched with fresh ginger juice, after which the parched Xiangfu can enter the spleen channel and act to regulate Qi and reduce phlegm.

There is a formula containing Xiangfu only but in different forms for treating female infertility. In the formula, Xiangfu is cut into many parts that have been processed with vinegar, liquor, salt separately, which can achieve a good therapeutic effect. This formula is effective for those women who suffer from infertility due to Qi and blood stagnation. However, this formula may not be effective for infertility due to the other causes. This suggests that Xiangfu can play different functions depending upon the processing methods; and if processed appropriately, it can work effectively.

Compatibility of Xiangfu

Xiangfu is an active herb. When it is used with Renshen or Baizhu, it can tonify Qi. Xiangfu regulates Qi, and consumes Qi, too. However, when used with herbs that tonify Qi, Xiangfu will reinforce the effects of regulating and tonifying Qi.

When used with Danggui and Dihuang, Xiangfu can regulate Qi on the one hand and reinforce the effects of enriching blood by Danggui and Dihuang on the other hand.

Xiangfu can become warm when used with the warm herbs, such as fresh ginger and Aiye (folium artemisiae argyi); and then, it can warm off the coldness of Qi and blood. It can help the warm herbs to give full play to their medical effects through relieving stagnation and regulating Qi; when used with the cold and cool herbs, such as Huanglian and Zhizi, Xiangfu can clear excess heat in Qi and blood and help the cold and cool herbs to give full play to their medical effects through clearing heat and regulating Qi.

Thus, it can be seen the symptoms involving cold, heat, deficiency or excess, to some extent, are involved with Qi stagnation and blood stasis. The human body should be in a balanced condition without abnormal heat, cold, deficiency or excess. However, Qi stagnation impairs the self-regulating functions of the human body, for which Xiangfu can help to regulate Qi circulation, and improve the self-regulation of the body. The effects of Xiangfu depend on its compatibility with other herb(s). Attention is also called that Xiangfu is severe dry in property, so misuse or long-term use will consume Qi and blood. As such, the compatibility and processing of Xiangfu is critical for its proper uses and effects.

Chuanxiong (ligusticum wallichii)

Chuanxiong is also called Xiongqiong (ligusticum sinense). Its leaves look like celery leaves, and its root can be used as medicine, which is shaped irregularly and hard in texture. It tastes pungent and slightly sweet.

Fuxiong and Chuanxiong

Xiongqiong produced in Jiujiang and Fuzhou cities in Jiangxi province of China is also named Fuxiong, which shows a lot pores after being sliced. The root of Chuanxiong is yellow or black outside and white inside. Fuxiong (or Xiongqiong) and Chuanxiong have the similar effects.

Comparing with Chuanxiong, Fuxiong has a stronger capacity to enter the Tri-jiao and relieve stagnation. Meanwhile, Fuxiong can also promote Qi and blood inter-communication and regulate Yin and Yang. Chuanxiong is more nourishing and widely used.

Properties and Contraindications of Chuanxiong

Chuanxiong is pungent, sweet, and slightly cold with ascending nature. It can enter the eight extra-channels and disperse wind cold in blood. Chuanxiong, aromatic in scent, always runs in disorder. Therefore, Chuanxiong needs assistance from some other herbs to protect it from running randomly in the body, or otherwise, it may impair Yin and the primordial Qi in blood.

Chuanxiong is a herb used for regulating Qi and dispelling the wind in blood. The stagnation/stasis in the blood system can be resolved with Chuanxiong. Besides, Chuanxiong is also an ascending herb that can be used to upbear the clear and disperse the dampness on the head. Chuanxiong can guide the medical effects of other herbs upwards to the head to cure all kinds of headache. Therefore, Chuanxiong is always used for curing headache with some other guiding herbs added based on the syndrome differentiation.

Herbs should be used according to the patients' characters. The inactive patients should use active herbs in order to activate the patient's Qi and blood. However, some others are active, so they should avoid using the active herbs.

Chuanxiong is a very active herb. It is used in the formula of **Siwu Tang**, in which Danggui, Baishao (sour in taste, playing a converging function) and Dihuang (nourishing and greasy) are all inactive, and only Chuangxiong is active. So, these four herbs in **Siwu Tang** can restrains each other so that they can reconcile their functions to an appropriate condition. Of course, in clinical practice, the dosage of each herb in this formula will have to be adjusted based on the syndrome differentiation. Chuanxiong in **Siwu Tang** helps activate the newly enriched blood to circulate in the blood vessel smoothly. However, in the period of menstruation or in the case of any bleeding symptom, try to control the dosage or avoid using Chuanxiong.

In addition, Chuanxiong tends to run upwards, so those who suffer the diseases of sore throat, oral ulcer and the like due to deficiency fire should avoid using Chuanxiong since it has dispersing effect that may further impair Yin and brings the deficiency fire upwards. Furthermore, Chuanxiong should also be avoided for the symptoms like vomiting, cough, high blood pressure, ephidrosis, and blood disorder, otherwise, the symptoms may be worsened.

However, blood disorder due to blood stasis is an exception, for which Chuanxiong is necessary. If there occurs menstrual disorder due to blood stasis for which herbs for removing blood stasis should be used for treatment with the basic formula of **Siwu Tang** plus Taoren, Honghua, Jiegeng and Niuxi (to make a new formula called *Xuefu Zhuyu Tang*) based on the syndrome differentiation. In this modified formula, Chuanxiong is used for promoting the blood circulation in order to eliminate the blood stasis. In brief, TCM attaches a great importance to the treatment based on syndrome differentiation in the clinical practice.

Examples of Proper Uses of Chuanxiong

Chuanxiong often has great clinical effects, for example, the symptoms of diarrhea, slip pulse, and greasy tongue coating with a swollen and teeth-marked tongue body, all these may attribute to dampness accumulation in the body. As such, based on the syndrome differentiation, a little Shenqu and Chuanxiong may be added in the formula for treatment, which will bring about great effects since Shenqu eliminates dampness and helps digestion, while Chuanxiong is for the blood system.

Another case is about the treatment of bloody flux, referring to diarrhea accompanied by intestinal bleeding and blood in the stools. After treatment, bloody flux can be cured, but stomachache may remain since bloody dysentery impairs Yin, resulting in Qi stagnation. Based on the syndrome differentiation, Chuanxiong added in the formula can relieve the stagnation and then the stomachache will disappear.

第五章　解郁药

我们继续讲两味芳香的药：香附和川芎。它们对人体的运化有很重要的作用。这两味药的作用都倾向于解郁：解气郁的是香附，解血郁的是川芎。

香附

香附是一种多年生的草本植物，在田野和水边都会有。它是一种草，根下面会结一两个子，长条型的，上面长了很多毛，这就叫"香附米"或"香附子"。细长的比较好。用的时候要把那一层毛去掉。香附以浙江金华产的最好。

香附的性能

香附辛温，微有甘甜。它归肝、肺、三焦经。实际上，香附是一味全身都走的药，归肝、肺、三焦的言外之意就是通行全身。肺主一身之气，解郁重在疏肝，调理肝肺之气，就能疏肝解郁。三焦是上焦、中焦、下焦，能通调水道，又是火府，是水火通调的场所，我们更倾向于认为三焦是我们整个的体腔，归三焦经的药往往能够行气、解郁。

肺主一身之气，解郁重在疏肝，调理肝肺之气，就能疏肝解郁。三焦是上焦、中焦、下焦，能通调水道，又是火府，是水火通调的场所，我们更倾向于认为三焦是我们整个的体腔，归三焦经的药往往能够行气、解郁。

香附是气分药，能通行十二经、奇经八脉的气分，也就是说它通行全身的气分。其实，入三焦经的药不多，一旦说某个药入三焦经，那言外之意就是它作用范围比较广，能够调理全身。

入肝经，还提示香附能入血分，能调节血中之气。它与入血分的药一起用，能把血分的药引到气分，然后来生血。所以，香附配当归则养血，配丹参则化瘀。

郁是什么

《黄帝内经》讲，天地有它的郁，东西南北方与五行都有它各自的郁。人体五脏六腑也有各自的郁，归纳起来，就气郁和血郁。气血在我们浑身是要上下通行、周流不息的，一旦不太通畅，就是郁了。但这种郁并不意味着完全停滞，只要有一点点的停滞，就叫郁。

治疗气郁和血郁，最终还是要以治气为主。

气和血是分不开的。气为血之帅，血为气之母。帅就是率领的意思，好比元帅，率领着军队往前走。气朝哪个方向走，血就会朝哪个方向走，人体的血液因此能够循环。血为气之母，气虽然在走，但要依附在血上。气和血是不可分割的。气属阳，血属阴，气血交抱在一起，有血就要有气，有气就要有血。如果没有气，光有血，血很快就凝滞了，成为瘀血，瘀血又进一步加剧气郁；如果有气没有血，或者气多血少，那就更不可想象。

气和血郁了，就要调气解郁，或者化瘀解郁，这是一个大法，香附正好有这种性质。不管什么郁，本源都在肝，所以解郁又要以疏肝为主。肝为将军之官，对人的情绪影响非常大，而气跟人的情绪也有很密切的关系，《黄帝内经》讲"怒则气上，喜则气缓，惊则气散，恐则气下"，情绪对气有直接的调节作用。比如呃逆，《黄帝内经》提供的治法之一就是突然吓唬他一下。这个方法我在生活中用过。有一次跟一个朋友走路，他老是呃逆。因为在路上，没有条件用药，当我们走到了一个稍微偏僻一点的地方的时候，我装作吓得魂不附体的样子，陡然一下拉起他就跑，他看到我那么害怕，也一下子被吓坏了，就跟着我赶紧跑，跑了几步之后我们站住了，他问我什么事，当时他的样子比我还害怕。我说没什么，就吓唬你一下，看看你还打不打嗝。后来他一上午都没再打嗝，为什么呢？因为他是被惊了一下，气乱了，但是乱了以后，马上又能顺过来，一乱再一定，气机就获得了重新调整。气顺了，就不会有呃逆。可见情绪对生理的影响之大。

越鞠丸

解郁必须以疏肝为主，肝木也特别容易郁。但肝木一郁，脾土的压力就大了，所以要解郁就必须健脾。解郁有一个很好的方剂，叫越鞠丸。

越鞠丸有五味药：香附、苍术、川芎、神曲、栀子。

中医常讲五郁：气郁、血郁、湿郁、食郁、火郁。气郁就是气行不通，这是根本；血郁，就是血行不畅；湿气太重也会导致气血的郁结，是为湿郁；食郁，就是吃多了食物，消化不通，脾胃升清降浊的功能受到了影响，导致人体的郁结；火郁，是体内有热，气机被热遏制住了，导致气血郁结。

越鞠丸的五味药，就是针对这五郁而来的：香附解气郁；苍术燥湿，解湿郁；川芎解血郁；神曲消食，解食郁；栀子清火，清三焦浮游之热，解火郁。哪里的郁比较重，哪个药就用得多一点。如果是没有食积，神曲就可以不用了；如果有寒像，栀子可以用炒栀子，甚至可以不用。总之在这个方子上加减。但越鞠丸不能久用，因为这五味药都是偏燥的，消耗正气，不滋润，所以不能经常用。我们在临床上，一般不会套用原方，而是根据具体情况取其中几味。

逍遥散

逍遥散解郁效果好，可以经常用。

逍遥散：柴胡、白术、白芍、当归、茯苓、甘草、薄荷。

柴胡是疏肝的。虽然我们经常讲疏肝解郁，但深究起来，疏肝是疏肝，解郁是解郁，它们之间是有差别的。为了解郁，我们不直接用解郁的药，转而用疏肝的药，也是一个策略。

疏肝的时候，我们要马上想到，肝木郁则克脾土，脾肯定要受影响，于是加个白术。《金匮要略》讲"见肝之病，知肝传脾，当先实脾"，就是这个意思。茯苓、甘草，也都是入中焦的药。茯苓利水，配白术能促进中焦气化；甘草甘缓养脾，还能调和诸药。

柴胡辛散，肝喜欢辛散，但过于辛散又会伤肝阴，所以叶天士讲柴胡"劫肝阴"。怎么办呢？通过醋炒，甚至鳖血炒等炮制方法，固然可以，但在组方的时候，我们可以用白芍反佐。白芍味酸，能入肝；性寒凉润泽，能泄肝火，柔肝养阴。白芍配当归，是一个养血生血的药对。疏肝不忘补肝阴，所以要加当归、白芍。何况有的肝郁就是因为肝阴虚引起的，所以当归、白芍更要用了。

薄荷是开表的，能调和表里，还能够帮助柴胡辛散解郁。

逍遥散与越鞠丸比起来，更加平和。它是通过调理五脏来达到解郁的目的。不仅通过疏肝来解郁，还兼顾了健脾、养阴，所以逍遥散的含义更加深远。

在逍遥散的基础上，如果是火郁，或者郁而生火，也可以加栀子，热象比较厉害，还可以再加丹皮，这叫丹栀逍遥散，也叫加味逍遥散。现在同仁堂产的加味逍遥丸便是。

如果有湿，苍、白术可以一起用；如果气滞，肝郁得非常厉害，也可以在逍遥散的基础上再加一味香附；如果血虚得厉害，当归、白芍还不够，可以再加川芎和生地，这样四物汤就凑齐了。

在临床上，逍遥丸是经常用的一个方剂，它的变化是无穷无尽的。现代人，有很多地方都是处在郁的状态，需要解郁，解郁了，气血就会更加通畅，气血一通畅，很多病自然就被化掉了。当气血不通的时候，哪怕开的药再对症，也没有用的，因此很多病在一开始都要用逍遥丸来打基础，把气血的郁结打开，把肝脾调和过来，尤其是要把肝气疏展开来，剩下的病就好治了；如果不打下这个基础，上来就化痰、化瘀，是化不动的。

为何女子多郁

在很多书里都讲香附是妇科仙药。为什么呢？因为女子多郁，女性比男性郁闷要多一些，当然郁闷既指心理上的郁闷，也指生理上的郁。当心里比较郁闷的时候，气血也会比较郁闷；当肝郁的时候，心情也是比较郁闷的；当心情郁闷的时候，肯定就会有肝郁，都是相通的。因此，妇科经常会用到香附来解郁。

女子为什么多郁呢？历代的医家有很多说法，有种比较常见的说法是，妇人多郁往往跟月经失血有关，因为每个月要失一次血，所以肝处在一种缺血的状态，肝阴一虚，肝阳就亢，肝处在阳亢阴虚的状态下就容易出现肝郁。

为什么有的女性在经期或月经前后容易烦躁，性格不稳定呢？因为这是气血不稳定的时候，或者说是失血比较多、肝郁比较严重的时候，往往还表现为乳房胀痛。所以，女子肝郁跟月经有很大的联系，这就要求男性必须多多的体谅。她的肝郁需要发泄，就要让她发泄。这比吃药疏肝的效果好。肝主疏泄，既有生理上的疏泄，也有情绪上的疏泄。

乳腺增生、乳腺癌、乳腺炎和那些妇科疾病，都是长期的郁结中慢慢形成的。因此，现代女性疏肝是非常重要的。加味消遥丸应该是一个必备的药。

香附的炮制

香附的使用是很讲究的。要让它充分发挥作用，就要掌握它的炮制和配伍。它全身都走，如果一味药它全身都走，就有点漫无目的，作用就会比较涣散，所以，在炮制上就尤其需要注意。

如果直接用生的话，它的作用是往上的，调胸肺之气，如果有胸闷之类的，或者体表需要解郁的话，就用生香附；用炒熟的，它就会往下走、走肝肾，是走腰部与脚部这些地方；如果你把它炒黑成炭，那么它就有理气止血的作用；如果用童便先泡再炒，那么它就能够补虚；用盐水来炒，它就走血分，能润燥；如果用青盐炒，它还能补肾气。青盐是一种特别的盐，它的颜色有点发青，是走肝肾的。如果用酒来浸炒，它就能上行，而且更偏行于经络；如果用醋来浸炒，它就入肝经更多一些，因为醋是酸的，酸能入肝，入肝它就能消肝里面的一些积聚，甚至入肝而解郁，就能够化瘀消积。比如肝硬化，需要理气的话，那么就要用醋香附。包括女子身上的一些疱块，乳房里面的一些结节，都要用醋香附。因为乳房是属于肝经的，乳腺炎或者乳房小叶增生是肝郁，也是积聚，要用醋制香附来让它们疏通，把积聚消掉。还有两胁痛，因为胁下也是肝经的循行部位。两胁痛也是肝气的郁结。那么，在辨证论治的基础上，方中也常用醋香附。

香附还可以用生姜汁来炒，炒过就会往脾经走，能理气化痰。

以前我在一本书里看到一个治女子不孕的方子。其实只用了一味药，就是香附，但是要把它分成很多份，分别用醋、酒、盐等不同的东西炮制，然后一起用，能达到很好的治疗效果。女子气血郁结引起的不孕不育，可以用这个方子。如果是因为其他的原因，用这个方子就不一定管用。当然，这提示我们，炮制的方法不同，香附的走向是有差异的。炮制方法得当的话，香附的作用会非常大。

香附的配伍

香附是一味比较活泼的药，它与人参、白术一起用，就能够补气。本来，香附是理气、耗气的药，跟补气的药一起，一边补，一边调，反而能让补气的作用更大。

香附它跟当归、地黄一起用，就能补血。当归、地黄是补血的，一边补血，一边理气，补血的效果会更好。

香附与生姜、艾叶这两味温药一起用，就是温的，能温气血之寒。通过解郁、理气，让温药的作用发挥开来；它与黄连、栀子这些凉药一起用的时候，又能清气血之热，边凉边理气，寒凉药的作用也会发挥的更好。

从这里我们可以看出，不管是寒热虚实，总跟气血的郁结有关。人体应该是一个平衡的整体，没有热也没有寒，没有虚也没有实。

出现了寒热虚实，都与气郁有关，气郁影响了人体自我调节机能。香附正好能调理气机，促进气化，调整人体的自我调节机能。它的作用取决于配伍，什么药与它一起，作用都会更强。当然话说回来，香附是比较燥烈的，用错或久用会耗气耗血，所以一定要注意它的配伍和炮制。

川芎

川芎又叫芎䓖，叶子很像芹菜。川芎入药的部位是根，根的形状不规则，坚硬，味道有点辣又微微甘甜。

抚芎与川芎

江西九江、抚州一带产的芎䓖叫抚芎。川芎跟抚芎区别是，川芎外边是黄或黑色，里面是白色的；抚芎最明显的特征是切成薄片后中间有孔。它们的作用是相近的，但又各有所长，有细微区别。

抚芎很多作用都和川芎很相似，唯独它直达三焦的作用更强一些，解郁的力度要强一些，而且它还能够沟通气血，调和阴阳。川芎则润一些，用的比较多。

川芎的药性及使用禁忌

川芎是辛甘微寒，有升浮之性，可以通奇经八脉，散血中风寒。它是非常香的，芳香就走窜，所以川芎需要用其他的药好好管一下，不能让它乱跑，如果它跑得没有方向和目的，就会伤阴，伤血中的元气。

川芎是血中的气药，也是血中的风药。如果血分有郁的话要用川芎来解。川芎是升浮之药，可以升清气，发散头上湿气，各种各样的头痛都可以用川芎来把药带到头上。所以，头痛必用川芎，再根据头痛的类型加上不同的引经药。

有的病人，天天坐在那里不动，用药就要用好动的药，让他的气血动起来。有的病人老是动，需要安静，就不宜给他用好动的药。川芎是一味好动的药，四物汤里就用到川芎，因为其中当归动得不怎么厉害，白芍酸收，不动，地黄滋腻，更不动。这个队伍里就是川芎动得比较厉害。这四个在一起就互相牵制了，就把动静调到了合适的程度，所以我们用药的时候要调它的剂量。四物汤里有了川芎才动起来，血一动起来，新血才能生，不然光补血，血补足了不动不行。来月经的时候，或者有其他出血的时候，不用或少用川芎。

川芎容易往上走窜，所以，虚火上炎类的病，就不要用它了。川芎耗散，会进一步伤阴，进一步把虚火往上带。还有呕吐、咳嗽也要慎用川芎，呕吐是肝胃之气上逆，再用往上升的药，恐加剧。高血压是血随气上，气血并走于上，如果还用川芎往上带，血压就可能会越来越高。汗多也要慎用川芎，血症也要慎用，用川芎动了血，血可能会出得更厉害。

当然，瘀血导致的血证除外。这种情况反而要用川芎。比如体内有瘀血，月经就老不干净，怎么治也不好，往往是因为有瘀血，活血化瘀，血就收住了。怎么化呢？四物汤的基础上加桃仁、红花，加桔梗、牛膝，这就成了血府逐瘀汤了，随症加进。这个方子里就用到川芎，川芎会帮助活血化瘀。中药在运用的时候，总要根据具体的情况而定。

川芎妙用举例

在临床上川芎经常有一些妙用。比如，腹泻，脉滑，舌苔腻，胖大有齿痕，这是因为体内有湿导致的，在辨证论治的基础上，在方子里加一点神曲、川芎，效果非常好。神曲化湿，而且消食，加了川芎，稍微兼顾一下血分，效果就大大提高了。

再比如，还有血痢，就是说拉血，拉出来的是红的，经过用药治疗以后，痢疾已经止住了，血也不再流了，但就是肚子疼。这是什么原因呢？这是因为血痢，拉血拉得太久，伤了阴了，伤阴就会气郁，所以也可在辨证论治的基础上，加一味川芎，气血的郁结就开了，肚子很快就不疼了。

Chapter 6 Medicines for Reducing Phlegm

This chapter will focus on T&T about reducing phlegm, dispersing stasis, and food digestion.

Only after understanding how to tonify the spleen (see the sections about Cangzhu and Baizhu), how to nourish the stomach and regulate Qi (see the sections about category of citrus genus), and how to regulate Qi and blood (see the sections about Houpo, Muxiang, Sharen, Chuangxiong and Xiangfu), can one start to learn how to reduce phlegm, disperse stasis and promote digestion.

Normally, the body fluid should be in proper T&T order. Otherwise, the body fluid may accumulate in the body, which might be transformed into phlegm. As it is always said that "life lies in movement", but in fact, the movement in life does not merely refer to sports, it also includes the microscopic movement of life. Reducing phlegm involves activating fluid, or promoting the body fluids to move smoothly in the body. Herbs that reduce phlegm do not merely function to get rid of phlegm, but also function to activate fluid movement without any obstruction within the body. All the internal organs accumulate phlegm in different forms, for which different herbs must be used for the treatment.

Banxia (Pinellia ternata) transforms the phlegm in the spleen channel; Nanxing (arisaema heterophyllum blume) transforms the phlegm in the liver channel; Beimu (fritillaria) transforms the phlegm in the lung channel; Shi Changpu (rhizoma acori graminei) transforms the phlegm in the heart channel. Kunbu (laminaria), salty in taste, enters the kidney to transform phlegm in the kidney channel; and Baijiezi (semen brassicae) transforms phlegm in between the skin and the underlying subcutaneous tissue. It is known that **Erchen Tang** is a formula for reducing phlegm, but it is just a basic formula. And one must know more herbs for reducing the phlegm in different locations in the body in order to resolve phlegm in clinical practice with high proficiency.

Banxia (Pinellia Ternata)

Banxia enters the spleen, which is the source where phlegm is induced.

Thus, the spleen should be considered first when phlegm is to be reduced. Furthermore, the spleen dominates the T&T functions, which also requires to take the spleen into consideration time and again. Banxia is the most important herb for reducing phlegm with a wide range of application.

Banxia seedlings start to grow around May according to the lunar calendar, and its root may be harvested and dried by the time of the Mid-Autumn festival, around the 15th August (the lunar calendar). Banxia has a relatively short growing period, and that is why it is so named in Chinese as Banxia (literally means half summer) since its growing period only lasts half of the summer season. It grows mostly through the growing summer (taking half summer) when the weather is very damp and hot. For all plants, they sprout in spring, grow in summer, transform in growing summer, get harvested in autumn and are stored up in winter. Banxia happens to grow through the "transforming" season (the growing summer). Therefore, Banxia is endowed with the properties to aid the transformation processes of human body. Furthermore, growing summer corresponds to the spleen, and Banxia enters the spleen. The growing summer is mostly characterized with more severe damp-heat pathogens. Dampness possesses similar features to phlegm in the human body. Hence, Banxia can transform phlegm in various forms in the human body.

Properties of Banxia

Banxia is severely dry in property. Some books claim that Banxia contains mucus and it is slippery. In fact, Banxia is slippery in texture, but dry in function. Therefore, in its processing, Banxia must be rinsed in clear water for seven days and nights, during which water must be changed on daily basis. This process is to rinse the mucus out of Banxia. And in the meantime, the rinsing process also allows Banxia to obtain the Yin and moistening property from water. Banxia is a combination of both dryness and moistness.

The spleen dislikes dampness, and Banxia with dry property can eliminate the dampness and tonify the spleen. The mucus of Banxia is like the phlegm in the body, assisting Banxia in its function to transform phlegm.

Banxia is pungent and warm, and it can play the nourishing and dispersing functions. As such, it can resolve the pathogens and promote bowel movements and urination. In the process of treatment based on syndrome differentiation, Banxia added to the prescribed formula will show its advantage of reducing phlegm, opening the orifices, and promoting the smooth bowel movement and urination.

Generally, the herb that is pungent in property will have a dispersing function, but Banxia is different since it is astringent though it is also pungent.

If one tries Banxia in the mouth, he may feel tingling and numb; or if he swallows a little Banxia, he may feel that the throat becomes blocked, even lose his tongue. There was a story of an officer in the south of China, who suddenly could not speak. The doctor advised him to eat fresh ginger, after which he gradually could speak again. Why was that so? The doctor told him that his trouble was caused by the partridge that ate Banxia, and the toxin of Banxia entered his body through the meat of partridge. Fresh ginger can detoxify Banxia and help him recover.

Banxia essentially reduces phlegm and promotes circulation of Qi. However, if used incorrectly, Banxia will cause troubles in the throat because of its double properties of pungency and astringency.

Banxia Resolves Various Phlegm

Banxia enters the spleen, stomach, and gallbladder channels, as well as the heart, lung, and large intestine channels. Every herb has the capacity to enter many different channels, but there is one leading channel that it enters. Banxia mainly enters the spleen channel, or the spleen and stomach channels, or the Middle Jiao.

Banxia is the principal herb for reducing phlegm, whatever type it is, for example, the damp phlegm that arises from accumulation of dampness in the body, which obstructs Qi circulation, and the body fluid is slowly transformed into phlegm; and the phlegm interacting with dampness makes one feel exhausted and sleepy. For such a symptom, Cangzhu and Fuling can be used with Banxia for treatment, in which Banxia resolves phlegm, Cangzhu dries dampness and tonifies the spleen, and Fuling excretes the dampness and alleviates the water retention through urination.

What if it is heat phlegm? It might be thought that Banxia is not suitable for treating the heat phlegm since it warm in property. However, it is not necessarily the case since the warm property of Banxia can be contained with some cool herbs such as Tianhua Fen (radices trichosanthis) and Huangqin (scutellaria baicalensis). Tianhua Fen is the root of Gualou (trichosanthes kirilowii maxim). Gualou Pi (peel of Gualou) can resolve phlegm, so can its root. Huangqin is bitter and cold, and it can clear lung heat. When used with herbs that resolve phlegm, Huangqin is helpful for reducing the heat phlegm.

Banxia used together with Nanxing (arisaema heterophyllum blume) can treat wind phlegm. The liver governs wind, and "wind often causes trembling and dizziness, all of which stem from the disorder of the liver". The wind phlegm originates from the liver. Wind and phlegm often co-exist. Wind may occur when Yang loses its Yin, while phlegm develops when Yin loses its Yang. Yin and Yang in the body essentially should hold together. In case Yin and Yang separate from each other, wind phlegm will then occur. In other words, the wind and phlegm will interwine together to replace the physiological Yin-Yang interacting status. Therefore, the wind phlegm needs to be transformed and eliminated, and then the interaction between Yin and Yang can be gradually restored. Banxia can promote the interaction between Yin and Yang so that Yin and Yang can hold together again to prevent the formation of wind phlegm. Furthermore, Banxia can dry the damp and tonify the spleen, after which the T&T function of the spleen will be intensified, and phlegm will surely not come into formation. Additionally, based on Banxia and Nanxing, Qianhu (radix peucedani) can also be added in the formula for treatment of wind phlegm.

Banxia used with Baijiezi and fresh ginger juice can treat cold phlegm (attributing to coldness). Baijiezi is warm and has a strong spurting effect. Fresh ginger juice is also warm in property.

In addition, there is also dry phlegm, resulting from dryness that dries up the body fluid. For treating the dry phlegm, Banxia should be used with caution, and can be substituted with Gualou and Beimu (fritillaria). In many cases, Beimu and Banxia can be substitute for each other, but they have different channel tropism. Beimu enters the lung channel, while Banxia enters the spleen and stomach channels. Beimu is divided into Zhe Beimu (thunberg fritillary bulb) and Chuan Beimu (bulbus fritillariae cirrhosae). The former is more powerful for resolving phlegm, while the latter is more powerful for moistening lungs, so, they can be used based on the specific symptoms. For example, for the patients who suffer from tuberculosis (TB), Chuan Beimu can be used to resolve phlegm on the one hand and cure TB on the other hand.

For the phlegm due to TB, the patient may be physically weak and suffer from impairment of both Yin and Yang, hence, Banxia should be used with great caution.

Eliminating Stagnation, Descending Qi and Arresting Vomiting

Banxia not only resolves phlegm, but also eliminates stagnation. As a matter of fact, many types of stagnation or stasis are involved with and attributed to phlegm. There are many herbs for eliminating stagnation. Some of them function to remove stasis through activating Qi, and some other herbs function to eliminate stagnation through dispersing blood stasis, while Banxia functions to eliminate stagnation through resolving phlegm.

Having strong descending effect, Banxia enters the Middle Jiao and descends Qi. It is often used to treat vomiting. However, it is not so simple to arrest vomiting with Banxia as it is imagined since one should make sure of the root causes of vomiting. It is related to the spleen, especially to the impairment of the stomach Qi descending, which is often accompanied by the presence of phlegm. For instance, some people vomit on account of car sickness. They always feel phlegmy sensation in their throats once they are in the car, which stirs in the throat and causes vomiting. Banxia can descend such phlegm. As it is known, the stomach Qi essentially tends to descend, and Banxia is endowed with the descending property, which helps the stomach Qi to descent. Therefore, it can relieve stagnation and regulates the Middle Jiao (the spleen and stomach) to arrest vomiting.

All the five internal organs may suffer from stagnation/ depression. Of these, the spleen stagnation is related to phlegm-damp. According to the **Wuxing**

Doctrine, the spleen is of the moist earth, and it dislikes phlegm-damp since too much phlegm-damp accumulation will result in the spleen stagnation, for which Banxia is especially focusing on. There is no doubt that when the spleen stagnation is eliminated, all the other stagnation or depression will be removed accordingly. This is the special effect of Banxia for removing stagnation/stasis.

The Three Contraindications of Banxia

There are three contraindications for using Banxia. Those patients who suffer from bleeding, frequent thirst and sweating should take great caution on using Banxia.

Bleeding conditions refer to all types of bleeding symptoms, like hematemesis, epistaxis, hemoptysis, bleeding gums, tongue bleeding, bleeding due to trauma and excessive loss of blood after delivery, hematuria, hematochezia etc. Under all the above circumstances, Banxia is contraindicated in order to prevent further damage to the blood since Banxia is dry in property, and it has the tendency to consume blood.

Those who always feel thirsty should also take great caution on using Banxia. For instance, Banxia is rarely used to treat diabetes mellitus since the patients feel thirsty, which means that there is fluid deficiency. Banxia is used often at the cost of consuming certain amount of body fluid. Hence, Banxia should not be used unless there is an obvious phlegm symptom.

It is normal to sweat in summer. However, those who suffer from abnormal and excessive perspiration not only in summer, but particularly in winter, or at night during sleep may suffer from the impairment of the body fluids. Under this circumstance, use of Banxia will cause further impairment to the body.

Nanxing (Arisaema Heterophyllum Blume)

Properties of Nanxing

Nanxing, also known as Tian Nanxing, is like Banxia, but its medicinal part is larger in size than that of Banxia. It is sometimes called Huzhang (literally means tiger paw) since the middle tuber of the herb is larger with some smaller ones around, and all the tubers combined look like a tiger palm.

Nanxing enters the liver, spleen, lung, and stomach channels, and it has an intensively warming function with toxicity stronger than Banxia. Nanxing, if kept in the mouth, will cause numbness. Also, it may cause dryness in the body like Banxia if not used appropriately, which indicates that Nanxing needs properly processing and appropriate compatibility of medicines. When used with Fangfeng (radix sileris), Nanxing may cause less numbness; when mixed with Niudan (ox bile), Nanxing will become less dry. Nanxing must be processed through parching before use, after which it can be detoxified. Raw Nanxing is rarely used except for external use as a sticking-plaster.

Nanxing and Banxia are quite similar in properties, but essentially, they are different in functions. Nanxing enters meridians and collaterals, so it is often used to direct the other herbs in the treatment of stroke and paralysis into the channels. Banxia mainly enters the intestines and stomach, so it is often used for treatment of vomiting and diarrhoea.

Processing and Uses of Dan Nanxing (Ox-bile Nanxing)

The Dan Nanxing refers to Nanxing that is processed with Niudan (ox bile). Nanxing is first rinsed over and again in clear water until the pungent and spicy taste is completely removed, after which it should be dried and crushed into coarse powder. Then, an equal proportion of ox bile or pig bile is added and mixed completely. The mixed Nanxing is cut into small pieces and dried in the shade. One year later, more ox bile is added and dried in the shade. Such a procedure is repeated for three times at an interval of one year, or even for nine times in sequence, in which case it is unnecessary to wait for a whole year in between each addition of ox bile. Such a processed Nanxing is called Jiuzhi Dan Nanxing (Nanxing that is processed with bile for nine times). It might be thought that this processing method is to use ox bile to restrain Nanxing. However, this process is different from the normal processing method. Dan Nanxing is the result of a combined effect from both ox bile and Nanxing, and two herbs of bile and Nanxing contained can bring out the best in each other and come into full play.

There are a lot of differences between Dan Nanxing and Nanxing. Dan Nanxing may become yellowish or blackish and bitter in taste after processing. The most critical change is that Dan Nanxing becomes cool in property rather than strongly warm.

After processing, the bile content in Dan Nanxing not only can clear gall-bladder heat, but also can promote the effects of Nanxing to go into the whole body to eliminate stagnation/stasis, tranquilize the mind, and nourish the liver. It is used as a reconciling herb with many similar medical effects to Niuhuang (calculus bovis).

Dan Nanxing is often used to treat stroke, mania, epilepsy, wind syndrome on the head, dizziness, and convulsions stemming from wind phlegm and gall-bladder heat. Nanxing can eliminate the wind phlegm mixed with gallbladder heat, and the bile can clear the gallbladder heat. In the clinical practice, Danpi (cortex moutan radices) and Zhizi (fructus gardeniae) can also be added to assist treatment.

Beimu (Fritillaria)

Beimu Enters the Lung and Reduces Phlegm

Beimu is an herbaceous plant whose root is used as a medicine. Beimu blooms in summer and its flower has six petals. Unlike many other flowers, Beimu's flowers hang down like bells. The human lungs also hang in the body like bells, suggesting that Beimu enters the lung to reduce phlegm. Beimu enters the Qi system of the lung channel, and the heart channel, too.

Beimu can reduce phlegm since it can eliminate the lung stagnation, remove stasis, purge heat, moisten the lungs and clear lung fire.

Chuan Beimu and Zhe Beimu

Beimu is classified into Chuan Beimu (bulbus fritillariae cirrhosae) and Zhe Beimu (thunberg fritillary bulb). Chuan Beimu is slightly bigger than pearl barley in size, looking like pearl barley in shape. Each piece of Beimu is the root of a whole plant. Thus, Chuan Beimu is extremely expensive. Zhe Beimu is bigger in size, and that produced in Xiangshan county, Zhejiang province of China, is the best in quality with strong medical effect.

Chuan Beimu is sweet and cold in properties with slight pungency and bitterness in tastes. The sweet taste suggests that it is moistening, and can moisten the lung dryness; its cold property suggests that it can clear the lung fire; its pungent taste suggests that it can eliminate the lung stagnation; and its bitterness can purge the heart fire. It can be concluded that Chuan Beimu, endowed with the function of eliminating the lung stagnation, is used to moisten the lung and reduce phlegm. Once the lung suffers from stagnation, there will arise heat, resulting in phlegm. Thus, fluid may not be distributed effectively throughout the body. The spleen upbears the clear, and the food nutrients ascend to the lungs, which will distribute the fluid to the whole body. The lung stagnation can generate heat, causing the fluid to fail to move from the lung to all parts of the body but accumulate in the lungs. As such, the heat in the lungs will refine the accumulated fluid into sticky or heat phlegm. The function of Beimu is to eliminate the lung stagnation, subsequently reducing and purging the lung fire. After that, the phlegm source is extinguished. In a word, Beimu is often used to reduce the dry and heat phlegm stemming from the lung Qi obstruction.

Zhe Beimu is not as sweet as it is bitter. Zhe Beimu has a stronger effect to eliminate the lung stagnation and resolve hard lumps, but it is not so effective as Chuan Beimu in respect of nourishing and moistening the lungs. Zhe Beimu is more expensive than Chuan Beimu. For resolving the thick phlegm, Zhe Beimu will work, but Chuan Beimu may be needed if there is an increasing risk of impairing the lung in the process of resolving phlegm and moistening the lung at the same time. Generally, whenever Chuan Beimu is needed, a dosage of 3 to 6g grams each time will be sufficient; but Zhe Beimu needs to be used with a larger dosage, at least 10 grams, or even 30 to 50 grams once based on the syndrome differentiation.

Besides, there is another herb in this family, called Ping Beimu, mainly produced in the northeast of China. Its size is in between that of Chuan Beimu and Zhe Beimu and its medical effect is the same as Chuan Beimu and Zhe Beimu.

Eliminating the Lung Qi Stagnation

The lung governs the skin and hair. In most cases, the ulcers on the skin are often related to lung Qi stagnation, affecting the permeation of the skin. Therefore, Zhe Beimu is used to remove the stagnation.

Zhe Beimu has come into use since ancient times. The ***Book of Songs*** says "Women feel depressed, so they go to pick Zhe Beimu from the mountains; Women are often sentimental, but each of them has her own reasons". Women are prone to stagnation, mainly the liver stagnation due to obstruction of Qi circulation. As it is known, the lung governs Qi of the whole body. When the lung suffers from stagnation, there will occur obstruction of Qi circulation, for which Zhe Beimu can be used to eliminate the lung Qi stagnation.

Xiaoyao San is also used for eliminating depression/ stagnation through dispersing the stagnated liver Qi, for which Zhe Beimu is often added in order to help the metal (i. e. , the lung) to soothe the wood (i. e. , the liver) since Zhe Beimu, with its function of eliminating the lung stagnation, can intensify **Xiaoyao San** to remove stagnation. Only when the liver and lung stagnation/depression is removed simultaneously, can Qi circulate smoothly in the body.

Dispersing Phlegm Stagnation

Where there is stagnation, there will be phyma and lumps, for which Zhe Beimu can be used for treatment since these phyma and lumps, such as the most common lobular hyperplasia in breasts, or mammitis, or even the more serious breast cancer, are all involved with stagnation and phlegm accumulation. Doctors often advise the patient who suffers from breast lumps to stay calm and stop anger since they know such lumps usually result from liver stagnation. Hence, the TCM doctors may prefer to prescribe **Xiaoyao San**, or **Jiawei Xiaoyao Pill** to soothe the liver. However, some patients find it effective, and some other patients find it ineffective since **Xiaoyao San**, or **Jiawei Xiaoyao Pill** is a ready-made medicine that cannot be modified. If raw herbs are used, Zhe Beimu can be added based on the formula of **Xiaoyao San**, or **Jiawei Xiaoyao Pill** to resolve the nodule.

Breasts are subsumed to the liver and lung meridians, and the nodules in breasts are also related to the lung Qi stagnation. Thus, Zhe Beimu should be added to the treatment formula with a larger dosage like 15 grams at least, or even up to 25 grams each time based on the syndrome differentiation. Besides, in clinical practice, Xiakucao (spica prunellae), as an effective herb for eliminating the heat stagnation, may also be added to the formula of **Xiaoyao San** according to the specific location of the breast nodules. For example, nodules above the nipple are often involved with fire; the nodules to the left part of the breast are more likely to be related to blood stasis (as the left side dominates blood); the nodules to the right part of the breast are more likely to be related to phlegm accumulation (as the right side dominates Qi). Therefore, addition of Zhe Beimu and Xiakucao to the formula of **Xiaoyao San** based on the specific symptoms can bring about a very good effect.

Beimu is often used with Jiegeng (platycodon grandiflorum) that can carry the medical effect to go upwards. Beimu moves downwards and enters the lung channel. Jiegeng can upbear the medical effect of Beimu to the lung first and hold it there for sufficient time to resolve phlegm and eliminate stagnation, and then let it move downwards. As such Beimu and Jiegeng can bring out the best in each other.

In addition, many women in suckling period may suffer from blockage of the milk ducts due to the obstruction of heat phlegm, causing distending breast pain. For such a case, Zhe Beimu and Jiegeng are often added to a formula for promoting lactation and eliminating the stagnation, after which milk will flow smoothly.

The Detoxifying Principle of Beimu

Beimu also has an antidotal function since it can guide heat to go downwards, as such, phlegm is reduced accordingly and Qi circulates smoothly. Once Qi is circulating smoothly, the body will become strong enough to remove the toxic influence arising from stagnation/stasis.

The liver is the detoxification organ, governing the catharsis of the body. Every day, food and emotional changes can produce toxins. The body has its own self-healing functions that are constantly clearing toxins, especially during sleep when blood returns to the liver, and detoxification function will work intensively. However, when stagnation occurs, toxins cannot be easily eliminated. Beimu is endowed with detoxifying effects, and it can also eliminate stagnation/stasis to activate the body to carry on detoxification naturally.

Beimu is often used with Lianqiao (fructus forsythiae) to eliminate the nodules, lumps, or nodule on the neck. Sometimes, Haizao (seaweed) and Kunbu (laminaria) may also be added when necessary. Both Haizao and Kunbu are endowed with the functions of eliminating stagnation and detoxification. Beimu is often used at a dosage of 3*qian* to 1 *liang*, or even more when necessary.

TCM always attaches great importance to the treatment based on syndrome differentiation, that is, the syndrome differentiation and formula are equally important. On the one hand, formulas must address the symptoms correctly; on the other hand, the appropriate herbs for specific disease should also be added to the formula as required. For example, Lianqiao and Beimu are the herbs for treating the nodule on the neck, therefore, if the nodule stems from the liver stagnation, these two herbs can be added based on the formula of **Xiaoyao San**; if the nodule stems from the dampness, the two herbs can be added based on the formula of **Pingwei San**.

Comparison between Beimu and Banxia

Both Bianxia and Beimu are principal herbs for reducing phlegm, however they differ greatly in many ways. Beimu, cold and partially dry in property, enters the lung channel to eliminate stagnation, while Banxia, warm in property, enters the spleen channel. Therefore, Beimu is used to resolve the fire and heat phlegm arising from the lung Qi stagnation, while Banxia is used to resolve the cold phlegm arising from the spleen Qi stagnation. When the fire and/or heat pathogen(s) in the body attacks the lungs, fluid will not be transformed and distributed properly, resulting in lung Qi stagnation that will then cause dry phlegm. For such a case, Beimu is suitable for treatment. When the spleen and stomach are in a cold and deficient state, fluid will remain in between the spleen and the lung to form damp phlegm that Banxia is suitable for treatment. However, when the phlegm sometimes is involved with both the lung and the spleen, Banxia and Beimu can be used together.

Beimu has a wide therapeutic application for treatment of various symptoms, such as dysphoria with smothery sensation, pulmonary abscess, the consumptive lung disease, pharyngitis, hemoptysis, hematemesis, dizziness due to consumptive disease, various phlegm, nodules, tumors, malignant sores, dystocia, and blockage of lactation.

Face Sores and Metaphysics

Regarding Beimu, there was a legend, saying that a person who had a sore looking like a human face on the arm. That sore was able to make faces and even able to ingest food. No one was able to cure the sore. A doctor suggested the patient to read herb names one by one to the face-like sore until it suddenly reacts to the name of Beimu and it started to frown and show a painful expression. And then, the doctor advised the patient to eat Beimu and feed the face sore on the arm with Beimu powder. And soon, the face-like sore disappeared.

This is only a legend, but the disease of face sore is indeed recorded in many ancient books. This type of disease may occur on the human face, arms and legs or other locations. It is a very weird disease. In fact, all weird diseases are attributable to phlegm, which can be treated with Beimu.

Changpu (Acorus Calamus)

Characteristics of Changpu and Its Selection

Changpu is an aquatic plant, including Shui Changpu (rhizoma calami) that grows in the ditches, and Shi Changpu (rhizoma acori graminei) that grows among the stones where water is flowing in mountain areas. They look alike, but they have some differences in properties due to their growing environment. For medical use, Shi Changpu is preferred.

Shi Changpu, also known as Jie Changpu (jointed Changpu), or Jiujie Changpu (nine-joint Changpu), usually has nine joints within one-inch length. As an herb, Shi Changpu can break stagnation/stasis.

After being dried up, Shi Changpu becomes tough and looks slightly reddish on the fracture surface. Such type of Shi Changpu is the best for medicinal use.

Opening the Orifices and Activating the Heart and Spleen

Shi Changpu looks slightly reddish, so, it can enter the heart. Having strong aroma, it has the effect of opening the heart orifice.

In case one suffers from obstruction of the normal Qi circulation, he or she may feel depressed and unhappy. The conditions of delight and depression are closely involved with one's psychological and physiological states. Shi Changpu has a function to make one feel delightful and can improve one's psychological state through improving his or her physiological conditions.

Shi Changpu, via its aromatic property, opens all the orifices of the body, through which phlegm can be discharged naturally. Phlegm is very common in the body. When it occurs in the pericardium, called "phlegm confusing heart" or "phlegm attacking the pericardium", one may become manic, saying nonsense, or remaining in delusions. Shi Changpu can open the heart orifice to allow phlegm to be eliminated, and thus, the patient will become clear-minded again. In brief, Shi Changpu can be used for treatment of psychological diseases.

Shi Changpu grows in water, indicating that it is water-resistant to some extent. It can dispel the water pathogen and remove the phlegm damp accumulated in between the heart and spleen. Shi Changpu can open orifices, indicating that it can drive out phlegm and dampness through certain channels. Besides, it is aromatic, suggesting that it can refresh the spleen and activate the spleen Qi. Shi Changpu can reinforce T&T functions of the spleen to its maximum potential. According to TCM theory, the heart fire may affect the spleen. Medicines that can take effects on the heart will surely be effective on the spleen. In addition, Shi Changpu's aromatic property can refresh the spleen. In conclusion, Shi Changpu can promote the T&T functions of the spleen.

Shi Changpu Used for Treating Cholera and Dysentery

Shi Changpu can be used for the treatment of cholera and dysentery. There is a famous formula called **Lianpu Yin** recorded in the book of "*Suixiju Reclassification of Cholera*" written by Wang Mengying, a medical scientist in the Qing dynasty.

Lianpu Yin contains the ingredient herbs of Huanglian (coptis chinensis), Houpo (mangnolia officinalis), Changpu (acorus calamus), Banxia (Pinellia ternata), Douchi (fermented soya beans), Zhizi (fructus gardenia).

Both Huanglian and Houpo used in this formula are for clearing damp heat in the spleen and stomach since the disturbance of the damp heat pathogens in the Middle Jiao can impair the spleen and stomach functions of upbearing the clear and descending the turbid. When the normal order of these ascending and descending functions is disturbed, cholera will then take place, causing vomiting and diarrhea. Changpu in the formula functions to promote the T&T functions of the spleen with its aromatic property, opens the orifices of the body, and assists in upbearing the clear and descending the turbid. Banxia tonifies the spleen. Douchi and Zhizi make up a sub-formula of **Zhizi Chi Tang**, which can clear the Upper Jiao.

Furthermore, long-lasting dysentery may be transformed into anorectic dysentery, which is always involved with deficiency of the speech, stemming from heat blocking the diaphragm. Generally, **Shenling Baizhu San** can be used for the treatment of this symptom. However, only **Shenling Baizhu San** is not so effective that Shi Changpu is added to the formula to improve the medical effects.

Shenling Baizhu San is for treating deficiency of the spleen, but the heat obstructs the Qi circulation, for which Shi Changpu is used for treatment in place of Muxiang (costustoot) since Shi Changpu is more effective for opening orifices. So, **Shenling Baizhu San** orally washed down with Shi Changpu decoction will be effective for anorectic dysentery. Furthermore, rice soup can also be used with **Shenling Baizhu San** since the patient who suffers from anorectic dysentery may have a very poor appetite. Rice soup can regulate the stomach Qi and replenish energy for the patient.

Compatibility of Changpu with Other Herbs

Shi Changpu, Shudi (radix rehmanniae praeparata) and Huangbai are used together to make into herbal pills to treat epicophosis due to the kidney deficiency. The ears are the orifices of the heart and the kidney. When blocked, deafness will occur. Therefore, on the one hand, the orifices need to be opened, and on the other hand, the kidney must be tonified. In this formula, Shudi nourishes the kidney Yin; Huangbai clears pathogenic fire in the kidney and reinforces the kidney; and Shi Changpu opens the ear orifices. Hence, the middle-aged persons can take such medicines to protect ears from hearing loss.

Changpu and Yuanzhi (polygala tenuifolia) are both dispersing in property, and often used to promote inter-communication between the heart and the kidney. Therefore, those who suffer from unconsciousness, psychosis and epilepsy may use these two herbs, but not too long or too much, and especially Changpu since it is very aromatic, dry and dispersing in properties, and long-lasting use of it may disperse the kidney Yin and Yang. However, the heart prefers the astringent action and dislikes the dispersing influence. Those who suffer from Yin deficiency should not use Shi Changpu at all. Besides, patients with excessive sweating should use Shi Changpu with much caution. In the decocting process, Shi Chang-pu must not be in contact with iron and steel utensils like spoon, pot, and chop-sticks etc. Otherwise, it may make the patient feel sick or even vomit. General-ly, decoction of herbs should be done with casserole, pottery pot or porcelain ware instead of metal wares.

Kunbu (Laminaria)

Kunbu and Haizao (Seaweed)

Kunbu, like a piece of big cloth, grows only in the sea, and it is tough in texture; Haidai (kelp) is smaller in size; Haizao is thin. Sometimes Haidai is al-so called as Kunbu by some people

Kunbu, Haidi and seaweed have the similar effects, all growing in the sea, salty in taste, softening hard masses, eliminating stagnation, nourishing the Low-er Jiao, clearing heat, and entering the kidney. Therefore, they may bring about good effects on resolving the tough-phlegm and phlegm stagnation, but long use may cause emaciation.

As a matter of fact, reduction of phlegm means to reduce fat tissue, after that, a fat person slims down. Therefore, there are many ways in TCM for losing weight, like tonifying the spleen to promote T&T functions, resolving phlegm to reduce fat tissue, using Shanzha to promote digestion of meat etc. , but all de-pend on the specific cases.

Haizao Yuhu Tang and Uses of Corrigent Medicines

Kunbu is very effective for the treatment of all kinds of scrofula, goiter and tumor, and agglutinating phlegm, but it is prohibited to use with Gancao since this combination is toxic, with only few exceptions, for instance, Haizao and Kunbu are used with Gancao in some formulas like **Haizao Yuhu Tang** recorded in the book of *Yizong Jinjian (Golden Mirror of Medicine)*.

Haizao Yuhu Tang contains the herbal ingredients of:

Haizao (seaweed) 1*liang*, Kunbu (laminaria) 5 *qian*, Beimu (fritillaria) 5 *qian*, Banxia (pinellia ternata) 3 *qian*, Qingpi (the green tangerine peel) 2 *qian*, Chenpi (pericarpium citri reticulatae) 3 *qian*, Danggui (angelica sinensis) 5 *qian*, Chuangxiong (ligusticum wallichii) 3 *qian*, Lianqiao (fructus forsythia) 3 *qian*, Gancao(liquorice) 2 *qian*.

Haizao Yuhu Tang is generally used for treatment of the Upper Jiao, especially the tough phlegm stagnation there, therefore, Haizao and Kunbu are used together in this formula.

For such tough phlegm, it is unclear whether it is attributed to coldness or heat; and whether it is subsumed to the spleen or the lung. As such, Beimu and Banxia are used together. Besides, the phlegm is stagnated and it needs to be softened and dispersed, for which the salty Haizao and Kunbu are suitable. In addition, Beimu in this formula plays a function of resolving hard lump through eliminating stagnation and resolving heat phlegm.

In the process of resolving phlegm, Qi and blood should also be taken into consideration simultaneously, therefore, Chenpi and Qingpi are used in this formula to regulate Qi and relieve the stagnant Qi so that phlegm will be resolved accordingly. When Qi starts to circulate, blood also needs to be activated. Hence, Danggui and Chuangxiong are used in this formula to promote the circulation of blood. Meanwhile, Lianqiao is used to clear heat arising from phlegm accumulation.

The medical effects of both Haizao and Kunbu in this formula move downward in the body, and Gancao can slow down the movement to hold the efficacy in the body for a longer time, which might cause an adverse rising action like vomiting for some patients. Thus, Banxia is used to calm the adverse-rising energy and arrest vomiting. After all, for the purpose of promoting Qi and blood circulation, Qingpi, Chenpi, Danggui and Chuangxiong are used in this formula and they can move very rapidly in the body. Therefore, Gancao used here will not cause harm to the body.

Without doubt, long phlegm stagnation will result in the occurrence of toxins. In a word, this formula can be modified based on the syndrome differentiation, for instance, Jinyinhua (honeysuckle flower) added to this formula can reinforce the effect of resolving phlegm stagnation.

Baijiezi (Semen Brassicae)

Baijiezi is the seed of medicinal mustard rather than the culinary mustard seed. The medicinal mustard has bluish-white leaves, and its seed is yellowish white, while the edible mustard has green leaves and the seed is purplish black.

Properties and Uses of Baijiezi

Baijiezi, pungent and hot in properties, enters the lung and stomach channels, dredges the channels, and resolves phlegm stagnation. Sometimes, phlegm may stay in the inner membrane, for which Banxia and Beimu are not effective, but only Baijiezi is workable due to its pungent and aromatic properties. Therefore, when phlegm stays in the limbs, or below the costal region, or in between the skin and the subcutaneous tissue, Baijiezi might be the only herb that can eliminate it. Particularly, when the overweight persons suffer from pains below the costal region, Baijiezi will be the more essential herb to choose.

Baijiezi exerts a strong influence on the channels, so it is often used to apply on the acupoints. For example, in case stasis and swelling occur due to strain or sprain, application of the paste of the crushed Baijiezi mixed with vinegar to the stasis and swelling part will bring about a very good medical effect. The raw egg white may be mixed into the paste so as to alleviate the irritating effect of Baijiezi and protect the skin from hurt, especially for children use because of their tender skin. By the way, such a paste may also be applied to the face to cure the toothache, or applied to the relevant acupoints to treat the pains in the internal organs, or applied to the arch of the foot to treat the diseases on the head and rheumatic disease. Of course, Baijiezi-soaked water can be used for foot bath, which is good for health.

Sanzi Yangqin Tang

The formula of **Sanzi Yangqin Tang** contains three types of ingredient seeds: Baijiezi (semen brassicae), Suzi (perilla seed) and Laifuzi (radish seed).

The elderly people often suffer from more phlegm that stays deep in the body, so Baijiezi is used in this formula to resolve the phlegm. Besides, the elderly people always suffer from adverse-rising Qi, for which Suzi is used to descend the Qi. And last, the elderly people are always suffering from the weakness of the spleen and stomach, easily resulting in dyspepsia, for which Laifuzi can help digestion. These three seeds should be slightly parched and crushed before they are decocted.

Sanzi Yangqin Tang is good for the eldly people. Although Baijiezi can resolve phlegm; Suzi can descend Qi; Laifuzi can help digestion and descend Qi, yet they should not be used with a large dosage or for a long time. Otherwise, they may consume the healthy Qi, or even cause some unexpected consequence. Hence, stop using **Sanzi Yangqin Tang** when it strikes the diseases.

第六章　化痰之药

从今天开始，我们讲运化的具体方面，即化痰、化瘀、化食等。

前面讲了苍术和白术，这是健脾的；后来又讲了橘类，这是养胃、理气的；接着又讲了厚朴、木香、砂仁，还有川芎、香附，这些都是调理气血的。要化痰、化瘀、化食化积，先得健脾，得调理气血，气血调了，大的格局定下来了，具体的化痰、化瘀等工作才好进行。

当人体的津液运行得非常好的时候，它就是津液，运行得不好的时候，津液聚集在那里，不活动了就成为痰了。所以说生命在于运动，这运动并不是单指体育运动，还有很多生命微观的活动。化痰就是让这些津液运行起来，或者说流通得更加通畅。化痰的药不但要把痰化掉，还要让津液在我们全身更通畅地运行开来。其实五脏六腑都有痰，这些痰并不单指我们吐出来的痰，根据痰所处脏腑的不同，用药也会有所差异。

半夏化脾经之痰，南星化肝经之痰，贝母化肺经之痰，石菖蒲化心经之痰。还有昆布咸入肾，化肾经之痰；白芥子化皮里膜外之痰。二陈汤是化痰的基础方剂，根据痰所在的部位，我们还要多掌握一些药，这样在用的时候才能更加的得心应手。

半夏

半夏入脾。脾为生痰之源，要化痰首先要考虑到脾；且脾主运化，也应该考虑到脾。半夏是化痰最主要的药，用途非常广。

农历五月，半夏苗生出，到了八月中秋节前后，采其块茎部位，晒干。半夏生长的时间比较短，之所以叫半夏，是因为它只得到了半个夏天的气，它是半夏而生。五月就是夏天过去一半了嘛。它的整个生长期基本处在长夏阶段，这是天地间是非常湿热的时候。春生夏长、长夏化、秋收冬藏。半夏正好生长在"化"的季节，所以天地也赋予它运化的机能。而且长夏对应的是脾，半夏也是走脾经的。长夏季节最明显的是湿热之邪比较重，湿与人体的痰有同气相求之处。所以生于一年之中最湿热季节里的半夏作用于人体，能化各种痰。

体滑而用燥，通阴阳

半夏得天之燥气而生，其性燥烈。还有的书上说它其中有黏液，性滑，其实这不矛盾，半夏是体滑而用燥。所以，炮制半夏，要放在清水里漂七天七夜，每一天一夜换一次水。换水时你会发现水有些黏了。这是为了把半夏里边的黏液漂出来。半夏放到水里边漂，也使它得到了水的阴气和滋润。所以半夏是燥和润的结合体。

半夏性燥，正好脾恶湿，燥就会化湿健脾。它的黏滑又跟痰涎同气相求，这也有利于它更好地化痰。

半夏辛温，味辛则能润能散，所以它能够化邪、利窍，能够通利大小便。在辨证论治的基础上，在方子里酌情加一味半夏来化痰涎、开窍，对大小便的通利都有好处，能够让大便变得干爽。

半夏味辛，通常味辛则散，但半夏不一样，它反而有涩性。

尝一尝生半夏，嘴里会发麻，如果能够吞一点下去，吞着吞着你就会发现，喉咙被它封上了，甚至说不出话来，这东西又麻又涩。从前有个故事，有一个在南方当官的，忽然嗓子肿了，渐渐说不出话，用了各种方法都治不好。后来有一位医生让他吃生姜。别人都会觉得生姜很辣，唯独他觉得生姜很甜很清爽，吃着吃着嗓子就开了，能说话了。这是怎么回事呢？医生告诉他，你这个病其实是吃多了山里的鹧鸪，而鹧鸪在这个季节吃半夏，所以鹧鸪有了半夏的毒，你吃多了鹧鸪，半夏的毒就结在你喉咙里了，喉咙就不通了，生姜可以解半夏的毒，嗓子自然就好了。

半夏本来是化痰的，化痰就能够让人体气机通畅。但如果用得不好的话，它能把喉咙给闭上。在五味上它是辛的，辛中带涩，能散能收，收中有敛，敛中有散，这是它的二重性。

半夏能化各种痰

半夏入脾经、胃经和胆经，兼入心经、肺经和大肠经。每味药都能归很多经，但它都有一个最主要的。半夏也入很多经，主要入脾经，或者说入脾胃、入中焦。

半夏是化痰的主药，不管化什么类型的痰都能用到半夏。比如湿痰，是体内有很多湿气，阻滞气机，使津液不断慢慢化成痰，痰和湿交织在一起，使人疲惫、贪睡，这时候用苍术、茯苓配半夏来治。半夏化痰，苍术燥湿健脾，茯苓渗湿利水，把湿渗掉一点，通过小便排出去。

如果是热痰怎么办？有人说半夏是味温药，用温药来治热痰是不是有点不好？也不一定，其温性可以用其他的凉药来牵制、反佐。比如，天花粉、黄芩。天花粉是瓜蒌的根。瓜蒌皮是化痰的药，瓜蒌根也是化痰的药。黄芩是一个苦寒的药，能清肺热，跟化痰的药一起则有助于化热痰。

半夏与南星一起能够治风痰。什么是风痰呢？肝主风，"诸风掉眩，皆属于肝"，风痰来源于肝。风和痰往往是并存的，阳不得其阴则为风，阴不得其阳则为痰。人体本来该是阴阳相抱在一起的，阴得其阳，阳得其阴，如果阴阳分离了，就不叫阴阳了，容易产生风痰，也就是风和痰搅合在一起，不再是阴阳交抱的生理状态。有了这些风痰，先要化掉，然后再慢慢地恢复人体阴阳交抱的能力。半夏能通阴阳，使阳得其阴、阴得其阳，自然能使风痰无法生成。同时半夏还能燥湿、健脾，脾的运化能力增强了，人也不会有痰。治风痰，在半夏和南星的基础上，还可以再加上前胡。

半夏与白芥子、生姜汁一起，可以治寒痰。寒痰是因寒而生的痰，我们就去温它，白芥子是一味温药，走窜的力度非常大，姜汁是生姜汁，也是温性的。

还有燥痰，是因为体内太燥，津液消耗干，走不动，就成了痰。治燥痰就要慎用半夏，改用花粉和贝母就可以了。贝母在很多情况下可以代替半夏用，但它们归经不同。贝母归的是肺经，半夏归的是脾胃，但是在不得已的时候，它们可以互相替代。贝母可以分川贝母和浙贝母。浙贝母化痰的力度大一些，川贝母润肺的力度大一些，要根据具体情况而选择使用。例如痨病，可以用川贝，一面化痰，一面修复肺部。

还有一种痰叫痨痰，是因为有虚劳，身体一直不好，伤了阴也伤了阳，同时又生了痰，这时候用半夏也要慎重一些。

散结解郁，降气止呕

半夏不仅能化痰，还能散结。其实很多结也跟痰有关，是痰导致的。散结的药有很多，有的药通过动气来散结，还有的药通过化瘀来散结，半夏就能够化痰来散结。

半夏走中焦而降，而且降的力度非常大，所以经常用来治呕吐。当然，半夏止呕的作用并不像我们想象的这么简单，让这些要呕吐出去的东西往下走它就往下走了？没那么简单。仍要追溯，病人为什么会呕吐呢？

跟脾有关，尤其跟胃气不降有关，其间往往有痰。比如，很多人晕车呕吐，他说只觉得一上车喉咙里就有口痰，吐掉了还有，痰在里面搅和，然后就吐了，半夏正好把这些痰往下降。胃气本降，半夏正好与胃的性质是一致的，能帮助胃气下降，所以它解郁调中，能够调脾胃，止呕吐。

五脏皆有郁，其中脾郁就跟痰湿有关系。脾为湿土，它已经很湿了，所以它就讨厌痰湿，如果痰湿积累得多了，脾就会郁。说半夏能解郁，其实就是解脾郁，当然很多时候脾郁解开了，其他的郁也跟着通了。半夏解郁的作用就在这里。

半夏三禁

有些情况是不能用半夏的，半夏有三禁：血家、渴家、汗家。意思就是说半夏在三种人身上应该是慎用的：

一种是老出血的。不管是出什么血，吐血、鼻血、咳血、牙龈出血、舌头出血、因为受伤出血、产后失血过多、还有尿血、便血，这些情况都不要用半夏，因为半夏是一味燥药，它本身就耗血，没有必要再让它耗了。

还有渴家，总是觉得渴，用半夏也要注意。比如，治糖尿病，用半夏的情况就非常少，因为他老渴，说明他津液不足，而用半夏要以消耗一定的津液为代价。只要不是明显的痰证，半夏都要慎用。

汗家是特别喜欢出汗的人。夏天出汗是正常的，如果冬天也出汗，晚上盗汗，刚一睡着身上的衣服就湿了。总之，过于喜欢出汗，必然损伤津液，再用半夏，就不好了。

南星

南星的性能

南星与半夏比较相似，又叫天南星。其入药部位比半夏大一些，还有个名称叫虎掌。它的块茎中间大，边上还有一些小的。合在一起，挺像老虎的掌。中间大的像老虎的掌心，边上小的像老虎的掌指。

南星归肝、脾、肺、胃这四经，大温，非常燥烈，它的毒性比半夏大，含在嘴里会麻，用得不好，也像半夏一样，会燥。这就需要有很好的药材炮制技术，还要有药材配伍的技巧。南星跟防风一起用，就不会令人发麻。用牛胆来拌，就能不会过于燥烈。南星有毒，炒一炒就能解毒。所以，用南星必须用炮制过的，生南星用得不多，除非做膏药外用。

南星和半夏如此相似，那么它们之间可以通用吗？也未必。南星和半夏有很多相似之处，但也有根本上的不同。南星是一味走经络的药，所以，中风、麻痹都以它为向导。半夏则专走肠胃，所以，呕吐、腹泻会经常用到半夏。

胆南星的制法和使用

现在我们常用的胆南星，是跟牛胆一起制过的南星。先把生南星放在清水里反复漂洗到没有麻辣味，再晾干，打成粗末，然后加入等量的牛胆汁，或者用猪胆汁，拌匀，切成小块阴干，一年后再加入牛胆汁，再阴干，再过一年再加入牛胆汁，再阴干。如此三遍。还有一连九遍的，就没必要一年一遍了。这就叫九制胆南星。人们可能会认为这样做是要用牛胆来反佐南星，其实不然，这跟普通的药物炮制不一样，胆南星是胆和南星共同发挥作用的结果。可以说，这一味药它包含着两味药：苦胆和南星。这两味药在一起相得益彰，一起发挥作用。

胆南星和南星有比较大的差异。胆南星因为是用牛胆制过的，所以颜色会变黄或变黑，味道会变苦，关键是它的性质会转凉，不再是大温的药了。

胆南星中的牛胆，与人的胆同气相求，它既能清胆热，又能使南星的药力在人的身上无处不到，能够散结气、镇静、养肝。这是一个调和之剂，在功效上很多时候跟牛黄相似。

胆南星经常用来治疗中风、疯癫、癫痫、头风、眩晕、抽搐等。这些病往往都是因为风痰、胆热。风痰夹杂着胆热，风痰用南星来化，胆热就用胆汁的苦来清。其中还可以加丹皮和栀子。

贝 母

入肺化痰

贝母是一种草，根部入药，夏天开花，花有六瓣。与别的花不同，它的花开了以后会倒垂下去。什么东西是倒垂的？钟是倒垂的，人的肺也像一口钟那样倒悬着，这也提示贝母是入肺的。贝母是入肺经的气分药，也入心经。贝母是入肺而化痰的。

贝母化痰，因为它能够解肺郁，能够散结、泻热、润肺、清火，这样就可以散痰化痰。

川贝母与浙贝母

贝母分川贝母和浙贝母。川贝母比薏米稍大一点，形状跟薏米有点相似，一颗贝母就是一株植物的根，所以川贝母特别的贵。浙贝母比较大，浙江象山县产的浙贝母最好，力度较大。

川贝母甘寒、微辛、微苦。甘就意味着滋润，能润肺燥；寒能清肺火，辛能解肺郁，苦能泻心火。所以川贝是用来润肺化痰的，有解肺郁的功效。肺一旦有郁就会生热，热就会生痰，津液就不能输布全身。脾主升清，把水谷之精微升到肺里边，再由肺输布津液，五经并行，使津液到达全身。肺郁生了热，津液就不能输布到全身，全郁在肺里边了，热把津液炼成了痰，这种痰往往是燥痰，或者是热痰。贝母的作用是解肺郁，解郁就能降火、散火。火一散开，痰的来源就没有了。所以贝母经常用来治因为肺气不通而产生的热痰、燥痰。

浙贝母甘少而苦多，其解肺郁、软坚散结的作用更强一些，养肺润肺的作用比川贝要弱得多。要化顽痰，用浙贝就可以了，而且浙贝还便宜。如果既怕伤了肺又要化痰又要润肺，就要用川贝，但川贝的价格很昂贵。一般是用川贝粉，每次用 3 到 6 克就够了。浙贝可以多用一点，最少用 10 克，多则可以用到 30 克或 50 克不等。

此外还有一种平贝，主要产于东北，其颗粒的大小在川贝和浙贝之间，作用也与二者相仿。

解肺气之郁

肺主皮毛，皮肤上的疮疡往往源于肺郁，肺气郁则皮肤不能通透，所以经常用浙贝来散郁。

浙贝是很早以前就开始使用的一种药，《诗经》里边就有这样的诗句："陟彼阿丘，言采其蝱。女子善怀，亦各有行。""蝱"就是贝母。这句诗的意思是，因为心情不舒服，所以到山上去采贝母。女子善怀，就是女子多愁善感，虽然各有原因，但总离不开一个郁字。女子多郁，主要是肝郁，肝郁又会导致气郁。肺主一身之气。肺郁了，气也就郁了，所以用贝母来解肺郁。

解郁，我们会想到逍遥散，这是用来疏肝解郁的，用逍遥散的时候经常加一味浙贝母，有佐金平木的作用。浙贝母能够帮助肺金来平肝木，让肝木的邪气平息下来。这个说法是讲得通的。还有更直接的说法，浙贝在解肺郁、解气郁。逍遥散再加一味解肺郁的贝母，解郁的力度就大大增强了。肝郁、肺郁一起解，气才能通。

散痰结

有了结，就会有各种肿块、包块，凡是因郁结产生的这些东西，都可以用浙贝母来化。因为这些包块有郁的成分，也有痰的成分在里边，最常见的包块，例如乳房小叶增生，或者说乳腺炎，更严重一点的就是乳腺癌。如果乳房里边有包块，医生会告诉你别生气，心情放舒适一些。他知道这是肝郁，特别喜欢给你开逍遥散、加味逍遥丸来疏肝，但是有人吃着有效，有人吃着无效，无效的更多一些，为什么呢？因为这是一个成药，不便加减。如果把它开成汤药的话，其中势必要加浙贝母，因为结节已经形成，这就不仅仅是肝郁了，所以要加浙贝母来散结。

乳房的部位固然属肝，但也属肺，因此乳房的结节跟肺郁也是有关的，所以必须加浙贝，而且用量还要大一些，至少是 15 克，甚至 25 克，要根据人、根据病情来加减。还可以加夏枯草，这也是一味散热结的好药，尤其是用于散乳房中的热结，效果非常好。在逍遥散的基础上加上这两味药，再根据结块的部位，例如结块是在乳头的上部，往往属火；如果左部偏多，左主血，那么可能跟瘀血有关；如果右部偏多，右主气，可能跟痰相关。据此继续进行加减，效果会非常好。

贝母经常与桔梗一起用。桔梗升提，能载药上行；贝母下行，又归肺经。为了让贝母能够充分地到肺里边，所以用桔梗先升提，让贝母在肺里边多停留一会，充分化痰散结，之后再肃降。一升一降之间，二者的作用会相得益彰。

因为肺经痰热郁阻，很多哺乳期的女子乳汁出不来，乳房会胀痛，在通乳的药里边加一些浙贝和桔梗，也能解郁，使乳汁自然出来。

贝母解毒的原理

贝母还有解毒的作用。因为贝母能够导热下行，热往下走，则不往上犯，痰也跟着减少，气就通了，气通则身体疏泄的能力就强了，毒就能解掉，因郁结产生的毒也就解掉了。

肝主疏泄，是人体解毒部位。人体每一天都在产生新的毒，饮食里边有毒，情绪太过不及都有毒。人体有自我修复的机能，无时无刻不在解毒，尤其是在睡觉的时候，血归于肝，正好进行大清扫。但在郁结的时候，毒是解不掉了。贝母能解毒，还能化痰、散结、解郁，能让人体舒畅起来，有能力把毒解掉。

贝母解毒，常配连翘，一般用于颈上的一些结块、结核，必要的时候加上海藻、昆布。海藻、昆布都是能开郁、散结、解毒的。贝母的用量可以用三钱到一两，如果有必要，还可以多用。

我们要有对证的方，也要有治病的药。我们常说辨证用药，其实辨证是辨证，用药是用药。方要与证对，在这个过程中可以加上治病的药，比如连翘和贝母，这是治病的药，用来治疗项上的结核，如果项上的结核是因为肝郁导致的，可以在逍遥散的基础上加上这两味药；如果是因为湿气导致的，可以在平胃散的基础上加上这两味药。

贝母与半夏的比较

半夏和贝母，都是化痰的主药，它们之间有很大区别。贝母解郁，走肺经；半夏偏燥，走脾经。贝母寒凉，半夏则温。所以贝母用来化火痰、热痰，半夏化偏寒的痰。当痰来自肺的时候，用贝母来化，当痰来自脾的时候，用半夏来化。当人体有火邪，有热邪，肺被火刑，水饮不化，肺气郁结就成了痰，此时的痰是燥痰，适合用贝母。当脾胃虚寒，水饮停积在脾肺之间不能通的时候，这是湿痰，适合用半夏。当然有时候也可以一起用，当痰既跟肺有关，也跟脾有关的时候，就可以半夏与贝母一起使用。

贝母治疗的范围比较广，虚劳的烦热、肺痈、肺痿、喉痹、咳血、吐血、目眩；还有各种痰结、各种瘤、恶疮；甚至难产、乳汁不通等都可以使用贝母。

人面疮与玄学

有一本书在讲到贝母的时候，顺便讲过这么个故事：说有人胳膊上长出了一张脸，这张脸能做出各种表情，还能吃东西，谁都治不好。后来医生教他对着这张脸念中药的名字，一个一个念下去，念其他药的时候，这张脸都不动声色，唯独念到贝母的时候，这个人面疮皱眉，表情很痛苦，医生就说：行了，你就服用贝母吧。于是，此人把贝母碾成粉，不仅自己服用，还往胳膊上这个小人嘴里灌，没多久，这张脸就消失了。

这种病叫人面疮，很多古书都有过记载。人面疮可能长在脸上，也可能长在四肢或其他地方。这属于怪病，而怪病皆属于痰，所以用贝母来治疗。

菖蒲

菖蒲的性状及选择

菖蒲是一种水草。生长在水沟淤泥里的叫水菖蒲，生长在山间流水石上的，叫石菖蒲。它们是很相近的，只是生长的环境不一样，性质就产生了差异。入药必须用石菖蒲。

石菖蒲又叫节菖蒲，或者叫九节菖蒲，中医临床上用的九节菖蒲是石菖蒲，节非常密，在一寸之内有九个节，这就是九节菖蒲，它也是一个能通的药。

石菖蒲干了以后，会很结实。把它折断，里面会微微的有点发红，这样的石菖蒲是最好的。

开窍而通心脾

石菖蒲有点微红，所以能够入心，同时它又有浓烈的芬芳，所以能够开心窍。

气闷住了，或气郁住了，人就不高兴了。开心与闷闷不乐，与人的心理有关，也与人的生理有关。石菖蒲能够通过作用于人的身体来影响人的心理，有令人喜悦的作用。

石菖蒲通过芳香，把人体内的各种孔窍打开，痰就能够自然排出去。人体到处都有痰，当心包络里面有痰的时候，叫痰迷心窍，或者叫痰犯心包，人往往就会神经病，乱说话，或者妄知妄见，看到的东西和平常人不一样，或者别人看不到的东西他看到了。石菖蒲把心窍打开了，把痰排出了，痰就不再扰乱人的心情了。这是石菖蒲的一个很重要的作用。所以，很多神志方面的疾病经常会用到石菖蒲。

石菖蒲是长在水里面的，它对水就有一定的抵抗力。所以，它能散水邪，还能通心脾之间的痰湿。它是开窍的，开窍就能够行痰、行湿，让痰湿有路可通、有路可去。它是芳香的，芳香能醒脾，能够开发脾气。脾主运化，它能让脾的运化功能进一步增强，甚至发挥到极致。因为心火生脾土。一个对心有作用的药肯定对脾有作用，何况芳香能够醒脾呢？所以，石菖蒲能够促进脾的运化。

菖蒲用于霍乱和痢疾

霍乱和痢疾都可以用到石菖蒲。王孟英《随息居重订霍乱论》里有一个很有名的方子叫连朴饮，其中就用到了菖蒲。

连朴饮：黄连、厚朴、菖蒲、半夏、豆豉、栀子

黄连、厚朴是清脾胃湿热的。当湿热之邪在中焦扰乱，让脾胃的升清降浊功能受到影响的时候，就会脾不升清、胃不降浊，升降失调就会导致霍乱，上吐下泻，所以用黄连、厚朴来清中焦的湿热。接着就用菖蒲，一则芳香化浊，二则促进脾的运化，三则打通体内的孔窍，也更有助于升清降浊。后面的半夏也是健脾的，豆豉和栀子为栀子豉汤，是清上焦的。

另外，痢疾，尤其是迁延时间较长而造成的噤口痢，跟脾虚有关，也因为热气阻闭在膈上。一般用参苓白术散，但效果差，加一味石菖蒲马上就不一样了。

参苓白术散作用于脾虚，但是热气把气机闭住了，用石菖蒲去打开会更好，因为石菖蒲的通窍作用比木香要大得多。所以，用石菖蒲熬汤，送服参苓白术散这个中成药就可以了。也可以再加一点米汤，米汤是调和胃气的。因为到了噤口痢的时候，人的食欲也会非常小，用米汤来调服这个药也算是给人增加一点能量。

菖蒲的其他配伍

石菖蒲与熟地、黄柏一块做成丸剂，可以治疗肾虚性的耳聋。耳为心肾之窍，清窍不通则耳聋，所以要来开窍。光开窍还不行，还得补肾。熟地是补肾阴的，黄柏清肾里面的邪火，还可以固肾。一个补真阴，一个清邪火，一个通窍，三个药用得非常精到。所以，人在中年，吃些这样的药，老来可以延缓听力减退。

菖蒲和远志都是散的，经常用来交通心肾，神志昏迷、精神病、癫痫可以用它，但不能用得太久，尤其是菖蒲，太香了，一香它就燥，一燥它就能散，能散人的真阴，也能散人的真阳。心喜欢收敛，它不喜欢散。阴虚不足的人，千万不要乱用石菖蒲，还有汗多的病人，在用石菖蒲的时候也要慎重。再有一个，石菖蒲熬药的时候千万不要用铁勺子去搅，更不要

用不锈钢锅熬带石菖蒲的药，否则就会让人有想呕吐的感觉，严重了就让人呕吐。一般来讲，熬药的时候要用砂锅，或者用陶罐、瓷器来熬，不要用金属器皿。

昆布

昆布和海藻

昆布，很像一匹很大的布，只长在海里面，比较硬，海带要小一些，海藻就是很细的了。有些时候海带和昆布也是相通的，也有人就把海带叫昆布。

昆布、海带、海藻，它们的作用很相似，都是海里面的，味咸，咸能软坚、能散结、能润下、能除热、能入肾。所以它们用来化顽痰、痰结会有比较好的作用。但是这不能久用，用久了就会使人消瘦。化痰就把脂肪都给消了，人就瘦了。所以经常有人问到中医怎么减肥，中医减肥的方法实在是太多了。健脾促进运化，可以减肥；化痰消脂肪，也能让人瘦；还有山楂也是让人瘦的，山楂是消肉食的，也能消肉，看情况而用。

化痰就把脂肪都给消了，人就瘦了。所以，中医减肥的方法实在是太多了。健脾促进运化，可以减肥；化痰消脂肪，也能让人瘦；还有山楂也是让人瘦的，山楂是消肉食的，也能消肉，看情况而用。

海藻玉壶汤及反药的运用技巧

昆布治疗一切的瘰疬、瘿瘤、顽痰胶结的效果很好。但它禁忌跟甘草一起用，会有毒。这就叫"藻戟遂芫具战草"，但也有的方子就是把海藻、昆布这些药跟甘草一起用。《医宗金鉴》里有个很有名的方剂，叫海藻玉壶汤。

海藻玉壶汤：

海藻一两，昆布五钱，贝母五钱，半夏三钱，青皮二钱，陈皮三钱，当归五钱，川芎三钱，连翘三钱，甘草二钱

海藻玉壶汤一般是治疗上焦的，尤其是上焦非常顽固的痰结。

这种顽固的痰结，你不清楚它是寒痰还是热痰，也不清楚是属脾还是属肺了。它既属脾又属肺，所以贝母和半夏一块用。痰已经结在那里了，所以要软坚散结。海藻、昆布，咸能散结；贝母通过解郁化热痰来软坚散结。

在化痰的同时，要兼顾气血，所以用陈皮、青皮来理气、破气，气行则痰化。同时，气行，血也要行，所以，加上当归、川芎来行血。既然痰已经结了，势必有热，用连翘来清。

海藻、昆布是往下走的，甘草是缓的，可以让海藻、昆布在人体停留的时间长一些，有的人可能会受不了，会呕吐，又有半夏降逆止呕。青皮、陈皮、当归、川芎是行气行血的，它们走得很快，有这些走得很快的药，加入一味甘草不要紧。

当然，痰结久了，就会产生毒，连翘后面还可以加一味金银花。还可以根据具体的情况来进行加减。这样化痰结的力度就非常大了。

白芥子

白芥子是药用芥菜结的种子，不是食用芥菜结的种子。药用芥菜的叶子是青白色的，子是黄白色；食用芥菜的叶子是青绿色，子是紫黑色的。

白芥子的性能和用法

白芥子是辛热的药，入肺、胃两经，可以通行经络，化痰，能够搜剔内外痰结。有时候，人体的痰就停留在内膜里，半夏化不了，贝母也化不了，唯独白芥子辛香走窜，专门走皮里膜外，所以当痰在四肢、胁下、在各种皮里膜外，只有用白芥子才能够搜刮到。尤其胖人的胁下痛，用白芥子更有必要。

白芥子能走窜经络，所以经常用它来敷贴穴位。比如摔伤了，有瘀肿，可以用白芥子捣碎，加上醋一起涂在患处，效果很好。如果直接涂抹，它的刺激性会很大，伤皮肤，可以跟鸡蛋清一起调，其性就会有所缓和，就不怎么伤皮肤了。如果不用鸡蛋清调的话，就千万不要给小孩用，小孩皮肤脆弱，很容易被灼伤。如果牙痛，可以把它敷在脸上；如果五脏痛可以将它敷在相应的穴位；如果是头上的病，可以把它贴在脚心；如果是风湿病，也可以把白芥子贴在脚心，或者用它泡水洗脚。

三子养亲汤

三子养亲汤，就是白芥子、苏子加莱菔子这三味药所组成的一个方子。

因为老年人总是多痰，而且痰藏得很深，所以用白芥子是用来化痰的；老人总是气往上逆，所以用苏子是来降气；老年人的脾胃虚了，有时稍微多吃了一点就会导致食积，所以用莱菔子来消食。用这三个种子，要把它们略微炒一炒，炒香了然后捣碎熬汤。

养亲汤，是用来孝敬父母双亲的，但也不能多用，用多了就会耗气。白芥子虽然化痰，化得没痰可化了，它就消耗人的正气了；苏子虽然是降气了，气降得差不多了，就不能继续降了，继续降下去人就没气了；莱菔子是消食的，消完了以后就不要再消，而且莱菔子也是降气的。多用久用，就会导致其他一些意想不到的后果。

Chapter 7   Medicines for Dispersing Blood Stasis

Overview of Blood Stasis

Blood stasis, as a pathological product, is formed when the normal blood circulation is disturbed. What does blood stasis look like? It looks like the pig or duck blood curd in the market.

Formation of Blood Stasis

Pig blood can be formed into curd (stasis) since it breaks away from the pig and cannot circulate in the body as it has, which suggests that "stasis occurs when blood stops circulating".

Blood stasis may also arise from heat, such as scald, it is always red. Besides, blood can stagnate too in case of coldness, or due to trauma or failure of blood to circulate in the vessels. In brief, blood stasis may stem from many reasons. In the body, where there is blood circulation, there is possibility of blood stasis.

Diseases and Syndromes Arising from Blood Stasis

Blood stasis may cause many different diseases, and many strange diseases could be treated based on diagnosis from the perspective of blood stasis.

A famous doctor named Luo Zan in Jiangxi province of China once met a young farmer suffering from manic syndromes as those recorded in the *Huangdi Neijing (the Internal Canon of Huangdi)*, such as to "climb to high places to sing, and to walk around nakedly", "swear at all people regardless of close relatives or strangers", for which the other doctors had treated him through the regular treatment of clearing fire and resolving phlegm, but failed. However, Luo Zan found that the patient had thin, weak thready and slow pulse, suggesting the patient suffered from deficiency of blood (showing thin pulse), and blood stasis (showing weak thready pulse) and no heat/fire (since the pulse is not rapid). And then, Luo Zan asked some details about the patient from his family and got to know that the patient had become manic after he came back home from a trip during which he tumbled and fell over. And finally, Luo Zan diagnosed the patient as having mania due to blood stasis, for which he prescribed **Taohe Chengqi Tang**, plus **Shixiao San** for eliminating the blood stasis. After that, the patient recovered very soon.

By the way, only serious blood stasis might result in mania. Besides, blood stasis at different locations can result in different consequences, for instance, some children have a fever that is not due to the common cold or flu or overeating. In such a case, it may be the result of blood stasis. Fever arising from blood stasis is quite common for children with the manifestations of a sudden fever, or dysphoria, or yellowish complexion, or deep fingerprint lines. All such manifestations suggest the blood stasis that may stem from recent tumbling or scare, for which **Xuefu Zhuyu Tang**, or **Xuefu Zhuyu Oral Liquid** can be used for treatment.

Blood stasis also has many other manifestations, such as dull yellow look, especially around the lips. Furthermore, the patients may dislike salty food since the salty taste enters the blood, and the overly salty food can impair the blood. Therefore, those who dislike the salty food might suffer from blood stasis.

New Stasis Shows Shaoyang Symptoms and Chronic Stasis Shows Yangming Symptoms

How can one differentiate the newly formed blood stasis and the long-lasting blood stasis? There is a rule for helping to make judgement, i. e. , "the newly formed blood stasis shows some symptoms (like bitter taste in the mouth with dry throat) that are like those of Shaoyang diseases, while the long-lasting blood stasis shows some symptoms that are like those of of Yangming diseases".

Shortly before, I met a patient who suffer from metrorrhagia and metrostaxis with a lot of Yangming symptoms such as uterine bleeding after around 5 p. m. till 11 or 12 hours at midnight. According to TCM theory, heat in Yangming meridian becomes vigorous after 5 p. m. and it will then cause bleeding. In fact, she was suffering from the long-lasting blood stasis.

The newly formed blood stasis can be treated with **Taoren Chengqi Tang**, while the long-lasting blood stasis can be treated with **Didang Tang**. Without doubt, every formula must be used based on the specific syndromes, especially the formula of **Didang Tang**, which contains the herbs like leech and gadfly. Generally, leech must not be used since it may revive to reproduce some small leeches in the stomach even it is crushed into powder in case that it is not properly processed prior to use. TCM always tries to avoid using the animal herbs unless there are no other choices. For the long-lasting blood stasis, it can also be treated with **Xuefu Zhuyu Tang** plus Danshen (radix salviae miltiorrhizae), Sanqi (notoginseng), Wulingzhi (trogopterus dung) and Raw Puhuang (raw cattail pollen).

Danshen (Radix Salviae Miltiorrhizae)

Danshen is a plant with its root being used as herb, and it is pungent, bitter, and slightly sweet, cool, and mild in properties. The peel of the root is red, indicating that it enters the blood and the heart. It is a special herb used for the blood system of the heart and pericardium. It enters the heart, liver, and kidney channels to promote blood circulation, remove blood stasis and clear the blood heat. Danshen can be used for the treatment of metrorrhagia, bloody flux (dysentery with bloody stool), oedema, ulceration, and blood stasis and stagnant heat in the chest and abdomen etc.

Equal Functions of Danshen to Siwu Tang

The experienced doctors of TCM all have a pet phrase, saying "a dose of Danshen has equal function to **Siwu Tang**".

Siwu Tang contains the four ingredient herbs of Danggui (angelica sinensis), Bai Shao (radix paeoniae alba), Chuangxiong (ligusticum wallichii) and Shengdi (radix rehmanniae recen). How can Danshen be used to achieve the same effects as those of **Siwu Tang**? Normally, Danshen is substituted for **Siwu Tang** when blood stasis arises, showing some symptoms of deficiency of blood. **Siwu Tang** may be used by some TCM doctors but it may not work well since the new blood is not regenerated under the influences of blood stasis. In that case, Danshen should be used instead to promote blood circulation to remove blood stasis, and after that, new blood will be regenerated. Otherwise, if **Siwu Tang** is used to enrich the blood without prior removal of blood stasis, it may worsen the stasis.

Fufang Danshen Tablets

Danshen is a mild herb for removing stasis, and it has a wide range of applications. For example, those who suffer from heart diseases may have blood stasis, so Danshen is often used in the treatment. There is a well-known patent medicine called **Fufang Danshen Tablet or Pill**, which is often used in the treatment of heart trouble.

The formula of **Fufang Danshen Tablet** contains the ingredient herbs: Danshen (radix salviae miltiorrhizae) 1 *jin*, Sanqi (notoginseng) 3 *liang* and Bingpian (borneol) 3 *qian*.

In this formula, Danshen is used with a large dosage for promoting blood circulation to remove stasis; Sanqi plays the same function as Danshen here; Bingpian is an aromatic herb used for opening orifices. These three herbs function together to make patients feel comfortable. However, this medicine cannot be used for too much long time. Otherwise, it may cause some impairment in the body.

Danshen having equal function to **Siwu Tang**, it has little effect for nourishing blood, and cannot enrich blood directly except that it promotes the circulation of blood to remove blood stasis. Therefore, stop using it when it strikes the diseases, otherwise, it may cause disorder of blood. Similarly, Bingpian cannot be used for long time, either, since it is aromatic with strongly dynamic nature, and it can disturb Qi and blood.

Sanqi (Notoginseng)

Sanqi is a famous herb that has a strong effect on treating blood trouble. It is the key ingredient in the **Yunnan Baiyao** (a famous and popular powdered medicine used for treatment of muscle injury) .

The original name of Sanqi is Shanqi, growing in the mountains. It is very effective for healing up wounds, acting like glue to close the cut, causing a cessation of bleeding immediately. In the past, those who practiced martial arts always carried some vulnerary with them, of which the key ingredient herb was Sanqi. Even in the army in the past, Sanqi was also popular for healing up wounds. As such, Sanqi is also called "Jinbuhuan" (literally means "not to be exchanged even for gold"), implying that Sanqi has a great potential for saving lives.

Varieties of Sanqi

Sanqi is produced in many places in China. Sanqi produced in Yunnan province of China is called Dian Shanqi, and Sanqi produced in the Tianlin county, Guangxi province of China is called Tian Sanqi. Both have very good medical effects in quality.

Sanqi is endowed with more bitterness than sweetness in tastes. It is like Renshen (ginseng) in shape and taste, so, Sanqi is also called Shen Sanqi. Sanqi produced in Yunnan province enjoys more sweetness, and has the functions of promoting blood circulation to remove stasis, which is accompanied with the effect of nourishing blood as well. Sanqi produced in Tianlin county of Guangxi province has more bitterness than sweetness, so it is mainly used for promoting blood circulation and remove blood stasis. The best medicinal part of Sanqi is its main root, which is usually irregular in shape with many nodules attached to it. Attached to the main root are many tiny rootlets and fibrils, which are sweeter and are less bitter than the main root, therefore, their therapeutic effect is much weaker.

In addition, there are some other types of Sanqi, like Zhujie Sanqi, specifically used for removing blood stasis; Bo Sanqi, yellowish-white in colour, akin to that of bone, used for curing wounds, invigorating the circulation of blood, and strengthening tendons and bones; and Teng Sanqi, which is a counterfeit form of Sanqi growing on vines, and to some degree, can promote blood circulation and remove blood stasis, too. However, these types of Sanqi are not so pure as Tian Sanqi in quality.

Sanqi Invigorates Blood Circulation without Causing Troubles and Stops Bleeding Without Causing Stasis

Sanqi enters the liver and stomach channels to treat various blood stasis, especially that resulting from wounds and scalds. It can invigorate the blood circulation and remove blood stasis. It can stop bleeding, but will not cause stasis. In a word, Sanqi can help the blood to return to its normal and optimal order.

The herbs that invigorate blood circulation and remove blood stasis can activate more bleeding, while the herbs that stop bleeding can slow down the blood circulation, leaving behind blood stasis once bleeding is stopped. Only Sanqi has the double functions of invigorating blood and stop bleeding without causing blood stasis. In the past, there was a method adopted to identify Sanqi, that is, mix Sanqi powder with coagulated pig blood, after which the blood curd would revert to its flowing/liquid state, proving the function of Sanqi.

Oral Administration of Sanqi

The elderly people are susceptible to blood stasis, and the age pigment on the face indicates the existence of blood stasis in the body. Therefore, the elderly people can take Sanqi powder on a regular base to remove the blood stasis. For such a purpose, Yunnan-produced Sanqi is the best since it is sweeter and it not only removes blood stasis, but also nourishes blood. For removing the chronic blood stasis, Yunnan-produced Sanqi is also effective.

Officers or clerks who are usually lack of physical exercises may also suffer from blood stasis. Hence, Sanqi powder is suitable to them, too. Besides, those who always do physical work may suffer from internal lesion caused by overexertion, which then results in blood stasis, to which Sanqi is also suitable.

Sanqi is extremely hard in texture. Of course, the harder, the better. The top-quality Sanqi shows the deep green color inside. By the way, Sanqi should be ground into powder and orally taken directly.

Honghua (Safflower Carthamus)

Cao Honghua (Safflower) and Zang Honghua (Saffron Crocus)

Honghua, as its name suggests, is a red flower, which covers Cao Honghua and Zang Honghua. These two come from different plants with different parts being used for medicinal use, but they have quite similar medical effects.

Cao Honghua grows all over China, but mainly in Sichuan, Jiangsu and

Zhejiang provinces. The whole flower can be used as medicine. Zang Honghua is planted in some European countries, such as Greece, and was introduced into China mainland through the region of Tibet, and thus, it is named Zang Honghua (literally means Tibetan red flower). Now, Zang Honghua is planted in Tibet, Shanghai, and other regions around China. In the plant of Zang Honghua, only the stigma can be used as medicine, and its output is quite limited, as such, it is very valuable.

Properties and Dosage of Honghua

Honghua is pungent, sweet, bitter, and warm in properties. Generally, the blood stasis arising from blood heat should be dispersed with the cool medicine, such as Danpi (the cortex moutan radices); if the heat symptom of the blood stasis is not so obvious, Honghua should be used instead. Honghua as a medicine can disperse the blood stasis if used in a larger dosage; and it can nourish blood too if used in a smaller dosage.

Honghua, a kind of flower as medicine, has a dispersing function like all the other flowers if used as medicines. Honghua, warm in nature, can promote the circulation of blood and disperse the blood stasis. However, Honghua is very particular about its dosage in each decoction. The larger dosage of Honghua can break blood stasis, and smaller dosage can nourish blood. Therefore, based upon syndrome differentiation, Honghua is sometimes used with a dosage of 3 or 4*qian*; sometimes with a dosage of 7 to 8 *fen* for soothing the liver with its aromatic scent and pungent taste; sometimes with a dosage of only 2 or 3 *fen* for purging the heart fire; and sometimes for some specific cases even a larger dosage may be used for greater effect of dispersing the blood stasis. Hence, different dosage should be used for different purposes with different effects.

When Honghua is used at a dosage of 3 to 4*qian*, it will have so strongly pungent and warming effects that it can activate the circulation of blood and disperse blood stasis. Therefore, Honghua is often used together with Sumu (sappanwood) to remove stagnated blood. Honghua is used with Rougui (cassia bark) in gynaecology to treat amenorrhoea due to coldness. Honghua used together with Danggui (angelica sinensis) and Chuangxiong (ligusticum wallichii) can treat stabbing pains all over the body, or the stabbing pain in the chest or abdomen.

Stabbing pains are often attributable to blood stasis. Thus, Honghua is used to promote the circulation of blood in order to stop the pains.

The best Cao Honghua should be purely red, in which there should be no yellow petals mixed since yellow color suggests that the petals had been picked before they were mature.

Zang Honghua

Cao Honghua has very good effects in most cases. Zang Honghua is extremely expensive, and practically, it is used for nourishing blood with a special effect, but it is less effective for removing blood stasis. Many books claim that Zang Honghua "can make one feel joyful if he or she uses it in a long run" since it can open the heart orifice.

Zang Honghua can also be used to tackle some heart troubles and psychological disorders since such troubles are all related to the blood.

In the surgical applications, Zang Honghua is often used in the formulas for injuries with blood stasis. In fact, such formulas usually contain a lot of herbs for promoting blood circulation to remove blood stasis, and Zang Honghua is used in these formulas to play a harmonizing function between the herbs for promoting blood circulation to remove blood stasis and the herbs for nourishing blood.

Taoren (Peach Kernel)

Taoren Used with Honghua

Taoren and Honghua are often used together. The Taoren used as medicine is from the wild peach that is small with a large peach pit, quite hard to crack open. The kernel inside the pit is also hard. Such type of Taoren is the best in quality.

Taoren, bitter and pungent in tastes, enters the liver, lung, and large intestine channels. Its pungent taste indicates that it can enter the lung, and its bitter taste indicates that it goes downwards. Bitterness and pungency can play the functions for opening and discharging purposes. Therefore, Taoren can eliminate blood stasis. Besides, Taoren also enjoys some sweet taste, helping to relieve the diseases of the liver and generate new blood.

As a matter of fact, all kinds of kernels have the functions of moistening dry-ness, and entering the large intestine to loosen/lubricate stool. Taoren can assist in the excretion of blood stasis via the bowel movement. Or put it in another way, Taoren can enter the six hollow organs, and remove blood stasis there. However, Honghua enters the five internal organs. Hence, Honghua and Taoren are often used together to treat the blood stasis in the viscera in the body. Furthermore, Taoren sinks and descends, while Honghua can disperse. They can bring out the best in each other when used together.

The formula of **Siwu Tang** can be modified into another formula called **Tao-hong Siwu Tang** by adding Honghua and Taoren. **Siwu Tang** nourishes blood, while Taoren and Honghua can break and remove blood stasis. Removing blood stasis often involves consumption of blood to some extent, so, **Siwu Tang** is used to nourish blood. Furthermore, **Siwu Tang can** guide the effects of Taoren and Honghua to the blood system to achieve better treatment outcomes.

Growing Vitality Exorcises Pathogenic Evil Spirits

Taoren also remind of the peach wood. It is said that the peach sword used by the Taoists can exorcise evil spirits, which may be the secondary reason. The key point is that peach wood possesses great growing vitality. In Spring, peach trees blossom early, exuberantly and vigorously. In summer, especially after rain, from the tree bark exudes resin that is called Taojiao (peach gum), which can be used as an herbal medicine, too. Peach resin also indicates the growing vitality of the tree, showing much stronger vitality than that of the other trees. Peach wood has higher level of growing Qi compared to the other trees. The strong growing vitality can repel pathogenic influence.

The growing vitality of the peach tree is concentrated in Taoren since it needs to store the life essence in order to sprout in the coming year. Taoren en-ters the liver to remove blood stasis. The liver possesses growing vitality, too; and with the help of such growing vitality, Taoren can generate new blood very quickly.

Taoren can exorcise evil spirits, too. Those who suffer from psychological disorders sometimes believe that they have seen a ghost. However, these psychological disorders are related to the liver blood stasis. Blood stasis in the six hollow organs can cause some hallucinations. For such cases, Taoren will be used in the treatment based on syndrome differentiation. Once the blood stasis is removed with Taoren, the patient will surely regain his or her consciousness, and hallucinations will be removed too. This is another aspect of peach wood that repels evil and ghosts. The benefits of Taoren in the treatment of such conditions involves both its content of high amounts of growing Qi and its effect of resolving blood stasis.

Puhuang (Cattail Pollen)

Properties of Puhuang

Puhuang is pollen from aquatic plant cattail that in summer produces a candle-like core with fluff inside and pollen on the surface. The pollen collected is called Puhuang. The fluff can be used as a medicine for external use for stopping bleeding of wounds and preventing fester. If applied properly, the wound will heal up perfectly even without a scar left.

Puhuang is a yellowish powder that needs to be wrapped up separately for decocting in order to avoid too much thick decoction. Puhuang, cool in property, enters the heart, liver, and spleen channels. Among so many herbs for invigorating blood circulation and eliminating stasis discussed in the previous sections, Puhuang is an exception since it enters the spleen channel via the heart and liver channels. Also, Puhuang has aromatic scent that can activate the spleen. As such, Puhuang has some special effects for cooling blood, invigorating blood circulation, eliminating blood stagnation and dispersing the blood heat, and even having some curative effects on various injuries to some extent.

Puhuang is classified into raw Puhuang and parched Puhuang. The raw Puhuang refers to the original cattail pollen without any processing, while the parched Puhuang refers to cattail pollen that is slightly fried until it turns yellowish-brown in color. Both raw and parched Puhuang can invigorate blood circulation and remove blood stasis, but the former is more slippery in property, and it can break blood stasis, subside swelling and promote circulation of blood while the latter becomes astringent in property without slippery property after frying, and particularly, it has a stronger effect for stopping bleeding, and removing blood stasis as well. Furthermore, the parched Puhuang has an intensified function to enter the spleen channel. Besides, the parched Puhuang is often used together with herbs for tonifying and invigorating the spleen to stop bleeding and strengthening the function of spleen to govern blood in order to control the blood to go where it should go.

Shixiao San

Puhuang can dredge meridians and collaterals, and relieve pains, with which a famous formula named **Shixiao San** is involved.

Shixiao San contains the ingredient herbs of Wulingzhi (trogopterus dung) and raw Puhuang.

Shixiao San is used for the treatment of pains, especially the chronic pain. Just as its name implies, the patient may break into laughter after using **Shixiao San**, which means that the patient feels rotten due to pain, but he or she will feel happy since the pain is relieved very soon after **Shixiao San** is used. The chronic pain is often involved with blood stasis. As it is always said that "smooth circulation results in no pain, while pains always remind of stagnation or obstruction". Stagnation usually refers to obstruction of either Qi or blood. The long-lasting obstruction of Qi will naturally result in blood stasis, and vice versa. Therefore, the long-lasting pain remind of the blood stasis, after which is removed with **Shixiao San**, the patient will suffer no pains and then burst into laughter accordingly.

The chronic pain may gradually extend into meridians and collaterals. Both Wulingzhi and raw Puhuang can be used to dredge the collaterals, and they are more effective for removing the stagnated blood. **Shixiao San** is not merely limited to the treatment of pains, and it can also be used for removing stagnation/stasis since long-lasting chronic blood stasis might not cause pain sometimes. By the way, parched Puhuang may be substituted for raw Puhuang in the formula of **Shixiao San** based on the syndrome differentiation.

Besides, Wulingzhi is used as a medicine of removing stasis, too, entering the blood system of the liver channel. In fact, Wulingzhi is the dung of trogopterus. The herbs of dung or excrement have a descending property. They can rapidly go downwards through the body, and then are discharged with stool. Wulingzhi can ensure proper downward flow of the blood and make the stasis excreted with the stool.

In a word, whatever the pains are, most of them are related to the liver and Qi, so the chronic pains can be treated with **Shixiao San**; and the acute pains can be treated with **Jinlingzi San** that contains only two herbs of Chuanlianzi (szechwan chinaberry fruit) and Xuanhusuo (corydalis turtschaninovii bess) (also known as Yanhusuo). Xuanhusuo can dredge both the blood and Qi systems to promote the circulation of blood and Qi, but principally for promoting the circulation of Qi, with a slight effect of removing blood stasis.

Apart from what have been discussed above, there are many other herbs for removing stagnation/stasis, such as Yimucao (motherwort) (it can be used by both males and females to cool blood and dredge the collaterals). In addition, Ruxiang (frankincense) and Moyao (myrrh) are used for eliminating the blood stasis in the Lower Jiao, and strengthening tendons and bones.

第七章　化瘀之药

瘀血概论

瘀血，是病理产物。当血不能正常运行的时候，就成了瘀血。瘀血是什么样子的呢？很容易看到。咱们吃的毛血旺，看到的猪血、鸭血，就是瘀血。这些血已经结成块了，成了巧克力色。

瘀血的形成

为什么你吃的猪血已经成了瘀血了呢？因为它脱离了这头猪，猪已经死了，血放出来了，血已经不能在动物的身上运行了，就成了瘀血，这就是"血不行则瘀"。

血遇到热也可能瘀，比如烫伤，烫伤的地方就会发红。血遇冷也会瘀，比如身体某个部位冻得发紫，一冻，血就行不通了，就成了瘀血。遇到跌打损伤，身上有的地方会出现青紫，这也是出现了瘀血。还有血不归经，也会导致瘀血。血应该在它本来血管里边走，现在它流到血管外面来了，没地方去了，也成了瘀血。所以导致瘀血的原因有很多，人体只要是血能经过的部位，都有可能出现瘀血。

瘀血导致的病症

瘀血会导致各种各样的病，有很多怪病都可以从瘀血来论治。

江西的名医罗瓒先生，有一次遇到一位青年农民，发狂一个星期了，跟《黄帝内经》讲的证状是一样的，"登高而歌，弃衣而走"，"骂詈不避亲疏"，不管是亲人还是不认识的人，见了就骂。前面的医生按照常规的治法，清火、化痰，都不管用。罗瓒先生诊他的脉，脉细、涩、不数。细，是血虚；涩，是有瘀血；不数，说明没有热。如果是有火，就应该会是数脉，跳得很快，或者脉很大，这个人的脉不是这样子的。他仔细地询问，病人家属说这个人曾经推车远行，不慎摔了一跤，回来以后就开始发狂了。罗先生于是诊断为瘀血的发狂症，给了桃核承气汤加上失笑散，瘀血化下来以后，狂症很快就好了。

瘀血瘀得非常多才能导致发狂，若瘀了一点点，或者瘀血的部位不一样，导致的症状也不一样。很多小孩发热，没有感冒，也没有吃多，也要考虑是否瘀血发热。瘀血发热的小孩很常见，它有哪些表现呢？比如，忽然发高热，烦躁不安；要么脸色发黄，其他的症状并不明显，都跟正常人一样；看他的手上的指纹，比较沉，看不太清。遇到小孩发热，有上面这些症状，你得问他最近是不是摔倒过啊，或者说受过惊吓。受惊吓也会影响血的运行，产生瘀血，导致瘀血发热。出现这种情况，可以用血府逐瘀汤，或者血府逐瘀口服液。

瘀血还有很多其他的症状，比如面色暗黄，尤其嘴唇周围发黄。还有，吃东西怕咸味。为什么怕咸味呢？因为咸入血，过咸就伤血，如果很讨厌吃太咸的菜，也跟瘀血有关。

新瘀似少阳，久瘀似阳明

有的瘀血，时间非常的长，有的瘀血则是刚刚形成的。该怎么判断呢？有一个规律，叫"新瘀血症似少阳，久瘀血症似阳明"。瘀血刚形成的时候，症状就像少阳病那样，出现口苦、咽干、目眩之类的；瘀血太久了，就有一些像阳明证。

前不久，我看一位崩漏的病人，她治了很长时间了，也是遍访名医，她就有很多阳明症状。比如，以前她一直是流血的，后来经过治疗一段时间，她就在下午大概五点以后就开始出血，一直出到晚上十一二点的时候才慢慢止住。阳明之热旺在申酉，也就是下午五点以后，热逼血出。其实这是一个久瘀症。

新瘀血症似少阳，可以用桃仁承气汤。久瘀血症似阳明，可以用抵挡汤主之。当然，方剂不必拘守，还得根据具体情况而定。尤其是抵挡汤，其中含有水蛭、虻虫之类的。水蛭，就是蚂蟥，这味药一般不要用。如果炮制不好的话，水蛭即使打成了粉还能复活，喝下去以后还能在你肚子里长出小蚂蟥，这是很可怕的。所以，能不用动物药，尽量还是不要用。久瘀血症，用血府逐瘀汤，再加上丹参、三七、五灵脂、生蒲黄这样的药，也是可以的。

丹参

丹参是一种植物，用它的根，根皮呈红色。红色就会入心、入血。这个药辛、苦，微微有些甘寒，性质也非常平和入心、肝、肾三经，是心和心包的血分药，能够行血、清血。行血就是让血动起来，行血才能活血化瘀。清血是能清血热。丹参可用于血崩、血痢、臃肿、各种疮疡，胸部、腹部的各种瘀血、瘀热等。

功同四物

老中医有个口头禅。"一味丹参，功同四物。"就是说，一味丹参的作用就相当于四物汤了。

四物汤是当归、白芍、川芎、生地这四味药。在什么情况下，用一味丹参，作用就相当于四物汤呢？就是在有瘀血的情况下。瘀血不去，新血不生，人就会有血虚的证状。一般的医生就会虚则补之，补血用四物汤，但是不管用。因为瘀血不去，新血不生啊。任凭怎么补血都补不进去。怎么办？就用丹参。丹参活血化瘀，把瘀血化掉，瘀血一去，新血自然就能生出来。所以一味丹参就有四物汤的功能。如果瘀血没有化掉，反而用四物汤来补，要知道瘀血忌补，它会越补越多的。

复方丹参片

丹参是一味非常平和的化瘀的药，运用的非常广泛。比如说心脏病有瘀血的，就经常用到丹参。我们都很熟悉一个药：复方丹参片、复方丹参滴丸。在心脏病的时候经常会用到这些。

尤其是复方丹参片，它的结构非常的简单：丹参一斤，三七三两，冰片三钱，只有这三味药。

丹参是活血化瘀的，用量非常的大，三七也是活血化瘀的，冰片是一味芳香的药，芳香就能开窍，瘀血化掉了，心窍打开了，人自然就会舒服。但是这个药不能久用，现在很多心脏不好的人，他只用复方丹参片，而且坚持用，吃了可以舒服一些，但是用得久了，确实不好。毕竟丹参是一个活血化瘀的药，虽说"一味丹参，功同四物"，但它养血的能力很小，不能直接补血，只活血化瘀，等到瘀血化得没有的时候，还继续活血化瘀就伤血了。冰片也不能久用，它芳香走窜，芳香开窍，因为它走窜所以能开窍，但是它走窜的太厉害了，也能够动气动血，所以说这药只能用于一时，而不可以长久的使用。

毕竟丹参是一个活血化瘀的药，虽说"一味丹参，功同四物"，但它养血的能力很小，不能直接补血，只活血化瘀，等到瘀血化得没有的时候，还继续活血化瘀就伤血了。冰片也不能久用，它芳香走窜，芳香开窍，因为它走窜所以能开窍，但是它走窜的太厉害了，也能够动气动血，所以说这药只能用于一时，而不可以长久的使用。

三七

三七是一味很有名的药，它治血的力度更大，我们现在用的云南白药，最主要的成分就是三七。

三七的原名叫山漆，是山里产的，能够合金疮，效果非常快，就像用漆把伤口粘住了一样，血就不再流了。过去的武林高手，都是治伤的高手，身上都带着伤药，其主要成分就是三七。过去在军队里也会经常用到这个药，用来疗伤止血。所以，三七又叫"金不换"，并不是说它有多昂贵，而是说它作用大，能救命。

各种三七

三七在很多地方都有生产，云南产的山漆叫滇山漆，广西出产三七的地方在田林，这里的三七也叫田三七。它们的质量都很好。

三七是一味甘苦的药，苦多一些，甘少一些，它的形状与味道都有一点像人参，所以又叫参三七。云南产的三七，甘甜的味道要多一些，于活血化瘀中略带养血功能。广西田林的三七就苦多甘少，主要用于活血化瘀。三七最佳的入药部位是主根，一般都是奇形怪状的，上面有很多瘤，这个活血化瘀的作用最好。主根上还有很多小根和须根，甘多苦少，药力薄得多。

此外还有竹节三七，是专门来化瘀的；还有亳三七，是黄白色的，像骨头那样，可以用来疗伤、活血、强筋壮骨。还有藤三七等，长在藤上，是三七的伪品，但也有一定的活血化瘀作用。这些三七，都不如田三七纯正。

活血不伤血，止血不留瘀

三七，甘苦微温，入肝、胃两经，治疗各种瘀血，尤其是治疗金疮、烫伤等。它可以活血化瘀，还能止血，止血又不留瘀。总而言之，它就是要让血回到它最佳的状态。

一般情况下，活血化瘀的药，能动血，让人出血更多；而止血的药，它能让血不运行，血止住了就会留下瘀血。唯独三七，能活血又能止血，止血又不会留下瘀血，这是它的特殊作用。过去鉴别三七有一个方法，就是把猪血取出来掺入三七末，猪血全化成血水，这就见证了三七化瘀的本领。

三七的服用方法

三七能活血化瘀，还能防止出血。老年人多瘀血，老年斑就是体内有瘀血在脸上的一种标志，所以老年人就可以经常用一些三七粉，化一化瘀。老人用云南三七是最好的，甘甜的多一些，化瘀之中偏于养血。对于慢性瘀血，效果也好。

经常坐办公室的人，由于缺乏运动，血行不通，也会有瘀血，需要经常化一化，常吃三七粉也很适宜。体力劳动过多，会造成劳伤，其间也有瘀血，也同样适宜用三七。

三七最好是打成粉，直接吃下去。三七非常的坚硬，象石头一样，越坚硬的越好。优质的三七，砸开里面是墨绿色的。

红花

草红花和藏红花

红花，顾名思义就是一种红色的花。它有草红花与藏红花之分，二者不是同一种植物，入药部位也不一样，但功效相近。

草红花，全国各地都有栽培，主要产于四川、江浙一带。全花入药；藏红花并不产于西藏，而是产于希腊等欧洲国家，经由西藏传入内地，所以叫"藏红花"，当然，现在西藏、上海等地也开始种植红花了。藏红花是花中小小的柱头入药，产量小，所以，非常珍贵。

红花的性能与用量

红花味辛、甘、苦，性温。如果瘀血是因为血热结成的，就要用一些凉性的药来散瘀，如丹皮之类；如果瘀血的热象不明显，就要用到红花了。红花是花入药，诸花皆主散，花作为药材一般都有散的作用，红花散血。红花性温，能够行血散血。但是，红花在用量上非常的讲究，有用到三四钱的（相当于10克到12克），有的用七八分（相当于2克），有的只用二三分（相当于1克），总体说来，红花就是多用则破血，少用则养血。

红花是花入药，诸花皆主散，花作为药材一般都有散的作用，红花散血。红花性温，能够行血散血。总体说来，红花就是多用则破血，少用则养血。但是，红花在用量上非常的讲究，有用到三四钱的，有的用七八分，是取红花芳香味辛，疏肝气的作用；有的只用二三分，主要是入心，散心火。在一些特殊的场合，红花还可以用得更多，这样它散血的作用会更大。所以用量不同，它的作用也不同。

当红花用三到四钱的时候，辛温的力度就非常的强大了，它能够使血运行起来，并且让瘀血散开，所以它经常配苏木来逐瘀血；在妇科上，跟肉桂一起用，可以治疗女子因为寒导致的闭经；与当归、川芎一起使用，还能治遍身的刺痛，或胸腹的刺痛。刺痛往往是因为有瘀血，这都是取红花活血的作用。

刺痛往往是因为有瘀血，这都是取红花活血的作用。

草红花以颜色清红者为佳，其中不宜夹杂过多黄色的花瓣，黄色的都是因为采收过早。

藏红花

通常，我们用草红花，效果就会非常好，没有必要非得用藏红花。藏红花太贵了，而且也有它适用的范围，它养血的作用大一些，祛瘀的作用要小一些。很多书讲藏红花"久服令人心喜"，就是说这个药吃久了就会让人高兴。因为它打开了心窍。

藏红花还能治疗心脏、神志方面的一些问题，这些问题又跟血有关。

在外科，就像武门的伤科的一些秘方里面会用到藏红花，受伤有瘀血。其实在这些方子里面，有大量活血化瘀或养血的药，而藏红花可以在活血化瘀和养血之间起到调和作用。

桃仁

桃仁配红花

桃仁红花经常一块用。入药的桃仁是用野桃子，那种桃子比较小，桃核却比较大，而且很难砸开，桃仁也很硬，这种桃仁才是比较好的。

桃仁入肝、肺、大肠经，味苦辛。辛能入肺，苦能往下走，辛苦开泄，能够泄瘀血。它还有甘味，能缓肝气、生新血。

所有的仁都能润燥，走大肠，通大便，桃仁能促使瘀血从大便排出。更进一步说，桃仁能走六腑，祛六腑瘀血。所以，我们经常讲，桃仁入六腑，红花走五脏，要治五脏六腑的瘀血，红花桃仁是常用的一对药。而且，桃仁是仁，是沉降的；红花是花，是发散的。也是相得益彰。

在四物汤的基础上加上红花和桃仁，叫桃红四物汤，四物汤养血，桃仁红花破血化瘀。化瘀要以消耗一定的血作为基础，所以配合四物汤养血；而且四物汤还能把桃仁和红花引到血分，更好的发挥作用。

生生之气能辟邪

看到桃仁我们就会想到桃木。道家用的桃木剑可以辟邪。有人说，桃木是红的，红色就可以辟邪，其实这倒在其次，主要是桃木有春天的生生之气。桃花开得早，而且开得比较盛，它的生生之气是很旺的。到了夏天，尤其是在雨后，桃树的皮只要破一点，就会流出很多树脂，这是桃胶，也是一味药。能流出这么多桃胶，也都是因为它的生生之气。桃木的生生之气比一般的树旺得多，生生之气旺就能辟邪。

桃树的生生之气主要集中于桃仁，这是因为它要封藏精华，以备下次发芽之用。桃仁能入肝，肝也是有生气的。所以，它能够逐瘀血，生新血。同时它的生生之气让新血更快地生成。

桃仁也能够辟邪。所以，有的有神智方面病的人，说见到了鬼，从生理上讲这些病都是跟肝血的瘀结有关。瘀血在六腑，就会导致妄知妄见，一会说见到鬼了，一会自己发狂了，这种情况，咱们在辨证论治的基础上，就要用到桃仁。桃仁把瘀化掉以后，人自然也就清醒了，这些鬼也就见到得少了。

蒲黄

蒲黄的性能

蒲黄是水生植物香蒲的花粉。香蒲生在水里，夏天结出像蜡烛那样的东西，里面是绒，表面有粉，收集起来就是蒲黄。那绒在我们那里叫刀割绒。被刀割了，用蒲黄的绒敷上，很快就能止血，不会化脓；如果绒敷得好，还不会留下伤疤。

蒲黄是黄色的粉末状，用的时候要单独包煎，否则会让药液变得浑浊。蒲黄生在水里，有凉性，是一个甘凉的药，入心、肝、脾三经。前面我们讲的那么多活血化瘀药，没有入脾经的，唯独蒲黄入脾经，它通过入心、肝之经，达到脾经；同时它气味芳香，也能够醒脾。因为入脾经，它才有一些特殊的作用。它能凉血、活血、散血，能够散除血热，对各种损伤也有一定疗效。

蒲黄有生蒲黄和炒蒲黄之分。生蒲黄就是直接用花粉，炒蒲黄就是把花粉略微的清炒一下，不加任何辅料，炒到黄褐色。虽然都是活血化瘀，但是生蒲黄性质比较滑，能够破血、消肿、行血；经过炒，性质就涩了，不滑了，止血的作用就要强一些，也能散瘀，但以止血为主。炒过后，入脾经的能力就强化了。所以炒蒲黄经常会与一些补脾、健脾的药一起用，达到止血的效果，加大了脾统血的作用，让血到它该去的地方。

失笑散

蒲黄通经脉，能够止痛。有一个名方叫失笑散。

失笑散：

五灵脂、生蒲黄。

失笑散是治痛的，而且是治久痛的。顾名思义，用过失笑散，能让人哑然失笑。本来痛得很难受，会愁眉苦脸，吃了药就笑了，说明很久的痛消失了。当然，久痛通常与血瘀有关，即使痛不是因瘀血引起的，痛得久了也会形成瘀血。通则不痛，痛则不通。是什么不通呀？要么是气不通，要么就是血不通。气不通久了，血自然也不通。血不通，气也会不通。所以，久痛有瘀血。把瘀血化掉，不痛了，病人就哑然失笑了，这就要归功于失笑散。

久痛入络，五灵脂、生蒲黄都是通络脉的，对瘀血比较久的，这两味药效果会比较好。它不仅仅局限于治痛，瘀血很久可以不痛，不痛也可以用五灵脂、生蒲黄。在这里它的功能就不是治痛，是化瘀了。失笑散在有的情况下用五灵脂和炒蒲黄，这要视情况而定。

五灵脂也是化瘀的药，入肝经血分。五灵脂是寒号鸟的粪便。粪便类的药可以往下走，也就是迅速地引血下行。它在人体内停留的时间也不会太长，能迅速地从大便当中排出体外。此时，瘀血也会随大便一起出来的。

不管什么痛，多数与肝有关，与气有关。久痛用失笑散，新痛则用金铃子散。金铃子散也是由两味药组成的：川楝子、玄胡索。玄胡索既通血分也通气分，行血也行气，主要还是以行气为主，兼有化瘀的作用。

化瘀的药还有很多。比如益母草，益母草并不是只有女性能用，男性也可以用，它可以凉血通络。还有比如乳香、没药，主要用来化下焦的瘀血，还可以强筋壮骨。

Chapter 8   Medicines for Removing Food Retention

Retention here refers to the accumulation of substances in the body over a long period. The accumulation could be phlegm or stagnated blood, finally resulting in disorder of normal circulation of Qi and blood, which will further induce phlegm and fire, causing various discomfort and threat to life eventually.

Long-lasting obstruction of Qi circulation will induce phlegm. In case of pathogenic fire and heat occurring in the body, it may cause the long-lasting phlegm to accumulate, and even result in the formation of subcutaneous nodule.

Impairment of blood circulation can cause blood stasis, and the prolonged blood stasis will then be formed into dried blood. According to *Jingui Yaolue (Synopsis of the Golden Chamber)*, the symptom of emaciation due to blood disorder can be treated with **Dahuang Zhechong Pill**.

Regardless of phlegm accumulation or blood stasis, the principle of treatment is still to resolve the phlegm, eliminate the stasis and stagnation. As for resolving the phlegm accumulation, Zhe Beimu (thunberg fritillary bulb) and Tianhua Fen (radices trichosanthis) and the like should be used. Zhe Beimu can eliminate the stagnation and remove the long-lasting phlegm accumulation. In addition, some herbs for softening the hard mass should also be added in order to remove the accumulated phlegm. Generally, the salty herbs have the functions to soften the hard masses, therefore, the herbs such as Haizao (seaweed), Kunbu (laminaria), Haige (sea clam) and the like can be used for eliminating the accumulated phlegm. As to the treatment of blood stasis, the herbs of removing stagnation or stasis can be used, plus some herbs of softening hard masses, such as the animal products.

Shanzha (Fructus Crataegi) and Other Herbs

Food retention refers to the accumulated food due to indigestion. In TCM, food retention always reminds of the medicine of **Dashanzha Pill**, whose main ingredient is Shanzha.

Shanzha Removes Meat Food Retention

Shanzha is the fruit from the hawthorn tree, which grows all round China, but for medical use, Shanzha produced in the north of China is taken as the best. Therefore, in the prescription, Shanzha, if needed, is often written as "Bei Shanzha (Northern Shanzha)".

Shanzha is sour, bitter, sweet in tastes and warm in property. It enters the liver, spleen, and stomach channels, having the grinding and eliminating effects. It can help to digest food, especially meat. Shanzha is roughly classified into two types: large-sized or small-sized. The small-sized and compact Shanzha is suitable for medicinal use since it is more sour, bitter, and warm in nature. However, the large-sized Shanzha is sweeter and less sour and bitter, especially much bitterer in taste. Therefore, medicinal Shanzha is slightly different from the Shanzha consumed in the diet, but they have the similar effects.

When Shanzha is used as medicine, the seeds are usually removed. In fact, the seed of Shanzha can be used as an herb, too, having the similar effects to Shanzha pulp. In addition to its food digesting function, the seed of Shanzha can be used to treat hernia and expedite child delivery. Shanzha can help digest meat and get rid of fat in the body. As a matter of fact, the fat is a sort of phlegm, too, which can be removed with Shanzha. Shanzha can enter the liver, suggesting it enters blood since the liver stores blood. Therefore, Shanzha also functions to remove blood stasis. Jiao Shanzha (parched Shanzha) refers to the Shanzha that is fried until it turns black, and it not only helps digest the accumulated food but also eliminates blood stasis. Those who keeps eating and drinking too much every meal are susceptible to blood stasis in the intestines and stomach, for which Jiao Shanzha is very suitable.

In the daily life, Shanzha can be used in many cases. For example, old hen meat is highly nutritious, but it is hard to stew it tender. Try to stew the old hen with a little Shanzha (not too much, otherwise it may spoil the taste), then one may find an amazingly tender, delicious, and digestible chicken dish.

Shanzha as Common Medicine Used in Pediatric Department

It is beneficial for children to take Shanzha now and then. Children usually have more vigorous liver Yang but relatively deficient spleen, which may result in hot temper and poor appetite. The sour taste can restrict the liver Yang and nourish the liver Yin. Therefore, it is necessary to nourish the liver Yin and purge the excessive liver fire. Little children often prefer the sour taste since that is what they need in the body. Shanzha, as an herb for food digestion, is essential for children when they suffer from food retention due to eating too much meat.

Shanzha also relaxes the muscles. It is used to treat hernia in pediatrics. Those children who suffer hernia may suffer from coldness in the Jueyin channel and the improper circulation of Qi and blood. When the imbalances of heat and coldness occurs in the body, coldness in the Jueyin channel and Qi and blood stagnation will then cause hernia. Therefore, treatment of hernia should involve warming the Jueyin channel, promoting the circulation of Qi, and mildly removing stagnation. For such a case, Shanzha may be used to eliminate the stagnation, and Xiaohuixiang (fennel), pungent and warm in properties, is used to warm the liver channel to promote the circulation of Qi. Shanzha and Xiaohuixiang can be broken into powder and made into pills, then taken orally with rice-cooked soup, which would have a great effect for treatment of the swelling hernia with bearing-down pain of one testis. Some doctors may use **Buzhong Yiqi Tang** for treatment of this symptom. However, it is not so effective sometimes, and the treatment should have to be done based on the syndrome differentiation. Xiaohuixiang and Shanzha are an herbal pair that may be used separately, or added to the other formula based on the specific symptom.

Besides, the poxes and rashes on children's skin, and especially the poxes would be terrible once they turn black. In that case, Shanzha and Zicao (radices lithospermi) can be added to the prescribed formula based on syndrome differentiation. Zicao, like Shanzha, enters the blood system and removes blood stasis. In addition, Shanzha relaxes the muscles so that toxins can be cleared out of the body. In brief, Shanzha is a commonly used herb in paediatrics.

Contraindications of Shanzha

Shanzha has many good effects, but it does not mean it is suitable for all the people. Those who suffer from deficiency of the spleen should not use Shanzha in case that they have not eaten too much meat. Furthermore, those vegetarians who never eat meat and who are underweight must not eat Shanzha either, since Shanzha can consume the stomach Yin, and prolonged intake of Shanzha will reduce appetite. Even the large-sized dietary Shanzha should not be eaten too much, either, since it warms the liver and the blood system, resulting in endogenous heat.

Parched Rice Bud and Wheat Malt

Rice and wheat food retention can be digested with parched rice bud, parched wheat malt and Shenqu (medicated leaven). In case of rice retention, the parched rice bud will work; in case of wheat food like noodle or steamed bun retention, fried wheat malt will do. It is not necessary to use the two of them simultaneously. Wheat malt enjoys growing vitality, which will remain even after they are parched. Meanwhile, the parched malt can enter the spleen because of its empyreumatic scent. Hence the parched wheat malt can eliminate the rice and wheat retention in the body.

The raw rice bud and wheat malt possess growing vitality, and they are often used to soothe the liver. Those who suffer from poor appetite and liver stagnation may use raw wheat malt to soothe the liver in case Chaihu is not suitable.

Shenqu (Medicated Leaven)

Shenqu is a product of fermentation, whose main ingredient is wheat flour, with the addition of the decoction of Chixiaodou (red phaseolus bean), Xingren (apricot kernel), Qinghao (artemisia apiacea), Cang'er (xanthii fructus), Yeliao (wild smartweed), etc. They are all mixed and fermented. Once they develop into a yellowish mildew on the top, they will then be dried and stored. The longer they are stored, the better they would be in quality.

Shenqu is like yeast, which can promote digestion. Food retention in the stomach can be fermented and become loose with Shenqu so that the accumulated food may be easily digested and then discharged out of the body.

Removing Liquor Retention

Too much drink may result in liquor retention that will occur in the forms of phlegm, damp-heat, blood-heat, etc., though it is intangible. Herbs that can eliminate liquor retention includeGegen (radix puerariae), Gehua (flos puerariae) and Zhijuzi (semen hoveniae).

Gegen (Radix Puerariae) and Gehua (Flos puerariae)

Ge (pueraria lobota) is a type of long vine, indicating that it must have a strong root system in order to distribute enough nutrition. Gegen sold in the pharmacy is diced. Many pores can be seen on the cut surface. In the growing process, the pores are filled with fluid, allowing Gegen to distribute the fluid absorbed from the earth to the vines above ground, signifying that Gegen can promote the flow of fluid. Gegen also has the ascending property that can stimulate the stomach Qi to go upwards. Therefore, Gegen can upbear the Yang, disperse fire and relax the muscle. Human being relies on stomach Qi to induce sweat. Once the stomach Qi is enhanced and Yang Qi is ascending and dispersing, the fire will surely be dispersed accordingly.

The liquor toxin can cause the spleen Qi to sink and produce damp-heat in the stomach. In such a case, Gegen is used to upbear the sinking spleen Qi and stimulate the stomach Yang, which then removes the damp-heat in the stomach.

Gehua refers to the strings of purple flower of puerariae vine. Purple color means it can enter the liver, and all flowers have dispersing efficacy. Gegen enters the stomach, while Gehua enters the liver. Both have ascending and dispersing effects, and they both can dispel the effect of liquor. Gegen and Gehua have something in common, but they have something different, too. They should be used based on the syndrome differentiation.

Zhijuzi (Semen Hoveniae)

For dispelling the effect of liquor, only ascending and dispersing are not workable, and the descending herb is also essential. For that purpose, Zhijuzi will be the best choice. Zhijuzi is the seed of an arbor plant that is mainly growing in the central China, like the jujube kernel in shape. Zhijuzi, sweet in taste, enters the lung, spleen and stomach channels, and it can promote the secretion of body fluid, relieve restlessness and dispel the effect of liquor.

Zhijuzi is sweet, and as a medicine, it should not be used too much. Or otherwise, it may result in damp-heat and breeding of roundworms in the body.

Uses of Medicines for removing the Effects of Liquor

Prolonged drinking of liquor can result in accumulation of liquor toxin in the body, which needs to be dispelled. The three herbs of Gegen, Gehua and Zhijuzi may be used together or separately based on the syndrome differentiation. In case of thin sloppy stool, Zhijuzi should be avoided since it may worsen the symptom. Gegen should be used with great caution in case of hypertension.

Those patients who have kept on drinking liquor for a long time should use the above-mentioned herbs now and then even if they have been free from the bottle. Without doubt, those who keep on drinking, Gehua and Zhijuzi may help them dispel the effects of liquor, but these herbs should not be used too much. Otherwise, they will become noneffective.

Removing Cigarette Toxin Accumulation

Smokers often inhale the cigarette smoke into the lung. The chain smokers always have gray or brown-colored smoke phlegm, indicating that there is much smoke accumulation in the lung, for which a formula called **Qianjin Weijing Tang** can be used.

As mentioned previously, the formula of **Qianjin Weijing Tang** originates from **Qianjin Yaofang** (**Thousand Golden Formulas**) written by Sun Simiao (medical scientist in the Tang Dynasty), and the original formula contains Lugen (rhizoma phragmitis), Dongguazi (seed of Chinese waxgourd), Taoren (peach kernel) and Yiyi Ren (coix seed). This formula was originally used for the treatment of lung abscess, but the accumulated smoke phlegm in the lung may result in lung Qi stagnation, which is, to a certain degree, a form of lung abscess. Hence, **Qianjin Weijing Tang** is used to clear the accumulated phlegm.

In the formula of **Qianjin Weijing Tang**, Lugen is used to promote the secretion of saliva or body fluid; Dongguazi plays descending and moistening functions; Taoren functions to remove stagnation or stasis and clear the lung, large intestine, and the liver; and Yiyi Ren is used to drive the pathogen in the lung downwards. These four herbs have a great effect on eliminating the heat phlegm in the Upper Jiao; and on the other hand, they can also wash away pathogenic factors in the lung. By the way, Yuxingcao (houttuynia cordata) can be added to the formula for clearing heat, removing swelling and apocenosis and clearing the lung. Furthermore, Gualoupi (peel of trichosanhes kirilowii maxim) and Zhe Beimu (thunberg fritillary bulb) may also be added to reduce phlegm. Zhe Beimu can resolve hard lumps, too, and especially it can enter the lung to descend lung Qi and disperse the stagnated phlegm in the lung. In a word, all these herbs together can eliminate the smoke retention in the lung.

Removing Fruit and Vegetable Retention

Caoguo (Amomum Tsao-ko) Removes Fruit and Vegetable Retention

Fruits and vegetables may also be stagnated in the stomach. The character for "蔬" (vegetable) is composed of "艹" (a symbol for grass) and "疏" (dredge), signifying that vegetables have the effects of soothing the liver and dredging the intestinal tract. As the saying goes "too much water drowns the miller", so, the effects will develop in the opposite direction when one eats excessive vegetable per meal, resulting in vegetable retention in the stomach. Furthermore, both vegetables and fruits are cold and damp in nature. Vegetable salad and fruits can easily cause the spleen to be trapped in cold-damp, impairing the normal T&T functions of the spleen.

Caoguo is pungent and warm in properties with pleasant aroma, and it enters the Middle Jiao. Its pungent property can help disperse the dampness; its warming property can help dispel the coldness; and its aromatic property can help invigorate the spleen to intensify the T&T functions. Hence, Caoguo can be a very effective medicine for eliminating fruit and vegetable retention.

Tao and Nature

Many people claim that he who wishes to learn TCM well must go into the classic formulas, so they believe that **Shanghan Lun (Treatise on Cold Pathogenic Diseases)** is much better than **Huangdi Neijing (the Internal Canon of Huangdi)**. As a matter of fact, those who do wish to learn TCM must attach great importance to both **Shanghan Lun** and **Huangdi Neijing,** especially the latter one. However, he who is just to hunt for formulas for learning TCM will surely find that **Shanghan Lun** is the best choice since it is a classic for TCM formulas that can function effectively and instantly in the treatment of diseases if they are used for treatment based on syndrome differentiation; in contrast, he who is trying to seek for the medical knowledge will find **Huangdi Neijing** is the best choice since it can make him understand the law of nature, theories of physiology and pathology, after which he tries to study the essence of TCM to know properties of medicines and then start to write prescriptions according to what he has learned.

Shanghan Lun is a great example of applying the principles of **Huangdi Neijing** in the clinical practice. **Shanghan Lun** is a classic, the *Tao* about formulas. But the learners should keep in mind that Lao Tseu said "the *Tao* follows nature". **Huangdi Neijing** not only discuss principles of medicine, but also the law of nature, and it instructs the learners to understand the nature. Therefore, he who begins with **Huangdi Neijing** to understand the TCM principles will be able to write their own effective prescriptions based on syndrome differentiation.

Shanghan Lun is a classic for clinical practice. However, if the TCM learners can view it from the perspective of the great nature, and try to broaden their horizon rather than confine themselves to the formulas in this classic, they may then begin with a broader scope of TCM learning, and give treatment of diseases in the way of nature rather than the doctrines.

第八章　消积之药

积，有积累的意思。言下之意是，体内的积是日积月累形成的一些东西。它们也是痰和瘀血形成的，它们导致气血不能周流，继续生痰、生火，给人体造成各种不适，最终甚至危及生命。

气经常不能周流就会形成痰，如果痰在体内长期存在，再加上体内有一些邪火邪热，把这些痰越烤越焦，又没有及时的排出去，那么就在体内形成了痰积，甚至形成了痰核。

血不行则成瘀，瘀血久了，又形成了干血。《金匮要略》就讲到干血痨，用大黄䗪虫丸来治。

不管是痰积还是血积，依然是要化痰、化瘀、散结，一边养一边化，这在前边我们已经讲过。化痰积，用浙贝母、天花粉之类，浙贝有散结的作用，能化掉积累了很久的痰结。还有必要加一些软坚的药，因为痰结已经结的很坚硬了。咸以软坚，用海藻、昆布、海蛤之类。血结也是这样的，用化瘀的药慢慢来化，加软坚、消磨之剂，最好用血肉有情之品、虫蚁搜剔之法。

山楂与消食积类药

食积，是因为食物不消化导致的积滞。说到食积，我们马上就会想到大山楂丸，其主要成分是山楂。

山楂消肉积

山楂是一种乔木，全国各地都有，以北方产的最好，所以开方常写"北山楂"。

山楂入肝、脾、胃三经，它的性质是酸、苦、甘、温，有消磨克化的作用。它能消磨食物，但它主要是能消磨肉食，一般吃多了肉就要用山楂来消化它。山楂有大、小两种，很小又很紧的那种适合入药。小而紧的酸多、苦多，性温，大的山楂甘甜的味道多一些，苦酸的味道略微小一些，尤其是苦味要小一些，这种就是我们平时吃的山楂，用来做糖葫芦的。所以，药用山楂和食用山楂还略有区别，但它们的作用都是相似的。

山楂入药用，一般要去核。山楂核也是一味药，它的作用和山楂比较相似，也有化食消积的作用，还能治疝气，能催生。山楂酸能入肝，能消肉食，消脂肪。脂肪其实是一种痰，山楂也能化痰。山楂入肝，入肝就是入血，因为肝藏血，所以山楂还能化瘀。把山楂炒黑，就成为焦山楂，它不仅能化食积，还能化瘀血。人如果暴饮暴食久了，也容易在肠胃中形成瘀血，用焦山楂非常适宜。

在平时也有很多场合下能够用到山楂，比如说，家里宰了一只老母鸡，老鸡营养价值比较高，但有一个缺点，就是肉太老，炖不烂，那么怎么办呢？在调料里边加一点山楂，肉就容易炖烂了，而且味道也好，吃了也容易消化。当然不要放的太多，太多就影响味道。

儿科常用药

小孩偶尔吃一些山楂，是有好处的。首先，肝体阴而用阳，小孩的肝阳比较旺，酸味能够对肝阳有制约作用，还能养肝阴。这就避免了肝木克脾土。小孩的肝木比较旺而脾土比较虚，木克土，导致脾气大而食欲差，所以要养肝之体，泻肝之用。小孩往往比较喜欢酸的，因为他的身体需要酸味；当然，也因为山楂具有消导化食的作用，小孩如果吃肉吃得多，山楂是必用的一味药。

山楂还能松肌肉。治小儿的疝气会用到山楂。健康的小儿一般是不会有疝气的，有疝气一方面是因为厥阴经有寒，另一方面也是因为气血不能周流。体内寒热不均，厥阴经有寒，气行不通就成了疝气了。所以要温厥阴经，行气，还要稍微化化瘀。我们可以用山楂来化瘀，再加一味小茴香，小茴香辛温，可以温肝经行气。把这两种药打成粉，做成小丸，用米汤服下，治偏坠的疝气效果会特别好。有的医生会用补中益气汤，但是光用这个是不行的，依然要辨证论治。小茴香和山楂是一个对药，可以单用，也可以根据具体情况加进别的药里面。

还有小孩的痘、疹，尤其是痘，一旦发黑，往往就不是什么好现象，那么也经常在辨证论治的基础上在方里边加入山楂和紫草。紫草是入血分的、化瘀的，山楂也入血分而化瘀，还能松肌肉，使毒能够清透出来，所以山楂是儿科经常用的一个药。

山楂的禁忌

当然，山楂也不是人人都适用。如果脾虚，吃肉又不多，没有肉积，就不要用山楂了。千万不要看到一个什么东西好就赶紧去吃，吃很多很多，这样就物极必反。尤其有些人是素食的，从来不吃肉，人又长得比较瘦，这时就千万不要吃山楂，在这种状况下，山楂只能去消磨胃本身，吃久了，人反而不爱吃饭了。即使是那种食用的大山楂，也不要吃的太多，吃太多容易上火，毕竟山楂温肝、温血分。

炒稻麦芽

炒稻麦芽是用来消米面食的，吃多了米饭、馒头、面条，导致的食积，可以用炒稻芽、炒麦芽、神曲之类的药来消。炒稻麦芽没有必要同时用，如果说他是吃多了饭，那就用炒稻芽，是吃多了馒头、面条，就用炒麦芽。麦子刚发芽的时候，还是有生生之气的，炒过之后，它的生生之气依然在，炒黄了它又焦香入脾。一则生生之气入肝，二则焦香之气入脾，两者加起来，足以消导米面在人体里面的积滞。

生稻麦芽有生发之性，所以，生麦芽经常用来疏肝。当病人不想吃饭又有肝郁，还不适合用柴胡的时候，疏肝就得用生麦芽。

神曲

神曲是通过发酵得来的，它的主要成份是面粉，里面加了赤小豆、杏仁、青蒿、苍耳、野蓼等熬的汁，放在一起发酵。等上面长了黄色的霉以后，再晾干保存，保存年头越久越好。

它相当于酵母片，也是用来消食的。食物到肚子里后成了食积，死死地积在那里排不出去。一发酵它就变松了，就容易化了。用神曲就是为了让积滞变松，以便更好地排出去。

化酒积

酒喝多了，会产生酒积，这是一个无形的东西，它也会以痰、湿热、血热等形式存在。化酒积的药有：葛根、葛花和枳椇子。

葛根和葛花

葛是一种植物，它的藤非常长，这意味着它的根必须有很强大的输布养分的能力。药店里卖的葛根会被切成丁，我们可以看到葛根的横断面上有很多小孔。在植物生长的过程中，这些小孔里面都是汁，是津液。正是通过这些小孔，葛根把从地下吸收来的水分往上输送，输送给长长的葛藤，这就意味着葛根能够行津液。而且葛根还有升腾的性质，能鼓舞胃气升腾，所以它能升阳散火、解肌。人要出汗，靠的是胃气，胃气振奋起来，阳气升发了，火也就顺势散掉了。

酒毒能让脾气下陷，让胃中产生湿热。脾气下陷可以用葛根来升它，胃中的湿热可以通过鼓舞胃气，让它往外升散，把胃的阳气鼓动起来，胃中的湿热自然容易化掉。

葛花是葛藤开的花，是一串一串的，紫色的小花，紫色入肝，而诸花皆散，葛根和葛花一个是入胃的，一个是入肝的，都有升散的作用，都解酒毒。它们有相通的地方，也有不同的地方，要根据具体情况来用。

枳椇子

解酒毒，仅有升散的还不行，还要有往下降的药，这就是枳椇子。枳椇子是一种植物的种子，形状与枣仁相似。这种植物是乔木，主要产于我国的中部。枳椇子入肺、脾、胃三经，味甘，能生津液、除烦、解酒毒。

枳椇子味甘，入药也不能用得太多，毕竟酒客不喜甘，用得太多太久的话就会助湿热，生蛔虫。

解酒毒之药的用法

如果长期喝酒导致酒毒的积滞，就要用这些解酒的药。这三种药可以同时用，也可以根据具体情况，用其中的一种或者几种。如果大便稀就不要用枳椇子了，枳椇子能让大便更稀。如果血压比较高，那么葛根就该慎用。

长期喝酒的人病了，即使后来他不喝酒了，也得经常用这几味药。当然正在喝酒的人，吃一点葛花、枳椇子也有解酒的作用。这些药不能喝多，喝多了就没有用了。

化烟积

吸烟是要吸进肺里的。经常吸烟的人会吐烟痰，这种痰是灰色的或者是褐色的，它说明肺里面有很多的烟积。所以得用一个方子，叫"千金苇茎汤"。

前面讲过，千金苇茎汤是孙思邈《千金方》里的，叫苇茎汤。千金苇茎汤是由四味药组成的，有芦根、冬瓜子、桃仁、薏苡仁。它本来是用来治肺痈的。当烟痰积在肺里边也会导致肺气壅滞，这也是某种意义上的肺痈，所以用千金苇茎汤来涤荡。

千金苇茎汤中，芦根是生津的，冬瓜子是降的、润的，桃仁能化瘀，还能通肺、通大肠，还通肝。薏苡仁能把肺里的邪往下引。这四味药用来化上焦的热痰，效果都会非常好。上焦之所以会有热痰，是因为肺被壅滞住了。那么，用千金苇茎汤一方面化上焦的热痰，一方面涤荡肺里面不好的东西。当然还可以加上鱼腥草，鱼腥草是一味清热解毒的药，有消痈、排脓的作用，也有洗肺的功能，能把肺里边一些不好的东西给洗涤出来。还可以加上栝蒌皮、浙贝母，这些是用来化痰的。浙贝母有软坚散结的作用，尤其是它入肺，能够降肺气，能散肺里边的痰结。

化果菜之积

草果化果菜之积

水果蔬菜吃多了也会有积滞。蔬菜的"蔬"，就是一个草字头下面一个疏通的"疏"，蔬菜有疏通的作用，能疏肝、疏通肠道。但物极必反，蔬菜吃得太多，它就不疏了，也会积在那里。此外，蔬菜、水果，本身就带有寒湿，当你凉着吃这些东西的时候，容易导致寒湿困脾，导致脾的运化不利。

草果是一味辛温的药，芳香怡人，走中焦。辛可以散湿，温可以祛寒，芳香醒脾，辛温健脾，它能加强脾的运化功能。所以，草果可以很好地化果菜之积。

思想与自然

很多人都说，学好中医，还是要回到经方，所以《伤寒论》比《内经》要好的多。其实，冷静地想起来，这个是寻找方子的人说的话。我觉得，《内经》和《伤寒论》两者都要重视，尤其要重视《内经》。有人学习中医是在寻找方子，那么《伤寒杂病论》必然是他最好的选择。经方只要对证，效如桴鼓。如果你学医是在寻求医道，那么《内经》是最好的选择，它让你明白自然之理，明白生理、病理。然后去格物致知，熟悉药性，勤修苦练，在此基础上开出方子。

　　《伤寒论》也是运用《内经》开方子的一个很好的范例，《伤寒论》是一部经典，是"道"。但是我们别忘了老子还说过一句话，叫"道法自然"。《内经》不但是讲医道的书，还是一部讲自然的书，它教我们怎么去认识自然。所以，如果以《内经》为基础去明理，那么你开出的方子。虽然可能你开出的方子，在《伤寒杂病论》里面没有，但是也会像《伤寒杂病论》的经方那么有效。

　　《伤寒论》作为一部临床的经典，但是如果把它放在自然的大背景下去考察的话，把眼光放宽一点，不局限于方子，我们学习中医的眼界会更广，所以要以思想去治病，而不要以方子去治病，有思想的方子才是活方子，当然这种思想不是教条的思想，而是自然的思想，是活泼的思想。

Epilogue

Here comes the end of *The Tao of Chinese Formulas and Medicines*, which covers some formulas and medicines, but still quite far from being complete, and even some very important formulas and medicines have not been included, yet. The properties of a certain medicine may have not been fully explained and even some unavoidable mistakes made in the book. However, it may be understood in another way that the specific knowledge can be learnt from any books. In the past, there was a saying that what the teacher should give to students is the "dried goods" (referring to the important outlines of learnings) like the dried eggplants or kidney beans that the consumers may soak for use before cooking. I do not quite agree with such a saying since "dried goods" in any case is dead and still limited in amount though it can be soaked with water to become loose. For learning TCM, what a book can cover is quite limited too, but what is unlimited is the idea that is like a living seedling. If the learners can plant a seedling in his or her mind and let it grow up into a big tree, it will bring about unlimited effects.

Therefore, from this book, the readers are requested not only to search for the "dried goods", but also try to understand and follow the natural Way/Tao of TCM. Of course, under the influence of modern science, many traditional concepts and methods have been ignored or neglected, but this book is trying to dig them out and put more stress upon them here.

When talking about a specific herb/medicine, this book adopts some different description methods and stylistic rules. Some are discussed based upon the TCM classics, some are analyzed from the perspective of the specific attributes of herbs, and some others are described from the angle of clinical practice, all of which are trying to initiate an idea or inspiring the readers to think about TCM in Way of the Nature.

结　语

　　方药之道到这里我们就全部讲完了，我们讲的药也不是太多，肯定是挂一漏万，还有很多方药没有讲到，甚至有很多非常重要的方药没有讲。某一味药的药性也还没有讲全，甚至有的还会有一些差错，这些都是难免的。但是话又说回来，这些具体的知识，我们都能从书本里面学习到，以前有一个说法，就是老师要给学生一些干货。不知道这种说法大家同意不同意，反正我是不同意的。干货就是菜市场上那些茄子豆角一晒，干了就是那些。你买回家用水一发就可以用了。但干货都是死的，干货用水来发，发的再多也只有那么多，毕竟课堂上的时间也少，他给你再多干货，也是有限的。所以给干货还不如给一些鲜活苗，把这些苗栽在我们心中，让它长成大树。

　　所以我们讲这个课，不仅仅要追求有干货，还要试图把尽可能多的正确思想方法，也就是中医的传统的思想方法体现出来，去影响大家，这是最重要的。当然很多的思想方法在现代科学的影响下，大家都不重视了，都不相信了。有很多传统，很多习俗，中医里面的很多讲究，现在都不讲究了，大家都忘了，我争取尽量把这些东西讲出来。我认为这才是比较重要的东西，也是别人不多讲的，所以我多强调一点。

　　在讲具体药物的时候，我们的方法、体例也不一样，有的是从经典入手，有的是从具体属性入手，有的则是从应用入手。这些都是在启发大家的思路。

Bibliography

Sun Xingyan. *Sheng Nong's herbal classic*. People's Medical Publishing House, 1963.01.

Qing Dynasty· Tang Rongchuan. *Medica Question and Answer*. Chinese Literature and Book Company, R. O. C. 1938.07.

Qing Dynasty · Xu Lingtai. *Shennong Herb through a Hundred Kinds of Records*. See *Xu Lingtai Medical Book*. China Press of Traditional Chinese Medicine Co. Ltd., 1999.08.

Qing Dynasty· Zhang Zhicong. Chinese Materia Medica Source. China Press of Traditional Chinese Medicine Co. Ltd., 1992.12.

Qing Dynasty· Zou Shu. Annotation to Sheng Nong's herbal classic. Academy Press Limited Company, 2009.09.

Tang Dynasty· *The Newly Revised Materia Medica*. Shang Zhijun. Edited and Corrected. Anhui Science & Technology Publishing House, 1981.

Qing Dynasty· Zhang Bingcheng. *Brief Reading of Chinese Materia Medica*. Shanghai Scientific & Technical Publishers, 1958.10.

Qing Dynasty· Zhou Yan. *Commentary on Materia Medica*. Beijing: People's Medical Publishing House, 1960.01.

Qing Dynasty· Yan Jie, et al., Compatibility of Materia Medica. People's Medical Publishing House, 2007.07.

Yuan Dynasty · *Summary of Herbal Properties of the supplementary Materia Medica to the Formulas of Heji Dispensary*. Traditional Chinese Medicine Ancient Books Publishing House, 1988.10.

R. O. C. Zhou Zhilin. Study on the Uses of Herbs. Chung Wha Book Company, Limited, 2nd Edition. 1949.06.

R. O. C. He Lianchen. Experimental Materia Medica. Fujian Science & Technology Publishing House, 2008.12.

Qing Dynasty · Wang Mengying. *Traditional Chinese Dietary Therapy in*

Daily Life. Jiangsu Science & Technology Publishing House, 1983.04.

Ming Dynasty· Li Shizhen. *Compendium of Materia Medica*. The Commercial Press, 1930, China Bookstore Press, 1988.

The Southern Dynasties· Lei Xiao. *Lei's Theory on Herbal Processing*. Jiangsu Science & Technology Publishing House, 1985.06.

Zhang Bingxin. *Review on the Evolution of Processed Chinese Medicine Products*. People's Medical Publishing House, 2011.01.

Qing Dynasty· Zhang Zhicong. Notes on the Inner Canon of Huangdi. Zhejiang Ancient Books Publishing House Limited Company, 2002.12.

Qing Dynasty· Ye Lin. Commentary on Explanation of Difficult Diseases. Shanghai Scientific & Technical Publishers, 1981.12.

Han Dynasty· Hua Tuo. *Zhongzang Jing*. Jiangsu Science & Technology Publishing House, 1985.07.

Sui Dynasty· Cao Yuanfang. *General Treatise on the Cause and Symptoms of Diseases*. People's Medical Publishing House, photoprint version, 1955.06.

Tang Dynasty· Sun Simiao. *Valuable Prescriptions for Emergency*. Traditional Chinese Medicine Ancient Books Publishing House, 1999.08.

Han Dynasty· Luo Longji, et al. , *Treatise on Supplementary Formulas to the Inner Canon of Huangdi*. Academy Press Limited Company, 2011.01.

Tang Rongchuan. *Treatise on Chinese and Western Medical Classics*. Chinese Literature and Book Company, R. O. C. 1936.

Hu Guangci. *New Conception on Treatment of Traditional Chinese Medicine Internal Miscellaneous Diseases and Syndromes*. Sichuan People's Publishing House, 1958.01.

R. O. C. Yao Guomei. *Compilation of Yao Guomei's Medical Lecture Notes*. People's Medical Publishing House, 2009.09.

R. O. C. Zhang Xichun. *Records of Tradition Chinese and Western Medicine in Combination*. Hebei Scientific & Technical Publishing House, 2002.

Qing Dynasty· Ye Tianshi. *Guideline to Clinical Practice with Medical Record*. Shanghai Scientific & Technical Publishers, 1959.02.

R. O. C. He Lianchen. National Famous Medical Examination Records. Fujian Science & Technology Publishing House, 2003.04.

Tang Wenji, Tang Wenqi. Remedial Notes on Disease Theory. Academy Press Limited Company, 2013. 05.

Song Dynasty· Zhu Xi, et al. The Four Books and The Five Classics. The world publishing company, 1936, Beijing Ancient Books Publishing House, Photoprint version.

Qing Dynasty· Huang Zongxi, et al. , Academic Thoughts in Song and Yuan Dynasties. Zhonghua Book Company, 1986. 12.

Qing Dynasty· Huang Zongxi. Academic Thoughts of Confucianism in Ming Dynasty. Zhonghua Book Company, 1985.

R. O. C. Qian Mu. Treatise on Modern Chinese Academics. SDX Joint Publishing Company, 2001. 06.

Giambattista Vico. The New Science, Translated by Zhu Guangqian. The Commercial Press, 1989. 06.

Northrop Frye. The Great Code. Translated by Hao Zhenyi, et al. Peking University Press, 1998. 01.

Jean-Henri Casimir Fabre. *Souvenirs Entomologiques* (*Insect Records*), 3rd version. 2011. 05.

参考书目

孙星衍. 神农本草经. 北京：人民卫生出版社，1963 年 1 月版。

清·唐容川. 本草问答. 中国文学书局，民国二十六年七月版。

清·徐灵胎. 神农本草经百种录. 见《徐灵胎医学全书》. 中国中医药出版社，1999 年 8 月版。

清·张志聪. 本草崇原. 中国中医药出版社，1992 年 12 月版。

清·邹澍. 本经疏证. 学苑出版社，2009 年 9 月版。

唐·新修本草. 尚志钧. 辑校. 安徽科技出版社，1981 年版。

清·张秉成. 本草便读. 上海科学技术出版社，1958 年 10 月版。

清·周岩. 本草思辨录. 人民卫生出版社，1960 年 1 月版。

清·严洁，等. 得配本草. 人民卫生出版社，2007 年 7 月版。

元· 增补和剂局方药性总论. 中医古籍出版社，1988 年 10 月版。

民国·周志林. 本草用法研究. 中华书局，民国三十七年 6 月再版。

民国·何廉臣. 实验药物学. 福建科学技术出版社，2008 年 12 月版。

清·王孟英. 随息居饮食谱. 江苏科学技术出版社，1983 年 4 月版。

明·李时珍. 本草纲目. 商务印书馆，1930 年版，中国书店 1988 年影印。

南朝·雷敩. 雷公炮制论. 江苏科学技术出版社，1985 年 6 月版。

张炳鑫. 中药炮制品古今演变述评. 人民卫生出版社，2011 年 1 月版。

清·张志聪. 黄帝内经集注. 浙江古籍出版社，2002 年 12 月版。

清·叶霖. 难经正义. 上海科学技术出版社，1981 年 12 月版。

汉·华佗. 中藏经. 江苏科技出版社，1985 年 7 月版。

隋·巢元方. 诸病源候论. 人民卫生出版社，1955 年 6 月影印版。

唐·孙思邈. 备急千金要方. 中医古籍出版社，1999 年 8 月版。

宋·骆龙吉，等. 增补内经拾遗方论. 学苑出版社，2011 年 1 月版。

唐容川. 中西汇通医经精义. 中国文学书局，民国二十四年版。

胡光慈. 中医内科杂病证治新义，四川人民出版社，1958 年 1 月。

民国·姚国美. 姚国美医学讲义合编，人民卫生出版社，2009 年 9

月版。

民国·张锡纯. 医学衷中参西录，河北科学技术出版社，2002 年版。

清·叶天士. 临证指南医案，上海科学技术出版社，1959 年 2 月版。

民国·何廉臣. 全国名医验案类编，福建科学技术出版社，2003 年 4 月版。

唐文吉，唐文奇. 重编时病论集注，学苑出版社，2013 年 5 月版

宋·朱熹，等注. 四书五经，世界书局 1936 年版，北京古籍出版社影印。

清·黄宗羲，等. 宋元学案，中华书局，1986 年 12 月版。

清·黄宗羲. 明儒学案，中华书局，1985 年版。

民国·钱穆. 现代中国学术论衡. 三联书店，2001 年 6 月版。

维科. 新科学，朱光潜译. 商务印书馆，1989 年 6 月版。

诺斯洛普·弗莱. 伟大的代码，郝振益等译. 北京大学出版社，1998 年 1 月版

法布尔. 昆虫记，2011 年 5 月第三版。

附录 1
Appendix 1

本书中药名称英汉对照表
Glossary of Chinese Medicines Mentioned in the Book

English Description	Chinese Description	Chinese Pinyin
moxa	艾绒	Airong
folium artemisiae argyi	艾叶	Aiye
Aiyecharcoal	艾叶炭	Aiyetan
croton	巴豆	Badou
defatted croton seed powder	巴豆霜	Badoushuang
morinda officinalis	巴戟天	Bajitiann
white lentils	白扁豆	Baibiandou
amomum cardamomum	白豆蔻	Baidoukou
alum	白矾	Baifan
white poria	白茯苓	Baifuling
rhizoma typhonii	白附子	Baifuzi
bletilla	白芨	Baiji
silkworm larva, stiff silkworm	白僵蚕	Baijiangcan
semen brassicae	白芥子	Baijiezi
radix ampelopsis	白蔹	Bailian
radix paeoniae alba, white peony root	白芍	Baishao
radix angelicae	白芷	Baizhi
rhizoma atractylodis macrocephalae, white atractylodes rhizome	白术	Baizhu

English Description	Chinese Description	Chinese Pinyin
radix stemonae	百部	Baibu
platycladi seed	柏子仁	Baiziren
radix isatidis, isatis root	板蓝根	Banlangen
pinellia ternata	半夏	Banxia
honewort	北柴胡	Beichaihu
fritillaria	贝母	Beimu
turtle shell	鳖甲	Biejia
areca – nut	槟榔	Binglang
borneol	冰片	Bingpian
mint	薄荷	Bohe
fructus psoraleae	补骨脂	Buguzhi
silkworm cocoon	蚕茧	Canjian
silkworm faeces, silkworm excrement	蚕沙	Cansha
xanthii fructus	苍耳	Cang'er
rhizoma atractylodis	苍术	Cangzhu
amomum tsao – ko	草果	Caoguo
cassia occidentalis	草决明	Caojueming
radix aconiti agrestis	草乌	Caowu
cacumen biotae	侧柏叶	Cebaiye
radix bupleuri	柴胡	Chaihu
cicada slough	蝉蜕	Chantui
acorus calamus	菖蒲	Changpu
semen plantaginis	车前子	Cheqianzi
pericarpium citri reticulatae, tangerine peel	陈皮	Chenpi
agilawood	沉香	Chenxiang
radix paeoniae rubra, red peony root	赤芍	Chishao
red phaseolus bean	赤小豆	Chixiaodou
szechwan chinaberry fruit	川楝子	Chuanlianzi

English Description	Chinese Description	Chinese Pinyin
radix cyathulae	川牛膝	Chuanniuxi
pangolin scales	穿山甲	Chuanshanjia
aconite root, monkshood	川乌	Chuanwu
ligusticum wallichii	川芎	Chuanxiong
tribulus terrestris	刺蒺藜	Cijili
fistular onion stalk	葱白	Congbai
semen sojae germinatum	大豆黄卷	Dadouhuangjuan
pericarpium arecae	大腹皮	Dafupi
rheum officinale	大黄	Dahuang
euphorbia pekinensis, circium japonicum	大戟	Daji
jujube	大枣	Dazao
cortex moutan radices, root bark of the peony	丹皮	Danpi
radix salviae miltiorrhizae, the root of red-rooted salvia	丹参	Danshen
lophatherum gracile	淡竹叶	Danzhuye
angelica sinensis	当归	Danggui
angelica sinensis tail	当归尾	Dangguiwei
codonopsis pilosula	党参	Dangshen
cortex lycii radices, the root-bark of Chinese wolfberry	地骨皮	Digupi
rehmannia	地黄	Dihuang
earthworm, lumbricus	地龙	Dilong
sanguisorba officinalis	地榆	Diyu
clove, syzygium aromaticum	丁香	Dingxiang
cordyceps sinensis	冬虫夏草	Dongchongxiacao
seed of Chinese waxgourd	冬瓜子	Dongguazi
fermented soya beans	豆豉	Douchi
sprouted black soybean	豆卷	Doujuan

English Description	Chinese Description	Chinese Pinyin
cardamun	豆蔻	Doukou
radix angelicae pubescentis	独活	Duhuo
eucommia ulmoides	杜仲	Duzhong
calcined calamine	煅炉甘石	Duanluganshi
donkey – hide gelatin	阿胶	E – jiao
folium sennae	番泻叶	Fanxieye
radix sileris	防风	Fangfeng
costazia bone	浮海石	Fuhaishi
poria cocos	茯苓	Fuling
poria cum ligno hospite	茯神	Fushen
radix aconiti carmichaeli	附子	Fuzi
licorice	甘草	Gancao
rhizome zingiberis	干姜	Ganjiang
euphorbia kansui	甘遂	Gansui
galangal	高良姜	Gaoliangjiang
radix puerariae	葛根	Gegen
flos puerariae, pueraria flower	葛花	Gehua
polished round – grained rice	粳米	Gengmi
gecko	蛤蚧	Gejie
fructus lycii	枸杞	Gouqi
pipewort	谷精草	Gujingcao
trichosanthes kirilowii maxim	瓜蒌	Gualou
cortex cinnamomic	官桂	Guangui
radix curcumae	广郁金	Guangyujin
tortoise plastron, tortoiseshell,	龟板	Guiban
tortoise plastron gelatin	龟板胶	Guibanjiao
cassia twig	桂枝	Guizhi
uncaria	钩藤	Gouteng

English Description	Chinese Description	Chinese Pinyin
Sea clam	海蛤	Haige
concha meretricis seu cyclinae	海蛤壳	Haigeqiao
lygodium japonicum	海金沙	Haijinsha
cuttlebone	海螵蛸	Haipiaoxiao
seaweed	海藻	Haizao
eclipta alba	旱莲草（墨旱莲）	Hanliancao（Mohanlian）
gypsum rubrum	寒水石	Hanshuishi
polygonum multiflorum	何首乌	Heshouwu
leadsulfide	黑锡	Heixi
safflower carthamus	红花	Honghua
mangnolia officinalis	厚朴	Houpo
fenugreek	葫芦巴	Huluba
walnut meat）	胡桃肉	Hutaorou
pricklyash peel	花椒	Huajiao
talcum powder	滑石粉	Huashifen
phellodendron amurense, amur corktree bark, golden cypress	黄柏	Huangbai
yellow lead	黄丹	Huangdan
coptis chinensis	黄连	Huanglian
astragali radix	黄芪	Huangqi
scutellaria baicalensis	黄芩	Huangqin
gardenia jasminoides	黄栀子	Huangzhizi
fructus sophorae	槐角	Huaijiao
achyranthes root	怀牛膝	Huainiuxi
foeniculum vulgare	茴香	Huixiang
fructus cannabis	火麻仁	Huomaren
ageratum	藿香	Huoxiang

English Description	Chinese Description	Chinese Pinyin
ageratum stem	藿香梗	Huoxianggeng
tribulus terrestris	蒺藜	Jili
caulis spatholobi	鸡血藤	Jixueteng
parched fructus crataegi, parched hawthorn fruit	焦山楂	Jiaoshanzha
platycodon grandiflorum	桔梗	Jiegeng
Isaria cicadae Miquel	金蝉花	Jinchanhua
szechwan Chinaberry fruit	金铃子	Jinlingzi
lysimachia christinae	金钱草	Jinqiancao
honeysuckle flower	金银花	Jinyinhua
schizonepeta	荆芥	Jingjie
schizonepeta spike	荆芥穗	Jingjiesui
hrysanthemum	菊花	Juhua
exocarpium citri rubrum	橘红	Juhong
tangerine pith	橘络	Juluo
cassia tora	决明	Jueming
cassia seed, cassia occidentalis	决明子	Juemingzi
fruit of chinaberry tree, chinaberry seed	苦楝子	Kulianzi
radix sophorae flavescentis	苦参	Kushen
flos farfarae	款冬花	Kuandonghua
laminaria, sea – tent	昆布	Kunbu
radish seed	莱菔子	Laifuzi
radix euphorbiae lantu	狼毒	Langdu
omphalia	雷丸	Leiwan
veratrum nigrum	藜芦	Lilu
fructus forsythiae	连翘	Lianqiao
sulfur	硫黄	Liuhuang
radix gentianae, felwort	龙胆草	Longdancao

English Description	Chinese Description	Chinese Pinyin
ossa draconis	龙骨	Longgu
longan aril, arillus longan	龙眼肉	Longyanrou
deer's testis and penis	鹿鞭	Lubian
rhizoma phragmitis, reed rhizome	芦根	Lugen
aloe	芦荟	Luhui
deer horn	鹿角	Lujiao
deer - horn gelatin	鹿角胶	Lujiaojiao
cornu cervi degelatinatum	鹿角霜	Lujiaoshuang
deer's sinew	鹿筋	Lujin
pilos antler	鹿茸	Lurong
sparrowgrass	芦笋	Luxun
Chinese starjasmine stem	络石藤	Luoshiteng
ephedra	麻黄	Mahuang
radix ophiopogonis	麦冬	Maidong
fructus viticis	蔓荆子	Manjingzi
mirabilite	芒硝	Mangxiao
couch grass root	茅根	Maogen
couch grass catkins	茅花	Maohua
couch grass shoot	茅针	Maozhen
butterflybush flower, flos buddlejae	密蒙花	Mimenghua
lithargite	密陀僧	Mituoseng
pawpaw	木瓜	Mugua
concha ostreae	牡蛎	Muli
akebiaquinata	木通	Mutong
costustoot	木香	Muxiang
myrrh	没药	Moyao
arisaema heterophyllum blume	南星	Nanxing
urine ice	尿冰	Niaobing

English Description	Chinese Description	Chinese Pinyin
ox bile	牛胆	Niudan
fructus arctii	牛蒡子	Niubangzi
calculus bovis	牛黄	Niuhuang
radix achyranthis bidentatae	牛膝	Niuxi
fructus ligustri lucidi, glossy privet fruit	女贞子	Nuzhenzi
soaked fructus evodiae	泡吴萸	Paowuyu
loquat leaf, folium eriobotryae	枇杷叶	Pipaye
arsenic	砒霜	Pishuang
zedoary	片姜黄	Pianjianghuang
fructus psoraleae	破故纸	Poguzhi
Glauber's salt	朴硝	Poxiao
cattail pollen	蒲黄	Puhuang
Chinese mugwort	蕲艾	Qiai
long – noded pit viper	蕲蛇	Qishe
radix peucedani	前胡	Qianhu
pharbitis	牵牛	Qianniu
semen pharbitidis	牵牛子	Qianniuzi
notopterygium root	羌活	Qianghuo
gentiana macrophylla	秦艽	Qinjiao
indigo naturalis	青黛	Qingdai
sabia japonica	清风藤	Qingfengteng
artemisia apiacea, sweet wormwood	青蒿	Qinghao
the green tangerine peel	青皮	Qingpi
autumn pear syrup	秋梨膏	Qiuligao
processed urine deposit	秋石	Qiushi
ginseng	人参	Renshen
depositum urinae hominis	人中白	Renzhongbai
rulvis glycyrrhizae extractionis sedilis	人中黄	Renzhonghuang

English Description	Chinese Description	Chinese Pinyin
cistanche	肉苁蓉	Roucongrong
nutmeg	肉豆蔻	Roudoukou
cassia bark, cortex cinnamomi	肉桂	Rougui
frankincense	乳香	Ruxiang
rhizoma sparganii	三棱	Sanleng
notoginseng	三七	Sanqi
notoginseng powder	三七粉	Sanqifen
cortex mori, the root bark of white mulberry	桑白皮	Sangbaipi
parasitic loranthus	桑寄生	Sangjisheng
mantis egg – case	桑螵蛸	Sangpiaoxiao
the mulberry fruits	桑葚	Sangshen
mulberry leaf, folium mori	桑叶	Sangye
mulberry twig	桑枝	Sangzhi
astragali complanati semen	沙蒺藜	Shajili
fructus amomi	砂仁	Sharen
radix adenophorae	沙参	Shashen
astragali complanati demen	沙苑蒺藜	Shayuanjili
Chinese yam	山药	Shanyao
fructus crataegi	山楂	Shanzha
cape jasmine	山栀	Shanzhi
Chinese herbaceous peony, paeonia lactiflora	芍药	Shaoyao
cornus officinalis (common macrocarpium fruit)	山茱萸（山英肉）	Shanzhuyu (Shanyurou)
musk	麝香	Shexiang
lycopodium clavatum	伸筋草	Shenjincao
medicated leaven	神曲	Shenqu
raw rheum officinale	生大黄	Shengdahuang
radix rehmanniae recen	生地	Shengdi

English Description	Chinese Description	Chinese Pinyin
radix rehmanniae recen, dried rehamnnia root	生地黄	Shengdihuang
rhizoma cimicifugae, rattletop	升麻	Shengma
raw malt	生麦芽	Shengmaiya
raw concha arcae	生瓦楞	Shengwaleng
raw ochre	生赭石	Shengzheshi
persimmon calyx	柿蒂	Shidi
quispualis indica	使君子	Shijunzi
halloysit	石脂	Shizhi
rhizoma acori graminei	石菖蒲	Shichangpu
gypsum	石膏	Shigao
dendrobe	石斛	Shihu
concha haliotidis	石决明	Shijueming
radix rehmanniae praeparata	熟地，熟地黄	Shudi, Shudihuang
uncaria laevigata	双钩藤	Shuanggouteng
rhizoma calami	水菖蒲	Shuichangpu
hydrargyrum	水银	Shuiyin
loofah sponge	丝瓜络	Sigualuo
caulis perllae	苏梗	Sugeng
sappanwood	苏木	Sumu
perilla leaf	苏叶	Suye
perilla seed	苏子	Suzi
wild jujube seed	酸枣仁	Suanzaoren
peach gum	桃胶	Taojiao
peach kernel	桃仁	Taoren
asparagus cochinchinensis, radix asparagi	天冬，天门冬	Tiandong, Tianmendong
radices trichosanthis	天花粉	Tianhuafen
gastrodia elata	天麻	Tianma

English Description	Chinese Description	Chinese Pinyin
tabasheer	天竺黄	Tianzhuhuang
tetrapanax papyriferus	通草	Tongcao
semen cuscutae, dodder	菟丝子	Tusizi
concha arcae	瓦楞子	Walengzi
hare dung	望月砂	Wangyuesha
radix clematidis	威灵仙	Weilingxian
centipede	蜈蚣	Wugong
cortex acanthopanacis	五加皮	Wujiapi
trogopterus dung	五灵脂	Wulingzhi
dark plum	乌梅	Wumei
aconite	乌头	Wutou
fructus schisandrae chinensis	五味子	Wuweizi
dutchmanspipe root	五香	Wuxiang
lindera aggregate	乌药	Wuyao
fructus evodiae	吴萸，吴茱萸	Wuyu, Wuzhuyu
rhinoceros horn	犀角	Xijiao
asarum	细辛	Xixin
spica prunellae	夏枯草	Xiakucao
rhizoma curculiginis	仙茅	Xianmao
rhizoma cyperi	香附	Xiangfu
elsholtzia ciliate	香薷	Xiangru
fennel	小茴香	Xiaohuixiang
herba cepbalanoplosis segeti	小蓟	Xiaoji
allium macrostemon	薤白	Xiebai
scorpion	蝎子	Xiezi
apricot kernel	杏仁	Xingren
realgar	雄黄	Xionghuang
radix dipsaci	续断	Xuduan

English Description	Chinese Description	Chinese Pinyin
inula flower	旋覆花	Xuanfuhua
corydalis turtschaninovii bess	玄胡索	Xuanhusuo
compound of glauber – salt and liquorice	玄明粉	Xuanmingfen
radix scrophulariae	玄参	Xuanshen
saltpeter	牙硝	Yaxiao
actinolite	阳起石	Yangqishi
rhizoma corydalis	延胡索	Yanhusuo
tuber fleeceflower stem	夜交藤	Yejiaoteng
wild smartweed	野蓼	Yeliao
bat dung	夜明砂	Yemingsha
motherwort	益母草	Yimucao
maltose	饴糖	Yitang
coix seed	薏苡仁	Yiyiren
bitter cardamom	益智仁	Yizhiren
oriental wormwood	茵陈	Yinchen
epimedium	淫羊藿	Yinyanghuo
radix curcumae	郁金	Yujin
houttuynia cordata	鱼腥草	Yuxingcao
radix polygonati officinalis	玉竹	Yuzhu
lilac daphne flower bud	芫花	Yuanhua
polygala tenuifolia	远志	Yuanzhi
jujubestone/kernel	枣仁	Zaoren
rhizoma alismatis	泽泻	Zexie
thunberg fritillary bulb	浙贝母	Zhebeimu
Pearl Powder	珍珠粉	Zhenzhufen
Concha margaritiferallsta, nacre mother of pearl	珍珠母	Zhenzhumu

English Description	Chinese Description	Chinese Pinyin
roasted radix astragali, roasted astragalus membranaceus	炙黄芪	Zhihuangqi
semen hoveniae	枳椇子	Zhijuzi
fructus aurantii	枳壳	Zhike
rhizoma anemarrhenae	知母	Zhimu
fructus aurantii immaturus, immature bitter orange	枳实	Zhishi
ochre	赭石	Zhishi
processed rhizoma cyperi	制香附	Zhixiangfu
fructus gardeniae	栀子	Zhizi
pig bile	猪胆汁	Zhudanzhi
cinnabar poria cum ligno hospite	朱茯神	Zhufushen
pig spinal cord	猪脊髓	Zhujisui
bamboo juice	竹沥	Zhuli
grifola	猪苓	Zhuling
bamboo shavings	竹茹	Zhuru
cinnabar	朱砂	Zhusha
bamboo leaf	竹叶	Zhuye
radices lithospermi	紫草	Zicao
placenta hominis	紫河车	Ziheche
purple perilla stem	紫苏梗	Zisugeng
purple perilla twig	紫苏旁枝	Zisupangzhi
xylosma twig	柞木枝	Zuomuzhi

附录 2
Appendix 2

中药计量单位换算表
Conversion of Weight Measurement Units in TCM

1 斤 = 16 两 = 500 克	1jin = 16 liang = 500 grams
1 两 = 31. 25 克	1liang = 31. 25 grams
1 钱 = 3. 125 克	1qian = 3. 125 grams
1 分 = 0. 3125 克	1 fen = 0. 3125 grams
5 分 = 1. 5625 克	5 fen = 1. 5625 grams
1 厘 = 0. 03125 克	1li = 0. 03125 grams
5 厘 = 0. 15625 克	5li = 0. 15625 grams
1. 5 钱 = 4. 6875 克	1. 5qian = 4. 6875 grams
2 钱 = 6. 25 克	2qian = 6. 25 grams
2. 5 钱 = 7. 8125 克	2. 5qian = 7. 8125 grams
3 钱 = 9. 375 克	3qian = 9. 375 grams
3. 5 钱 = 10. 9375 克	3. 5qian = 10. 9375 grams
4 钱 = 12. 5 克	4qian = 12. 5 grams
4. 5 钱 = 14. 0625 克	4. 5qian = 14. 0625 grams
5 钱 = 15. 625 克	5qian = 15. 625 grams
6 钱 = 18. 75 克	6qian = 18. 75 grams
7 钱 = 21. 875 克	7qian = 21. 875 grams
8 钱 = 25 克	8qian = 25 grams
9 钱 = 28. 125 克	9qian = 28. 125 grams